The Dental Specialties

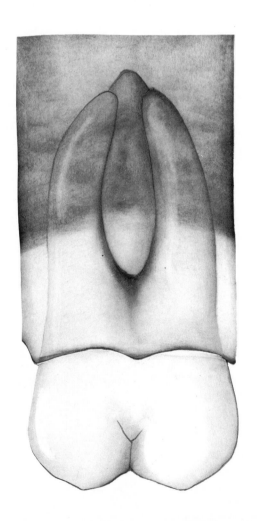
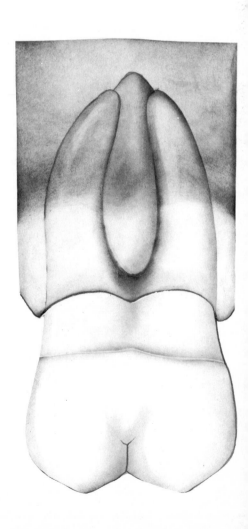

in General Practice

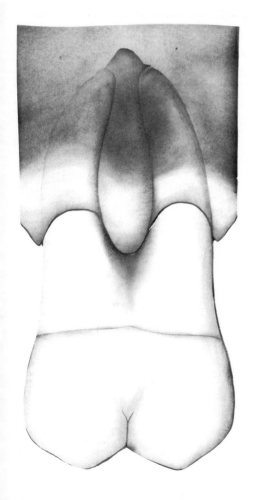

Alvin L. Morris, D.D.S., PH.D.

Professor, Dental Care Systems and Oral Medicine
Associate Vice President Health Affairs-Government Relations
University of Pennsylvania, School of Dental Medicine

Harry M. Bohannan, D.M.D., M.S.D.

University of North Carolina, School of Dentistry

Daniel P. Casullo, D.M.D.

Division of Advanced Dental Education,
  General Practice Fellowship Program,
School of Dental Medicine, University of Pennsylvania

1983

W. B. SAUNDERS COMPANY

PHILADELPHIA/LONDON/TORONTO/MEXICO CITY
RIO DE JANEIRO/SYDNEY/TOKYO

W. B. Saunders Company: West Washington Square
Philadelphia, PA   19105

1 St. Anne's Road
Eastbourne, East Sussex BN21 3UN, England

1 Goldthorne Avenue
Toronto, Ontario M8Z 5T9, Canada

Apartado 26370—Cedro 512
Mexico 4, D.F., Mexico

Rua Coronel Cabrita, 8
Sao Cristovao Caixa Postal 21176
Rio de Janeiro, Brazil

9 Waltham Street
Artarmon, N.W.S. 2064, Australia

Ichibancho, Central Bldg., 22-1 Ichibancho
Chiyoda-Ku, Tokyo 102, Japan

Library of Congress Cataloging in Publication Data
Main entry under title:

The dental specialties in general practice.

1. Dentistry—Practice. I. Morris, Alvin L.,
1927–   . II. Bohannan, Harry M., 1927–
III. Casullo, Daniel P. [DNLM: 1. General practice,
Dental. 2. Specialities, Dental. WU 100 G326]
RK58.G46   1983   617.6   82-42609
ISBN 0-7216-6572-1

The Dental Specialties in General Practice   ISBN 0-7216-6572-1

Last digit is the print number: 9   8   7   6   5   4   3   2   1

DEDICATED TO

Lester W. Burket

*Clinician, educator, scientist,
administrator, statesman*

*Whose commitment to excellence
set an example for us all*

CONTRIBUTORS

DANIEL P. CASULLO, D.M.D.
Associate Professor, Department of Form and Function of the Masticatory System, Director of the Division of Advanced Dental Education, General Practice Program, and Director of the General Practice Residency Program, University of Pennsylvania, School of Dental Medicine; Head of Restorative Dentistry, Hospital of the University of Pennsylvania; Head of Periodontics, Methodist Hospital, Philadelphia, Pennsylvania; Consultant in Periodontics and Restorative Dentistry, The Graduate Hospital, Philadelphia, Pennsylvania

GORDON J. CHRISTENSEN, D.D.S., M.S.D., Ph.D.
Adjunct Professor, Brigham Young University; Clinical Professor, University of Utah; Co-Director, Clinical Research Associates; Attending Prosthodontist, Surgical Specialty Staff, Utah Valley Hospital, Provo, Utah

D. WALTER COHEN, D.D.S.
Professor of Periodontics and Dean, School of Dental Medicine, University of Pennsylvania

EMMETT R. COSTICH, D.D.S., Ph.D.
Professor of Oral Surgery, University of Kentucky, College of Dentistry; Attending Oral Surgeon, University Hospital, University of Kentucky Medical Center

HENRY W. FIELDS, D.M.D., M.S., M.S.D.
Associate Professor of Pedodontics and Orthodontics, University of North Carolina at Chapel Hill, School of Dentistry

GERALD N. GRASER, D.D.S., M.S.
Chairman, Department of Prosthodontics, Eastman Dental Center; Associate Professor of Clinical Dentistry and Dental Research, The University of Roch-

MILTON I. HOUPT, D.D.S., M.D.S., M.Ed., Ph.D.
Professor and Chairman, Department of Pedodontics, and Director of Postgraduate Program, University of Medicine and Dentistry of New Jersey, Dental School

ester, School of Medicine and Dentistry; Senior Attending Dentist, Department of Dentistry, The Genesee Hospital, Rochester, New York; Senior Associate Dentist, Strong Memorial Hospital, Rochester, New York

ALVIN L. MORRIS, D.D.S., Ph.D.
Professor of Dental Care Systems and Oral Medicine, and Associate Vice President, Health Affairs–Government Relations, University of Pennsylvania, School of Dental Medicine

WILLIAM R. PROFFIT, D.D.S., Ph.D.
Professor and Chairman, Department of Orthodontics, University of North Carolina at Chapel Hill, School of Dentistry

LOUIS W. RIPA, D.D.S., M.S.
Professor and Chairman, Department of Children's Dentistry, State University of New York at Stony Brook, School of Dental Medicine

NORMAN H. STOLLER, D.M.D.
Professor and Chairman of Periodontics, University of Colorado, School of Dentistry

LEIF TRONSTAD, D.M.D., Ph.D.
Professor of Endodontics and Chairman, Department of Endodontics, University of Pennsylvania, School of Dental Medicine

CONTENTS

ix

INTRODUCTION

During the past decade, primary care has emerged as the most important and most desired component of the nation's health care delivery system. In dentistry, it is the general practitioner who serves as the primary care dentist, around whom the nation's dental care delivery system is built. There is the clear expectation by those who receive and purchase dental care that the general dentist will provide services that are advanced and comprehensive in their scope. The profession has entered an era when the challenges and the satisfactions of serving as a general practitioner in dentistry have never been greater.

PURPOSE AND ORIENTATION

This book is intended to provide a compilation, under one cover, of techniques of a specialty nature that rightfully belong in the hands of the enlightened, progressive, and conscientious general practitioner. In seeking to reflect the most common needs and interests of general dentists, a conscious effort has been made to develop a text that is practical, useful, and applicable in day-to-day practice.

During the past decade, many excellent books related to dentistry have been published. Routinely, however, these books have been directed toward individuals with a particular interest in one special area of clinical dentistry. The general practitioner has been forced to turn to many texts in order to increase his competence and confidence in providing diversified care for his or her patients. It is to such sources that the reader of this book should turn if a discourse on fundamentals or an interpretation of the literature relevant to a specialized field is needed. This book, however, emphasizes practical applications of knowledge and the integration of information from different disciplines on behalf of individual patients.

DESCRIPTION OF THE READER

General Practice Residents. Increases in formal training opportunities in general practice represent the most rapidly expanding aspect of dental education. With increasing frequency, graduating dental students enter hospital-based general practice residency programs or advanced educational programs in general dentistry associated with other institutions. The Task Force on Advanced Dental Education of the American Association of Dental Schools has recommended that such training opportunities be increased to accommodate approximately one half of all dental graduates by the mid-1980s. It is to the students of such programs that this text is specifically targeted.

Members of the Academy of General Dentistry. The Academy of General Dentistry is one of the most dynamic, progressive, and rapidly growing organizations in dentistry. Its status within the profession reflects both its high principles and the emergence of the general practitioner to a position of high stature within the dental work force. A hallmark of the Academy is its commitment to continued learning and professional development. It is for the present and future members of the Academy that this book has special relevance.

Senior Dental Students. Dental students in the upper classes of those schools that place special emphasis on comprehensive patient care will find this book a useful adjunct to other educational resources.

Specialists in Dentistry. A significant proportion of current dental specialists entered specialty training with a background in general dentistry obtained through private or military practice. The dominant pattern today, however, is one of direct admission to specialty training from dental school. Specialists who follow such a pattern but who recognize the value of being able to relate to their referring dentists with more understanding will find this text useful.

ORGANIZATION OF CHAPTERS

Each chapter begins with a concise statement of objectives, e.g., what the author intends to accomplish through presentation of the chapter. In addition, this introductory section explains what the reader will be able to do on behalf of his or her patients after reading the chapter.

There is a limit to the extent that the presentation of material of all disciplines can and should conform. Except where the format is not applicable or is awkward to use, however, chapters cover the following topics: management of the patient, principles of therapy, biological considerations, illustrative techniques, and complications.

As an aid to the reader, each chapter ends with a list of basic questions that a general practitioner would want to be able to answer and that can be answered through reading of the chapter. The questions are straightforward and relate directly to the care of patients. Answers are provided at the end of the text.

LOUIS W. RIPA

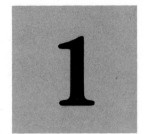

THE PREVENTION OF DENTAL CARIES IN GENERAL PRACTICE

Although the prevention of dental caries does not constitute a dental specialty, a vast amount of information has been published on this subject. The belief that all generalists should include preventive procedures in their practices is the rationale for reviewing caries prevention in this book.

The caries-preventive methods described in this chapter will generally be those that have been proved to inhibit dental caries in controlled clinical trials. Although they have been substantiated in trials involving large groups of individuals, the methods discussed will be applicable to individual patients in private programs of preventive care rather than to large groups of patients in public health programs.

For the dentist, a practical approach is to classify cariostatic methods into those that involve the treatment of the patient in the dental office and those that must be performed by the patient in his own home (Table 1–1). Even though these latter procedures are not professionally administered, it is the dental professional who should recommend or prescribe them and who should instruct the patient in their use.

TABLE 1–1   Caries-Preventive Methods

Methods Performed in the Dental Office
   Occlusal sealants
   Professionally applied topical fluoride

Methods Performed in the Patient's Home
   Diet control
   Maintenance of oral hygiene and use of a
     therapeutic dentifrice
   Self-applied topical fluoride
   Dietary fluoride supplementation

Before the methods listed in Table 1–1 are described, however, it is important to discuss those mechanisms that occur in the human mouth, often without direct intervention from either the dentist or the patient, that inhibit the carious process. By recognizing that some cariostatic mechanisms occur naturally in the mouth, practitioners will have a broader understanding of the concepts of caries prevention.

NATURALLY OCCURRING CARIOSTATIC MECHANISMS

It is important for the dentist who practices preventive dentistry to realize that there are biochemical processes occurring in the mouth that not only can alter the progress of a carious lesion but also can arrest the lesion so that it reverts to a clinically sound status.

The concepts of lesion *reversal* and *remineralization* have gained acceptance through systematic investigation only during the last two decades. A reversal is a clinical observation. Specifically, a tooth surface that is diagnosed as carious at one visit is, when the same diagnostic criteria are applied, called sound at a subsequent visit. This change can occur only if the area of the tooth that was undergoing demineralization becomes hardened, or remineralizes.

Reversal of Carious Lesions

The earliest clinically recognizable stage of dental caries is the "white spot" lesion (Fig.

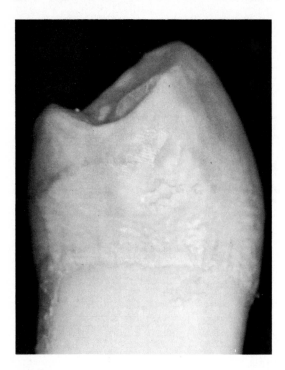

FIGURE 1–1 Clinical appearance of an early carious "white spot" lesion. At this stage, the surface is intact and the principal area of demineralization is beneath the surface.

1–1). White spots are the result of demineralization, usually occurring beneath dental plaque, in which calcium phosphate salts are dissolved out of the tooth, leaving behind microscopic spaces. Because these small spaces become filled with air and water, which have a lower refractive index than normal enamel, the demineralized area assumes a paper-white appearance. This opaque whiteness is easily distinguished from the translucent whiteness of normal enamel, especially when the tooth is dried; hence, the dentist diagnoses the surface as carious.*

Although the popular term for a carious lesion is "cavity," it is important to realize that at the white spot stage the surface of the enamel is still intact. The principal area of demineralization is actually beneath the surface. Figure 1–2 is a microradiograph of a histologic section prepared through a white

---

*Carious white spots must be distinguished from developmental white spots, which represent *hypo*mineralized rather than *de*mineralized areas. Developmental white spots usually have a different distribution throughout the mouth than carious white spots and are found on areas of the teeth that usually do not decay, such as incisal edges of incisors.

spot. The subsurface radiolucency overlaid by a radiopaque surface layer is characteristic of the historadiographic appearance of the lesion at this stage.

Several clinical studies of caries in humans have demonstrated that before the carious lesion has progressed to the stage of cavitation, it may arrest, that is, become hard, and may even disappear so that the surface of the tooth appears clinically sound.[1–10] In some of these reports, the alteration of the progress of the lesion occurred when therapeutic agents such as fluoride rinses, calcium phosphate and fluoride solutions, or a xylitol chewing gum were used.[5, 6, 10] In others, the reversals occurred without any direct therapeutic intervention and were, presumably, caused by the remineralizing effect of the saliva itself.[4]

The two reports that are most often cited as evidence of the remineralization of white spot lesions in the human mouth are those of Backer-Dirks[4] and of von der Fehr and coworkers.[6] Backer-Dirks conducted longitudinal dental examinations on 90 school

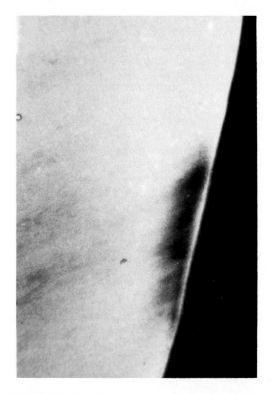

FIGURE 1–2 Microradiograph through a proximal "white spot" carious lesion. The surface of the lesion is radiopaque, indicating that it is less demineralized than the radiolucent subsurface area.

children in the Netherlands at yearly intervals from age 7 or 8 until age 15.[4] The mesial surfaces of the maxillary and mandibular first molars were examined exclusively on bite-wing radiographs. As he anticipated, he found that a number of lesions that were limited initially to the enamel advanced to the dentin as the children got older. However, he remarked that an unexpected number of lesions did not progress beyond the enamel. In fact, 50 per cent showed no progress 4 years after first being detected on radiographs; 33 per cent showed no progress after 6 years; and 26 per cent had not progressed after 8 years when the study was terminated. This suggested to Backer-Dirks that the lesions had arrested, although he could not predict whether this was a temporary or permanent condition.

Backer-Dirks also conducted visual and tactile examinations on the buccal surfaces of the first and second permanent molars in the same children. One hundred eighty-four buccal surfaces were examined on maxillary first molars when the children were 8 years old. At that time the surfaces were diagnosed as being sound, having a white spot, or having a cavity. Seven years later, the same surfaces were reexamined. Of 72 white spots found at the first examination, 9 had progressed to the stage of cavitation and 26 were still diagnosed as white spots, but 37 had disappeared and the surfaces were judged to be sound (Fig. 1–3). Backer-Dirks attributed this change to "remineralization, or a process of recrystallization, or both."

Von der Fehr and coworkers evaluated the effect of cariogenic and caries-protective

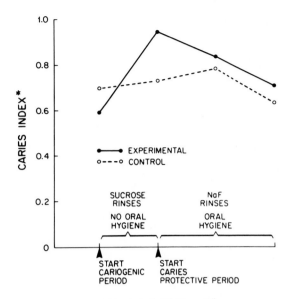

FIGURE 1–4 The effect of a cariogenic challenge on "white spot" formation in humans. During the cariogenic period, the experimental group ceased all oral hygiene procedures and rinsed nine times a day with a sucrose solution. During the caries protective period, they practiced meticulous oral hygiene measures and rinsed daily with a 0.2 per cent NaF solution. The control group maintained their usual routine. (After von der Fehr, R. F., Loe, H., and Theilade E.: Experimental Caries in Man. Caries Res., 4:131–148, 1970.

factors in the mouths of six volunteer dental students. Another six dental students served as control subjects. The experimental group ceased oral hygiene procedures for 23 days. During this period they rinsed their mouths with a 50 per cent aqueous sucrose solution. Rinsing was performed nine times a day for 2 minutes each time using 10 ml of solution. During the 23 days, two dozen buccogingival white areas developed on the enamel surfaces of the teeth. Following this cariogenic period the teeth were cleaned and polished, meticulous oral hygiene measures were reinstituted, and the subjects rinsed daily with a 0.2 per cent NaF solution. One and 2 months after reinstituting the oral hygiene measures and starting the fluoride rinses, the buccal surfaces of the teeth were reexamined. Figure 1–4 shows the changes in Caries Index Scores[11] for the experimental group of students compared with the control group during the cariogenic and caries-protective periods. The return of the Caries

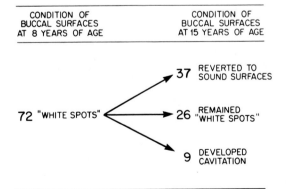

CONDITION OF BUCCAL SURFACES AT 8 YEARS OF AGE	CONDITION OF BUCCAL SURFACES AT 15 YEARS OF AGE
72 "WHITE SPOTS"	37 REVERTED TO SOUND SURFACES
	26 REMAINED "WHITE SPOTS"
	9 DEVELOPED CAVITATION

FIGURE 1–3 The fate, after seven years, of buccal "white spot" carious lesions on the maxillary first permanent molars of children.

Index Scores to near baseline levels in the experimental group indicates that the enamel surfaces had reverted to a clinically sound status. The disappearance of the white decalcified areas during the caries-protective period was attributed to "remineralization."

Remineralization

The carious process in enamel is believed to involve not just a series of demineralizing attacks, but rather periods of demineralization alternating with periods of remineralization and arrest. Demineralization occurs when plaque pH falls following carbohydrate ingestion. When the pH rises, some of the calcium and phosphate that dissolved from the enamel during the period of demineralization reprecipitates into the lesion and onto its surface. Calcium, phosphate, and other minerals that are present in the saliva and plaque may also precipitate on the surface of the lesion as the pH changes.

The histologic appearance of the early carious white spot lesion is consistent with a process that involves both demineralization and remineralization. Rather than being homogeneous, a cross section of the lesion shows it to consist of several zones (Fig. 1–5).[12–15] These zones all contain less mineral than normal enamel, yet they differ from each other in their extent of demineralization. As already mentioned, the surface zone is relatively more mineralized. The immediate underlying zone, called the "body" of the lesion, shows the greatest mineral loss.

Other zones within the lesion usually exhibit a degree of demineralization intermediate between these two areas. The zone pattern is believed to occur as enamel dissolved during demineralization; the dissolved mineral diffuses through the lesion, and then the mineral reprecipitates, especially in the surface layer, as the pH within the lesion rises.

Evidence that the surface of demineralized enamel can be remineralized comes from both in vivo[16] and in vitro investigations.[17–21] Surfaces that have been etched with phosphoric acid during bonding procedures, but to which a dental resin was subsequently not applied, remineralize in the presence of saliva.[22, 23] Blocks of enamel whose surfaces have been made soft either by demineralization in the mouth or with an acid in the laboratory become hard again when exposed to saliva or to "mineralizing solutions" containing calcium and phosphate.[16, 24–26]

The Role of Fluoride in Remineralization

During the remineralization process, fluoride acts in at least two ways.[27] First, in the presence of fluoride ions, remineralization is accelerated. Second, as mineral is reprecipitated back into the enamel, if fluoride is present, it is also incorporated into the remineralized tissue. In this way, white spot enamel will accrue more fluoride than will sound enamel.[28] Because of this fluoride enrichment, the white spot areas become more resistant to further caries attack than does sound enamel.[29] Koulourides has coined the

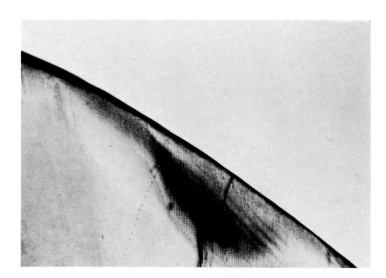

FIGURE 1–5 Longitudinal section through a proximal "white spot" carious lesion. The affected area consists of zones that are demineralized to different degrees. The body of the lesion shows the most demineralization.

term "cariogenic priming" for the process whereby cariously demineralized enamel that has been exposed to fluoride becomes converted to a state of higher caries resistance.[29]

Clinical Implications of Caries Reversal and Remineralization

The concept that through a process of remineralization early carious lesions can arrest or even revert to a clinically sound status has profound implications for the clinician. Previously, the goal of caries prevention was limited to inhibiting the formation of new lesions; now the goal can be expanded to include treating existing lesions by preventing them from progressing. It is evident that all areas of a tooth diagnosed as carious need not be treated by restoring the involved surface with a filling. If a lesion has not progressed to the stage of cavitation, it may be amenable to remineralization.

Whether new lesions develop or existing ones progress to cavitation depends upon the balance that exists at the plaque–tooth surface interface between caries-promoting factors and caries-protective factors (Fig. 1–6). If the frequency and duration of the cariogenic challenge supersedes the resistance afforded by the caries-protective factors, a lesion will develop and cavitation will occur.

Saliva is a natural remineralization agent[27, 30, 31] and will act to inhibit lesion development and progression. There are a number of ways, however, in which the dental profession and the patient can intervene

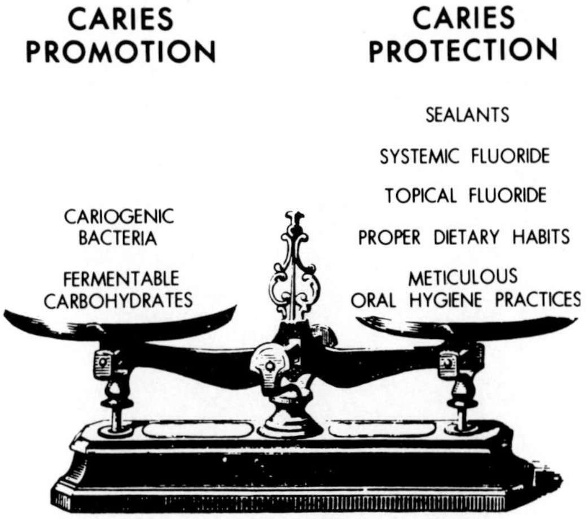

FIGURE 1–6 The oral balance: The initiation and progression of the carious lesion is dependent upon the balance between caries-promoting and caries-protective factors.

to tip the intraoral balance in favor of the caries-protective factors. The cariogenic challenge can be reduced by diet modification and by meticulous oral hygiene practices that remove plaque from the teeth. The caries-protective factors can be enhanced by chemically altering the tooth's solubility to acids with systemic and topical fluoride administration, by promoting remineralization through the use of frequently applied fluoride agents, and by physically occluding the pits and fissures from the rest of the oral environment with sealants. These methods of caries prevention will be discussed in the following sections.

Office Procedures

OCCLUSAL SEALANTS

Every dentist is aware of the disproportionate number of restorations that are placed in occlusal surfaces compared with the other surfaces of the teeth. The impression that occlusal surfaces are the most caries-susceptible sites in the mouth is substantiated by clinical research.[32–35] Not only is there a high incidence of occlusal caries, but the initiation and progression of the lesion also occurs quite rapidly. Thus, Miller and Hobson have reported that 40 per cent of occlusal surfaces of permanent teeth develop caries within 12 to 18 months after eruption,[36] and Backer-Dirks found that most of the occlu-

sal surfaces of first and second permanent molars were carious by 9 and 14 years of age, respectively.[37]

It is the pits and fissures of the occlusal surfaces that predispose them to decay. Located in depressions between the cusps of the teeth, pits and fissures form narrow cul-de-sacs in which bacteria and food debris accumulate, favoring the initiation of dental caries.[38, 39] Since the enamel at the base of most fissures is quite thin (Fig. 1–7), the developing lesion can progress rapidly into the dentin.[40]

Although fluoride reduces the incidence of dental decay, the occlusal surfaces are least protected by topical or systemic fluo-

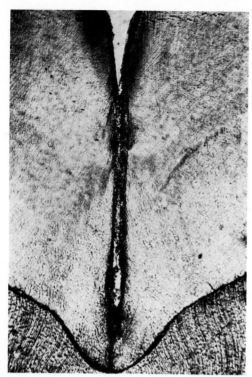

FIGURE 1–7 An occlusal fissure. The fissure is constricted, providing a shelter for oral bacteria. There is a thin layer of enamel separating the base of the fissure from the dentin. (Courtesy of Dr. M. Buonocore.)

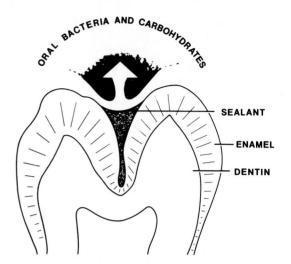

FIGURE 1–8 The purpose of a sealant is to physically occlude the pit or fissure.

Available Sealant Systems

Most, if not all, of the sealants currently marketed have a base formulation of dimethacrylates, which represent the reaction product of bisphenol A and glycidyl methacrylate (BIS-GMA) (Fig. 1–9). The BIS-GMA system also forms the base of the anterior composite restorative materials. A diluent, such as methyl methacrylate, is added to make sealants less viscous and, therefore, able to flow more readily into the pits and fissures of the occlusal surfaces.

There are two principal types of BIS-GMA sealants currently marketed: autopolymerizing and ultraviolet light–polymerizing sealants. Autopolymerizing sealants are polymerized chemically, usually by the addition of benzoyl peroxide. Ultraviolet systems employ long-wavelength ultraviolet light emitted by an ultraviolet lamp to activate benzoin methyl ether, which, in turn, initiates polymerization. Other differences between commercial products are that some are tinted or opaque while others are clear and that some contain inert filler particles while others are unfilled.

The choice of which commercial sealant to use is largely based on the personal preference of the operator, since most marketed sealants have been accepted or provisionally accepted by the Council on Dental Materials and Devices of the American Dental Association.[46] The advantages of an autopolymerizing sealant are its simplicity and ability to harden within a specified time after mixing. Conversely, the advantage of the ultraviolet

rides.[41–43] For instance, the caries reduction from community water fluoridation on smooth surfaces has been reported to be as high as 70 per cent, while the concomitant occlusal caries reduction was only 20 per cent.[44] Recently, Ripa and coworkers reported that elementary school children who had participated in a school-based fluoride mouthrinsing program for up to 4 years had a 68 per cent reduction in proximal caries compared with a 35 per cent reduction of caries of the occlusal surfaces.[45] Thus, the use of fluoride cannot be relied upon as the sole method for preventing decay of occlusal surfaces.

Sealants were developed specifically to prevent caries of the occlusal surfaces. In the sealant procedure, a resinous material is placed over the pits and fissures, isolating them from the rest of the oral environment. Since sealants contain no active therapeutic agent to make the enamel more resistant to decay, the coating acts as a physical barrier, preventing oral bacteria and their nutrients from forming the acid conditions necessary to initiate the carious process (Fig. 1–8).

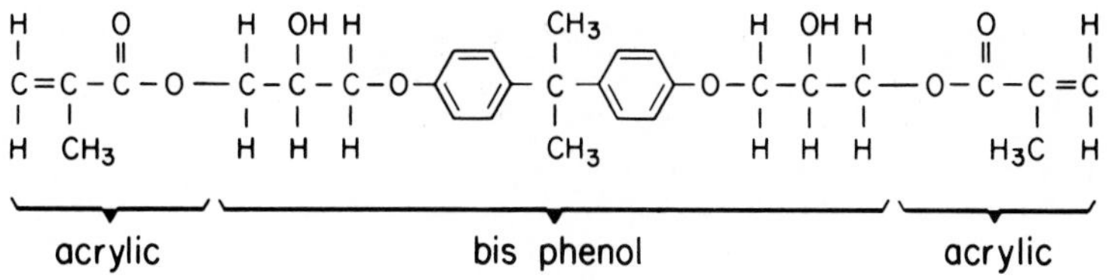

FIGURE 1–9 The bisphenol A glycidyl methacrylate (BIS-GMA) molecule.

acrylic   bis phenol   acrylic

system is that the operator initiates setting only when he or she feels the sealant has been adequately applied. Tinted and opaque products offer the advantage of better visibility when checking for their presence at recall visits, while a semifilled sealant resists occlusal abrasion more than unfilled sealants.

Indications for Use of Sealants

The first step toward deciding whether a tooth should receive a sealant is to perform a visual and tactile examination of the occlusal surface. With the use of a dental explorer, the caries status of the surface is determined. If caries is found, the tooth should not be sealed but must be restored. If the occlusal surface is sound, it *may* be sealed. The determination of whether a sound surface should receive a sealant is based upon several considerations. These include the caries status of the proximal surfaces, the occlusal morphology, tooth age, general caries activity in the mouth, and use of other caries-preventive methods. Sealant protection is limited to the pits and fissures. Thus, in or-

der to achieve the greatest possible caries reduction, sealants should be used in conjunction with other caries-preventive methods such as systemic and topical fluorides, sound dietary habits, and good oral hygiene procedures, which include the use of fluoride-containing dentifrices. The use of sealants together with other methods of caries prevention is especially important in patients who are highly susceptible to decay. The various factors to be considered when deciding whether or not to seal a tooth are outlined in Table 1–2.

Occasionally a dentist cannot decide whether an occlusal surface is carious or sound. Since a surface for which a definite caries diagnosis is lacking should not be restored, the treatment in the past was to "watch" it. This approach was acceptable at a time when there was no appropriate therapy for such surfaces. It is, however, no longer acceptable. Provided the proximal surfaces of the tooth are sound, an occlusal surface with a questionable caries diagnosis should definitely be sealed in order to prevent the surface from developing a frank

TABLE 1–2 Indications and Contraindications for Occlusal Sealants

Diagnosis of Occlusal Surface	Clinical Considerations	Do Seal	Do Not Seal
Caries-free	Occlusal morphology	Deep, narrow pits and fissures	Broad, well-coalesced pits and fissures
	Tooth age	Recently erupted teeth	Teeth that have been caries-free for 4 years or longer
	Status of proximal surface(s)	Sound	Carious
	General caries activity	Many occlusal lesions, few proximal lesions	Many proximal lesions
Questionable	Status of Proximal surface(s)	Sound	Carious
	General caries activity	Many occlusal lesions, few proximal lesions	Many proximal lesions
Carious	Occlusal Anatomy	If pits or fissures are discrete and separated by a transverse ridge, a sound pit may be sealed	Carious pits or fissures are not to be sealed

carious lesion. This approach is justified, since it has been shown that if caries is inadvertently sealed, the lesion will not progress but, instead, should arrest.[47, 48]

From Table 1–2 and the foregoing, it is evident that sealants are indicated for children, not adults. Since the permanent premolars and molars erupt between 6 and 13 years of age (exclusive of third molars), 6 to 16 years constitutes the general age range when sealants should be applied. Primary molars may also be sealed. However, when these teeth first erupt, the child is usually too young to sit quietly and allow adequate isolation of the teeth. Conversely, in the older child, the occlusal surfaces of some primary molars may have already decayed, while those that remain noncarious may be caries-resistant and not require sealing.

Application Technique

Sealants may be applied by a dentist or a dental auxiliary. The state dental practice acts of approximately 30 states allow hygienists and, of 13 states, allow dental assistants to apply sealants under appropriate supervision.

Figures 1–10 through 1–22 demonstrate the application of an autopolymerizing sealant system. The steps involved when using an ultraviolet light–polymerizing system are similar, and both depend upon the strict maintenance of a dry field.

Sealant-treated teeth should be examined at each 6-month recall visit. If some or all of the sealant is missing, it should be replaced by repeating the procedure outlined above (provided the tooth is caries-free). If, at the recall visit, the sealant is intact and cannot be

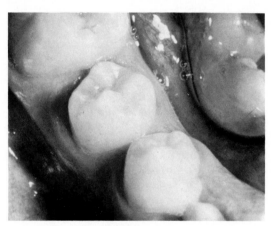

FIGURE 1–10

Step 1: Selection. Teeth are selected for sealing based on the indications previously discussed. In this case, the second premolar and distal portion of the occlusal surface of the first premolar are going to be sealed. The first molar was treated when the child was younger. The mesial portion of the first premolar is smooth and therefore does not require sealing. (Courtesy of Johnson & Johnson Dental Products Company, East Windsor, New Jersey.)

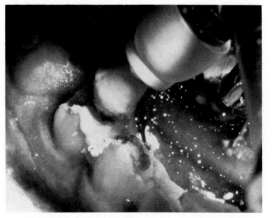

FIGURE 1–11

Step 2: Prophylaxis. A fluoride-free prophylaxis paste is used to clean the occlusal surfaces. An aqueous slurry of flour of pumice is recommended. The prophylaxis removes soft debris and plaque from the occlusal surfaces. (Courtesy of Johnson & Johnson Dental Products Company, East Windsor, New Jersey.)

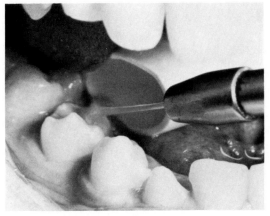

FIGURE 1–12

Step 3: Rinsing. The occlusal surfaces are thoroughly washed with a water spray. (Courtesy of Johnson & Johnson Dental Products Company, East Windsor, New Jersey.)

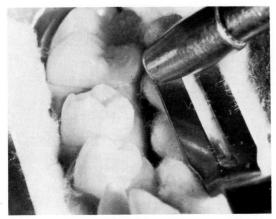

FIGURE 1–13

Step 4: Isolation and Drying. The quadrant is isolated with cotton rolls. Each tooth is air dried for 30 seconds. The air spray must contain no moisture or droplets of oil. (Courtesy of Johnson & Johnson Dental Products Company, East Windsor, New Jersey.)

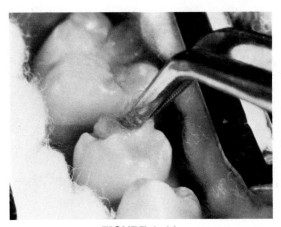

FIGURE 1–14

Step 5: Acid Etching. The cleaned and dried occlusal surface is etched with phosphoric acid (35 to 50 per cent) for 60 seconds. The acid is applied by gently wiping the surface with a small pledget of cotton. The acid etching should be confined to the occlusal portion of the teeth. (Courtesy of Johnson & Johnson Dental Products Company, East Windsor, New Jersey.)

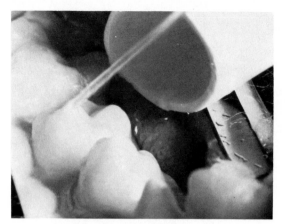

FIGURE 1–15

Step 6: Rinsing and Drying. The etched surface is thoroughly rinsed with a water spray and then dried with air. The air line must be free of contaminants. *From this point until the sealant is placed, saliva must not contact the etched surface of the tooth.* If cotton rolls require changing, the change must be accomplished without the teeth becoming contaminated with saliva. (Courtesy of Johnson & Johnson Dental Products Company, East Windsor, New Jersey.)

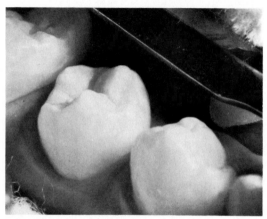

FIGURE 1–16

Clinical Appearance of Etched Surface. A properly etched surface will have a dull matte appearance, in contrast to the glossy surface of nonetched enamel. (Courtesy of Johnson & Johnson Dental Products Company, East Windsor, New Jersey.)

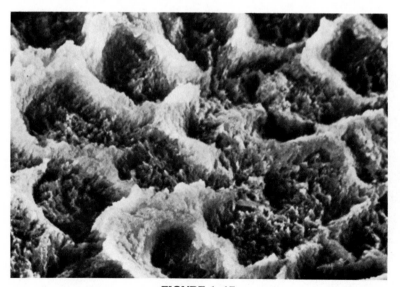

FIGURE 1–17

Microscopic Appearance of Etched Surface. Etching creates a preferential pattern of demineralization at the surface and dissolves mineral from the first 25 to 50 microns of the enamel, producing spaces into which the sealant will flow. (Courtesy of Dr. A. J. Gwinnett and Johnson & Johnson Dental Products Company, East Windsor, New Jersey.)

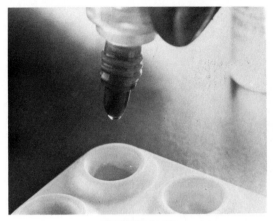

FIGURE 1–18

Step 7: Mixing the Sealant. The liquid catalyst and base are mixed according to the manufacturer's directions. (Courtesy of Johnson & Johnson Dental Products Company, East Windsor, New Jersey.)

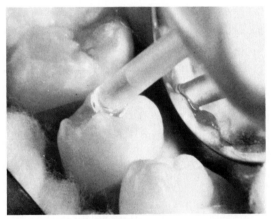

FIGURE 1–19

Step 8: Sealant Application. The sealant is applied to the etched surface to cover all of the pits and fissures. (Courtesy of Johnson & Johnson Dental Products Company, East Windsor, New Jersey.)

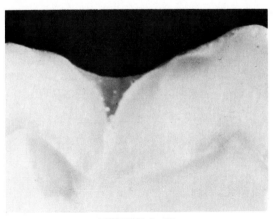

FIGURE 1–20

Cross Section of Sealant-treated Tooth. The sealant lies over the pits and fissures and on the internal slopes of the cusps of the teeth. Retention is obtained by covering as large a surface area of the tooth as possible.

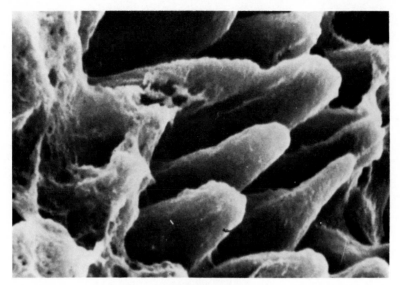

Microscopic Appearance of Sealant Undersurface. Extensions of sealant, called "tags," penetrate the pores in the enamel created by the etching procedure. Upon polymerization, the tags form a strong physical bond with the tooth and thus retain the sealant. (Courtesy of Dr. A. J. Gwinnett and Johnson & Johnson Dental Products Company, East Windsor, New Jersey.)

FIGURE 1–21

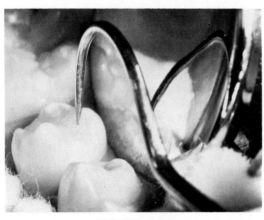

FIGURE 1–22

Step 9: Postapplication Check. After the sealant hardens, it is checked with an explorer. The margins should be smooth, and there should be no surface porosities. If there is a porosity created by an air bubble at the surface of the sealant, it should be filled with a new mix of sealant. An attempt should be made to dislodge the sealant with the tyne of the explorer. A properly placed sealant will not dislodge. If the sealant comes off, new sealant should be reapplied, omitting the prophylaxis step and reducing the etching step to 10 seconds. If an unfilled sealant was used, occlusion need not be checked. The patient's own occlusion will abrade any excess. If a semifilled sealant is used, reduction of occlusal interferences is indicated. (Courtesy of Johnson & Johnson Dental Products Company, East Windsor, New Jersey.)

dislodged with an explorer, no further treatment is indicated.

It was believed initially that sealants were not retained as well on primary teeth as they were on permanent teeth, and it was suggested that the occlusal surfaces of the primary teeth be etched for more than 60 seconds or that a thin layer of occlusal enamel be ground off before etching. Recent studies, however, have failed to confirm a difference between the retention rate of sealants on primary and permanent teeth.[49] Therefore, the application of sealants to the primary teeth should employ the same 60-second etch procedure used for the permanent teeth, and the results should be expected to be similar.

Results Using Sealants

An assessment of the clinical success of sealants involves a determination of the occlusal caries reductions obtained by their use and an evaluation of the clinical retention of the sealant after placement. Retention is especially important, because the ability of sealants to prevent decay is dependent upon their adherence to the tooth surface, where they continue to act as a physical barrier between the caries-susceptible pits and fissures and the rest of the oral environment.

There have been at least three dozen reports in which sealants have been evaluated on the permanent or primary teeth.[49, 50] Table 1–3 summarizes the findings for the per-

TABLE 1–3   Use of BIS-GMA Sealants on the Permanent Teeth: Retention and Occlusal Caries Reduction

Years After Sealant Application	Number of Reports	% Retention*		Number of Reports	% Occlusal Caries Reduction	
		Range	Average		Range	Average
1	19	18–99	77	11	65–100	83
2	12	3–87	59	10	14–99	67
3	3	33–70	47	2	68–73	71
4	3	25–50	41	3	22–45	37
5	1		42	1		37

*Completely covered teeth only.
Adapted from Ripa, L. W.: Occlusal Sealants: Rationale and Review of Clinical Trials. Int. Dent. J., 30:127–139, 1980.

manent dentition. Most of the studies involved a single application of the sealant followed by 6- or 12-month recall examinations. The longest study reported results 5 years after sealant placement.[51] This study found 42 per cent of the teeth still completely covered with sealant and an occlusal caries reduction of 37 per cent.

Since sealants contain no active cariostatic agent but depend upon the maintenance of a physical barrier for their effect, success is especially dependent upon the operator's technique and the clinical conditions at the time of placement. Probably the greatest cause of failure is the inability of the operator to maintain a dry field. Salivary contamination of the enamel surface after it has been etched will prevent tag penetration of the sealant into the underlying enamel, and thus retention will be poor. It is not surprising that retention is poor in younger children whose behavior may be difficult to control or that clinically less experienced operators are not as successful with the use of sealants as are more experienced ones. Also, teeth that have just erupted and the more posterior molars, especially in the maxillary arch, are very susceptible to loss of sealant because they are difficult to isolate and to keep dry during the sealant procedure. These different factors are undoubtedly responsible for the wide range of retention rates and caries reductions listed in Table 1–3.

PROFESSIONAL TOPICAL FLUORIDE THERAPY

Professional topical fluoride therapy refers to the application of concentrated fluoride agents to the erupted teeth of a patient by a dentist or dental auxiliary. While the mechanism of action of this treatment method is still incompletely understood, the most commonly accepted hypothesis is that the fluoride reacts with the hydroxyapatite of the enamel, forming calcium fluoride and fluorapatite. The calcium fluoride is quickly lost from the surfaces of the teeth; however, the fluoride that is bound as fluorapatite remains and makes the enamel more resistant to dissolution by the acids produced by the bacteria in dental plaque.

Topical Fluoride Compounds and Vehicles

Since the 1940s, different fluoride compounds have been studied as potential topical agents. The first clinical investigations employed aqueous solutions of neutral sodium fluoride (NaF), and the ability of this compound to inhibit dental caries was confirmed in numerous clinical trials conducted on children residing in fluoride-deficient communities. In the 1950s, stannous fluoride (SnF_2) gained acceptance as a topical fluoride compound, and in the next decade an acidulated form of sodium fluoride (acidulated phosphate fluoride, or APF) became available. The rationale for the formulation of APF was based on the known information that acidic fluoride solutions deposited more fluoride into enamel than did neutral solutions. By the addition of phosphate to the acidified solution, the degree of enamel dissolution was controlled, and the formation of fluorapatite over calcium fluoride was enhanced.[52] Another compound, amine fluoride, is used as a topical fluoride agent in other countries but is not available in the United States. Table 1–4 lists the fluoride concentrations of the three most commonly used fluoride compounds.

Initially, only aqueous solutions were available for topical fluoride application. In

TABLE 1–4   Fluoride Concentrations of Professionally Applied Topical Fluoride Compounds

Compound*	Fluoride Ion Concentration	ppm F
2.0% NaF	0.9% F⁻	9040
8.0% SnF₂	2.0% F⁻	19,360
APF	1.2% F⁻	12,300

*NaF = Sodium fluoride; SnF₂ = Stannous fluoride; APF = Acidulated phosphate fluoride.

an effort to expedite the treatment procedure, topical fluoride compounds have been incorporated into prophylaxis pastes and gels. Fluoride aqueous solutions and fluoride gels have been found to be effective in inhibiting dental caries. However, clinical studies have failed to justify using a fluoride-containing prophylaxis paste as the *sole* agent when performing a topical fluoride treatment, although it may be used in conjunction with other agents.

Fluoride has also been incorporated into varnishlike materials that are painted on the teeth and remain adherent to the enamel surface for 12 hours or longer. A varnish will increase the exposure time of the fluoride to the teeth without increasing chair time. Because of the longer contact, the uptake of fluoride by the enamel is significantly increased. Two commercial fluoride varnishes, one containing NaF and the other containing an organic fluoride, difluorosilane, have been tested in laboratory and clinical studies and are available in several countries, although not in the United States. While fluoride uptake is enhanced by the use of these products, sufficient clinical evidence is not available to demonstrate that

fluoride applied in this form is superior to the use of fluoride in aqueous solutions or gels.

Indications for Professional Topical Fluoride Therapy

Because it is realized that a single topical fluoride treatment imparts little lasting benefit to the teeth, the question is not whether a patient should receive one treatment, but whether topical fluoride applications should be routinely applied for several years.

Three interrelated factors influence the decision to routinely recommend professional topical fluoride applications for a patient. These are (1) the patient's age, (2) the concentration of fluoride in the drinking water, and (3) the patient's caries status. No matter what their caries status is, patients who are in their caries-susceptible years (approximately 17 and younger) are candidates for professional topical fluoride treatments if they reside in a fluoride-deficient community. On the other hand, if they reside in an optimally fluoridated community, they require topical fluoride treatments only if they present with active carious lesions, especially of the smooth surfaces of the teeth. Patients older than 17 years, regardless of the concentration of fluoride in the drinking water, require topical fluoride therapy only if they are caries-active. These recommendations are summarized in Table 1–5.

Choice of Fluoride Compounds and Vehicles

Sodium fluoride, SnF₂, and APF all appear to be equally effective in reducing den-

TABLE 1–5   Indications for Professionally Applied Topical Fluoride Therapy

Patient's age	Community Water Fluoride Concentration	Patient's Caries Status*	Need for Professionally Applied Topical Fluoride Therapy
17 Years and Younger	F-deficient (F≤0.7 ppm)	Caries active	Yes
		Caries inactive	Yes
	Fluoridated (F>0.7 ppm)	Caries active	Yes
		Caries inactive	No
Older than 17 Years	F-deficient (F≤0.7 ppm)	Caries active	Yes
		Caries inactive	No
	Fluoridated (F>0.7 ppm)	Caries active	Yes
		Caries inactive	No

*Caries active: Patient presents with one or more new carious lesions. Caries inactive: Patient presents with no new lesions at two or more consecutive recall visits.

tal caries.[53] Nevertheless, largely because of the convenience of application and patient acceptance, most dental practitioners use APF for professional topical fluoride treatments. Advantages of the APF formulation include its stability and indefinite shelf life when kept in a plastic container, and the fact that it has no untoward intraoral side effects, such as staining the teeth or causing gingival irritation. Although the low pH gives the formulation a bitter taste, some of the commercial products are flavored to make them more acceptable to patients.

Both APF aqueous solutions and gels contain 1.2 per cent fluorine ion, from NaF and HF, buffered with orthophosphoric acid to a pH of 3.0 to 3.5. Gels contain a hydroxyalkyl cellulose that increases the viscosity. Recently thixotropic gels have been introduced. Thixotropy refers to the property of becoming fluid when agitated and relatively firm when at rest. This property is useful when using trays to apply the fluoride gel to the teeth. All commercially available APF gels contain coloring and flavoring agents that make them more acceptable to patients.

Topical fluoride applications using an aqueous solution involve a relatively time-consuming paint-on technique, wherein the topical fluoride is applied to each tooth surface using a cotton-tipped applicator. Since the fluoride should remain in contact with the teeth for 4 minutes, the paint-on technique can take 16 minutes if each quadrant of the mouth is treated separately or 8 minutes if one half of the mouth is treated at a time. Because a gel allows treatment to be accomplished in a convenient tray application, in which the whole mouth can be treated simultaneously in 4 minutes, a fluoride gel is the most often used vehicle for topical fluoride applications.

Application Technique

Since the first studies in the 1940s, the technique of professional topical fluoride application has involved two steps. In the first step, the teeth are cleaned using a prophylaxis paste and dental floss. This procedure removes materia alba, plaque, and other natural coatings from the surfaces of the teeth, which could prevent fluoride uptake by the enamel. Next, the topical fluoride agent is applied. Although the need to perform a *thorough* prophylaxis before applying the topical fluoride has been questioned, currently there is no clinical evidence indicating that this step should be omitted.

After the trays are removed, the patient may expectorate but is asked not to eat or drink for 30 minutes. While this admonition is somewhat empirical, Richardson has shown in an in vitro study that the length of time between a topical fluoride application and washing the teeth significantly affects fluoride uptake.[59]

Professional topical fluoride applications are usually performed at 6-month or yearly intervals. A 6-month treatment interval appears to be more effective than a yearly one. For individual patients in whom the caries activity is especially high, treatments may be performed even more frequently.

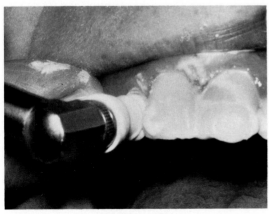

FIGURE 1–23

Step 1: Prophylaxis. All accessible surfaces of the teeth are cleaned by applying a dental prophylaxis paste in a rotating rubber cup. Since a pumice paste abrades a thin layer of fluoride-rich surface enamel,[54–56] a paste with a less abrasive cleaning agent such as silicone dioxide should be used.[57] Use of a fluoride-containing prophylaxis paste is also recommended, since it may replace some of the enamel fluoride lost from the surface by abrasion.[57]

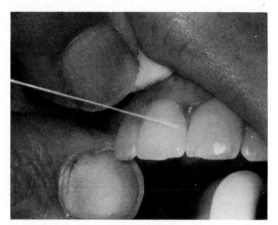

FIGURE 1–24

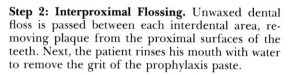

Step 2: Interproximal Flossing. Unwaxed dental floss is passed between each interdental area, removing plaque from the proximal surfaces of the teeth. Next, the patient rinses his mouth with water to remove the grit of the prophylaxis paste.

Step 3: Tray Preparation. A variety of disposable commercial trays are available, including polystyrene, wax, and vinyl trays with paper or foam inserts. Objective comparisons of the different tray types are unavailable; nevertheless, the operator should choose a tray that can be easily modified to fit different size arches, which allows the fluoride gel to cover all surfaces of the teeth and prevents the gel from seeping into the mouth.

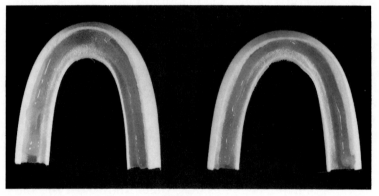

First, the trays should be tried in the mouth. They must fit over all of the teeth in each arch. If a tray is too long, its ends should be cut with scissors. A thin ribbon of gel is squeezed into the trays. Enough is added to cover the teeth, but not enough to flow out when inserted into the mouth.

FIGURE 1–25

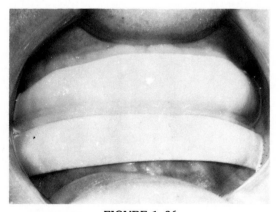

FIGURE 1–26

Step 4: Topical Fluoride Application. The teeth are air-dried of saliva and the maxillary and mandibular trays are inserted simultaneously. A saliva ejector may be used if excess saliva accumulates, as the presence of saliva on the teeth can reduce fluoride uptake by as much as 25 per cent.

The patient closes his mouth on the trays so that all of the teeth are immersed in the fluoride. The trays are worn for 4 minutes, and the patient is reminded to flex the oral musculature to stimulate the gel to flow interproximally. This is especially necessary with a thixotropic gel, since the intermittent pressure induces the fluidity of the product.

During the treatment, any excess gel that exudes from the trays is aspirated by the saliva ejector or expectorated into a paper napkin held by the patient.

Results of Professional Topical Fluoride Therapy

During the past 40 years, numerous clinical trials have evaluated the caries protection afforded by the professional application of NaF, SnF$_2$, and APF. The caries inhibition from the use of these agents has generally been accepted to be between 30 and 40 per cent.[60] In a report by Ripa in which 35 clinical trials involving 74 treatment groups using these three agents were reviewed, the average reductions were between 28 and 32 per cent.[53] All of the studies reviewed employed aqueous solutions of the fluoride compounds and were conducted on children residing in fluoride-deficient communities.

Since the use of gels is a relatively recent innovation, there are fewer published clinical studies evaluating the gel-tray mode of application. Ripa also reviewed studies employing gel trays and found most of these studies were positive, indicating that this method is also effective in reducing dental caries.[53]

Most clinical trials testing professional topical fluoride application have been conducted on the permanent teeth of children residing in fluoride-deficient areas. Although topical fluoride treatments inhibit dental decay in these circumstances, there are other clinical situations in which the efficacy of topical fluoride treatments should be known. These include application to the teeth of children who are lifetime residents of an optimally fluoridated community, application to the primary dentition, and application in adults. Since the number of clinical trials that have tested topical fluoride treatments in these clinical situations has been relatively small, statements on efficacy in these circumstances are probably less universally accepted.

A review of studies designed to provide information about the efficacy of professionally applied topical fluorides in the aforementioned clinical situations leads to the following conclusions. Evidence is lacking to prove that professional topical fluoride treatment significantly reduces dental caries in groups of children who are already receiving the benefits of community water fluoridation. This suggests that professional topical fluoride treatments should *not be routinely performed* on children who are lifetime residents of an optimally fluoridated community. However, individual patients with high caries activity, despite a history of communal water fluoride contact, and persons who previously resided in a fluoride-deficient community are candidates for professional topical fluoride therapy. Topical fluoride applications are effective in the primary dentition; however, the caries reductions are generally not as great as those reported for the permanent teeth. Topical fluoride treatments are also effective in adults, although the need to prevent enamel lesions may be less, since the teeth of older patients are believed to be less susceptible to decay. Older patients begin to develop carious lesions of the roots of the teeth. Fluoride is taken up by the cementum,[61, 62] and, on this basis, it is expected that topical fluoride treatments in patients with exposed roots would be effective in inhibiting cemental lesions.

COMBINED USE OF OCCLUSAL SEALANTS AND PROFESSIONAL TOPICAL FLUORIDE THERAPY

From the foregoing, it is evident that the two preventive office treatments, occlusal sealants and professional topical fluoride application, will provide maximal protection when used concomitantly. By performing topical fluoride treatments at 6-month intervals, all of the tooth surfaces should benefit. However, maximal protection will be afforded to the smooth surfaces, while the pit and fissure surfaces will be least protected. By also treating the same patient with sealants, the pit and fissure surfaces will be provided maximal caries protection. Sealants should be used not only on the occlusal surfaces but also anywhere that a deep pit or fissure exists. Thus, lingual pits on maxillary lateral incisors, buccal pits on mandibular molars, and lingual grooves on maxillary molars should all be treated with sealants if they are judged susceptible to decay because of their deep or constricted morphology.

The sealant application and professional topical fluoride treatment may be done at the same appointment or at different appointments. Whether they are performed together or separately should depend upon the total dental treatment that a patient is to receive.

If quadrant restorative dentistry treatment is planned for a patient, then sealants can be included in the quadrant approach to care. As each quadrant is restored, teeth in that quadrant for which sealing is indicated would be treated at the same visit. At the final visit, all of the restorations can be polished and the prophylaxis and topical fluoride treatment performed.

If little or no restorative care is indicated, it is usually more practical to perform the prophylaxis, topical fluoride treatment, and sealant applications at the same visit. When performing these procedures together, the sequence is very important. At one time,

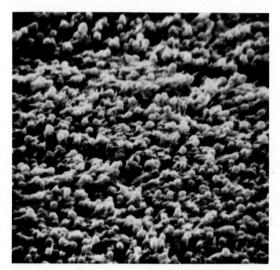

FIGURE 1–27   An etched enamel surface following topical treatment with sodium fluoride. The contaminating globular layer, which is believed to be reaction products between the calcium of the tooth and the topical fluoride, obscures the preferential demineralization pattern created by etching. Surface contamination is also found when stannous fluoride and acidulated phosphate fluoride are the treatment agents. When this layer is present at the interface, the bond strength between the sealant and tooth is decreased. (SEM, 10,000×) (Courtesy of Dr. Zia Shey.)

some people thought it desirable to apply sealants over occlusal surfaces immediately after they had been treated with fluoride. It was believed that the sealant would "lock in" the fluoride and, should the sealant be lost, the prolonged contact of the fluoride with the enamel would provide that surface with a greater resistance to decay. However, treating with fluoride immediately before a tooth is sealed is detrimental to the retention of the sealant. This is especially true if the fluoride is applied between the etching and sealant application steps. Topical fluoride reacts with the enamel to result in calcium fluoride reaction products that adhere to the tooth surface and physically occlude the porosities created by etching.[63] An example of these reaction products covering an etched tooth surface is seen in Figure 1–27. The presence of this contaminating layer weakens the bond strength between the sealant and tooth surface, and the sealant is more likely to fail.[64] The correct sequence when sealant application and professional topical fluoride therapy are done at the same visit is:

First, perform a thorough prophylaxis of all the tooth surfaces, including the occlusal surfaces, that are to be sealed. Use flour of pumice rather than either a fluoride-containing prophylaxis paste or another commercial product with coloring and flavoring additives, whose ingredients might leave a contaminating coating on the teeth that could be potentially detrimental to bonding.

Second, apply the sealants. This is done on a quadrant by quadrant basis, following the steps outlined in the section on occlusal sealants.

Third, apply the topical fluoride. If a fluoride gel is applied in trays, the entire mouth will be treated in the same application.

Home Procedures

DIET CONTROL

When discussing the relationship between food and caries, two terms are frequently confused: nutrition and diet. *Nutrition* is the process by which food is ingested and assimilated by the body in order to promote the growth and repair of tissues. *Diet* is what a person eats or drinks. Nutrition may have a systemic effect on the teeth as they are de-

veloping; diet may have a local effect on the teeth after they have erupted.

The Effect of Nutrition on Dental Caries

Whether a nutritionally adequate diet promotes the caries resistance of teeth is not known. People in developing countries frequently subsist on nutritionally inadequate diets. These individuals show signs of mal-

nourishment, including rachitic bones and dysplastic teeth. Yet, rampant caries is not endemic in malnourished populations. This fact has been cited as evidence that nutritional status during tooth development does not influence caries resistance or susceptibility. However, malnourished populations generally do not eat diets that are highly caries-promoting. The degree of caries resistance of the teeth cannot be determined accurately in the absence of a significant cariogenic challenge. There is some evidence, however, in both animals and human beings, that a protein-calorie deficiency during the period of tooth development, coupled with a cariogenic challenge, can result in caries levels that are higher than normal.[65–67] Even if this relationship is substantiated, in the United States one would not expect malnutrition to play a significant role in the caries susceptibility of the population because the nutritional level of American children generally is high.

The principal effect of nutrition on dental caries is through the ingestion of fluoride. When present at appropriate levels during development of the teeth, fluoride reduces dental caries by about 50 per cent. While other trace elements such as strontium, boron, lithium, and molybdenum may also alter the caries susceptibility of teeth,[68, 69] the magnitude of their effect does not appear to be as great as that of fluoride. The use of systemic fluoride supplements will be discussed in detail in a later section of this chapter.

The Effect of Diet on Dental Caries

An individual's dietary habits have a direct effect on caries activity. Of the three major dietary components, fats and proteins do not appear to have a significant influence on dental decay. However, there is a direct relationship between the ingestion of carbohydrates and caries. In order to control the cariogenic potential of a diet, the types of carbohydrates ingested, the physical form of the carbohydrates, the frequency of carbohydrate ingestion (snacking frequency), and the amount of carbohydrate ingested must all be considered.

Type of Carbohydrates. Most articles detailing food-caries interrelationships have stressed that sucrose, common table sugar, is the major cariogenic item in the human diet.[70–72] Sucrose, a disaccharide, and glucose and fructose, the monosaccharides that compose the sucrose molecule, can all be easily metabolized by plaque bacteria to yield acids that cause demineralization. In addition, sucrose can be used by plaque bacteria to form sticky polymers (dextrans and levans) that help the bacterial plaque adhere to the teeth.

Although there has been an increase in the use of fructose corn syrup in the preparation of soft drinks and candy, the principal sugar constituent in the human diet is still sucrose. Americans consume approximately 100 pounds of sucrose a year, much of which is contained in commercially prepared foods and confectionary items.[73]

Form of Carbohydrate. The physical form in which the carbohydrate is eaten and its retention in the mouth are major factors in promoting dental decay. In one investigation in Sweden, when sticky candies such as toffee and caramel were added to the diet, subjects experienced a marked increase in caries activity. When the basic diet was supplemented with sugar in solution, in which the retentive quality is low, there was a minimal increase in tooth decay. Sugar supplements with intermediate oral clearance activity were associated with intermediate levels of caries increase.[74]

Frequency of Carbohydrate Ingestion. A quantity of carbohydrate consumed over several snacking sessions is potentially more cariogenic than if the same amount were consumed at one session.[75, 76] This is believed to be related to the changes in plaque acidity that accompany ingestion of certain sugars. The pH of the dental plaque is normally neutral. When a sugar, such as sucrose, is ingested, there is a rapid pH drop to approximately 5.0, at which acid dissolution of the tooth occurs.[77] When a sucrose-containing food is consumed at a single session, there will be only one drop in the pH curve and, therefore, only a single acid attack. However, if the food is divided and consumed at several sessions, there will be several drops in pH and several periods during which enamel dissolution can occur.

When sugar is available for long periods because of its retentive quality or because of the frequency with which it is ingested, the acid attack on the teeth will be prolonged, and the tooth will undergo demineralization. In addition, the period during which the developing lesion can remineralize will be curtailed. The prolonged acid attack and the

shortened period of potential remineralization favor the initiation and development of carious lesions.

Amount of Carbohydrate. Of the four factors that can influence the ability of dietary carbohydrates to produce dental decay, the amount of carbohydrate consumed was always considered to be the least important. This is because, in human studies, attempts to link the amount of carbohydrate ingestion to caries activity have generally failed. However, these results were contrary to animal studies that demonstrated that as the percentage of sugar in the diet was increased, the caries activity was increased. The recent view is that the amount of sugar ingested by humans does influence caries activity; however, the relationship is not as direct as it is in animals, in which the diet can be completely manipulated by the investigator. It is believed that very low levels of sugar, e.g., sucrose, in the human diet are not conducive to caries or result in a low clinical decay activity. This is because at low sucrose dietary concentrations, sufficient extracellular polysaccharide production does not occur for the primary cariogenic bacteria, *Streptococcus mutans,* to colonize on the teeth in large numbers. As the amount of sucrose increases in the human diet, insoluble extracellular polysaccharide production increases, allowing significant adherence of plaque to the teeth and the production of acids that dissolve the enamel. Finally, a point is reached in the human diet at which still further increases in sugar consumption will no longer be related to a proportionate caries rise because caries activity is at a maximum.

Figure 1–28 illustrates the presumed relationship between the amount of sucrose in the diet and caries activity in an individual with a frequent snacking habit. Caries activity rises after a "threshold level" of sugar in the diet is reached. When a sugar saturation level is attained, the patient is in a rampant caries status, and further increases in dietary sugar do not significantly alter the clinical picture.

Dietary Advice

For patients with a high caries incidence, including those with rampant caries, special dietary counseling is necessary. For most other patients, a single session explaining the pertinent food-caries relationships should suffice to make them informed. This is especially true for patients who are caries-free or have low caries activity. Presumably, their dietary practices are already sound, or else they would not present with such a low level of decay.

It has been stated that the wife or mother should be especially targeted as the recipient of dietary advice, since she is the one who usually purchases the food, plans the menus, and prepares the meals for the other members of the household. However, Shaw has pointed out that, within the last generation, more and more people are eating their meals away from home.[73] Hence, the woman's role as the "gatekeeper" of the household diet has diminished significantly, making it more important than ever that all members of the family receive dietary advice.

A receptive recipient of dietary advice has always been the *new* mother. Dental studies in Sweden have shown that dietary advice to new mothers can produce positive results.[78, 79] Preventive dental education programs, including dietary advice, to new mothers resulted in lower caries scores in their children compared with the children of nonparticipating families. While fluoride supplements

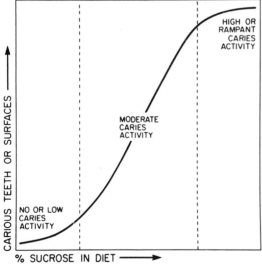

FIGURE 1–28 The effect of amount of dietary sucrose coupled with frequent snacking. Relatively low amounts of sucrose may not produce clinically detectable carious lesions. However, increasing the amount of dietary sucrose will eventually result in demonstrable lesions. Large amounts of sucrose in the diet, coupled with a habit of frequent snacking, can result in rampant caries.

were included in these programs, compliance was poor, and the principal factor associated with the lower caries scores was believed to be the reduced frequency of sugar ingestion.

For the average patient the diet advice session should take no more than 30 minutes. The presentation may be made by the dentist or by a trained member of the office staff. While the format of the program will vary between offices and may include audio-visual materials, informational handouts, or brochures, the following information should be common to all programs: (1) a description of the carious process, emphasizing the role of carbohydrates; (2) a discussion of the factors that contribute to the cariogenicity of carbohydrates in the diet; and (3) general dietary recommendations, including which foods to avoid and which are acceptable. A typical lesson plan follows.

The Carious Process

The patient should be told that dental caries is a disease in which local etiologic factors predominate. Three factors are essential for decay to occur: (1) a tooth surface that can be dissolved by acid; (2) bacteria, adherent to the tooth surface, that produce acids that dissolve the tooth; and (3) food that the bacteria use to make the acids. The foods used by the bacteria are carbohydrates. Carbohydrates consist of starches and sugars. Bacteria metabolize starches slowly, whereas simple sugars are acted upon quickly. Therefore, it is the simple sugars in the diet, especially table sugar (sucrose), that are most harmful to the teeth.

It is helpful to show the patient the following formulas, which illustrate the relationship between the teeth, bacteria, and sugar in the carious process.

$$\text{Bacteria} + \text{Sugar} \longrightarrow \text{Acid}$$
$$\text{Acid} + \text{Tooth Enamel} \longrightarrow \text{Dental Caries}$$

Contributing Dietary Factors

It must be stressed that, in addition to the type of sugar, the retention of the food in the mouth, the frequency with which it is consumed, and the amount consumed are also important. Sugar must be available numerous times per day and consumed for approximately 60 to 100 minutes per day for carious lesions to occur.[73]

The graph in Figure 1–29 can be used to emphasize the importance of frequency of consumption (between-meal snacking) and retention of sticky sugar-containing foods in the mouth. A single sugar challenge will lower the pH of the plaque to a level at which demineralization can occur for about 20 minutes. Thereafter, the pH slowly returns to neutrality. Each time there is a sugar challenge, there is another 20-minute period during which demineralization of the tooth can occur and a "cavity" can develop. A prolonged sugar challenge, such as from a sticky candy or a hard candy that is meant to be sucked for a long period, will provide a reservoir of sugar to the cariogenic bacteria of the plaque. There will be a prolonged lowering of the pH curve, and consequently the demineralization period will be extended.

Dietary Recommendations

The preceding dietary information should serve as a basis for making general dietary recommendations to patients. When a patient does not have a severe dental problem, the objective of this part of the discussion should be to reinforce the patient's present dietary habits and to make substitutions where appropriate. Potentially cariogenic

FIGURE 1–29 The effect of frequency of sucrose consumption on caries. Sucrose ingestion results in a drop in the plaque pH to a level that will dissolve the tooth. The pH slowly returns to the resting level; however, a habit of frequent snacking will produce multiple acid attacks on the tooth.

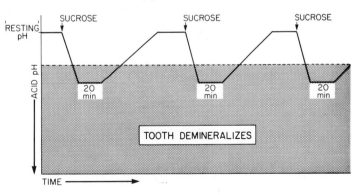

TABLE 1–6 Examples of Foods That Are Potentially
Cariogenic

Chocolate milk	Cakes, cookies, pies, doughnuts
Milk shakes and malts	Candy, caramels, mints
Commercially prepared yogurt	Sugar-containing gum
Powdered drink mixes	Cough drops, lollipops
Canned sweetened fruit juices	Presweetened cereals
Honey, syrup, molasses	Dried fruits
Ice cream	Canned sweetened fruits
Popsicles	Jam, jelly, preserves
Sherbet	Glazed meats or vegetables
Jell-O, pudding	

foods in the diet should be identified (Table 1–6) as well as those that are less cariogenic or noncariogenic (Table 1–7). The following dietary recommendations, which are intended to promote good dental health, should be made to all patients:

1. Sucrose, common table sugar, should be reduced in the diet and replaced by less cariogenic carbohydrates or other foodstuffs. Snacking with potato chips, a starch, or peanuts, primarily protein, is a far less cariogenic practice than snacking with candy, cookies, or cake.

2. "Sugar-free" candy and chewing gum are available in stores. These confections do contain a sugar, usually sorbitol or mannitol; however, these sugars are believed to produce very little acid in the dental plaque. Xylitol is another sugar that is not metabolized by plaque bacteria. Patients should be encouraged to use these "sugar-free" items.

3. Flour and most breads are not highly cariogenic. Bread is sticky because it contains gluten in addition to starch. Bread may influence caries principally by aiding in the retention of sugar on the teeth. Therefore, bread spread with butter or margarine should be substituted for bread with jam or jelly.

4. Because presweetened breakfast cereals can contain between 30 and 50 per cent sucrose (by weight) and therefore may have a

high cariogenic potential, their elimination from the diet, especially as a dry snack, is recommended.[80]

5. Soft drinks are far less cariogenic than the amount of sugar (sucrose and/or fructose) they contain would indicate because of the rapid oral clearance of sugar in liquid form. Soft drinks, in moderate amounts, can be tolerated in the diet, although low-calorie "sugar-free" drinks are preferred.

6. Ice cream has a total sugar concentration of approximately 30 per cent.[81] Eating ice cream as a mealtime dessert is not considered dentally hazardous. Because of its sugar content, however, the frequent ingestion of ice cream as a between-meal or bedtime snack can be considered potentially cariogenic, even though the intraoral retention of ice cream is short.

7. Sugar-containing foods should be consumed at mealtime as the dessert. It is preferable even in this situation that the teeth be cleaned within 5 minutes after eating to remove the cariogenic substrate from the mouth.

8. The frequent exposure of teeth to sticky foods containing high amounts of sugar is the factor most responsible in a diet that promotes dental decay.

Diet Counseling

Patients with high caries rates, including those with rampant caries, should receive a detailed diet evaluation in order to determine the dietary factors that are contributing to their dental problem. The dietary analysis should include what the individual is eating, when he is eating it, and why. Modification of the diet should then be made, which would include restriction of some foods and substitution of others. Generally, dietary counseling will require several sessions.

TABLE 1–7 Examples of Foods That Are
Noncariogenic

Milk	Popcorn, potato chips, tacos
Unsweetened fruit juices	Corn chips, wheat chips, pretzels
Plain yogurt	
Sugar-free soft drinks	Nuts, olives, pickles
Fresh fruits and vegetables	Butter, peanut butter
Cheese, cottage cheese	Toast
Eggs	Luncheon meats and sandwiches
Sugarless gum	Pizza

Several methods of dietary counseling have been described, to which the reader is referred.[82–84] Generally, these have a nutritional as well as a dietary component. The primary objective of the counseling sessions should be the modification of the patient's diet in order to improve dental health. However, the recommendations should also be consistent with good nutrition so that the general health of the patient is maintained. Additionally, the recommendations must reflect the patient's dietary preferences, lifestyle, and economic situation; otherwise, they will not be accepted by the patient.

ORAL HYGIENE PROCEDURES AND THE USE OF THERAPEUTIC DENTIFRICES

The two dental diseases, gingivitis and dental caries, result from the presence of bacterial plaque on the teeth. Hence, removal of plaque is essential to prevent or limit these diseases. Because plaque can reestablish itself as early as 24 hours after a complete cleaning, oral hygiene procedures that remove or limit the growth of plaque must be performed daily. When plaque removal was deliberately stopped, histologic changes in the gingiva appeared after 2 days[85] and clinical gingivitis after 2 weeks.[86] After ceasing oral hygiene procedures and performing frequent sucrose rinses, white spot carious lesions developed within 23 days.[6] In the absence of plaque, the lesions did not form.

The most common methods of removing plaque are by brushing and flossing the teeth. In order to improve the effectiveness of mechanical plaque removal, several designs of toothbrushes and toothbrush bristles have been developed and a variety of toothbrushing techniques have been advocated. Dental floss is available in different diameters and may be waxed or unwaxed.

Manual Toothbrushes. Manual toothbrushes have different design characteristics that are believed by their manufacturers to improve their effectiveness. Toothbrushes can be purchased that are straight or bent, presumably to reach the posterior teeth better. Handles are plain or have a contour grip in an effort to enhance the dexterity of the brusher. The greatest variety in design occurs in the head and bristles of the brush. The head may have multiple tufts of bristles or may have separated bristles. The bristles may be arranged in two or more rows; may be soft or hard and nylon or "natural" (usually hog hair); may have a round, flat, or tapered end; and may vary from approximately 0.007 to 0.013 inches in diameter.

There are no clinical studies that have evaluated the effect of toothbrush design on the prevention of dental caries, although there have been numerous reports that have assessed the cleaning ability of different toothbrushes or the effects of the bristles on the gingiva.[87–91] Based upon these reports, toothbrushes that have soft nylon bristles with rounded ends arranged in multiple tufts are generally recommended. These brushes appear to be most effective in removing dental plaque, are nontraumatic to the gingiva, and are long lasting.

Brushing Techniques. The variety of brushing techniques is almost as great as that of toothbrush designs. Based upon the hand movement involved, brushing techniques are categorized into the horizontal or horizontal scrub method, the vertical method, the circular (Fones) or roll methods, and the vibrating (Bass, Stillman, Charters) methods.

No study has attempted to evaluate the effect of brushing technique on the incidence of dental caries. While a number of reports have evaluated and compared the ability of different toothbrushing methods to remove plaque from the teeth,[88, 89, 91–94] no one method has proved superior. Because the dexterity of the brusher is an important determinant of effectiveness, it is generally felt that a technique that is appropriate for one age group may be unsuitable for another. The horizontal or horizontal scrub method is generally advocated for young children because it is a technique that is easily mastered, whereas a more complicated vibrating technique, such as the Bass or Charters method, is preferred for adults.

Flossing. The pits and fissures of the occlusal surfaces and the proximal surfaces of the teeth are usually inaccessible to the bristles of the toothbrush. The use of dental floss has been advocated as an effective method for cleaning the interproximal areas of the teeth, and, indeed, Keller and Manson-Hing demonstrated that manual toothbrushing followed by flossing was the most effective means of cleaning the proximal tooth surfaces.[95]

One study has evaluated the effectiveness of interproximal flossing in reducing dental decay. In that study, Wright and co-workers demonstrated a 50 per cent caries reduction in proximal caries of 5- and 6-year-old children who participated in a school program in which their teeth were regularly flossed by dental assistants.[96, 97]

While flossing is effective in cleaning between the teeth and appears to be beneficial in reducing caries on the proximal surfaces, the technique requires a high degree of dexterity and is quite time-consuming. Young children cannot use dental floss by themselves. If they have tight contacts that require flossing, their parents must do it for them. Older children and adults can floss for themselves but frequently lack the motivation to do so.

Automatic Cleaning Aids. Since the 1960s, automatic cleaning aids such as electric toothbrushes and water jets have been available. The effectiveness of these devices has been reviewed for their ability to remove dental plaque[98, 99] but not for their ability to control dental caries. It is generally agreed that manual and electric toothbrushes have a comparable plaque-removing potential and that the quality of brushing is a reflection of the skill of the brusher rather than the type of brush used. For this reason, electric toothbrushes have been especially recommended for handicapped patients who lack the usual manual skills. Water jets will not remove adherent plaque or pellicle; therefore, use of a water jet is not a substitute for toothbrushing, although it may be an adjunctive procedure.

Oral Hygiene Status and Dental Caries. Since plaque is essential for the development of gingivitis and dental caries, the logical corollary is that by reducing the level of plaque on the teeth, there will be a concomitant reduction in gingivitis and dental caries. Numerous studies have demonstrated a correlation between oral hygiene status and gingivitis. Improving oral hygiene by various tooth-cleaning procedures that control the level of dental plaque reduces the incidence and severity of gingival disease. A similar relationship has not been established between oral hygiene and dental caries.

The relationship between toothbrushing and dental caries has been reviewed in several publications.[100–102] The results of these reviews indicate that a definitive relationship between patients' oral hygiene status or their frequency of toothbrushing and dental caries could not be confirmed. Indicative of this situation are the reports by Ripa, Barenie, and Leske.[103–105] These investigators compared the relationship between toothbrushing frequency, oral hygiene, gingivitis, and dental caries in 9- to 13-year-old children. Although a trend toward decreased caries scores with increased brushing frequency was observed, there was no statistically significant relationship between either toothbrushing frequency or oral hygiene status and dental caries. Both Horowitz and co-workers[106] and Silverstein and co-workers[107] conducted school-based plaque control programs. These programs lasted from 20 to 29 months. Neither produced a statistically significant difference in caries incidence compared with control groups of children.

Therapeutic Dentifrices. The common methods of mechanical tooth cleaning as practiced by most patients do not appear to be sufficient to control dental caries. The time, effort, and degree of dexterity needed for complete plaque removal may exceed the ability of the average patient, and only for the well-motivated patient who is willing to spend the amount of time necessary to conduct meticulous tooth cleaning may plaque control actually be successful in limiting dental caries. However, by using a therapeutic dentifrice when brushing, patients can reduce their level of dental decay.

Historically, the primary function of a dentifrice is to clean and polish the accessible surfaces of the teeth. By the addition of active ingredients to the formulations, dentifrices can be used therapeutically to reduce the incidence of dental caries and not merely to provide a cosmetic function.[108, 109]

All currently marketed therapeutic dentifrices contain fluoride. However, just because a dentifrice has fluoride does not mean it is effective against dental caries. Early fluoride-containing dentifrices were not effective because the fluoride reacted with other ingredients in the dentifrice formulation, specifically the abrasive system, and was therefore unavailable for reaction in the mouth. The American Dental Association conducts a review of therapeutic dentifrices. A dentifrice is *Accepted* by the American Dental Association's Council on Dental Therapeutics when there is adequate evidence of its safety and effectiveness.

As of this writing, there are five dentifrices that have been classified as *Accepted*:

TABLE 1–8   Fluoride-containing Dentifrices Classified "Accepted" by the American Dental Association

Brand	Manufacturer	Therapeutic Agent*	Abrasive
Aim	Lever Brothers Company	Na_2PO_3F	silica
Aquafresh	Beecham Products	Na_2PO_3F	calcium carbonate/silica
Colgate with MFP Fluoride	Colgate-Palmolive Company	Na_2PO_3F	dicalcium phosphate dihydrate
Crest	Procter & Gamble Company	NaF	silica
Macleans Fluoride	Beecham Products	Na_2PO_3F	calcium carbonate

*Na_2PO_3F = sodium monofluorophosphate
NaF = sodium fluoride

Crest, Colgate MFP, Macleans Fluoride, Aquafresh, and Aim. Table 1–8 lists these dentifrices together with their active ingredients and compatible abrasive systems. Notice that four of the five dentifrices contain sodium monofluorophosphate as the active ingredient and one contains sodium fluoride. While the first Accepted dentifrice (Crest) originally contained stannous fluoride as the active ingredient, the formulation of this dentifrice has recently been changed to the one listed in the table.

Used regularly, a fluoride-containing dentifrice can reduce dental caries by 15 to 30 per cent. Because it is a proven cariostatic method, dentists must recommend the use of American Dental Association Accepted dentifrices to their patients.

SELF-APPLICATION OF TOPICAL FLUORIDE

With the exception of fluoride-containing dentifrices, fluoride has been applied topically to patients' teeth by dentists or hygienists, usually in the dental office. Within the last 20 years, however, self-application methods, whereby patients apply topical fluoride to their own teeth, have been studied extensively. While the investigation of these methods was prompted by their usefulness in caries-prevention public health programs, they can also be used for caries-susceptible patients in individual programs of caries prevention.

For individual patients, the advantage of applying topical fluoride to their own teeth is that they can treat themselves more frequently than is possible by the traditional method of professional application. The greater number of fluoride contacts should impart a higher level of caries protection to the teeth.

Methods of Self-Application

Three methods of self-application have been studied: toothbrushing, mouthrinsing, and the use of mouthtrays.

Toothbrushing. A fluoride solution or gel or a fluoride-containing prophylaxis paste is applied to a toothbrush with which the patient brushes his teeth. This method was once very popular in school-based caries prevention programs. However, because of the relative costs of the procedure, the time and materials involved, and the equivocal results that were obtained, it has generally been superseded by methods that are less costly and give more consistent results. Nevertheless, for very young patients, toothbrushing can be a useful method to provide the teeth with topical fluoride, as will be described later.

Mouthrinsing. The patient swishes a measured amount of fluoride mouthrinse in the mouth. Depending on the fluoride concentration and rinse formulation, the level of fluoride in the drinking water, and whether the patient is already taking a systemic fluoride supplement, the rinse may be either swallowed (see section on dietary fluoride supplements) or expectorated.

Mouthrinsing is easy to perform and is relatively inexpensive. Currently, it is the most frequently used method in school-based programs and is probably also the most popular home-based self-application topical fluoride technique. Because some commercial fluoride mouthrinses can be purchased without a prescription, rinsing is also the most accessible self-application method for the individual patient.

Mouthtrays. Custom-fitted trays are prepared, into which several drops of fluoride gel are placed. The patient positions the trays in his mouth, and the gel remains in contact with the surfaces of the teeth for several minutes.

Compared with the other self-application methods, this method has produced the highest caries reductions in a school-based program.[110] Nevertheless, it has not been adopted in schools because it is a time-consuming, relatively complicated, and costly procedure.[111] This approach, however, does have application in a caries-prevention program for an individual patient, especially when the patient is highly susceptible to caries.

Indications for Self-Application Methods

All patients who, at their initial examination or recall visit, present with new carious lesions are candidates for a home program of self-applied topical fluoride. If lesions have advanced to the stage of cavitation, the involved teeth must be restored, and the objective of the caries-prevention procedures is to inhibit the development of new lesions. If the lesions are incipient and their surfaces are judged to be intact, the objectives of fluoride therapy are to prevent new lesions from forming and to arrest the existing ones, thus possibly avoiding having to prepare and restore the involved teeth.

Patients who are caries-free need not be placed on a self-applied topical fluoride program. Caries-free patients include those who have only sound teeth with no restorations and those who have fillings but who present to the dentist at their 6-month or 1-year recall visit with no new lesions.

Certain special patients should be recognized by the dentist as candidates for self-applied topical fluorides. These include preschool children with nursing bottle caries, teenagers and others with rampant caries, and older patients with exposed cementum who are developing carious lesions of the roots. Patients who are undergoing orthodontic treatment, for whom complete plaque removal is difficult, should use self-applied topical fluorides. Patients with reduced salivary gland function, such as those undergoing head and neck radiation therapy or those being administered anti-anxiety drugs with anticholinergic activity, should also be

TABLE 1–9 Patients for Whom Self-applied Topical Fluoride Therapy Is Indicated

Caries-active Patients
  Incipient lesions
  Cavitated lesions
Patients with Special Caries Problems
  Nursing bottle caries
  Rampant caries
  Root caries
Potential Caries-active Patients
  Orthodontic therapy
  Xerostomia
    Radiation
    Anti-sialogogues

routinely placed on self-applied topical fluorides. Table 1–9 lists the several types of patients for whom self-applied topical fluorides are indicated.

Use of Self-Application Methods

The determination of which technique to use for a particular patient must be based on considerations of the efficacy and practicality of the method and the ability of the patient to master the technique. Additionally, successful self-application topical fluoride therapy depends on the cooperation of the patient and, if the patient is a child, on the patient's parent to follow the dentist's recommendations conscientiously.

Preschool Children (5 Years and Younger)

Most preschool children cannot rinse properly and may not be able to accept custom trays; therefore, for the preschooler, brushing is the preferred method of self-application.

Dentists may dispense a commercial fluoride gel that is packaged for individual use. One supplier, Hoyt Laboratories, has a flavored APF gel (1.2 per cent F) in a small, 7.0 gm dispensing tube and an APF gel and a neutral gel (each 0.5 per cent F) in 60 mg polyethylene bottles.* The parent is instructed to brush the child's teeth once a month with the gel. Before bedtime, the parent should first brush the child's teeth using a dentifrice. Then the gel should be ap-

---

*Luride Topical Gel, 7.0 gm tubes; Thera-Flur Topical Gel Drops and Thera-Flur-N Topical Gel Drops, respectively; Hoyt Laboratories, Needham, Massachusetts.

plied to the bristles of the child's brush, and the parent should brush the teeth for approximately 4 to 5 minutes. Since the child will swallow most of the gel, *only enough gel to wet the ends of the toothbrush bristles should be used.* After the fluoride application, the child may expectorate but should not rinse.

School-Aged Children (6 to 13 Years)

School-aged children can master either a rinsing or a tray technique. However, a 6- to 13-year-old is in the mixed dentition stage of dental development. Exfoliation of primary teeth and eruption of permanent teeth contraindicate the long-term use of custom trays in this age group, since frequent reconstruction would be required. Consequently, for a school-aged child in the mixed dentition stage, the mouthrinsing technique is recommended.

The rinsing technique for patients at home involves daily rinsing with a 0.05 per cent NaF solution.[112] The child is instructed to rinse each evening for 60 seconds after first brushing the teeth. One teaspoonful (5 ml) is swished throughout the mouth and then the solution is expectorated.

A number of neutral 0.05 per cent NaF rinses are available (Table 1–10). A dentist may either prescribe a commercial rinse that the patient purchases from a pharmacy or dispense the rinse from the dental office. Most rinses of this concentration are packaged in 480 or 500 ml bottles and will last for approximately 3 months. Some commercial rinses, containing sodium or stannous fluoride, are also available without prescription, and these are also listed in Table 1–10.

If the 6- to 13-year-old child who is placed on a home rinse program should also need a dietary fluoride supplement, an *oral rinse supplement* may be prescribed. One teaspoonful of a 0.044 per cent NaF solution (usually as APF) will provide 1 mg systemic fluoride if swallowed. By recommending an oral rinse supplement that can be swished and then swallowed, the patient will receive both a topical and a systemic benefit from the same fluoride agent.

Adolescents and Adults

For the patient with all of his permanent teeth erupted (exclusive of third molars), the use of custom trays is recommended. This method should provide the greatest protection against caries.

Horseshoe-shaped mouthtrays for the maxillary and mandibular arches are custom-made using polyvinyl mouthguard material that is vacuum-adapted to casts of the patient's teeth. The patient is given an APF or neutral gel* and is instructed to place five to ten drops in both mouthtrays, which are held in contact with the teeth every day for 5 minutes.

If the patient will not comply with routine tray applications, he should be placed on daily fluoride rinsing. Orthodontic appliances may make use of a mouthtray difficult. The patient identified for orthodontic therapy can use a mouthtray daily for approximately 4 to 6 weeks before the appli-

---

*E.g., Thera-Flur Topical Gel Drops or Thera-Flur-N Topical Gel Drops, Hoyt Laboratories, Needham, Massachusetts.

TABLE 1–10   Fluoride Mouthrinses for Home Rinsing Programs

Brand	Manufacturer	Type of Fluoride*	Sodium Fluoride Concentration (%)
Prescription Rinses			
Kari Rinse	The Lorvic Company	NaF	0.05
Monoject Fluoride Mouthrinse	Monoject	NaF	0.05
NaFrinse, 0.05% Neutral	Orachem Pharmaceuticals	NaF	0.05
Fluorinse, 0.05%	Cooper Laboratories	NaF	0.05
Nonprescription Rinses			
Fluoriguard	Colgate-Palmolive Company	NaF	0.05
Stan Care	Block Drug Company	SnF$_2$	†
Oral Rinse Supplements			
NaFrinse Acidulated Oral Rinse and Systemic Supplement	Orachem Pharmaceuticals	APF	0.044
PHOS-FLUR Oral Rinse Supplement	Hoyt Laboratories	APF	0.044

*NaF = Sodium fluoride; SnF$_2$ = Stannous fluoride; APF = Acidulated phosphate fluoride.
†0.1% stannous fluoride
All products listed in this table are Accepted by the American Dental Association.

TABLE 1–11   Recommendations for Self-Applied Topical Fluoride Methods

Brushing	Rinsing	Mouthtrays
For Preschool Children (Primary Dentition)	*For Young School-aged Children (Mixed Dentition)*	*For Adolescents and Adults (Permanent Dentition)*
Parent brushes the child's teeth for 5 minutes once a month with a neutral or APF gel.	Patient rinses for 60 seconds once a day with 1 teaspoonful (5 ml) of 0.05 per cent NaF solution.	Patient applies neutral or APF gel once a day in custom mouthtrays held against teeth for 5 minutes.

ance, bands, or bonded devices are inserted. Once orthodontic therapy is begun, the patient should continue with a regimen of daily fluoride rinsing until the therapy is completed. Patients with radiation- or chemical-induced xerostomia may also begin their treatment with a 4- to 6-week program of daily mouthtray application, which is then followed by daily rinsing. If the xerostomia is permanent, the patient must stay on the home topical fluoride program indefinitely. Once the patient is free of new carious lesions for two consecutive recall visits, the dentist should consider suspending the home topical fluoride treatments. The recommendations for the use of self-applied topical fluoride methods are summarized in Table 1–11.[113]

Results of Self-Application Methods

Generally the self-application methods have been monitored in school-based programs rather than in programs involving individual patients for whom these techniques were specifically indicated. As already mentioned, the brushing method has produced equivocal results. However, fluoride mouthrinsing is a recognized caries-preventive method[114] with an expected caries reduction of 30 to 40 per cent. Additionally, mouthrinsing appears to be effective in fluoridated communities[115–119] as well as fluoride-deficient ones. Mouthtrays have also proved to be highly effective in a fluoride-deficient community where, after 2 school years of daily application (an average of 245 self-treatments), the caries reductions were 64 to 67 per cent.[110] In a fluoridated community, the use of mouthtrays produced a 29 per cent caries reduction.[120] Several reports have also indicated that various self-applied topical fluoride methods used by patients with xerosto-

mia not only prevent the occurrence of new lesions but also reharden existing ones.[10, 121, 122]

DIETARY FLUORIDE SUPPLEMENTATION

Children consuming a therapeutically optimal amount of fluoride in their drinking water experience 50 to 60 per cent less dental decay than children using fluoride-deficient water. Currently, about one half of the population of the United States is drinking water containing optimal fluoride levels. For children who are not, an alternative is the use of dietary fluoride supplements.

Fluoride supplements include sodium fluoride drops, tablets, and lozenges, fluoride-containing vitamin preparations, and oral fluoride rinse supplements. Because these products are swallowed, they provide a systemic benefit before the teeth erupt into the mouth. Ingested fluoride is rapidly absorbed into the bloodstream and circulates throughout the body. A small amount deposits in the enamel of developing teeth. Enamel formed in the presence of fluoride is less soluble in acid, presumably accounting for its greater resistance to tooth decay.

Dosage of Dietary Fluoride Supplements

Dietary fluoride supplements are available to the patient only upon prescription from a physician or dentist. The proper dosage is determined by the concentration of fluoride in the drinking water and the patient's age.

Water Fluoride Concentration.   Traces of fluoride are naturally present in all drinking water; furthermore many communities have added fluoride to their water supply in order to prevent dental decay. If a community's water supply contains natural or controlled amounts of fluoride at a concentration of 1.0 ppm (part per million) fluoride, it is considered to be optimally fluoridated.* Children living in optimally fluoridated communities do not require dietary fluoride supplements. *Children consuming drinking water containing 0.7 ppm F or less should be placed on dietary fluoride supplements.*

Children's Age. Because there is little evidence that prenatal supplements protect the teeth against caries, it is not recommended that they be prescribed during pregnancy.[123–125] Dietary fluoride supplements should be started at birth, since all of the primary teeth and some of the permanent teeth (first molars) are forming. It is recognized that during the period between crown formation and tooth eruption, systemic fluoride can still continue to accrue in the enamel of the tooth. Therefore, fluoride supplements should be continued not only until all of the permanent tooth crowns have formed, which is about age 8 years, but also until all of the permanent teeth have erupted. Excluding third molars, this will be until approximately 13 years of age.[126]

Dosage Schedule

To avoid the possibility of enamel fluorosis, which occurs if too much fluoride is consumed during the period of tooth development, the recommended dosage of fluoride has been adjusted empirically to accommodate the variability of natural fluoride levels in the water supplies of the different communities in the United States.[126–128]

Table 1–12 presents the daily dosage

---

*The optimal level of fluoride in the drinking water for a community varies according to the average maximum daily air temperature. Water supplies located in hot climates, where the residents would drink more, require a lower fluoride concentration than those located in colder climates. The range for optimal community water fluoridation is 0.7 to 1.2 ppm F.

schedule for dietary fluoride supplements. Notice that there are two levels of supplementation based on the concentration of water-borne fluoride, and there are three tiers within each schedule that consider the child's age. The maximum fluoride supplement is 1 mg F per day. Thereafter, the dosage decreases according to the child's age or the concentration of fluoride in the drinking water.

Dosage Form

All fluoride supplements are provided as sodium fluoride. In most cases the sodium fluoride has a neutral pH, but acidulated phosphate fluoride tablets, lozenges, and oral rinse supplements are available.

Fluoride supplements should be prescribed in a vehicle that is compatible with the individual child's ability to master the technique. For instance, infants from birth to 24 months should receive fluoride in liquid form, as fluoride drops, or fluoride-vitamin drops. Two- to 3-year-olds should also have fluoride prescribed in a liquid vehicle. Depending upon the skill of the individual child, at some time between 3 and 6 years, the child should be switched to either fluoride tablets or an oral rinse supplement.

The recommended procedure for tablet supplementation is to have the child chew it for 30 seconds, rinse with the resulting salivary mixture for an additional 30 seconds, and then swallow. When an oral rinse supplement is used, the child swishes the solution throughout the mouth for 60 seconds and then swallows. The preliminary chewing and swishing steps provide *topical* fluoride contact to the teeth that have already erupted. Swallowing provides *systemic* fluoride contact to the teeth that have not yet erupted. Thus, participation in a tablet program involving chewing, swishing, and swallowing, or a rinse-supplement program in which the so-

TABLE 1–12 Daily Dietary Fluoride Supplement Schedule

Fluoride in Water (ppm)	Age		
	Birth to 24 Mos.	*25 to 36 Mos.*	*37 Mos. to 13 Yrs.*
Less than 0.3	0.25 mg F	0.50 mg F	1.00 mg F
0.3 to 0.7	0.0 mg F	0.25 mg F	0.50 mg F
Greater than 0.7	0.0 mg F	0.0 mg F	0.0 mg F

Note: A 2.2 mg NaF tablet provides 1.0 mg F.
Modified from Ripa, L. W.: The role of the pediatrician in dental caries detection and prevention. Pediatrics, *54*:176–182, 1974.

TABLE 1–13 Dosage Forms and Amounts of Fluoride
Available in Dietary Fluoride Supplements

Dosage Form	How Provided
Fluoride drops	0.125 mg/drop 0.25 mg/drop 0.50 mg/drop
Fluoride-vitamin drops	0.25 mg/drop 0.50 mg/drop
Fluoride tablets and lozenges	0.25 mg/tablet 0.50 mg/tablet 1.0 mg/tablet*
Fluoride-vitamin tablets	0.50 mg/tablet 1.0 mg/tablet*
Oral rinse supplement	1.0 mg/5.0 ml (teaspoonful)†

*A 2.2 mg NaF tablet provides 1.0 mg F.
†The concentration of oral rinse supplement is 0.044 per cent NaF.

lution is rinsed and swallowed, provides the child with both topical and systemic fluoride benefits. The combined systemic and topical benefit that is obtained from the same vehicle makes both tablets and rinse supplements very versatile methods of providing fluoride to the teeth.

Prescribing Dietary Fluoride Supplements

Fluoride supplements are available not only in different dosage forms but also in different concentrations. For instance, different brands of fluoride drops provide 0.125, 0.25, or 0.50 mg F per drop, and fluoride tablets may provide 0.25, 0.50, or 1.0 mg F. Table 1–13 lists the amounts of fluoride provided by the different fluoride products available. Since the concentration of fluoride in a particular product may be changed by the manufacturer, it is important that the dentist consult a current issue of *Accepted Dental Therapeutics* or *Physician's Desk Reference* or check with the local pharmacist before prescribing a fluoride supplement.

Figures 1–30 to 1–36 are sample prescriptions for fluoride supplements that correspond to the fluoride dosage schedule presented in Table 1–12. Samples of fluoride-vitamin preparations are not included, since it is presumed that they would be prescribed by a physician rather than a dentist. The prescriptions are for generic drugs, although when writing prescriptions for fluoride supplements, it might be less confusing to use brand names. Notice that when prescribing a fluoride supplement, one is actually writing a prescription for sodium fluoride.

Less Than 0.3 ppm in Water Supply

R

Sodium Fluoride drops
0.25 mg F/drop

Dispense 24 ml

Sig: One drop each day

Birth to 24 Months. Sodium fluoride drops are packaged with calibrated dispensers. The drops may be given plain, in water, or in fruit juice, but should not be given in milk, which binds the fluoride and slows absorption.

FIGURE 1–30

R

Sodium Fluoride drops
0.5 mg F/drop

Dispense 50 ml

Sig: One drop each day

FIGURE 1–31

25 to 36 Months. Children of this age should still receive fluoride in drops.

R

Sodium Fluoride tablets
2.2 mg NaF/tablet

Dispense 100 tablets

Sig: One tablet before
bedtime. Chew for 30
seconds, swish for 30
seconds, and swallow.

FIGURE 1–32

37 Months to 13 Years. As soon as the child can master the technique, he should be placed on tablets that can be chewed and swished before being swallowed or an oral rinse supplement that is swished and then swallowed. These regimens allow both a topical and systemic benefit to the teeth.

Most pharmaceutical firms supply fluoride tablets in bottles of 100 or 120 for home use. The American Dental Association recommends that, for safety, no more than 120 tablets be prescribed at one time. The warning, "Keep out of reach of young children" should be placed on all prescriptions.

R

Oral fluoride rinse supplement
acidulated phosphate fluoride
0.044 % NaF

Dispense 500 ml

Sig: One teaspoonful before bedtime. Rinse for 60 seconds and
swallow.

FIGURE 1–33

One teaspoonful (5 ml) of an oral rinse supplement having a concentration of 0.044 percent NaF provides 1 mg of fluoride when swallowed. The dentist should check that the local pharmacist stocks an oral supplement before prescribing it.

0.3 to 0.7 ppm F in Water Supply

FIGURE 1–34

25 to 36 Months. A child this age receives fluoride in liquid form. The dosage is half that for a child of comparative age living in a community with virtually no fluoride (less than 0.3 ppm) in the drinking water.

FIGURE 1–35

37 Months to 13 Years. Notice that half-strength tablets are prescribed. If the drugstore does not stock 1.1 mg NaF tablets, *scored* full-strength (2.2 mg NaF) tablets can be prescribed but must be halved before using.

FIGURE 1–36

One-half teaspoonful of an oral rinse supplement can be measured with a baking spoon measure. Some recommendations allow the child to rinse and swallow one teaspoonful every *other* day. In practice, it is too easy for the child to forget on which day he should take the fluoride, and this, therefore, is not the desired recommendation.

Results of Dietary Fluoride Supplement Programs

Several reports have recently reviewed the efficacy of dietary fluoride supplementation.[129–132] They emphasize that supplement programs have been instituted either in the patients' homes, in which the children begin supplementation as infants, or in school, in which they start at 5 or 6 years of age. When the children enter the program as infants, the level of caries protection achieved is similar to that achieved with community water fluoridation—namely, 50 to 60 per cent.[129] When the program is started at school age, the level of caries reduction is approximately 30 to 40 per cent.[133–134]

The success of a home-based dietary supplement program depends upon the motivation and cooperation of the parent and child to continue regular daily intakes for 12 to 13 years. Several investigators, however, have indicated that cooperation wanes after a few years.[135–137] Periodic encouragement and reinforcement from the dentist and office staff are necessary to continue patient and parent compliance for the long period of time necessary for this technique to be maximally effective.

COMBINATION OF CARIES-PREVENTIVE METHODS

The success of an individual program of caries prevention requires a dentist who is knowledgeable in the field of preventive dentistry and a patient who is motivated to adopt the behavioral changes required for the preventive program to work. Additionally, from even a casual reading of the methods described in this chapter, it should be evident that no single technique will completely eliminate dental caries. However, by the combined use of several techniques that are appropriate for a particular patient, a maximal preventive result can be achieved (Fig. 1–37).

Rationale for a Combination Approach

As demonstrated in patients with hereditary fructose intolerance, the almost complete elimination of easily fermentable carbohydrates results in almost no dental decay.[138] However, such a drastic dietary change is not a realistic approach for the average patient. Modest dietary restrictions, described in this chapter, should reduce the incidence of dental caries but will not completely eliminate it. The use of systemic and topical fluorides will protect the teeth further against decay, but the surfaces least protected by fluoride are the occlusal surfaces. By the addition of sealants to the preventive regimen, a maximum protection to the teeth should be achieved.

Both Bagramian and coworkers[139] and Fischman and coworkers[140] evaluated comprehensive preventive programs for children that included oral hygiene instruction, prophylaxis and topical fluoride applications, occlusal sealants, and restorative care either directly or through referral. Even

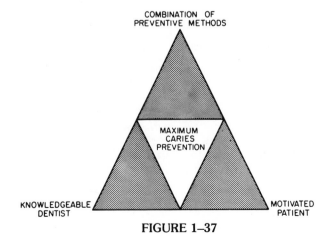

FIGURE 1–37

though both programs were conducted in fluoridated communities, further caries reductions were reported, indicating that additional caries protection can be obtained for individuals who are already receiving benefits of systemic fluoride. In both studies, the major impact on the prevailing decay rate was achieved by the use of occlusal sealants.

Indications for Combination Caries-Preventive Therapy

Every patient should be the beneficiary of a combination approach to caries prevention. The specific combination indicated for a particular patient who will follow the dentist's advice conscientiously depends upon the patient's age, the concentration of fluoride in the drinking water, and the patient's caries status.

Age

The patient's age affects the choice of caries-preventive procedures in several ways. It influences acceptance and mastery of the preventive technique. For instance, a preschool child may not allow a professional topical fluoride treatment to be performed and cannot use a rinse technique. The patient's age is an indicator of his degree of dental development, thus determining whether a dietary fluoride supplement is indicated. If all of the permanent teeth are erupted, there is no need for a fluoride supplement. The patient's age is also a determining factor in whether sealants will be used. In a young child it may be difficult to maintain the strict conditions of dryness necessary to apply sealants, and their use may have to be deferred. Conversely, in an adult, sealants are generally not indicated, since it is unlikely that the occlusal surfaces that have remained caries-free will decay.

Water Fluoride Concentration

The concentration of fluoride in the drinking water determines whether a child should have dietary fluoride supplements and if so, in what dosage (see Table 1–12). The concentration of fluoride in the water also influences whether professional topical fluoride applications should be given. Generally, professional topical fluoride applica-

tions should not be performed *routinely* on patients who reside in an optimally fluoridated community unless a patient's caries activity is high.[141, 142]

Caries Status

Whether of a child or an adult, the patient's caries status is an important consideration in determining the preventive program on which the patient should be placed. Patients with a high caries rate should be considered for all of the preventive regimens discussed in this chapter. A diet analysis should be performed to determine the possible cause of the high caries activity, and the patient should receive dietary counseling to reduce the cariogenic potential of the diet. Professional and self-applied topical fluorides are indicated in order to increase the frequency of topical fluoride contacts to the teeth. The routine use of a fluoride-containing dentifrice is also indicated. Sealants must be considered, but their use will be influenced indirectly by the proximal caries experience of the patient. The use of dietary fluoride supplements would depend on the patient's age and the water-borne fluoride concentration.

Patients with moderate caries activity usually do not require a diet analysis but should receive general dietary advice. However, all of the other preventive methods used for the patient with a high caries rate should be considered for the patient with moderate caries activity.

Even the patient who is caries-free should be on a caries-preventive program. Minimally, this should include the use of a fluoride-containing dentifrice and dietary fluoride supplements if the patient is a child who resides in a fluoride-deficient community.

It is impossible to provide caries-preventive recommendations using a combination approach that would include every patient in every exigency. The dentist must determine what preventive methods are indicated for each patient. The information contained in this chapter will help to determine the most appropriate therapy for a particular patient. When a knowledgeable dentist recommends appropriate preventive therapy that will be conscientiously applied by the patient, a near 100 per cent reduction of dental caries is possible.

QUESTIONS

1. What is meant by the reversal of a carious lesion, and how is remineralization involved in this process?

2. In the early stages of caries development, where is demineralization principally occurring? For control of the lesion, why is it advantageous to have demineralization occur in this area?

3. Discuss the role of fluoride in enamel remineralization.

4. Discuss the relative importance of sealants and fluoride in the prevention of occlusal lesions.

5. What is the base formulation of most commercial sealant systems? List the differences between sealant products.

6. In what circumstances should sealants be placed on occlusal surfaces that are sound? carious? questionable?

7. List and describe the steps of sealant application. What is the importance of a dry field? At what point in the application procedure is dryness critical?

8. List the three compounds available for professional topical fluoride treatments. Why is APF the most popular compound for use in the dental office?

9. List and describe the steps in professional topical fluoride application. How often should topical fluoride be administered?

10. What are the expected results of topical fluoride treatments on patients in a fluoride-deficient community? in an optimally fluoridated community?

11. If occlusal sealants and professional topical fluoride therapy are provided at the same visit, list the sequence in which the clinical steps should be performed. How can an improper sequence adversely affect the results?

12. Distinguish between nutrition and diet. Which appears to be the more important determinant of the carious status of a patient?

13. List and discuss the four factors of the diet that determine cariogenicity.

14. Distinguish between the type of patient who should receive dietary advice and the type who should receive dietary counseling.

15. List the fluoride-containing dentifrices that have been Accepted by the Council on Dental Therapeutics of the American Dental Association. What is the therapeutic ingredient of each?

16. List the three methods of fluoride self-application. Which method is most often used in a school-based program? Which is the most convenient for use in a home-based program? Which has given the greatest caries reduction?

17. For what types of patients are self-applied fluoride methods indicated? Which method is preferred for a preschool child? a school-aged child? an adolescent or adult?

18. Distinguish between a fluoride rinse and an oral fluoride rinse supplement.

19. Reproduce the dietary fluoride supplement dosage schedule.

20. At what age should dietary fluoride supplementation begin? When is it no longer indicated? Are prenatal fluoride supplements beneficial?

See answers in Appendix.

REFERENCES

1. Groenveld, A., and Purdell-Lewis, D. J.: The Origin and behavior of white spot enamel lesions. Neth. Dent. J., *85* (Suppl. 15):6–18, 1977.

2. Marthaler, T. M.: Clinical-visual and radiographic grading of dental caries. *In* Methods of Caries Prediction, B. G. Bibby and R. J. Shern (eds.). Washington, D.C. Information Retrieval, Inc., 1978, pp. 281–284.

3. Kleinberg, I., Chatterjee, R., Domokos, A., et al.: An ultraviolet photographic technique for the early detection of carious lesions. *In* Methods of Caries Prediction, B. G. Bibby and R. J. Shern (eds.). Washington and London, Information Re-

trieval, Inc., 1978, pp. 271–279.

4. Backer-Dirks, O.: Post-eruptive changes in dental enamel. J. Dent. Res., *45*:503–511, 1966.

5. Scheinin, A., Makinen, K. K., Tammisalo, E., and Rekola, M.: Turku sugar studies. XVIII. Incidence of dental caries in relation to 1-year consumption of xylitol chewing gum. Acta Odontol. Scand., *33* (Suppl. 70):307–316, 1975.

6. von der Fehr, F. R., Loe, H., and Theilade, E.: Experimental caries in man. Caries Res., *4*:131–148, 1970.

7. Levine, R. S.: An initial clinical assessment of a mineralising mouthrinse. Br. Dent. J., *138*:249–253, 1975.

8. Loe, H., von der Fehr, F. R., and Schiott, C. R.: Inhibition of experimental caries by plaque prevention. The effect of chlorhexidine mouthrinses. Scand. J. Dent. Res., *80*:1–9, 1972.

9. von der Fehr, F. R.: Maturation and remineralization of enamel. Adv. Fluor. Res., *3*:83–95, 1965.

10. Johansen, E., and Olsen, T. O.: Topical fluorides in the prevention and arrest of dental caries. *In* A.A.A.S. Selected Symposia Series No. 11, Continuing Evaluation and Use of Fluorides, E. Johansen and T. O. Olsen (eds.). Boulder, Colorado, Westview Press, 1979, pp. 61–110.

11. von der Fehr, F. R.: The effect of fluorides on the caries resistance of enamel. Acta Odontol. Scand., *19*:431–442, 1961.

12. Darling, A. I.: Studies on the early carious lesion of enamel with transmitted light, polarized light, and radiography. Br. Dent. J., *101*:289–297, 329–341, 1956.

13. Gustafson, G.: The histopathology of caries of human dental enamel with special reference of the division of the carious lesion into zones. Acta Odontol. Scand., *15*:13–55, 1957.

14. Silverstone, L. M.: Structure of carious enamel, including the early lesion. Oral Sci. Rev., *3*:100–160, 1973.

15. Silverstone, L. M.: Structural alterations of human dental enamel during the incipient lesion development. *In* Proceedings of a Symposium on Incipient Caries of Enamel, N. H. Rowe (ed.). Ann Arbor, University of Michigan Press, 1977, pp. 3–50.

16. Koulourides, T., and Cameron, B.: Enamel remineralization as a factor in the pathogenesis of dental caries. J. Oral Pathol., *9*:255–269, 1980.

17. ten Cate, J. M., and Arends, J.: Remineralization of artificial enamel lesions *in vitro*. Caries Res., *11*:277–286, 1977.

18. ten Cate, J. M., and Arends, J.: Remineralization of artificial enamel lesions *in vitro*. II. Determination of activation energy and reaction order. Caries Res., *12*:213–222, 1978.

19. ten Cate, J. M., and Arends, J.: Remineralization of artificial enamel lesions *in vitro*. III. A study of the deposition mechanism. Caries Res., *14*:351–358, 1980.

20. ten Cate, J. M., Jongebloed, W. L., and Arends, J.: Remineralization of artificial enamel lesions *in vitro*. IV. Influence of fluorides and diphosphonates on short- and long-term remineralization. Caries Res., *15*:60–69, 1981.

21. Silverstone, L. M., Wefel, J. S., Zimmerman B. F., et al.: Remineralization of natural and artificial lesions in human dental enamel *in vitro*. Effect of calcium concentration of the calcifying fluid. Caries Res., *15*:138–157, 1981.

22. Albert, M., and Grenoble, D. E.: An *in vivo* study of enamel remineralization after acid etching. J. So. Calif. State Dent. Assoc., *39*:747–751, 1971.

23. Arana, E. M.: Clinical observations of enamel after acid etch procedure. J. Am. Dent. Assoc., *89*:1102–1106, 1974.

24. Koulourides, T.: Dynamics of tooth surface—oral fluid equilibrium. Adv. Oral Biol., *2*:149–171, 1966.

25. Gelhard, T. B. F. M., ten Cate, J. M., and Arends, J.: Rehardening of artificial enamel lesions *in vivo*. Caries Res., *13*:80–83, 1979.

26. Koulourides, T., Phantimvanit, P., Munksgaard, E. C., and Housch, T.: An intraoral model used for studies of fluoride incorporation in enamel. J. Oral Pathol., *3*:185–195, 1974.

27. Silverstone, L. M.: Remineralization phenomena. Caries Res., *11* (Suppl. 1):59–84, 1977.

28. Weatherell, J. A., Deutsch, D., Robinson, C., and Hallsworth, A. S.: Assimilation of fluoride by enamel throughout the life of the tooth. Caries Res., *11* (Suppl. 1):85–115, 1977.

29. Koulourides, T., Keller, S. E., Manson-Hing, L., and Lilley, V.: Enhancement of fluoride effectiveness by experimental cariogenic priming of human enamel. Caries Res., *14*:32–39, 1980.

30. Wei, S. H. Y.: Remineralization of enamel and dentin—a review. J. Dent. Child., *34*:444–451, 1967.

31. Johansson, B.: Remineralization of slightly etched enamel. J. Dent. Res., *44*:64–70, 1965.

32. Grainger, R. M., and Reid, D. B. W.: Distribution of Dental Caries in Children. J. Dent. Res., *33*:613–623, 1954.

33. Walsh, J. P., and Smart, R. S.: The relative susceptibility of tooth surfaces to dental caries and other comparative studies. N Z Dent. J., *44*:17–35, 1948.

34. Hennon, D. K., Stookey, G. K., and Muhler, J. C.: Prevalence and distribution of dental caries in preschool children. J. Am. Dent. Assoc., *79*:1405–1414, 1969.

35. Graves, R. C., and Burt, B. A.: The pattern of the carious attack in children as a consideration in the use of fissure sealants. J. Prev. Dent., *2*(3):28–32, 1975.

36. Miller, J., and Hobson, P.: Determination of the presence of caries in fissures. Br. Dent. J., *100*:15–18, 1956.

37. Backer-Dirks, O.: The distribution of caries resistance in relation to tooth surfaces. *In* CIBA Foundation Symposium Caries Resistant Teeth, G. E. W. Wolstendholme and M. O'Conner (eds.). Boston, Little, Brown & Co., 1965, pp. 66–83.

38. Gwinnett, A. J.: The scientific basis of the sealant procedure. J. Prev. Dent., *3*(2):2–15, 1976.

39. Galil, K. A., and Gwinnett, A. J.: Three-dimensional replicas of pits and fissures in human teeth: scanning electron microscopy study. Arch. Oral Biol., *20*:493–495, 1975.

40. Galil, K. A.: Scanning and transmission electron microscopic examination of occlusal surface plaque following toothbrushing. J. Can. Dent. Assoc., *41*:499–503, 1975.

41. Ast, D. B., Smith, D. J., Wachs, B., and Kantwell, K. T.: Newburgh-Kingston caries fluorine study. XIV. Combined clinical and dental radiographic

dental findings after 10 years of fluoride experience. J. Am. Dent. Assoc., 52:314–325, 1956.

42. Marthaler, T. M.: Caries-inhibiting effect of fluoride tablets. Helv. Odontol. Acta, 13:1–13, 1969.

43. Englander, H. R., Carlos, J. P., Senning, R. S., and Mellberg, J. R.: Residual anticaries effect of repeated topical sodium fluoride applications by mouthpieces. J. Am. Dent. Assoc., 78:783–787, 1969.

44. Backer-Dirks, O.: The assessment of fluoridation as a preventive measure in relation to dental caries. Br. Dent. J., 114:211–216, 1963.

45. Ripa, L. W., Leske, G. S., Sposato, A. L., and Rebich, T., Jr.: Supervised weekly rinsing with a 0.2% neutral NaF solution: results of a demonstration program after four school years. J. Am. Dent. Assoc., 102:482–486, 1981.

46. Council on Dental Materials and Devices. Certification and classification programs for dental materials and devices. J. Am. Dent. Assoc., 98:272–282, 1979.

47. Handelman, S. L., Buonocore, M. G., and Schoute, P. C.: Progress report on the effect of a fissure sealant on bacteria in dental caries. J. Am. Dent. Assoc., 87:1189–1191, 1973.

48. Handelman, S. L., Washburn, R., and Wopperer, P.: Two-year report of sealant effect on bacteria in dental caries. J. Am. Dent. Assoc., 93:967–970, 1976.

49. Ripa, L. W.: Sealant retention on primary teeth: A critique of clinical and laboratory studies. J. Pedodont., 3:275–290, 1979.

50. Ripa, L. W.: Occlusal sealants: Rationale and review of clinical trials. Int. Dent. J., 30:127–139, 1980.

51. Horowitz, H. S., Heifetz, S. B., and Poulsen, S.: Retention and effectiveness of a single application of an adhesive sealant in preventing caries: Final report after five years of study in Kalispell, Montana. J. Am. Dent. Assoc., 95:1133–1139, 1977.

52. Brudevold, F., Savory, A., Gardner, D. E., et al.: A study of acidulated fluoride solutions. I. *In vitro* effects on enamel. Arch. Oral Biol., 8:167–177, 1963.

53. Ripa, L. W.: Professional (operator) applied topical fluoride therapy: A critique. Int. Dent. J., 31:105–120, 1981.

54. Vrbic, V., Brudevold, F., and McCann, H. G.: Acquisition of fluoride by enamel from fluoride pumice pastes. Helv. Odontol. Acta, 11:21–26, 1967.

55. Zuniga, M. A., and Caldwell, R. C.: The effect of fluoride-containing prophylaxis pastes on normal and "white spot" enamel. J. Dent. Child., 36:345–349, 1969.

56. Stookey, G. K.: *In vitro* estimates of enamel and dentin abrasion associated with a prophylaxis. J. Dent. Res., 57:36, 1978.

57. Mellberg, J. R., Nicholson, C. R., Ripa, L. W., and Barenie, J.: Fluoride deposition in human enamel *in vivo* from professionally applied fluoride prophylaxis paste. J. Dent. Res., 55:976–979, 1976.

58. Ericsson, Y.: The distribution and reactions of fluoride ions in enamel-saliva environment, investigated with the radioactive fluorine isotope [18]F. Acta Odontol. Scand., 16:127–141, 1958.

59. Richardson, B.: Fixation of topically applied fluoride in enamel. J. Dent. Res., 46:87–91, 1967.

60. Carlos, J. P.: Currently available preventive methods. *In* Prevention and Oral Health, DHEW Pub. No. (NIH) 74–707, Washington, D.C., U.S. Government Printing Office, 1974, Chapter 3, pp. 21–26.

61. Mellberg, J. R., and Shulman, L.: The treatment of human teeth with fluoride for replantation and allotransplantation. J. Dent. Res., 53:844–846, 1974.

62. Shannon, I. L., Buchanan, W. E., Jr., and Mahan, C. J.: *In vitro* treatment of human root surfaces with fluorides. J. Public Health Dent., 36:201–206, 1976.

63. Gwinnett, A. J., Buonocore, M. G., and Sheykholeslam, Z.: Effect of fluoride on etched enamel surfaces as demonstrated by the scanning electron microscope. Arch. Oral Biol., 17:271–278, 1972.

64. Sheykholeslam, Z., Buonocore, M. G., and Gwinnett, A. J.: Effect of fluorides on the bonding of resins to phosphoric acid etched bovine enamel. Arch. Oral Biol., 17:1037–1045, 1972.

65. Navia, J. M., DiOrio, L. P., Menaker, L., and Miller, S.: Effect of undernutrition during the perinatal period on caries development in the rat. J. Dent. Res., 49:1091–1098, 1970.

66. Menaker, L., and Navia, J. M.: The effect of undernutrition during the prenatal period on caries development. II, III, IV. J. Dent. Res., 52:680–687, 688–691, 692–697, 1973.

67. Infante, P. F., and Gillespie, G. M.: Enamel hypoplasia in relation to caries in Guatemala children. J. Dent. Res., 56:493–498, 1977.

68. Losee, F. L., and Ludwig, T. G.: Trace elements and caries. J. Dent. Res., 49:1229–1235, 1970.

69. Curzon, M. E. J., and Losee, F. L.: Dental caries and trace element composition of whole human enamel: Eastern United States. J. Am. Dent. Assoc., 94:1146–1150, 1977.

70. Makinen, K. K.: The role of sucrose and other sugars in the development of caries: A review. Int. Dent. J., 22:363–386, 1972.

71. Newbrun, E.: Sucrose, the arch criminal of dental caries. J. Dent. Child., 36:239–248, 1969.

72. Nizel, A. E.: Dental caries: Proteins, fats, and carbohydrates: A literature review. NY State Dent. J., 35:71–81, 1969.

73. Shaw, J. H.: Changing food habits and our need for evaluations of the cariogenic potential of foods and confections. Pediatr. Dent., 1:192–198, 1979.

74. Gustafsson, B. E., Quensel, C. E., Lanke, L. S., et al.: Vipeholm Dental Caries Study. Acta Odontol. Scand., 11:232–364, 1954.

75. Weiss, R. L., and Trithart, A. H.: Between-meal eating habits and dental caries experience in preschool children. Am. J. Public Health, 50:1097–1104, 1960.

76. Duany, L. F., Zinner, D. D., and Jablon, J. M.: Epidemiologic studies of caries-free and caries-active students. II. Diet, dental plaque, and oral hygiene. J. Dent. Res., 51:727–733, 1972.

77. Stephan, R. M.: Changes in hydrogen ion concentration on tooth surfaces and in carious lesions. J. Am. Dent. Assoc., 27:718–723, 1940.

78. Holst, K., and Kohler, L.: Preventing dental caries in children: Report of a Swedish program. Dev. Med. Child Neurol., 17:602–604, 1975.

79. Holm, A. K., Blomquist, H. K., Grossner, G.-G., et al.: A comparative study of oral health as related to general health, food habits and socio-economic conditions of 4-year-old Swedish children.

Community Dent. Oral Epidemiol., *3*:34–39, 1975.

80. Shannon, I. L., and McCartney, J. C.: Presweetened dry breakfast cereals: Potential for danger. J. Dent. Child., *48*:215–218, 1981.

81. Shannon, I. L.: Ice cream: Potential dental hazard. J. Dent. Child., *47*:251–254, 1980.

82. Katz, S.: A diet counseling program. J. Am. Dent. Assoc., *102*:840–845, 1981.

83. Nizel, A. E.: Personalized nutrition counseling. J. Dent. Child., *39*:353–360, 1972.

84. Young, C. M.: Nutrition counseling for the dental patient. J. Am. Dent. Assoc., *63*:469–472, 1961.

85. Loe, H., Theilade, E., Jensen, S. B., and Schiott, C. R.: Experimental gingivitis in man. The influence of antibiotics on gingival plaque development. J. Periodont. Res., *2*:282–289, 1967.

86. Loe, H., Theilade, E., and Jensen, S. B.: Experimental gingivitis in man. J. Periodontol., *36*:177–187, 1965.

87. Bay, I., Kardel, K. M., and Skougaard, M. R.: Quantitative evaluation of the plaque-removing ability of different types of toothbrushes. J. Periodontol., *38*:526–533, 1967.

88. Sangnes, G.: Effectiveness of vertical and horizontal toothbrushing techniques in the removal of plaque. J. Dent. Child., *41*:119–123, 1974.

89. Gibson, J. A., and Wade, A. B.: Plaque removal by the Bass and roll brushing techniques. J. Periodontol., *48*:456–459, 1977.

90. Robertson, N. A. E., and Wade, A. B.: Effect of filament diameter and density in toothbrushes. J. Periodont. Res., *7*:346–351, 1972.

91. Hansen, F., and Gjermo, P.: The plaque removing effects of four toothbrushing methods. Scand. J. Dent. Res., *79*:502–506, 1971.

92. Frandsen, A. M., Barbano, J. P., Suomi, J. D., et al.: The effectiveness of the Charters', scrub and roll methods of toothbrushing by professionals in removing plaque. Scand. J. Dent. Res., *78*:459–463, 1970.

93. McClure, D. B.: A comparison of toothbrushing techniques for the preschool child. J. Dent. Res., *33*:205–210, 1966.

94. Frandsen, A. M., Barbano, J. P., Suomi, J. D., et al.: A comparison of the effectiveness of the Charters', scrub and roll methods of toothbrushing in removing plaque. Scand. J. Dent. Res., *80*:267–271, 1972.

95. Keller, S. E., and Manson-Hing, L. R.: Clearance studies of proximal tooth surfaces. Parts III and IV. *In vivo* removal of interproximal plaque. Ala. J. Med. Sci., *6*:399–405, 1969.

96. Wright, G. Z., Banting, D. W., and Feasby, W. H.: Effect of interdental flossing on the incidence of proximal caries in children. J. Dent. Res., *56*:574–578, 1977.

97. Wright, G. Z., Banting, D. W., and Feasby, W. H.: The Dorchester Dental Flossing Study: Final Report. Clin. Prevent. Dent., *1*(3):22–26, 1979.

98. Ash, M. M., Jr.: A review of the problems and results of studies on manual and power toothbrushes. J. Periodontol., *35*:202–213, 1964.

99. Parfitt, G. J.: Therapeutic devices. Ann. NY Acad. Sci., *135*:360–373, 1968.

100. Bibby, B. G.: Do we tell the truth about preventing caries? J. Dent. Child., *33*:269–279, 1966.

101. Sutton, R., and Sheiham, A.: The factual basis of dental health education. Health. Educ. J., *33*:49–55, 1974.

102. Ripa, L. W.: The effectiveness of oral hygiene methods in the control of dental caries. *In* Oral Hygiene in Oral Health, H. J. V. Goldberg and L. W. Ripa (eds.). Springfield, Ill., Charles C Thomas, 1977, Chapter 10, pp. 283–308.

103. Ripa, L. W., Barenie, J. T., and Leske, G. S.: The relationship between oral hygiene and dental health: An epidemiological survey. NY State Dent. J., *43*:530–535, 1977.

104. Leske, G. S., Ripa, L. W., and Barenie, J. T.: Comparisons of caries activity of children with different daily brushing frequencies. Community Dent. Oral Epidemiol., *4*:102–105, 1976.

105. Barenie, J. T., Ripa, L. W., and Leske, G. S.: The relationship of frequency of toothbrushing, oral hygiene, gingival health, and caries experience in school children. J. Public Health Dent., *160*:37–49, 1973.

106. Horowitz, A. M., Suomi, J. D., Peterson, J. K., and Lyman, B. A.: Effects of supervised daily dental plaque removal by children. II. 24 months' results. J. Public Health Dent., *37*:180–188, 1977.

107. Silverstein, S., Gold, S., Heilbron, D., et al.: Effect of supervised deplaquing on dental caries, gingivitis, and plaque. J. Dent. Res., *56* (Spec. Issue A):A85, 1977.

108. von der Fehr, F. R., and Moller, I. J.: Caries-preventive fluoride dentifrices. Caries Res., *12* (Suppl. 1):31–37, 1978.

109. Dentifrices. *In* Preventive Dental Services, Practices, Guidelines and Recommendations. Ottawa, Canada, Minister of National Health and Welfare, Cat. No. H 39–4/1980E, Sept. 1974, pp. 103–109.

110. Englander, H. R., Keyes, P. H., Gestwicki, M., and Sultz, H. A.: Clinical anti-caries effect of repeated topical sodium fluoride applications by mouthpieces. J. Am. Dent. Assoc., *75*:638–644, 1967.

111. Heifetz, S. B.: Cost-effectiveness of topically applied fluorides. *In* The Relative Efficiency of Methods of Caries Prevention in Dental Public Health Programs, B. A. Burt (ed.). Ann Arbor: University of Michigan, 1978, pp. 69–104.

112. Ripa, L. W.: Fluoride rinsing: What dentists should know. J. Am. Dent. Assoc., *102*:477–481, 1981.

113. Ripa, L. W.: Self-application of topical fluoride: Review and recommendations for use in a private office program. Quintessence Int. Dent. Digest, *7*(11):51–58, 1976.

114. Council on Dental Therapeutics: Council classifies fluoride mouthrinses. J. Am. Dent. Assoc., *91*:1250–1252, 1975.

115. Heifetz, S. B., Franchi, G. J., Mosley, G. W., et al.: Combined anticariogenic effect of fluoride gel-trays and fluoride mouthrinsing in an optimally fluoridated community. J. Clin. Prev. Dent., *6*(1):21–23, passim 28, 1979.

116. Radiake, A. W., Gish, C. W., Peterson, J. K., et al.: Clinical evaluation of stannous fluoride as an anticaries mouthrinse. J. Am. Dent. Assoc., *86*:404–408, 1973.

117. Laswell, H. W., Packer, M. W., and Wiggs, J. S.:

Cariostatic effects of fluoride mouthrinses in a fluoridated community. J. Tenn. Dent. Assoc., 55:198–200, 1975.

118. Kawall, K., Lewis, D. W., and Hargreaves, J. A.: The effect of a fluoride mouthrinse in an optimally fluoridated community. Final two year results. J. Dent. Res., 60 (Spec. Issue A):471, 1981.

119. Driscoll, W. S., Swango, P. A., Horowitz, A. M., and Kingman, A.: Caries-preventive effects of daily and weekly fluoride mouthrinsing in a fluoridated community: Findings after 18 months. J. Dent. Res., 60 (Spec. Issue A):471, 1981.

120. Englander, H. R., Sherrill, L. T., Miller, B. G., et al.: Incremental rates of dental caries after repeated topical sodium fluoride applications in children with lifelong consumption of fluoridated water. J. Am. Dent. Assoc., 82:354–358, 1971.

121. Westcott, W. B., Starcke, E. N., and Shannon, I. L.: Chemical protection against postirradiation dental caries. Oral Surg., 40:709–719, 1975.

122. Dreizen, S., Brown, L. R., Daly, T. E., and Drane, J. B.: Prevention of xerostomia-related dental caries in irradiated cancer patients. J. Dent. Res., 56:99–104, 1977.

123. Thylstrup, A.: Is there a biological rationale for prenatal fluoride administration? J. Dent. Child., 48:103–108, 1981.

124. Driscoll, W. S.: A review of clinical research on the use of prenatal fluoride administration for prevention of dental caries. J. Dent. Child., 48:109–117, 1981.

125. Stookey, G. K.: Perspectives on the use of prenatal fluorides: A reactor's comments. J. Dent. Child., 48:126–127, 1981.

126. Fluoride compounds. In Accepted Dental Therapeutics, 38th Ed. Chicago, American Dental Association, 1979, pp. 316–358.

127. American Academy of Pediatrics, Committee on Nutrition. Fluoride supplementation, revised dosage schedule. Pediatrics, 63:150–152, 1979.

128. Ripa, L. W.: The role of the pediatrician in dental caries detection and prevention. Pediatrics, 54:176–182, 1974.

129. Driscoll, W. S.: The use of fluoride tablets for the prevention of dental caries. In International Workshop on Fluorides and Dental Caries Reductions, D. J. Forrester and E. M. Schulz, Jr. (eds.). Baltimore, University of Maryland, 1974, pp. 25–93.

130. Binder, K., Driscoll, W. S., and Schutzmannsky, G.: Caries-preventive fluoride tablet programs. Caries Res., 12 (Suppl. 1):22–30, 1978.

131. Fluorides. In Preventive Dental Services, Practices, Guidelines and Recommendations. Ottawa, Canada, Minister of National Health and Welfare, Cat. No. H 39–4/1980E, 1979, pp. 172–225.

132. Mellberg, J. R., and Ripa, L. W.: Dietary fluoride supplements. In Fluoride in Preventive Dentistry: Theory and Clinical Applications, J. R. Mellberg and L. W. Ripa (eds.). Chicago, Quintessence, in press.

133. Driscoll, W. S., Heifetz, S. B., and Kortz, D. C.: Effect of chewable fluoride tablets on dental caries in school children: Results after six years of use. J. Am. Dent. Assoc., 97:820–824, 1978.

134. Driscoll, W. S., Heifetz, S. B., and Brunelle, J.: Treatment and posttreatment effects of chewable fluoride tablets on dental caries: Findings after 7½ years. J. Am. Dent. Assoc., 99:817–821, 1979.

135. Fanning, E. A., Cellier, K. M., Leadbeater, M. M., and Somerville, C. M.: South Australian kindergarten children: Fluoride tablet supplements and dental caries. Aust. Dent. J., 20:7–9, 1975.

136. Gray, A. S., and Gunther, D. M.: Supplemental fluorides. A community health centre project in preventive dentistry. Can. J. Public Health, 67:55–58, 1976.

137. Richardson, A. S.: Parental participation in the administration of fluoride supplements. Can. J. Public Health, 58:508–513, 1967.

138. Newbrun, E.: Substrate: Diet and caries. In Cariology, E. Newbrun (ed.). Baltimore, Williams & Wilkins Co., 1978, pp. 76–96.

139. Bagramian, R. A., Graves, R. C., and Srivastava, S.: A combined approach to preventing dental caries in school children: Caries reductions after three years. Community Dent. Oral Epidemiol., 6:166–171, 1978.

140. Fischman, S. L., English, J. A., Albino, J. E., et al.: A comprehensive caries control program—design and evaluation of the clinical trial. J. Dent. Res., 56 (Spec. Issue C):C99–103, 1977.

141. Horowitz, H. S.: A review of systemic and topical fluorides for the prevention of dental caries. Community Dent. Oral Epidemiol., 1:104–114, 1973.

142. Wei, S. H. Y.: The potential benefits to be derived from topical fluorides in fluoridated communites. In International Workshop on Fluorides and Dental Caries Reductions, D. J. Forrester and E. M. Schulz, Jr. (eds.). Baltimore, University of Maryland, 1974, pp. 178–240.

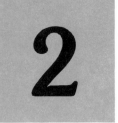

MILTON I. HOUPT

PEDODONTICS IN GENERAL PRACTICE

Child patients are the building blocks of most developing general dental practices. A parent frequently takes a child to a new dentist before seeking care for the whole family. Consequently, it is important that the general practitioner develop the requisite knowledge and skill to treat children. This chapter reviews the practice of pedodontics. It provides information that will assist the reader who treats child patients to manage behavior in the dental operatory; perform a clinical examination and plan treatment; administer local anesthesia; perform restorative treatment; perform pulp therapy; remove primary teeth; and manage traumatic injuries.

BEHAVIOR MANAGEMENT

Child patients are the cornerstone for developing family dental practices. Nevertheless, there are many practitioners who fear treating children; they seek magical drugs for child management or do not treat children at all. Many practitioners fear giving children local anesthetic injections and instead attempt to use nitrous oxide as an analgesic. Too frequently they fail, because nitrous oxide does not take the place of local anesthesia, and a severe management problem results. It is important to note that pedodontists who routinely manage difficult behavioral problems do not use drugs to do so. Their patients are usually managed without premedication, conscious sedation, or general anesthesia; therefore, it would be instructive to examine the manner in which pedodontists manage their patients.

The aims of child management are twofold: (1) management of the child so that dental treatment can be performed comfortably, and (2) management of the child so that the child develops a positive attitude toward dentistry, which motivates good dental hygiene.

Children come to the dental office with general anxieties and specific fears that are quite normal. The general anxieties are due to basic personality traits and are influenced by parents, siblings, or peers. A child may have a specific fear caused by previously undergoing a painful dental procedure or from hearing siblings, peers, or parents speak of unpleasant experiences. The anxieties or specific fears lead children to display differing behaviors according to their developmental age. Frankl categorized child behavior according to degree of cooperation:

1. *Definitely negative* behavior. The child refuses treatment, cries forcefully, is fearful, or demonstrates any other overt evidence of extreme negativism.

2. *Negative* behavior. The child is reluctant to accept treatment or is uncooperative; some evidence of negative attitude exists but is not pronounced, e.g., sullenness, withdrawal.

3. *Positive* behavior. The child accepts treatment, is at times cautious, or is willing to comply with the dentist with reservation, but generally follows the dentist's directions cooperatively.

4. *Definitely positive* behavior. The child has a rapport with the dentist, is interested in the dental procedures, and laughs and enjoys the situation.

This classification describes children who may be cooperative, apprehensive, fearful, stubborn, or defiant. Additionally, children may be physically, mentally, or emotionally handicapped or perhaps emotionally immature (e.g., the very young child with whom it is difficult to communicate). The various behaviors may be managed with a variety of techniques, including:

Nonpharmacologic techniques
1. Tell, show and do.
2. Voice control.
3. Hand over mouth exercise.

Pharmacologic techniques
1. Nitrous oxide conscious sedation.
2. Oral premedication.
3. General anesthesia.

The tell, show, and do technique is used with all patients, as is voice control. The hand over mouth exercise is reserved for children 3 to 6 years of age who are mature enough to understand basic communication but exhibit stubborn or defiant behavior. Nitrous oxide conscious sedation is used with fearful children, particularly those with generally anxious personality traits. Oral or intramuscular premedication is used in patients with extreme anxiety and in those with whom it is difficult to communicate, such as children under 2 years of age or mentally retarded individuals. General anesthesia is reserved for those children requiring extensive treatment or those with whom other pharmacologic methods have been unsuccessful.

Nonpharmacologic Methods

Tell, Show, and Do Technique

The tell, show, and do technique is a method in which dental procedures are introduced in a manner that gains the child's acceptance. The child should be told everything in words appropriate for the child's age. What, why, and how the procedure is to be done should be explained simply (Fig. 2–1). It is not necessary to explain each and every instrument, but rather the few major instruments to be used, for example, the mirror, the tooth counter (explorer), the toothbrush (prophylaxis handpiece), the vacuum cleaner (suction), the raincoat (rubber dam), and the water gun (water syringe).

Terminology appropriate for a 3-year-old is very different from that used for a 6- or 8-year-old. Similarly, the degree of explana-

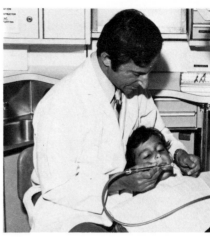

FIGURE 2–1 Using the "tell, show, and do" approach to introduce the handpiece.

tion varies according to the child's interest.

It is important that the dentist *tell* the child what will be done rather than ask for permission. Asking permission allows the child to say "no," presenting a major problem. Voice control is important when telling about a procedure. If one speaks softly, the child tends to be quieter in order to listen. The dentist should speak in a slow, soothing, reassuring voice, preferably over a short distance; that is, the dentist should be as close to the child as possible. The voice should display confidence, for if the dentist acts positively, the patient will react positively, whereas, if the dentist is unsure, the child will sense the uncertainty and react accordingly. The manner of speech often conveys more meaning than the words themselves.

While the child is being told about the procedure, instruments should be *shown* to the child. Some practitioners suggest that the child use a mirror to observe the procedure. The child should be allowed to touch, feel, and smell those things that are to be placed in the mouth.

The practitioner should always use positive suggestion in describing the sensation an instrument will produce. The funny sensation of a prophylaxis cup on marginal gingiva could be interpreted as discomfort. However, if the dentist describes that feeling as "ticklish," the child will react positively. The dentist could describe the explorer as the tooth counter to a young child who is asked to listen as the instrument taps the teeth, rather than stress the idea of a point being pushed into the teeth. The *"do"* part of the tell, show, and do technique should follow the telling and the showing smoothly, with no break in time, and the dentist should do what was said and shown.

The tell, show, and do technique is a method whereby the child can be trained in small increments to cooperate with the dentist. The technique may progress quickly or slowly, depending on the situation. Often ideal cooperation is not achieved, but it is important that something be achieved and the child thanked and praised for that amount of cooperation. The child should not be left with the feeling that he or she has controlled the environment and has not allowed the appropriate procedures to be performed.

Praise and thanks are essential to reinforce good behavior, whereas unacceptable behavior should not be tolerated. Consequently, at the outset of treatment, if the child is told to straighten his or her feet and doesn't listen, it is important to precipitate the crisis of cooperation at its beginning. If the dentist allows the child to disobey at this point, he sets the stage for lack of cooperation during the more difficult phases of treatment. If, on the other hand, the child does cooperate and is praised for that cooperation, the stage is set for complete cooperation throughout treatment. It is most important not to ask permission to do a procedure but rather to tell the child what is to be done; thus, in small increments the child is trained to observe the rules of the environment.

It is also essential that the beginning appointment not be viewed as a game with the child playing with the equipment. When the suction equipment, air and water syringes, and automatic chair are demonstrated to the child, it should not be in the context of a game. If so, the child may at some future time choose not to play any longer and a behavior management problem develops. Most children are rather curious, and the dentist can benefit from that curiosity by explaining the various procedures. When there is a behavioral problem, it is important that some communication be maintained continuously, particularly during a difficult procedure. When an injection is being given, the operator should talk and continuously praise the child for cooperating rather than remain silent, which allows the child's anxieties to build. If for some reason the dentist must leave the operatory, the assistant should continue the communication so that the child does not feel abandoned. When the visit is completed, the dentist should prepare the child for the next visit by explaining that the next visit will be just as easy as this one.

At the conclusion of the visit, the child should be offered a small token as a gift or reward for cooperation. The gift is not to be used as a bribe, for it will fail, but rather it is used as a reward. Even if a child has exhibited rather negative behavior, some aspect of that behavior should be selected for positive reinforcement. If the dentist thanks the child for some aspect of cooperation, the dentist can expect that the cooperation will be even greater at the next visit.

Voice Control

Voice control is the intentional raising of one's voice in an attempt to demonstrate a firm attitude to the child (Fig. 2–2). The dentist should speak in a loud voice in order to startle a child from disruptive behavior or simply to be heard when a child is screaming. When the dentist gains the child's attention, he should speak more softly, adjusting his voice to the activity of the child. Voice control should be used in an objective manner, and the dentist should not raise his or her voice because of anger. If an operator is

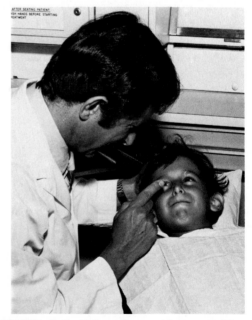

FIGURE 2–2 Being firm with a recalcitrant child.

not able to control him- or herself and begins to lose control of the situation, it is best to abort the procedure and attempt to complete something minor rather than fail at a more involved procedure.

Hand Over Mouth Exercise

When a child is screaming and out of control, it is difficult to establish communication, as the child cannot hear any commands. The hand over mouth exercise (HOME) is used if voice control has failed. Its primary objective is to cover the child's mouth in order to quiet the screams so that the child can hear the dentist talking. Its secondary objective is to serve as an aversive stimulus that will be removed when the child cooperates by quieting down.

The technique is used for those patients who are able to understand; consequently, it is not used for children under the age of 2½, for mentally retarded individuals, or for children sufficiently premedicated as to be unable to comprehend. The dentist places the hand firmly over the child's mouth to muffle the noise (Fig. 2–3) but does not obstruct the airway by pinching the nostrils.

He then talks to the child in a rather quiet manner with his mouth close to the child's ear. The child is told that the hand will be removed if the screaming stops. This is repeated until the crying lessens. Then the hand is removed and the child thanked for cooperating. Frequently the crying begins again and the hand is immediately replaced until the crying lessens. When the child realizes that the dentist is in control of the situation, the temper tantrum usually ends, and the child becomes a cooperative patient. If crying starts again, a gentle but firm reminder that the hand will be replaced is usually enough to make the child reconsider. The technique is an excellent aversive conditioning procedure to modify undesirable behavior. However, although the hand over mouth technique is used by most pedodontists, it is seldom needed, and most patients are suitably managed with appropriate use of the tell, show, and do technique and voice control.

A major question in child management is what should be done with the parent while a young child receives dental care. Children under 2 years of age should be examined while sitting in the parent's lap (Fig. 2–4). If

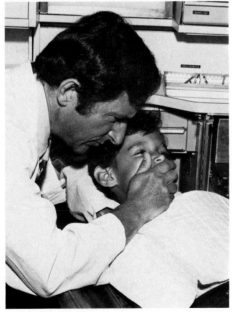

FIGURE 2–3 Using the HOME (hand over mouth exercise). Note the position of the dentist speaking close to the child's ear. The dentist's hand covers the mouth but not the nose, thus cutting off the child's sounds but leaving the airway open.

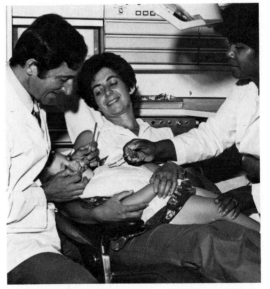

FIGURE 2–4 Examining an infant in the lap of a parent. Note that the parent cradles the child and restrains the hands. The assistant restrains the feet with one hand while assisting with the other, and the dentist secures the child's head between his arms and his body.

comprehensive treatment is required, it will usually be performed under premedication and without the presence of the parent. Children aged 3 to 5 years may benefit from the parent's presence during the first visit. However, many practitioners prefer that the parents remain in the waiting room during treatment visits. When the parent is not present, the child can devote complete attention to the dentist and will quickly learn to accept the authority of the dental environment. Five guidelines for management proposed by Starkey are: (1) leave the parent in the reception area, (2) be honest with the child, (3) reject unacceptable behavior at its inception, (4) praise the child for good behavior, and (5) be friendly.

Pharmacologic Methods

Pharmacologic methods include the use of nitrous oxide conscious sedation, oral and intramuscular premedication, and general anesthesia.

Nitrous Oxide Conscious Sedation

Nitrous oxide conscious sedation is a useful adjunct in controlling anxiety in children; however, it should not be used routinely for most children, and those who receive it should be weaned from its use as treatment progresses and anxiety is lessened. Nitrous oxide conscious sedation is not a substitute for local anesthesia, as it often does not produce adequate analgesia; consequently, local anesthesia should routinely be used. Rubber dam application will aid in controlling mouth breathing, thus promoting the effect of the nitrous oxide. This technique is beneficial for those with real fears, as it will lessen fear and anxiety, raise the pain threshold, improve patient cooperation, and reduce the gag reflex. However, nitrous oxide sedation is not useful for defiant or recalcitrant children exhibiting temper tantrums. Its method of administration (Fig. 2–5) is similar to that used with adults, but for children, a 5 or 6 liter flow and a nitrous oxide concentration of between 25 and 50 per cent are used. Nausea will occur if excessive concentrations are used or if the concentration of nitrous oxide is changed frequently during the procedure. It is essential that an appropriate scavenging system nasal inhaler be used.

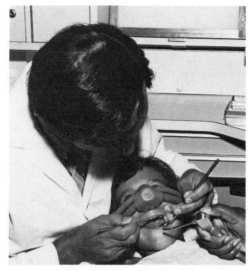

FIGURE 2–5   Preparing to work with nitrous oxide analgesia. Note the use of a scavenging system nasal hood.

Oral Premedication

Oral or intramuscular premedication is used in the very young, the mentally retarded, or those others with extreme apprehension, and it is frequently an alternative to general anesthesia. Such premedication will produce a child who is calm and perhaps in arousable sleep; however, it should not be confused with general anesthesia, and excessive drug dosages producing general anesthetic effects should not be used. The child who is premedicated will often require restraint in a pediwrap, Papoose board (Fig. 2–6), or similar type of restraint. A mouth prop is routinely used together with rubber dam isolation. The general practitioner will usually use only oral premedicants. Frequently used oral premedicants are chloral hydrate (Noctec), hydroxyzine hydrochloride (Atarax, Vistaril), diazepam (Valium), promethazine hydrochloride (Phenergan), and meperidine hydrochloride (Demerol). It is best that the practitioner become completely familiar with a few drugs rather than have a superficial knowledge of many drugs.

The very young child will frequently be managed with chloral hydrate administered alone or administered together with promethazine. The older child will best be managed with hydroxyzine, diazepam, or a combination of meperidine and promethazine. Drug dosages are somewhat arbitrary and are usually based on body weight: chloral

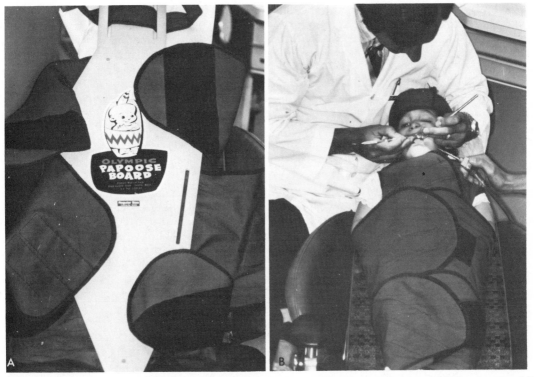

FIGURE 2–6 *A,* The Papoose Board restraining device. *B,* The cloth sides are folded over the child and secured with Velcro fasteners.

hydrate, 25.0 mg/lb; hydroxyzine, 0.5 mg/lb; diazepam, 0.15 mg/lb; promethazine, 0.5 mg/lb; meperidine, 1.0 mg/lb. However, children frequently require greater amounts for the desired effect, and the appropriate dose is sometimes determined by trial. If a dose is administered and the desired effect is not achieved, it is best to abort the procedure and continue at a second appointment with an altered dose rather than add a second dose at the same appointment as the first administration.

Oral premedication is best administered in the morning when the patient has less food in the stomach. At other times the patient should have nothing by mouth for 3 to 4 hours before the administration of the drug. This speeds the absorption of the medication and reduces the possibility of nausea and vomiting. The premedication should be administered approximately 45 minutes before the onset of treatment. This is best done in the dentist's office, where the amount of drug taken can be observed. The child should then be kept continually in the presence of the parent or a responsible adult and observed periodically. Although the

drugs are quite safe in proper dosage, resuscitation equipment and positive-pressure oxygen should always be readily available. Fifteen to 20 minutes following administration of the drug the child will become drowsy and perhaps irritable. It is not uncommon for the very young child to cry and be quite agitated until arousable sleep finally ensues after 45 minutes. Local anesthesia is routine and nitrous oxide sedation is frequently used as an adjunct. The sedation may permit treatment procedures for 1 to 2 hours, but the child will probably sleep for several hours following the procedure, and a parent or a responsible adult should plan to observe the child accordingly.

General Anesthesia

General anesthesia is usually performed in a hospital operating room or other specially equipped facility. Because of the complexity and associated risk of general anesthesia, it is used as a last resort for controlling behavior. Its use is usually limited to mentally retarded persons, very young children, and children with extreme apprehension in whom premedication techniques have failed. Patients requiring general anesthesia should be referred to an appropriate specialist for treatment.

EXAMINATION, TREATMENT PLANNING, AND CASE PRESENTATION

History

The clinical examination of a child should be performed in a thorough and orderly manner so that a complete examination is accomplished. The examiner should take the time to gather a complete history with information that might affect treatment. Specifically, information describing any serious illness or abnormal conditions the child might have experienced, the presence of any bleeding tendencies or allergies, and any previous abnormal reactions to any drugs administered should be noted. A sample history appears in Figure 2–7.

Clinical Examination

The examination begins with unobtrusive observations during the first contact with the patient. The child's stature, gait, dress, level

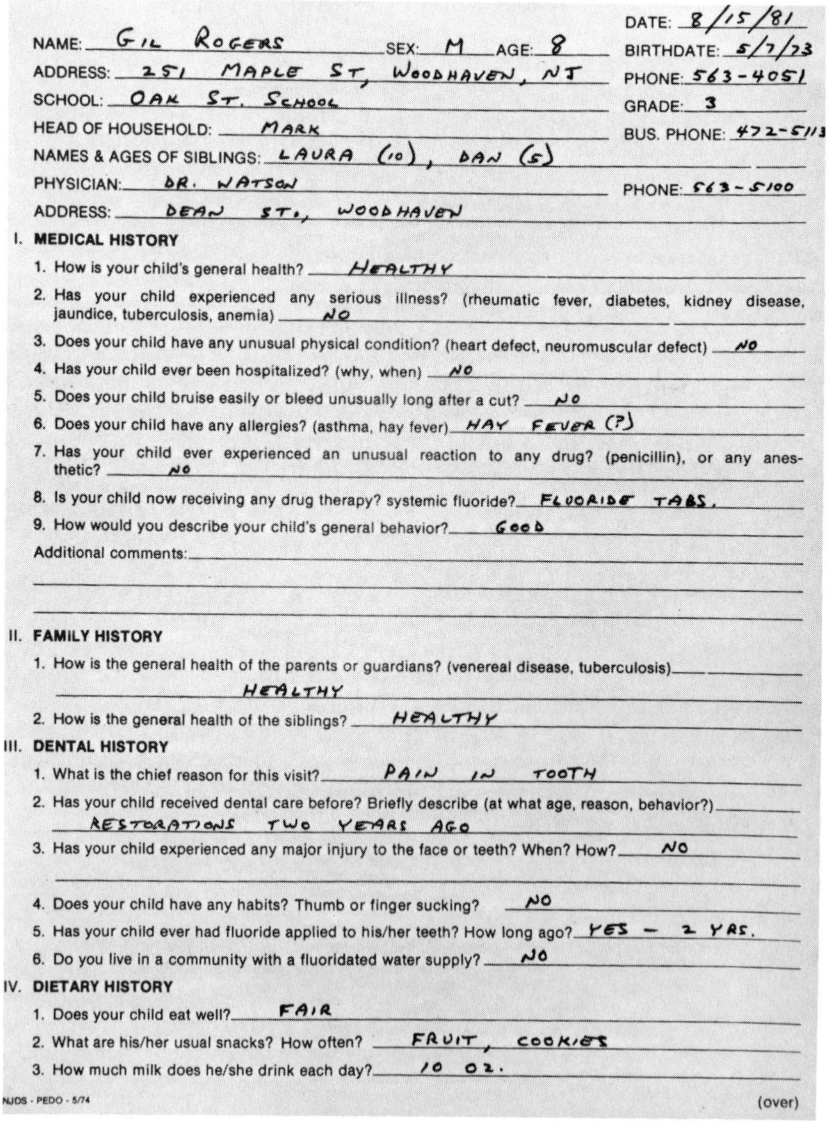

DATE: 8/15/81
NAME: GIL ROGERS SEX: M AGE: 8 BIRTHDATE: 5/7/73
ADDRESS: 251 MAPLE ST, WOODHAVEN, NJ PHONE: 563-4051
SCHOOL: OAK ST. SCHOOL GRADE: 3
HEAD OF HOUSEHOLD: MARK BUS. PHONE: 472-5113
NAMES & AGES OF SIBLINGS: LAURA (10), DAN (5)
PHYSICIAN: DR. WATSON PHONE: 563-5100
ADDRESS: DEAN ST., WOODHAVEN

I. MEDICAL HISTORY

1. How is your child's general health? HEALTHY
2. Has your child experienced any serious illness? (rheumatic fever, diabetes, kidney disease, jaundice, tuberculosis, anemia) NO
3. Does your child have any unusual physical condition? (heart defect, neuromuscular defect) NO
4. Has your child ever been hospitalized? (why, when) NO
5. Does your child bruise easily or bleed unusually long after a cut? NO
6. Does your child have any allergies? (asthma, hay fever) HAY FEVER (?)
7. Has your child ever experienced an unusual reaction to any drug? (penicillin), or any anesthetic? NO
8. Is your child now receiving any drug therapy? systemic fluoride? FLUORIDE TABS.
9. How would you describe your child's general behavior? GOOD

Additional comments:

II. FAMILY HISTORY

1. How is the general health of the parents or guardians? (venereal disease, tuberculosis) HEALTHY
2. How is the general health of the siblings? HEALTHY

III. DENTAL HISTORY

1. What is the chief reason for this visit? PAIN IN TOOTH
2. Has your child received dental care before? Briefly describe (at what age, reason, behavior?) RESTORATIONS TWO YEARS AGO
3. Has your child experienced any major injury to the face or teeth? When? How? NO
4. Does your child have any habits? Thumb or finger sucking? NO
5. Has your child ever had fluoride applied to his/her teeth? How long ago? YES — 2 YRS.
6. Do you live in a community with a fluoridated water supply? NO

IV. DIETARY HISTORY

1. Does your child eat well? FAIR
2. What are his/her usual snacks? How often? FRUIT, COOKIES
3. How much milk does he/she drink each day? 10 OZ.

NJDS - PEDO - 5/74 (over)

FIGURE 2–7 Sample chart illustrating medical history questions.

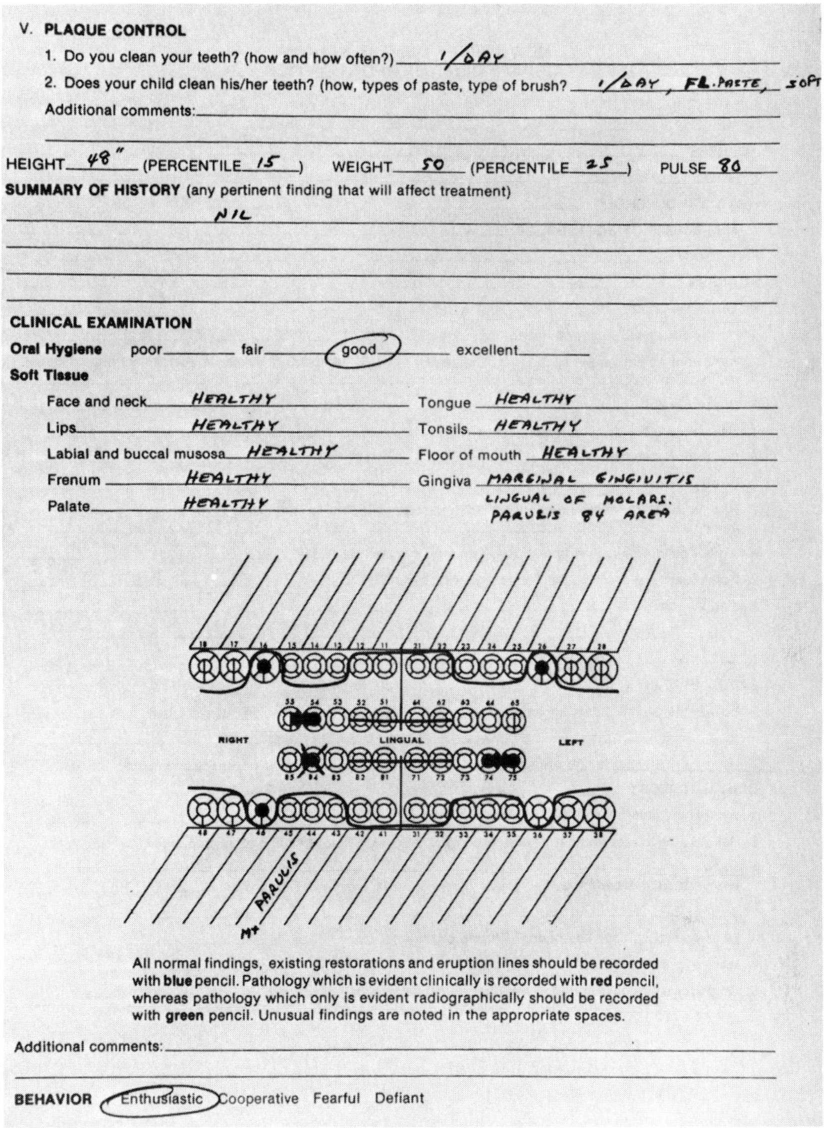

V. **PLAQUE CONTROL**

　　1. Do you clean your teeth? (how and how often?)_____ *1/DAY* _____

　　2. Does your child clean his/her teeth? (how, types of paste, type of brush? _____ *1/DAY, FL-PASTE, SOFT*

　　Additional comments:_____

HEIGHT___*48"*___(PERCENTILE _*15*_)　WEIGHT___*50*___(PERCENTILE _*25*_)　PULSE _*80*_

SUMMARY OF HISTORY (any pertinent finding that will affect treatment)

　　　　　　　　　　NIL

CLINICAL EXAMINATION

Oral Hygiene　　poor_____　fair_____　(good)_____ excellent_____

Soft Tissue

　　Face and neck___*HEALTHY*___　　Tongue___*HEALTHY*___

　　Lips___*HEALTHY*___　　　　　　Tonsils___*HEALTHY*___

　　Labial and buccal musosa___*HEALTHY*___　Floor of mouth___*HEALTHY*___

　　Frenum___*HEALTHY*___　　　　Gingiva___*MARGINAL GINGIVITIS*___

　　Palate___*HEALTHY*___　　　　　　*LINGUAL OF MOLARS.*
　　　　　　　　　　　　　　　　　　PARULIS 84 AREA

All normal findings, existing restorations and eruption lines should be recorded with **blue** pencil. Pathology which is evident clinically is recorded with **red** pencil, whereas pathology which only is evident radiographically should be recorded with **green** pencil. Unusual findings are noted in the appropriate spaces.

Additional comments:_____

BEHAVIOR (Enthusiastic) Cooperative　Fearful　Defiant

FIGURE 2–8　Sample chart showing diagrammatic representation of teeth.

of awareness, and manner of speech should be observed. The extraoral examination should include observation of head size, shape, and symmetry, skin color and hair texture, size and symmetry of the eyes, ears, and nose, and the glands and lymph nodes in the neck. Intraorally, all soft and hard tissues should be observed to note any deviation from normal. Dentists err by looking first for carious lesions in teeth, which are relatively easy to see, and, consequently, many soft tissue lesions are overlooked. The lips, labial and buccal mucosa, frenum, palate, tongue, tonsils, floor of the mouth, and gingiva all should be closely examined for

any signs of abnormality. The results of the clinical examination are included with the history in the patient's records (Fig. 2–8).

When the teeth are examined, existing restorations should be charted in addition to new carious lesions. An eruption line should be drawn to indicate which permanent teeth have erupted in the mouth. The occlusal examination records any rotations or displacement of teeth, the anteroposterior, vertical, and transverse relationships of the arches, and the function of the mandible (Fig. 2–9). When necessary for orthodontic problems, a mixed-dentition space analysis will have to be completed.

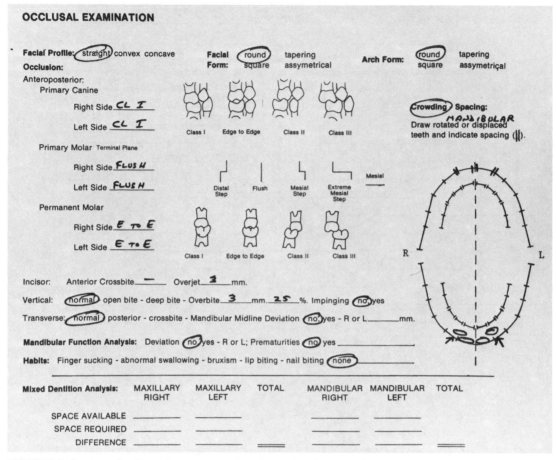

FIGURE 2–9 Sample chart illustrating occlusal examination notations.

Radiographic Examination

Radiographs are important diagnostic aids in pedodontics, providing information concerning the presence of pathologic conditions in both developing and erupted teeth. Nevertheless, radiographs are no longer advocated as part of a routine examination unless they contribute information that will affect treatment. Previously, it was routine in pedodontics to take a full mouth survey for each new patient regardless of age and regardless of the presence or absence of pathologic conditions. It was argued, for example, that radiographs in a 4-year-old might show missing teeth. However, such knowledge is of academic interest only, since no treatment is performed for the patient as a result of that knowledge. Because of the profession's increasing concern with unnecessary use of ionizing radiation, a more conservative approach to the use of x-irradiation with children is suggested. The following guidelines should determine when and which radiographs should be taken:

1. In the primary or mixed dentition, when contacts between posterior teeth are open and there is no clinical abnormality, no radiographs should be taken.

2. When contacts between posterior teeth are closed, bite-wing radiographs are indicated. These should be taken every 6 months in a patient with active caries but delayed to 12- or 18-month intervals in patients with no recent active lesions. The interval can be even longer in children with no previous caries.

3. Whenever an abnormality is present, the appropriate radiograph should be taken. For example, a periapical view is necessary if pulp therapy is to be performed, if a tooth is to be extracted, if a tooth has been traumatized, or if a suspected supernumerary is delaying the eruption of a permanent tooth.

4. Full mouth surveys should not be taken

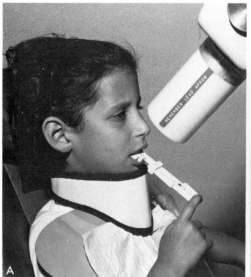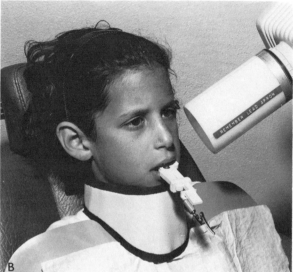

FIGURE 2–10   Obtaining radiographs of maxillary teeth. Note that the patient is protected with a lead body apron and a lead thyroid shield and that the Rinn Snap-A-Ray holder is used to hold the film in place. *A,* Anterior periapical exposure. *B,* Posterior periapical exposure.

routinely. However, they are indicated when carious teeth are present in all quadrants; they are also indicated prior to orthodontic treatment.

5. Posttreatment films are rarely necessary. They should not be taken to submit to third-party payers to record treatment.

Radiographic techniques with children are similar to those with adults, except that the procedure should first be explained to children with the "tell, show, and do" approach. The taking of radiographs can serve as an excellent training tool for new patients when the dentist directs the child to hold still and praises the child for cooperating. The child should be protected with both the lead body apron and the thyroid collar (Fig. 2–10), and the operator should stand behind an appropriate shield.

When many films are to be taken, the anterior views should be taken first, as they are the easiest for the patient. For an apprehensive preschooler, it is advisable to begin with a mock anterior occlusal film to prepare the child for the more difficult posterior views. The edges of the film may have to be rolled to prevent soft tissue impingement. This precaution is particularly appropriate with

TABLE 2–1

Type of View	Size of Film	Vertical Angulation of Central Ray to Film
Primary Dentition		
Maxillary anterior topographic occlusal	#2	+60°
Mandibular anterior topographic occlusal	#2	−60°
Maxillary posterior periapical	#0	+20°
Mandibular posterior periapical	#0	−10°
Bite-wing	#0	+ 8°
Mixed Dentition		
Maxillary anterior periapical	#0	+45°
Mandibular anterior periapical	#0	−35°
Maxillary posterior periapical	#2	+35°
Mandibular posterior periapical	#2	−10°
Bite-wing	#2	+ 8°

bite-wing views, which should be taken last. Gagging is usually controlled by talking to the child through the procedure. Occasionally the film surface may be wetted with cold water or coated with a small amount of flavored prophylaxis paste to control gagging. Children under 3 years are usually radiographed while sitting on the parent's lap with the parent holding the film in place.

The Rinn Snap-A-Ray film holder is advocated for all periapical views. If the patient's occlusal plane is placed parallel to the floor, then the vertical angle settings in Table 2–1 can be used for the machine head, with the horizontal angulation perpendicular to the film.

Interpretation of radiographs should follow an orderly progression. The radiographs should be viewed with a hand magnifying glass on a lighted viewbox and studied to answer the following questions:

1. Was the film adequately positioned to show all required anatomic structures?

2. Is any bone pathology present?

3. Are all the permanent teeth present and developing normally?

4. Is any disease evident within or around the roots of the teeth?

5. Is any disease evident within or on the surface of the crowns of the teeth? By directing attention from the general to the specific, complete interpretation may be accomplished.

Treatment Planning

After all the required data have been collected, a comprehensive treatment plan is formulated. Emergency treatment should be scheduled first; otherwise, treatment should

TREATMENT PLAN   PATIENT *GIL ROGERS*   CHART NO. *5103*

Apt. No.	Tooth or Area	PROCEDURE	Fee	Completed
1		TBI, Rx Fl. tabs		
	L6	O amal		
	E|	adapt band, impression		
2	6|	O amal		
	D|	ext.		
	E|	cement spacer		
3		Check hygiene		
	|D	DO amal		
	|E	MO amal		
4	6|	O amal		
	E|	MO amal		
	D|	DO amal		
		Check spacer		
5		Check hygiene		
		Polish amal		
		Prophy & fl.		
			TOTAL	

FIGURE 2–11 Sample treatment plan.

start with the initiation of the preventive program. Restoration of teeth should be scheduled with the most advanced lesions being treated first. Whenever possible, quadrant dentistry should be performed, making complete treatment easier for the patient and faster for the operator. A sample treatment plan appears in Figure 2–11.

Case Presentation

At the beginning of the second appointment, the clinical findings and plan of treatment should be presented to one parent or, in complicated cases, to both parents. If very young, the child should be occupied with some activity, such as toys or a coloring book, so that the dentist has the parent's undivided attention. General findings should be discussed as well as a brief explanation of the etiology of abnormalities and methods of prevention. The type and extent of treatment should be described in detail, including the probable cost and number of appointments. Future disagreements can be prevented if the parent has a complete understanding of what will be done for the child. A payment schedule should be determined, and the parent should sign and receive a copy of the case presentation summary. A case presentation summary appears in Figure 2–12.

PREVENTION

The major reason for care of primary teeth is prevention of future problems for the child. Consequently, it is understandable that a major activity of the pedodontist is involvement in preventive procedures. Routine practice is the use of fluoride, fissure sealants, and plaque control programs. (These procedures are described in Chapter 1.) Brushing and flossing methods for teenagers are similar to those for adults described in chapter 5. Children under the age of 8 or 9 years usually lack the manual dexterity to use such techniques, and parents must assist with hygiene procedures. Parents are taught to brush the child's teeth with the scrub technique each night following the child's attempt to do so. The child leans back comfortably with the head placed in the parent's lap for good visibility. Conscientious parents can be taught to floss the interproximal areas of posterior teeth.

Parents should be advised that they will be successful in motivating proper oral hygiene practices in their children only if they adopt "do as I do" rather than "do as I say" behavior. Two- and 3-year-old children delight in copying their parents and playing with the toothbrush. They should be encouraged to develop daily toothbrushing habits together with their parents. Consequently, practition-

---

CASE PRESENTATION SUMMARY

1. Diagnosis a. Cranio-facial development ___HEALTHY___

    b. Supporting bone ___HEALTHY___

    c. Occlusion ___NORMAL   E TO E, SOME LOWER CROWDING___

    d. Soft tissues ___MARGINAL GINGIVITIS, PARULIS___

    e. Dentition: ___RECURRENT DECAY___

    defs__8__ DMFS __3__ (e or M=3 surf). Caries Activity: extensive (moderate) minimal nil

2. Treatment a. Preventive___Rx Fl, TBI___

    b. Restorative: No. Teeth ___7___ No. Surfaces ___11___

    c. Pulp therapy ___—___

    d. Space maintenance___1 BAND/LOOP___

    e. Special procedures ___1 EXT.___

3. Prognosis ___GOOD___

4. Total estimated fee_____ Approximate number of appointments ___5___

    Parent or Guardian___Barbara Rogers___ Date___9/2/81___

FIGURE 2–12 Sample of case presentation summary form.

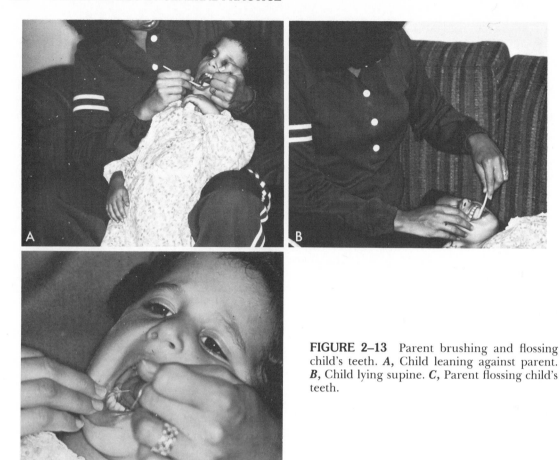

FIGURE 2–13 Parent brushing and flossing child's teeth. *A,* Child leaning against parent. *B,* Child lying supine. *C,* Parent flossing child's teeth.

ers teaching children oral hygiene techniques should involve parents in learning and practicing these same techniques on themselves.

LOCAL ANESTHESIA

The proper management of pain and discomfort is of utmost importance in dentistry for children. There is no greater cause of behavior problems in children than the infliction by the dentist of psychologic or physical pain. Such behavior problems are the principal reason children are referred to pedodontists for treatment, and pedodontists frequently find that the behavior problems resulted from treatment being attempted with little or no anesthesia. Treatment without local anesthesia is a frequent error made by apprehensive dentists in an attempt to avoid a confrontation with an apprehensive child or because of a belief that primary teeth require less anesthetic than permanent teeth, which is fallacious. The child experiencing pain loses the ability to cooperate with the dentist, who then is forced to compromise treatment by inadequate cavity preparation and incomplete caries removal. The child who is comfortable will be a cooperative patient. A smooth injection technique allows treatment to be painless and to proceed in a more relaxed and efficient manner.

Preparation

Good local anesthetic technique should be preceded by a suitable medical history, preparation of the necessary equipment, and proper positioning of patient, operator, and assistant.

An appropriate *medical history* should be taken to determine the presence of conditions affecting the administration of local anesthetic, such as allergy, bleeding or cardiac disorders, and kidney or liver problems. *Topical anesthetic* is routinely used prior to infiltration injections in the mucobuccal fold. The tissue should first be wiped dry and the topical anesthetic placed only on the small area to be penetrated. Allowing excess anesthetic to drip around the mouth is distasteful for the patient and invites problems. If topical anesthetic is used, the appropriate amount of time specified by the manufacturer must elapse in order for it to take effect (30 seconds to 1½ minutes).

An *aspirating syringe* and the use of an aspiration technique are essential to prevent inadvertent intravascular injection.

Disposable needles ensure sterility as well as avoid the use of reused needles whose tops may be blunted. The 27-gauge needle is the thinnest needle that still allows aspiration of blood, and, consequently, it is used routinely. Occasionally a 30-gauge needle is used for the anterior maxillary region in young, apprehensive children. The length of the needle recommended for all injections in children is 1 inch, whereas a 1¼ inch needle is used for block injections in teenagers.

Local anesthetic solutions are of two types: ether derivative (e.g., Novocain) or amide derivative (e.g., Xylocaine, Carbocaine, and Citanest). The duration of anesthesia desired dictates the choice of anesthetic agent and whether it should contain a vasoconstrictor. For example, one may choose a short-acting (Citanest; 45 minutes), medium-acting (Xylocaine with 1/100,000 epinephrine; 90 minutes), or long-acting agent (Carbocaine with 1/20,000 Neo-Cobefrin; 120 minutes).

Preparation of the child, regardless of age, is of great importance. The local anesthetic procedure may be unnecessarily traumatic if the child is not told in understandable language what will actually happen. For example, a preschooler would be told, "I'm going to put your tooth to sleep, not you, just your tooth. I'm going to squirt some sleepy water beside your tooth and you may feel a little mosquito bite, like this." (The dentist then demonstrates with a little pinch on the child's hand.) The child should never be told that "nothing will hurt" but rather to expect a "pinch." Words such as "needle," "shot," or "hurt" should be avoided because of their negative connotations. Words such as "numb" have little meaning to a preschooler, but "funny feeling" does communicate. The dentist should talk in a calm, friendly, and confident manner. Uncertainty in the operator causes anxiety in the child.

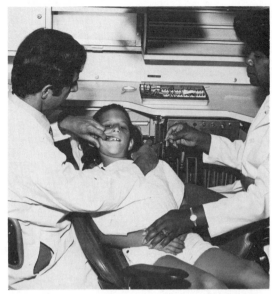

FIGURE 2–14 Assistant passing syringe from behind and out of sight of child. Note that assistant rests her hand on child's hands to prevent any unexpected sudden arm movement.

The operator, assistant, and patient should be positioned for efficient four-handed, sit-down dentistry. The child should be in a reclined, comfortable position. The assistant is seated opposite the operator with one hand gently restraining the child's hands, preventing any sudden movement during the injection, while the other hand passes the syringe unobtrusively to the operator from behind and under the patient's chin (Fig. 2–14). A

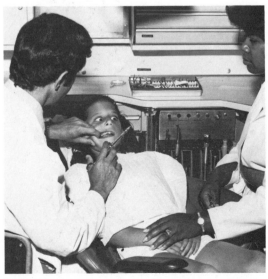

FIGURE 2–15 Unnecessarily producing fear by holding syringe in front of child's face.

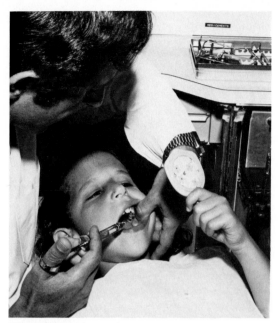

FIGURE 2–16 Child observing injection procedure with small hand mirror.

needle in front of the child's face will produce unnecessary fear (Fig. 2–15).

The child should be instructed to hold still during the procedure, which should be carried out in a slow, deliberate, and smooth manner. Once the procedure begins, the operator should not hesitate, and it is important to talk to the child continually during the injection, which distracts the child and reinforces appropriate behavior, saying, for example, "You're being such a good helper!"

Occasionally with some patients, some operators prefer that the child hold a mirror and watch the complete procedure (Fig. 2–16). This can be a successful technique as long as the child has been prepared appropriately for the procedure.

Anesthetizing Mandibular Teeth

The inferior alveolar block injection (Fig. 2–17) is used routinely to anesthetize mandibular teeth in children, although occasionally infiltration techniques are used. The inferior alveolar block injection anesthetizes the inferior alveolar and lingual nerves, providing anesthesia for the mandibular teeth and soft tissue in that quadrant. Anatomic landmarks are first located with the index finger (or thumb) by palpating the mucobuccal fold beside the molar teeth. The finger is moved posteriorly along the external oblique ridge and up the anterior border of the ramus until the deepest concavity is reached. The concavity is in line with the mandibular foramen and is the level for penetration of the needle. The finger is moved medially to the internal oblique ridge and then slightly laterally, allowing the penetration of the needle to be in the depression between the pterygomandibular raphe and the internal border of the mandible.

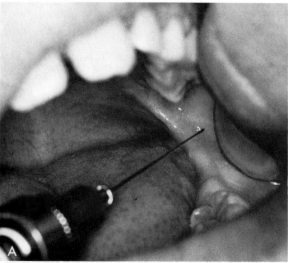
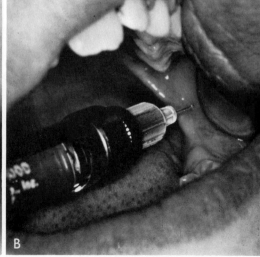

FIGURE 2–17 The inferior alveolar nerve block injection. *A,* Positioning the needle. *B,* Inserting the needle short of the hub.

The mandible should be supported by placing the thumb (or index finger) behind the ramus.

The syringe is brought from the opposite side of the mouth and directed parallel to the occlusal plane, with the barrel of the syringe lying across the opposite primary molar area and the needle bisecting the thumbnail on the anterior border of the ramus. Slight pressure by the finger on soft tissue will distract the patient from the penetration of the needle, as topical anesthetic is not routinely used. The needle is inserted approximately three quarters of an inch, contacting bone in the mandibular foramen area. (The needle should not be injected completely to the hub. Rarely, the needle may break at the hub, and injecting short of the hub leaves part of the needle exposed for retrieval.) A little solution is deposited and the syringe is slightly aspirated. If no blood is aspirated, approximately 1 ml (slightly more than half of the Carpule) of the solution is deposited to anesthetize the inferior alveolar nerve. The solution is injected slowly (for approximately 30 seconds) to minimize any pain of injection. The needle is then withdrawn halfway and an additional .50 ml (¼ Carpule) is deposited to anesthetize the lingual nerve. The syringe may then be used for the buccal nerve injection; otherwise it is removed, and the mouth is rinsed. Anesthesia will be profound if tongue and lip symptoms extend to the midline and there is no pain during treatment.

The buccal nerve is anesthetized whenever surgery is performed on the posterior teeth, and optionally for placement of the rubber dam clamp. The mucobuccal fold distal to the second molar is stretched with the thumb or index finger, and the needle is inserted one-quarter inch toward the external oblique ridge. When bone is contacted, approximately .25 ml is injected slowly. The syringe is then removed, and the mouth is rinsed.

Anesthetizing Maxillary Teeth

Infiltration techniques are routinely used to anesthetize maxillary teeth in children, although occasionally nerve block injections are used. The maxillary infiltration (Fig. 2–18) is used to anesthetize the posterior, middle, or anterior superior alveolar nerve, providing anesthesia for the maxillary teeth in that quadrant. Following the routine use of topical anesthetic, the cheek is pulled out to stretch the mucobuccal fold in the area to be injected. The needle is directed just above the attached gingiva toward the apex of the tooth being anesthetized, with the syringe at a 45 degree angle to the maxillary teeth. If two adjacent teeth are being anesthetized, the needle is directed between the teeth. (If a permanent first molar in a teenager is being anesthetized, two injections are required, one mesially and one distally on either side of the zygomatic process.) The needle is inserted approximately one-half inch, a few drops of solution are deposited, and the syringe is slightly aspirated. If no blood is aspirated, approximately 1 ml of solution is injected slowly (for approximately

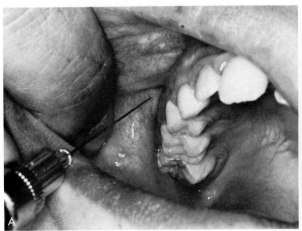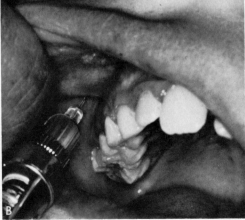

FIGURE 2–18   The maxillary infiltration injection. *A,* Positioning the needle. *B,* Inserting the needle short of the hub.

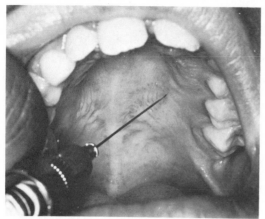

FIGURE 2–19 The anterior palatine injection.

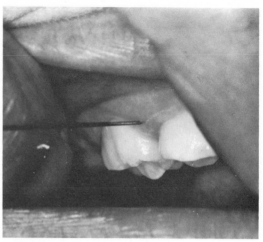

FIGURE 2–21 Injecting into the interdental papilla.

30 seconds) to minimize any pain of injection. The syringe may then be used for palatal infiltration if required. Otherwise, it is removed and the mouth rinsed.

The palatal injection is used to anesthetize the anterior palatine or nasopalatine nerves supplying the soft tissue palatal to the maxillary teeth (Figs. 2–19 and 2–20). The injection is used routinely for surgery and frequently for rubber dam placement. The syringe is directed 90 degrees to the palate lingually to the tooth, and approximately one-quarter inch from the margin of the papilla toward the midline of the palate. The needle is inserted about one-eighth inch until bone is contacted, and a few drops of solution are injected slowly until the tissue blanches. The syringe is then removed and the mouth rinsed.

In apprehensive children, a modified technique should be used in order to lessen any pain associated with the palatal injection. Following maxillary infiltration buccal to the tooth, a few drops of solution are injected in the interdental papilla from the buccal toward the palatal side (Fig. 2–21). Then the needle may be injected into the palatal tissue, which is already anesthetized. The profundity of anesthesia of maxillary teeth can be tested only by observing the patient's response to treatment. Unfortunately, it cannot be determined adequately before treatment.

Postoperative Instructions

Following anesthesia, and again when treatment has been completed, the patient should be cautioned not to bite the cheek or lip. This caution should be repeated to the parent, who should particularly observe the young child to prevent cheek biting. Otherwise, a painful ulcer lasting several days might occur (Fig. 2–22).

RESTORATIVE DENTISTRY

Morphology of Primary Teeth

There are many morphologic differences between primary and permanent teeth that influence restorative techniques for children. Primary teeth are smaller with proportionately larger pulp chambers and higher pulp horns than permanent teeth. Consequently, cavity preparation must be shal-

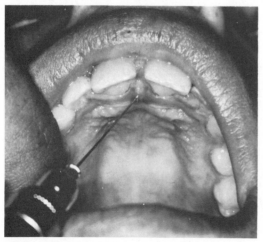

FIGURE 2–20 The nasopalatine injection.

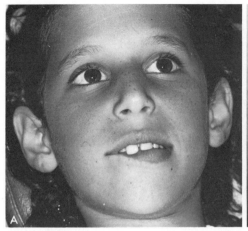 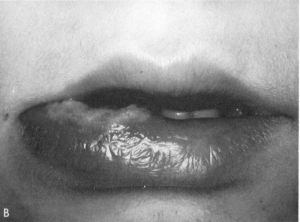

FIGURE 2–22 Postoperative lip biting following the inferior alveolar injection. *A,* Lip biting. *B,* Resulting ulcer.

lower and performed with care. The enamel is thinner and of more uniform depth throughout the crown, so that when preparations are approximately 1.5 mm deep, they are just beneath the dentinoenamel junction. Molar crowns are short and squatty, with a greater mesiodistal dimension relative to the height of the crown and with prominent cervical bulges. These anatomic differences influence crown preparation for stainless steel crowns. The buccal and lingual surfaces converge occlusally, and the contact areas are broader and flatter than in permanent teeth. The enamel rods at the cervical margin of the crown slope horizontally or occlusally, so it is not necessary to bevel the gingival cavosurface margins in Class II preparations. Primary teeth are lighter in color then permanent teeth, and this factor must be considered when anterior teeth are restored with composite resin.

Rubber Dam Application

Rubber dam is used routinely in dentistry for children to provide a dry isolated field as well as to aid in management of the patient. Although many dentists do not use rubber dam for restorative procedures, most pedodontists do because they find its use saves time, improves the quality of treatment, and controls many management problems. It is not infrequent to find an apprehensive preschooler sleep through restorative treatment because of rubber dam placement!

Rubber dam placement can be mastered easily when a minimum number of teeth are isolated. For a Class I or Class V restoration, only the teeth to be restored are isolated. For Class II restorations, one tooth anterior and, where possible, one tooth posterior to the tooth being restored are isolated. A 5-inch square piece of dark heavy rubber dam is used (Fig. 2–23) and punched with the largest hole for the tooth to be clamped and the permanent molars, the middle hole for the primary molars and permanent incisors, and the smallest hole for primary incisors and canines. The most posterior hole is punched first at a point midway between the top and bottom of the dam and one third the distance in from the side edge. Additional holes are punched 2 mm apart in an

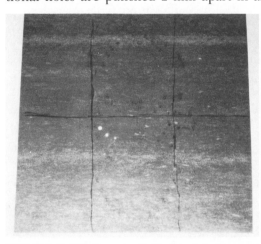

FIGURE 2–23 Dam is divided into halves vertically and thirds horizontally. Hole for permanent molar is punched at the intersection of the lines. Hole for primary second molar is punched about 5 mm from that point.

arc toward the midline and top or bottom of the dam. If the teeth are spaced or mal-aligned, the holes are adjusted accordingly.

Many different types of clamps are available, but the operator should use a minimum number of different ones; for example, for second primary molars No. 14 or No. 27, and for permanent molars No. 14A, No. 5, or No. 8A. A length of dental floss is tied around the bow of the clamp and it is tried on the tooth. There are different ways to carry the clamp, dam, and frame to the mouth. Perhaps the simplest is to use wing-less clamps. The clamp is carried to the tooth with the rubber on the bow of the clamp; the frame can then be inserted in the rubber. Alternately, with winged clamps, the clamp could be placed into the dam, the dam mounted on the frame, and the complete assembly carried to the tooth.

The rubber should be stretched over the teeth, and waxed floss should be used to pull the dam interproximally. One edge of the rubber dam septum is pulled through first rather than all the rubber pulled through at once. The floss is then pulled buccally or lin-gually but not occlusally. The teeth are dried as air is blown at the gingival areas; the edge of the rubber is everted into the sulcus with a plastic instrument. If the tooth surfaces are not dried, the rubber will keep popping up, and the edges will not evert easily. If the rubber is held away from the clamped tooth, the clamp is opened slightly to allow the rubber to slide under the jaws of the clamp. Ligatures and wedges are used whenever inter-proximal preparations are to be made because

they keep the gingiva and the dam away from the cutting instruments (Fig. 2–24). In addition, ligatures are used to stabilize the dam of the most anterior tooth when posterior teeth are isolated or for the most posterior tooth when anterior teeth are isolated.

If the rubber obstructs the patient's nostrils, the top corner of the dam is folded over and hooked at the middle of the side of the frame. Excess rubber at the bottom of the frame is folded and hooked at the middle of both sides of the frame, forming a pouch in which the saliva ejector is placed to remove any excess water that escapes the high-velocity suction. The saliva ejector is not usually placed in the mouth, as it stimulates salivary flow, but periodically throughout the procedure any saliva not swallowed is suctioned. Rarely, a patient cannot breathe through the nose and feels restricted from breathing through the mouth by the dam. In such instances, a few air holes can be punched in the middle of the dam to relieve any feeling of discomfort.

When the dam is to be removed, the ligatures and wedges are removed first. The rubber is then stretched buccally and each interproximal septum is lifted and cut with scissors. The clamp is then removed from the mouth together with the dam and the frame. The interproximal areas should be checked to ensure that no pieces of rubber or floss remain. The dam should be examined by laying it on a flat surface to see if all rubber between the holes has been removed. The soft tissue in the areas of the clamp is massaged, and the mouth is then rinsed.

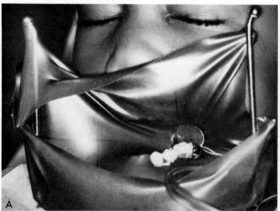 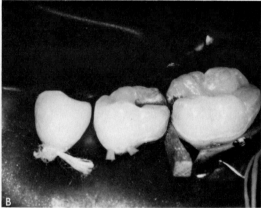

FIGURE 2–24 Rubber dam in place. *A,* Note the fold of the dam pulling it away from the patient's nose and the lower fold of the dam forming a pouch to gather excess water from the water spray. *B,* Interproximal wedges and ligatures in place.

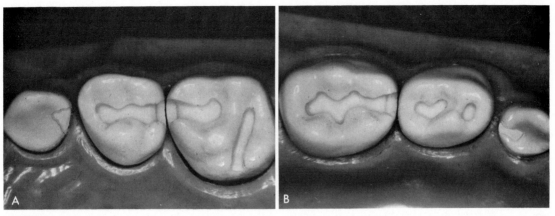

FIGURE 2–25 Typical cavity preparations in primary molars. *A,* Maxillary teeth. *B,* Mandibular teeth.

Restorative Techniques for Children

The principles of cavity preparation and restoration with amalgam alloy and composite resin materials for children are similar to those for adults with a few differences attributable to the morphologic differences between primary and permanent teeth. Cavity preparations (Fig. 2–25) are shallower because primary teeth are smaller, and there is no gingival cavosurface bevel because of the slope of the enamel rods. Because preparations are shallower, thick bases are not used and only shallow occlusal anatomy is carved into amalgam restorations.

A minimal number of instruments are

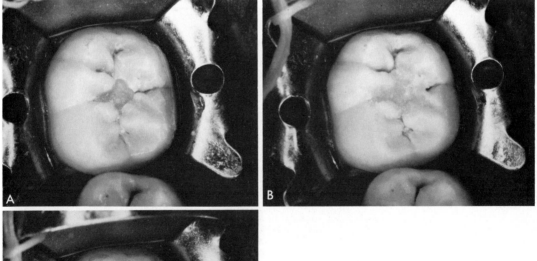

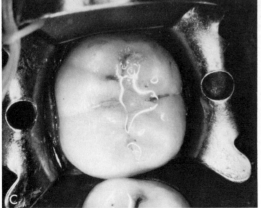

FIGURE 2–26 Conservative cavity preparation of occlusal surface of permanent molar. *A,* Before restoration. *B,* After restoration with composite. *C,* After sealant application.

used: a No. 330 pear-shaped bur for cavity preparation; one double-ended hatchet or chisel to smooth proximal walls; a cleoid/discoid and a Hollenback carver to carve amalgam; and a ball burnisher to burnish amalgam margins after carving. A variety of matrices can be used for Class II restorations, including the T band, the spot-welded matrix, and bands with matrix retainer. Criteria for cavity preparation are listed below.

External Occlusal Outline Form. The tooth structure should be conserved, particularly at the cusp incline. Pits and fissures are removed with a minimal width (1 mm) between cusps and an isthmus width one-third to one-half the intercuspal width.

Internal Occlusal Outline Form. Buccal and lingual walls should converge slightly occlusally with no undermining of marginal ridges. Walls should be relatively smooth, and internal line angles should be rounded.

Depth. Pulpal floor depth should be just past the dentinoenamel junction (1.5 mm from the tooth surface). Axial wall depth should be just past the dentinoenamel junction (1 mm from the proximal tooth surface). Gingival seat depth should be just be-low the contact area as checked with the tip of an explorer.

Proximal Box Extension. The buccal and lingual walls should be extended only so that the tip of an explorer can just barely reach all margins.

Damage to Adjacent Tooth. Care should be observed with interproximal preparation so that the adjacent tooth is not damaged by the bur.

Recently a conservative approach to restoring minimal or moderate occlusal carious lesions in permanent teeth has been advocated. In order to conserve tooth structure the cavity preparation involves only removal of caries and undermined enamel with no extension for prevention (Fig. 2–26). A composite restoration is placed followed by a layer of sealant, so that pits and fissures are sealed and conserved rather than removed for prevention.

When a primary anterior tooth is severely decayed, simple celluloid matrices are insufficient. The tooth is prepared for full crown coverage, and a composite resin is constructed with a fitted celluloid crown matrix and acid-etch technique (Fig. 2–27).

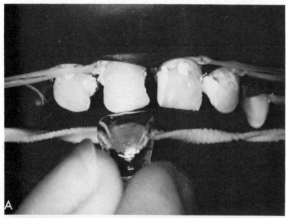
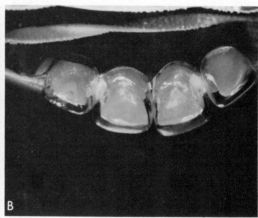
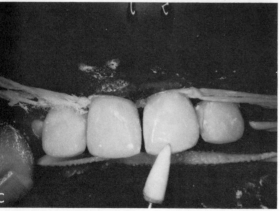

FIGURE 2–27 Restoration of primary incisor. *A,* Selecting correct size crown form. *B,* Matrices trimmed and in place. *C,* Polishing finished restorations. (Courtesy of Dr. Zia Shey, Newark, New Jersey.)

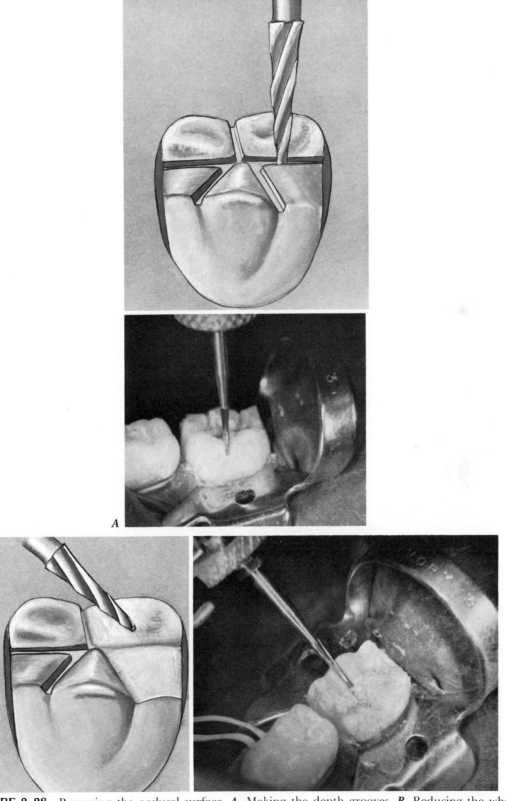

FIGURE 2–28 Preparing the occlusal surface. *A,* Making the depth grooves. *B,* Reducing the whole surface.

Stainless-steel Crown Restoration

The stainless-steel crown is used to restore molar teeth when the tooth is too weak to receive an amalgam restoration. The procedure involves four major tasks: tooth preparation, pulp protection, crown preparation, and crown cementation. It begins with anesthesia and isolation of the tooth with rubber dam and interproximal placement of wedges. The tooth is prepared with a small tapered carbide (No. 169L) or a diamond bur at high speed with water spray as a coolant. Depth cuts are placed 1.0 to 1.5 mm in the occlusal grooves (Fig. 2–28), and then the remaining occlusal surface is uniformly reduced 1.5 mm, roughly maintaining the occlusal outline of the crown.

The proximal surface is reduced with the bur held slightly convergent to the long axis of the crown. The bur is swept buccolingually starting occlusally about 1 mm from the proximal surface and moving gingivally

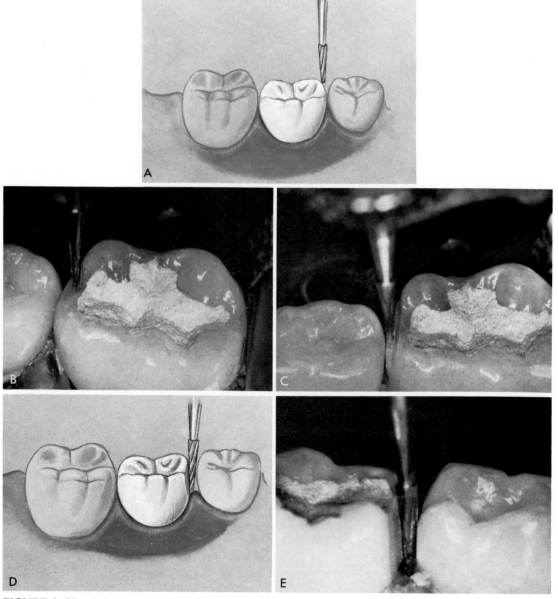

FIGURE 2–29 *A* through *E,* Preparing the proximal surface.

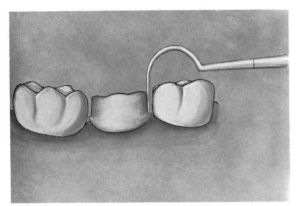

FIGURE 2–30 Checking the cervical margin for any ledging.

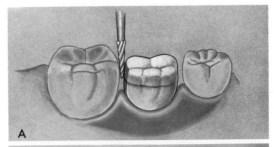

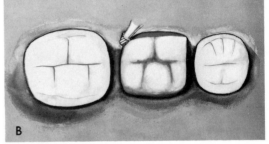

FIGURE 2–32 *A* and *B,* Rounding all line angles.

just past the contact area (Fig. 2–29). The reduction should be relatively uniform, following the tooth contour and extending out to the buccal and lingual line angles. Care should be taken so that a ledge (Fig. 2–30) is not created at the gingival aspect and the adjacent teeth are not damaged. Optionally, the occlusal third of the buccal and lingual surfaces may be reduced slightly (Fig. 2–31). Any excessive cervical bulge may also be reduced; however, some undercut should remain for retention of the crown. All line angles should be rounded, removing any sharp corners that might interfere with seating of the crown (Fig. 2–32). Any remaining caries is removed, and pulp protection or other appropriate pulp therapy is performed.

Preparation of the crown begins with crown selection. Beginning with the middle size, various precontoured crowns are tried until the crown that most closely restores the mesiodistal width of the tooth being restored is selected. Normal spacing (e.g., the primate space) should not be closed. The selected crown is pressed gingivally onto the prepared tooth to establish a preliminary occlusal relationship, and with the tip of a scaler or enamel hatchet, a line is scribed on the crown at the gingival margin. If necessary, the crown is trimmed to 1 mm below the scribed line with crown-and-bridge scissors

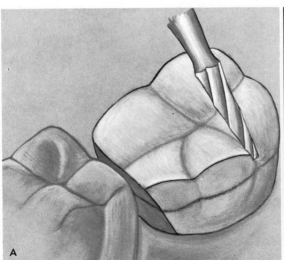

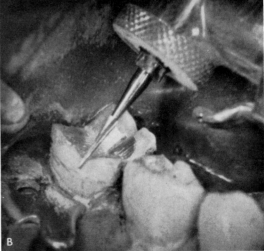

FIGURE 2–31 *A* and *B,* Reducing the buccal and lingual surfaces.

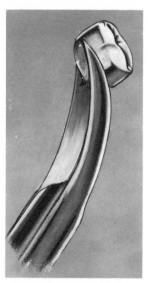

FIGURE 2–33 Cutting the margins with the crown-and-bridge scissors.

(Fig. 2–33), because a crown that is too long will cause gingival irritation or traumatic occlusion. Optionally, the rubber dam is removed to check the occlusion. If necessary, the gingival third of the crown may be contoured with No. 114 contouring pliers placed mainly on the buccal and lingual surfaces, bending the crown slightly inward (Fig. 2–34). Additional contouring of the gingival margin can be performed with the crown-crimping pliers (Unitek No. 800-417) (Fig.

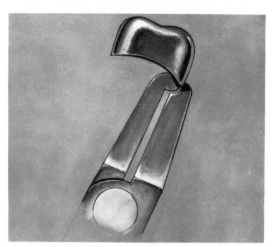

FIGURE 2–35 Contouring the margins of the crown with crown-crimping pliers.

2–35). Occasionally there is insufficient contact with the adjacent tooth, and the proximal surface can be recontoured with the No. 112 ball-and-socket pliers (Fig. 2–36).

The crown is seated on the tooth from the lingual to the buccal aspect for mandibular teeth and in the opposite direction for maxillary teeth. Firm resistance should be encountered when the crown is seated, and it should snap into place (Fig. 2–37). Rarely, the preparation extends beyond the cervical margin of the longest available crown, and banding material may be spot-welded to ex-

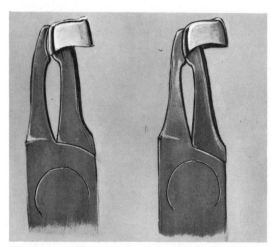

FIGURE 2–34 Contouring the margins of the crown with No. 114 pliers.

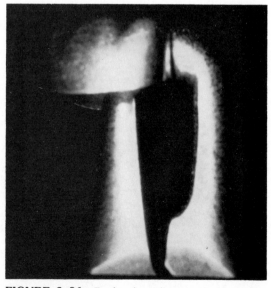

FIGURE 2–36 Reshaping the proximal surface with ball-and-socket pliers.

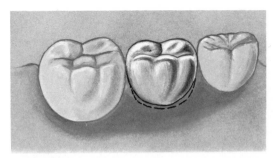

FIGURE 2–37 Crown seated 1 mm below gingival margin.

tend the margin. Those margins of the crown that were cut and contoured should be finished with a heatless stone and polished with a rubber wheel (Fig. 2–38).

The tooth is washed, and, if the rubber dam was removed, the tooth is isolated with cotton rolls, and any required additional pulp protection is placed. A zinc phosphate or polycarbonate cement is mixed according to the manufacturer's instructions and is poured into the crown to contact all crown margins. The crown is seated with firm pressure, and after the occlusion is checked, the patient bites on a wooden tongue blade until the cement sets. Excess cement is removed with explorers and scalers, and dental floss with a small knot is pulled through to clean the interproximal space. Air is then blown into the gingival sulcus to make sure that all excess cement was removed. A prophylaxis cup may be used to shine the crown surface.

Fracture Repair

When an incisor crown is fractured, the broken segment is replaced by a composite resin with the acid-etch technique (Fig. 2–39). The procedure is rather simple and can be performed immediately after the trauma if the time is available. Anesthesia is not required, but rubber dam isolation is beneficial and pulp protection should be placed. The enamel at the fracture edge is beveled slightly with a suitable diamond or carbide flame-shaped bur in order to remove loose enamel rods. Beveling also provides a better edge for and improves the appearance of the restoration. A celluloid or metal corner matrix is cut to fit 2 mm beyond the edge of the enamel preparation. The enamel is prepared in the usual manner (clean, wash, and dry; etch, wash, and dry). Following placement of the bonding agent, the composite is placed according to the manufacturer's instructions. Light-polymerized materials (e.g., Nuvafil) will not set until polymerized by a suitable accompanying light source, whereas the self-polymerizing materials (e.g., Adaptic) will polymerize after mixing. Following polymerization, the matrix is removed and the restoration is polished according to the manufacturer's instructions. A glaze can be added to the surface, improving the initial appearance of the restoration. If marginal discoloration develops after a few years, the surface discolora-

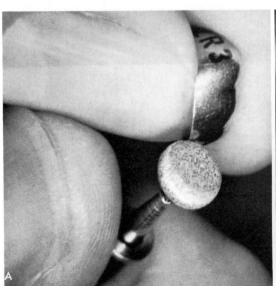
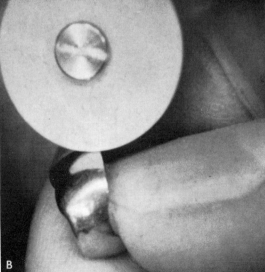

FIGURE 2–38 Finishing the crown margins **A,** with a stone and **B,** with a rubber wheel.

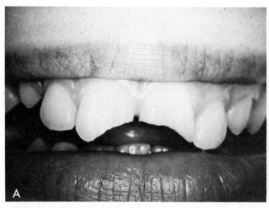
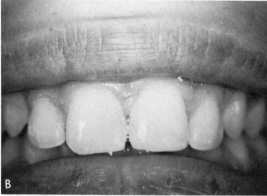

FIGURE 2–39 Restoration of fractured incisor with the acid-technique. *A,* Before repair. *B,* After repair. (Courtesy of Dr. Melvyn Oppenheim, Scarsdale, New York.)

tion can be trimmed and a new layer of composite added.

PULP THERAPY

The fundamental purpose of pulp therapy is to maintain pulp vitality. The dental pulp in young children is highly vascularized, with a great potential for healing following treatment. When dentin is stimulated by thermal, bacterial, chemical, or mechanical irritants, odontoblasts react by forming new reparative dentin. Pulp therapy includes pulp protection, indirect and direct pulp treatment, and formocresol and calcium hydroxide pulpotomy. (The pulpectomy procedure will also be described in this section since it deals with the consequence of pulp death.)

Pulp response to frequently used dental materials differs when the material is placed on dentin or directly on exposed pulp tissue. *Calcium hydroxide* placed on dentin stimulates new reparative dentin formation by the pulp, and it may stimulate sclerosis or hypermineralization of the existing underlying dentin. When placed on exposed pulp tissue, calcium hydroxide initially produces a thin zone of necrosis, followed by bridging with reparative dentin formation. Frequently in primary teeth the new bridge formation is followed by internal resorption or pulp necrosis or both. Pulp calcification also occurs, sometimes obliterating the root canal. *Zinc oxide–eugenol* cement placed on dentin sedates the pulp and allows reparative dentin formation. However, when it is placed directly on exposed pulp tissue, zinc oxide–

eugenol cement causes chronic inflammation and necrosis of pulp tissue.

Many signs and symptoms should be used to diagnose pulp health. When *pain* is present, its characteristics should be determined. A short-lasting, localized, stimulated, sharp type of pain usually indicates an irritation of an otherwise healthy pulp, for example, thermal stimulus of exposed dentinal tubules under a broken restoration. A longer lasting pain indicates pulp inflammation. An unstimulated, long-lasting, generalized, dull pain indicates necrosis of the pulp with periapical involvement. Pain on percussion indicates periapical involvement, although exfoliating primary teeth may also be painful to percussion. The absence of pain does not indicate absence of pulp pathology, and when pulp tissue in primary teeth degenerates, there is frequently no pain present.

Swelling of soft tissue, whether by cellulitis (Fig. 2–40) or parulis formation (Fig. 2–41), usually indicates necrosis and periapical or

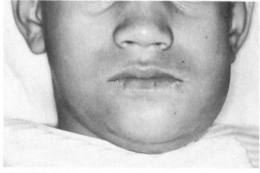

FIGURE 2–40 Cellulitis due to necrotic pulp in a primary molar.

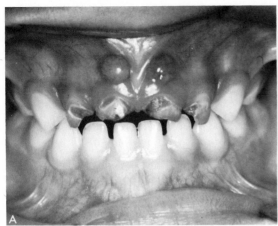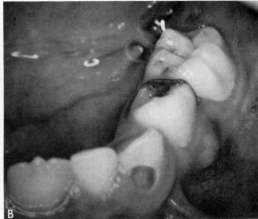

FIGURE 2–41 Parulis due to necrotic pulp. *A,* Primary incisor. *B,* Primary molar.

furcation involvement. The tooth should be examined for *color* changes, which could indicate pulp changes, and *mobility,* which would indicate periapical involvement. *Vitality tests* should be used in doubtful cases, although their results are not reliable in children. *Radiographs* should be carefully examined for evidence of calcification in the pulp chamber, internal or external resorption, and radiolucency in the furcation or apical areas. The periapical view is used to examine the roots (Fig. 2–42), but the bitewing view should be used to examine the proximity to the pulp horns of a deep carious lesion (Fig. 2–43). If available, a radiograph of the antimere should be used to distinguish between pathologic and normal anatomic appearance.

Pulp Protection

Purpose. Pulp protection is performed to protect the dental pulp when the dentinal tubules and odontoblastic processes have been exposed through cavity preparation or traumatic injury.

Indication. Pulp protection is usually indicated whenever dentin is exposed, although in shallow amalgam restorations it is sometimes omitted. Cavity varnish may be used to reduce leakage and to provide protection from chemical stimuli. Calcium hydroxide can provide thermal and chemical protection. Zinc oxide–eugenol provides thermal protection as does zinc phosphate cement placed over a cavity liner.

Procedure. When the decay has not penetrated deeply into the dentin and the cavity

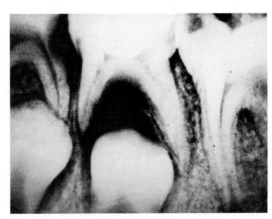

FIGURE 2–42 Radiograph of primary molar with external root resorption due to periapical infection.

FIGURE 2–43 Radiograph of primary molar with furcation involvement.

preparation is shallow (1 to 2 mm into dentin), a thin layer of medicament (varnish or calcium hydroxide) is used. All exposed dentin is covered. If the decay has penetrated deeply into dentin, a thicker layer of calcium hydroxide should be used to provide thermal insulation. Alternatively, a zinc oxide–eugenol or zinc phosphate base could be placed on top of a thin calcium hydroxide liner. *Calcium hydroxide is preferred to zinc oxide–eugenol in deep preparations in the event that a clinically undiagnosed microexposure is present.*

Indirect Pulp Treatment

Purpose. Indirect pulp treatment is used to treat primary and permanent teeth when a carious lesion has penetrated so deeply that the pulp will probably be exposed if all caries is removed. The treatment involves the removal of superficial carious dentin and placement of a medicament over the residual caries, allowing the pulp to form reparative dentin between the lesion and the pulp. This is not the "gross caries removal" or "excavate and sedate" procedure used for initial caries control when multiple extensive carious lesions are present. Rather, it is the meticulous removal of all caries except that which would cause pulp exposure. The carious dentin removed is decalcified, soft, infected, and nonvital. The remaining leathery dentin is the transitional zone of the lesion. It is decalcified but still vital, and following treatment it may become remineralized or sclerotic.

Indications and Contraindications. Indirect pulp treatment is used only for lesions that radiographically approximate the pulp with the possibility of pulpal exposure if all caries is removed. The tooth should otherwise appear normal radiographically with a normal lamina dura, a normal periodontal membrane space, and no furcation or apical radiolucency. The tooth should not be mobile, and the gingival tissue approximating the tooth should appear healthy. Although a mild, intermittent pain might be stimulated when eating, prolonged or unstimulated pain should not be present, and the tooth should not be sensitive to percussion.

The procedure is contraindicated if there are any signs or symptoms of advanced pulpal pathology, such as prolonged pain, tooth mobility, sensitivity to percussion, negative response to vitality tests, a parulis on the gingiva, or radiographic radiolucency adjacent to the tooth roots. Indirect pulp treatment is also contraindicated if the carious lesion radiographically appears to definitely penetrate the pulp, in which case a pulpotomy would be indicated.

Procedure. Following local anesthesia and rubber dam application, a typical cavity preparation is performed, with the exception of deep caries removal. Although indirect pulp treatment is not a sterile procedure, surgically clean techniques should be used to avoid additional bacterial contamination of the pulp. The rubber dam should be wiped with a disinfectant and sterile instruments should be used. Caries removal is carefully accomplished with a slowly rotating large round bur (No. 4 or No. 6) or a large spoon excavator. If the excavator is used, a gentle scraping rather than a digging motion must be employed to prevent pulp exposure. The soft, mushy caries is removed until the firmer leathery dentin is encountered, and 1 mm of carious dentin is left over the pulp. If firm dentin is not present, indirect pulp treatment cannot be performed. Only caries that overlies the pulp should be left. Caries at the dentinoenamel junction should be removed.

The dentin is then covered with a 1-mm layer of radiopaque calcium hydroxide. Although other medicaments could be used (e.g., zinc oxide–eugenol), calcium hydroxide is preferred in the event that a minute, clinically undetected pulp exposure is present. A restoration of choice is then placed, sealing the cavity. Some practitioners prefer to re-enter the area at some later time to determine if active caries remains; however, this re-entry is not usually performed.

Treatment Results. Prognosis is excellent with proper diagnosis and treatment. When indirect pulp treatment fails, it is usually due to inadequate caries removal or a faulty restoration with excessive leakage. When the treatment is successful, the residual carious dentin becomes sterile, remineralized reparative dentin forms, and the pulp remains vital.

Direct Pulp Treatment

Purpose. Direct pulp treatment is used to treat pinpoint exposures of the pulp caused by mechanical exposure in primary or permanent teeth, or carious exposure in permanent teeth. The prognosis following direct treatment is usually not as good as more radical forms of treatment, and, consequently, it is performed only when all factors are ideal.

Indications and Contraindications. Direct pulp treatment should be performed only when the exposure is mechanical because of trauma, minute in size, relatively clean, and in a tooth free of caries. It can be attempted for small carious exposures in permanent teeth in an attempt to conserve pulp vitality. The tooth should be asymptomatic with a healthy pulp. Any sign of pulp pathology contraindicates direct pulp treatment as does a larger or a contaminated exposure of the pulp. Carious exposures of primary teeth are treated more radically because of better results with the pulpotomy procedure.

Procedure. The tooth should be isolated properly, and, if necessary, the exposure site should be washed gently and dried with a sterile cotton pellet. A few layers of hard-setting, radiopaque calcium hydroxide should be applied to the exposure site and the surrounding dentin, forming a 1-mm base covering the exposure. Optionally, an additional zinc phosphate base can be added followed by appropriate final restoration of the tooth.

Treatment Result. If the treatment succeeds, a dentinal bridge forms at the exposure site, and the pulp remains vital and healthy. The apex of a developing tooth will close in a normal manner. If the treatment fails, either bridging did not occur, or following bridging, internal resorption or pulp necrosis or both occurred. In primary teeth, internal resorption frequently occurs when calcium hydroxide is applied directly on the pulp tissue (Fig. 2–44).

Pulpotomy

Purpose. A pulpotomy is the surgical excision of diseased tissue from the pulp chamber, leaving healthier tissue in the root canals, upon which is placed an appropriate medicament. The pulpotomy is based on the premise that the coronal pulp is too diseased to respond favorably to more conservative pulp treatment and that because of its distance from the site of the infection the pulp tissue in the canal is less diseased and can remain vital following treatment.

There are two types of pulpotomies categorized according to the medicament used. The formocresol pulpotomy is used in primary teeth with large mechanical or carious exposures of a vital pulp. The calcium hydroxide pulpotomy is used in immature permanent teeth with large exposure of the pulp due to trauma. In both types of pulpotomy the tissue remaining in the root canals must be vital for the procedure to succeed.

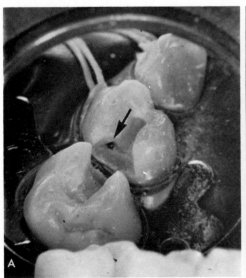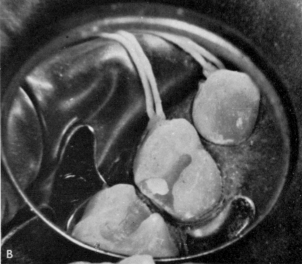

FIGURE 2–44 Mechanical exposure in axial-gingival line angle. *A* and *B*, Before and after direct pulp treatment with calcium hydroxide.

Formocresol Pulpotomy

Indications and Contraindications. The formocresol pulpotomy is usually performed on primary teeth with infected vital pulps. Radiographically a normal lamina dura and a normal periodontal membrane space should be evident with no radiolucency adjacent to the tooth roots and no internal resorption in the pulp canals. A large carious lesion, probably exposing the pulp, will be evident in the radiograph. Clinically, the tooth should be relatively asymptomatic with only infrequent (if any) episodes of unstimulated pain. Mobility should not be present and the soft tissues should appear healthy. Any sign or symptom of complete pulp necrosis contraindicates the pulpotomy procedure. Tooth mobility, the presence of a parulis, negative response to vitality tests, prolonged unstimulated pain, or pain on percussion all indicate pulp necrosis with furcation or periapical involvement. Although the pulpotomy procedure may eliminate acute symptoms with a nonvital pulp, it should not be used as a final treatment, because chronic infection will result.

Procedure. Following local anesthesia and rubber dam application, the stainless-steel crown preparation is completed with the exception of deep caries removal. (Alternatively, the pulpotomy could be completed before the crown preparation.) Although the pulpotomy is not a sterile procedure, surgically clean techniques should be used to avoid additional bacterial contamination of the pulp. The rubber dam should be wiped with a disinfectant and sterile instruments should be used. With a slowly rotating large bur (No. 4 or No. 6), the caries is removed, except for the last amount, which would expose the pulp. Then, with a high-speed fissure or pear-shaped bur, the enamel and dentin overlying but not penetrating the roof of the pulp chamber are removed. Finally, with a fresh sterile bur, the roof of the pulp chamber is removed by first penetrating the chamber in the area of a pulp horn and then moving the bur laterally to the other pulp horns, encircling the pulpal roof so that the remaining island of dentin may be lifted out of the cavity with college pliers. Overhanging ledges are removed with the bur, and care should be taken so that the base of the chamber is not perforated.

The coronal pulp is excised with a large sharp spoon excavator or a large round bur down to the level of the entrance into the pulp canals. Residual tags of tissue are excised rather than pulled from the canals. The chamber is filled with warm water to remove any debris, and a dry cotton pellet is used to clean and dry the chamber. A moist pellet placed over the stump with slight pressure will usually control the hemorrhage after a few minutes. If the hemorrhage persists, pulp tissue tags may remain in the chamber and should be removed. The chamber should be inspected to ensure that all canals are exposed, that no tissue tags are remaining, and that the chamber floor has not been perforated. A cotton pellet moistened with formocresol is placed into the pulp chamber with slight pressure applied to the pulp stumps; it should not have excessive formocresol flowing out of the cavity onto the gingiva. The pellet is left in place for 5 minutes, after which the pulp stumps,

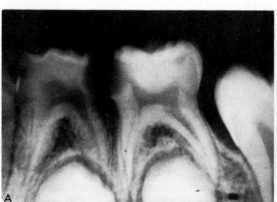 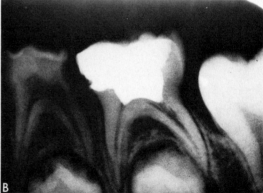

FIGURE 2–45 Radiograph of primary molar in which a formocresol pulpotomy is indicated. **A,** Before treatment. **B,** After treatment.

appearing dark and clotted, are covered with 2 to 3 mm of a thick mix of zinc oxide–eugenol cement containing eugenol and formocresol at a ratio of 1:1. (Some practitioners use diluted formocresol for the 5-minute application and do not add any formocresol to the zinc oxide–eugenol cement.) A stainless-steel crown is usually placed following the pulpotomy procedure (Fig. 2–45).

Treatment Result. Histologic examination of a formocresol pulpotomized pulp demonstrates three zones: (1) a zone of "fixed" tissue immediately underlying the cement; (2) a broad zone of coagulation necrosis in the middle third of the tooth, and (3) a zone of vital pulp or vital granulation tissue at the apex of the root. The ingrowth of granulation tissue occurs in approximately 7 weeks.

Treatment is very successful (80 to 95 per cent depending on whether criteria are histologic, radiographic, or clinical). The treated tooth is usually asymptomatic and should be examined clinically every 6 months and radiographically each year. When treatment fails, it is usually because the technique was used on a nonvital pulp. The tooth might become mobile, and a parulis or fistula might develop. If the treatment fails, a pulpectomy should be performed or the tooth should be extracted. A chronically infected primary tooth should not be retained as it might damage the permanent successor.

Calcium Hydroxide Pulpotomy

Indications and Contraindications. The calcium hydroxide pulpotomy is performed on young permanent teeth with incompletely formed apices in which a vital pulp is exposed by trauma or caries. It is an interim treatment to allow apical closure, after which a complete pulpectomy may be performed. Radiographically and clinically the pulp should appear healthy, and any signs or symptoms of pulp necrosis contraindicate the pulpotomy procedure.

Purpose. The procedure is similar to the formocresol pulpotomy described above, except that the dried pulp stumps are covered with a 1 mm–thick layer of radiopaque calcium hydroxide instead of formocresol. The calcium hydroxide is then covered with a layer of cement (zinc oxide–eugenol or zinc phosphate), and the tooth is restored.

Treatment Result. The calcium hydroxide initially produces a surface zone of ne-

crosis followed by reparative dentin formation bridging the canal openings. Beneath the dentinal bridge the pulp remains vital and healthy. Spontaneous calcification in the root canals frequently occurs following calcium hydroxide pulpotomy, and canal obliteration may occur. For this reason many practitioners prefer to perform a complete pulpectomy once the root apex has fully developed. In primary teeth, internal resorption frequently develops following calcium hydroxide pulpotomy. Consequently, formocresol is routinely used instead of calcium hydroxide for pulpotomy in primary teeth.

Pulpectomy

Purpose. Whenever the pulp is in such an advanced state of degeneration that a pulpotomy will not be successful, or when the pulp is completely necrotic, a pulpectomy must be performed. The total contents of the pulp canal are removed, and the canal is cleansed and then sealed appropriately. Pulpectomy in primary molars has long been advocated (Fig. 2–46); however, difficulties are present. The canals in primary molars, particularly in children over 5 years of age, are thin and tortuous. There are numerous accessory canals, and the root apex usually ends with a broad, elongated opening. Consequently, it is difficult to manipulate the instruments used to seal the canals. The apex is also in close proximity to the developing permanent tooth bud, presenting a potential for permanent damage from instruments or materials used in the primary molar canal. Nevertheless, if the pulpectomy is carefully performed, a successful result can be obtained.

Indications and Contraindications. The pulpectomy procedure is performed in primary teeth when signs or symptoms indicate pulp necrosis. However, this indication is related to other factors, such as the strategic importance of the tooth, the length of time the tooth will remain in the mouth, the restorability of the crown, the condition of the periapical tissues, and the amount of root remaining. Excessive tooth mobility, a large furcation or periapical involvement, internal root resorption, and external resorption leaving less than two thirds of the root remaining are all contraindications to pulpectomy procedures for primary teeth. In addition, the procedure is contraindicated in children with certain systemic diseases or ab-

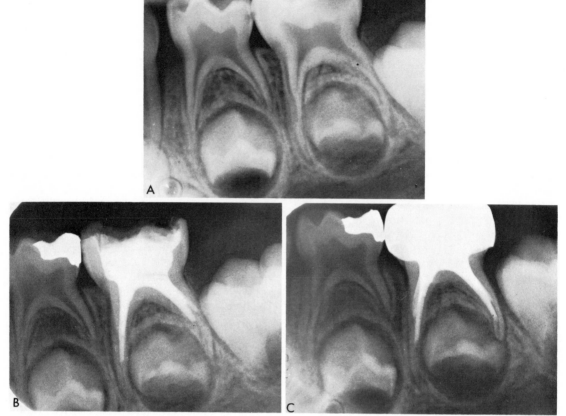

FIGURE 2–46 Radiograph of primary molar in which pulpectomy was performed. *A,* Before treatment. *B,* After treatment. *C,* After stainless-steel crown placement.

normal conditions; for example, in children with cardiac defects, in whom chronic infection would create a particular risk.

Procedure. The pulpectomy procedure for primary teeth is similar to that for permanent teeth except that it is usually performed in one appointment, the degree of biomechanical cleansing is less, and the canal is sealed with a resorbable paste. Following local anesthesia and rubber dam isolation, the pulp chamber is opened and cleansed in a manner similar to the pulpotomy procedure.

Any remaining pulp tissue is removed from the canals with a small barbed broach. The canals are then irrigated with sodium hypochlorite, and after canal length has been determined radiographically, the canals are instrumented to three or four sizes larger than the first file reaching the apex. Following biomechanical cleansing, the canals are dried and sealed with a creamy mix of zinc oxide–eugenol cement or other re-

sorbable root canal sealer to approximately 1 mm short of the apex. The cement is placed with a pressure syringe (Pulpdent Corporation of America Brookline, Mass.) or a long amalgam condenser. If the condenser is used, the paste can be pushed farther into the canals by pushing on a cotton pellet placed in the pulp chamber. Care must be taken not to overfill the canal. If the canal is underfilled, additional cement can be added. However, if it is overfilled, the cement pushed into the developing permanent tooth bud may damage it.

If the patient presents with acute symptoms, a two-appointment procedure should be used. Formocresol medicament should be sealed in the pulp chamber for 3 to 7 days in order to allow acute symptoms to subside. When there is no pain or prolonged drainage, the canals can be sealed. The tooth is then appropriately restored. Nonvital primary molars are usually restored with a stainless-steel crown.

Treatment Results. If all canals are successfully instrumented and sealed, the tooth should remain asymptomatic until exfoliation, which might occur slightly earlier than normal. The tooth should be examined clinically every 6 months and radiographically each year for signs of failure, which include pain, mobility, gingival swelling, furcation or periapical radiolucency, or premature root resorption.

Apexification

Purpose. Apexification is a procedure used to promote continued root development in immature permanent teeth with nonvital pulps (Fig. 2–47).

Indication. Whenever immature permanent teeth with incompletely formed apices become nonvital, apexification should be attempted prior to complete seal of the root canal.

Procedure. The canal is opened and instrumented in a manner similar to routine endodontic treatment except that files are instrumented 1 mm short of the apex. After the canal has been cleansed and dried, a mixture of calcium hydroxide and sterile distilled water, to which barium sulfate is added for increased radiopacity, is placed into the canal. The pressure syringe is used with the largest needle that reaches the root apex to fill the canal. Care should be taken not to overfill the root apex.

At 6 and 12 months, the patient is recalled and a radiograph is taken. If there is no evidence of continued root formation after 1 year, the cleansing and calcium hydroxide seal procedure is repeated. However, in the majority of cases, some evidence of root closure with cementumlike tissue will be evident at 6 months. Once root closure begins, the canal is instrumented carefully so as not to disturb the root apex and sealed with gutta percha in the usual manner.

Treatment Results. Following routine gutta percha seal, the tooth has an excellent prognosis, similar to that of teeth treated with regular endodontic therapy.

EXODONTICS

A common misconception held by practitioners who do not regularly treat children is that extracting primary teeth is a difficult procedure and is traumatic to the child. However, the procedure is frequently simpler than routine restorative treatment, and, when it is explained properly, the child accepts it as such. The child is not told, "I'm going to pull out your tooth, so hang on!" but rather, "Your tooth has a big hole and is full of germs, and we have to move it out of the way so it doesn't harm your new tooth. It's a strong tooth and I have to push on it just like this to make it loose." (The dentist demonstrates by pushing on the child's shoulder.) "You feel me pushing, but it doesn't hurt; it's just pushing. You'll feel the

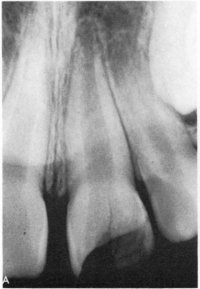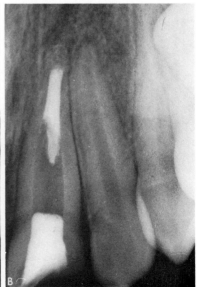

FIGURE 2–47 Apexification of traumatized incisor. *A* and *B*, Before and after treatment. (Courtesy of Dr. Steven Wechsler, Newark, New Jersey.)

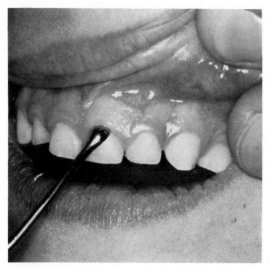

FIGURE 2–48 Using a surgical spoon to sever gingival attachment.

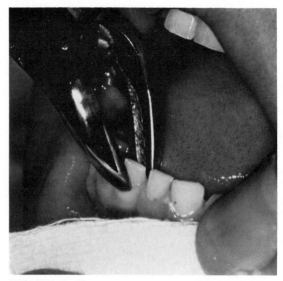

FIGURE 2–50 Placement of forceps to remove mandibular anterior primary tooth.

same with your tooth. It won't hurt because it's sleeping, but you'll feel lots of pushing. Then you can help me. After I push on your tooth, you can help me move your tooth out of the way. Now here is my pusher." (The dentist holds the forceps beaks and shows the child the handle of the instrument, then engages the tooth and manipulates it slightly.) "Do you feel me pushing?" (The dentist then luxates the tooth, and when it is ready

to be removed from the mouth, invites the child's assistance.) "Okay, we are finished pushing. Now you can help me move the tooth out of the way. Put your hand on my arm, and now help me move the tooth." In a smooth manner the dentist extracts the tooth. The child feels pressure initially, but then almost nothing as the tooth is removed. Most importantly, the child is made to feel a participant in the procedure. The child

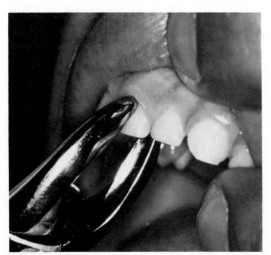

FIGURE 2–49 Placement of forceps to remove maxillary anterior primary tooth.

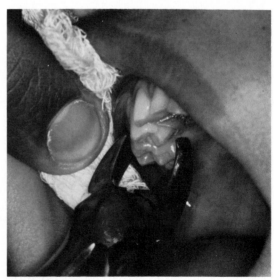

FIGURE 2–51 Placement of forceps to remove maxillary primary molars.

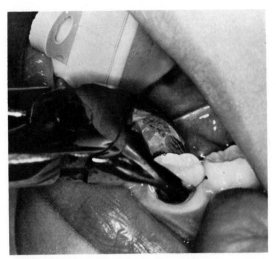

FIGURE 2–52 Placement of forceps to remove mandibular primary molars.

helps the dentist remove a tooth; thus, the connotation of the dentist pulling a tooth from a helpless child is not present.

The extraction procedure is performed with little trauma to the patient. It presumes profound anesthesia has first been achieved. The gingival attachment is severed with a surgical spoon excavator or periosteal elevator (Fig. 2–48). The forceps are then engaged at the neck of the tooth. Anterior teeth are pushed apically, slightly rotated mesially and distally, breaking the periodontal ligament, and then removed (Figs. 2–49 and 2–50). Molar teeth are pushed apically, and then slightly buccally and lingually (Figs. 2–51 and 2–52). The force is slowly increased in both directions, with no jerking movements, until the tooth is loosened, after which it can be removed along the path of least resistance. When two adjacent molars are extracted, an interproximal suture is used occasionally.

Primary teeth of older children usually have partially resorbed roots, and it is quite common for these to fracture. If the root tips are small and difficult to locate, it is best to allow them to resorb rather than risk injuring the developing permanent tooth. The parent should be informed of that decision.

Most bleeding should have stopped before the child is dismissed; this is accomplished by having the child bite on a 2×2 inch square of gauze. Extra gauze squares are provided in case of continued bleeding, and the child is cautioned not to eat anything hard or too hot during the day. Healing is usually uneventful.

SPACE MAINTENANCE

Whenever a primary tooth is lost prematurely, space maintenance procedures should be considered. The various types of space maintainers, as well as their indication for use, appear in Chapter 7, Orthodontics in General Practice.

TRAUMATIC INJURIES

Injuries with broken or displaced teeth produce great anxiety. Both parent and child experience feelings of guilt because of an accident that might have been prevented. Both are concerned about the child's appearance, and it is important for the dentist to allay this anxiety.

Incidence

The incidence of injuries to anterior teeth is usually reported to be between 5 per cent and 10 per cent, although a few studies have suggested a higher incidence. Males experience more injuries than females, and children with protruding incisors have the highest risk of injury. Injuries in the primary dentition occur most frequently around the age of 2 years when children begin to walk. Injuries in the permanent dentition occur in children most frequently between 6 and 12 years of age. Blows to teeth with low-mass objects at high velocity tend to fracture teeth. Blows to teeth with high-mass objects at low velocity tend to produce displacement of teeth rather than fracture.

Diagnosis

Before any treatment is rendered, a thorough history and careful examination should be conducted to establish a correct diagnosis.

History. A medical history should be taken in order to evaluate the health status of the patient. For example, significant medical problems might affect treatment in a child requiring antibiotic coverage for a cardiac defect. In order to determine the type and prognosis of treatment, it is important to determine how, when, and where the accident occurred. Previous injuries to the mouth and teeth may affect prognosis of treatment. Subjective complaints of pain, sensitivity to heat and cold, or soreness to touch also determine the type and prognosis of treatment.

Examination. The involved tooth and the adjacent hard and soft tissues should be carefully *examined* to determine the type and extent of injury. It is not infrequent for tooth fragments or debris to become embedded in soft tissues and for adjacent or opposing teeth to sustain injury that eludes notice. The injured and neighboring teeth should be carefully *manipulated* to determine degree of mobility and any sensitivity to light pressure indicating periodontal trauma and root fracture or both. *Percussion* of the tooth with the mirror handle may also demonstrate periodontal trauma. When the sound of a percussed injured tooth is duller than that of neighboring teeth, ankylosis of the root may have occurred. The crown should be *transilluminated* by reflecting light through it from the lingual aspect to observe subtle pulp changes or enamel cracks. *Vitality* tests should be used as an aid to diagnosis, although they are not completely reliable. Frequently an injured tooth gives false readings as do healthy primary or young permanent teeth. Uninjured adjacent teeth should be used for control responses. *Radiographic examination* is performed in order to reveal root fracture, amount of root development, and injury to supporting structures.

Treatment of Permanent Teeth

Children who have received deep contaminated soft tissue injuries require protection against tetanus. A tetanus booster should be administered if it has been more than 5 years since the previous booster.

Concussion. A tooth receiving a concussion may or may not sustain pulp death. If the tooth remains vital, no treatment is required. If it is nonvital, routine pulpectomy is performed with apexification when there are incompletely formed roots. Care must be taken when labeling a tooth nonvital, and definite signs or symptoms should be present. If the only sign is a negative response to vitality tests, endodontic treatment should be delayed, because concussed teeth frequently give false negative vitality readings for months following injury.

Coronal Fracture. Treatment of coronal fracture depends on how much of the crown is lost and entails (1) a consideration of pulp protection by covering exposed dentinal tubules, and (2) restoration of function and appearance by replacing the missing fragment. Of immediate concern is protection of exposed dentin. Restoration of appearance can be performed at the same visit if time permits and if the patient is amenable to treatment. Otherwise, any medicament placed is protected with a layer of bonded composite and the restoration is performed at a more suitable time. If the fracture involves enamel only, there is no dentin to be protected and the incisal edge can be either slightly reshaped or repaired with the acid-etch technique. When dentin is exposed by fracture, the tooth is usually hypersensitive to thermal changes or air applied to the fractured edge. After the area has been carefully cleansed, a layer of radiopaque calcium hydroxide is applied to all exposed dentin and the missing fragment is restored with the acid-etch technique. If the pulp is exposed by the fracture, it is important to determine the time of injury and the size of exposure. Small pinpoint exposures examined within a few hours after injury can be treated by direct pulp therapy with a mix of radiopaque calcium hydroxide. If the exposure is large, relatively dirty, or long standing, a more radical type of treatment is indicated.

If the apex is closed, complete pulpectomy is performed. However, with an open apex, only a partial pulpectomy or a pulpotomy is performed. The tooth can then be restored with the acid-etch technique or full-crown coverage. If the complete crown is fractured, a suitable crown with a post and core will have to be constructed following endodontic treatment.

Root Fracture. The location of the root fracture usually determines the prognosis of treatment; apical fractures have a good prognosis, whereas cervical fractures have a poor prognosis. If excessive mobility is present, the tooth should be splinted for approximately 6 to 8 weeks. Many types of splints are available (Fig. 2–53), but perhaps the easiest to fabricate consists of a piece of slightly curved 0.030 stainless steel wire bonded with the acid-etch technique to the mobile tooth and two abutment teeth. Healing will occur with dentin, cementum, connective tissue, or bone. Granulation tissue develops between the fractured segments

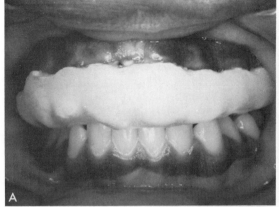

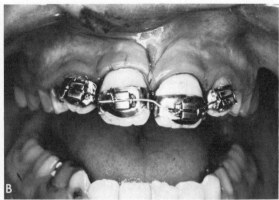

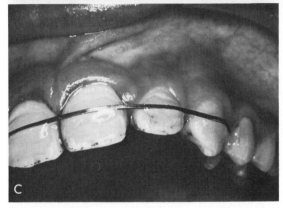

FIGURE 2–53 Types of splints for anterior teeth. **A,** Acrylic splint. **B,** Orthodontic bands and brackets. **C,** Bonded stainless steel wire.

when infection occurs in the pulp chamber and apicoectomy is indicated. When no mobility is present, no treatment is required. The tooth, however, should be examined at regular 6-month intervals to determine if pulp vitality is maintained.

Displacement. Teeth displaced laterally or labiolingually or extruded should be repositioned and splinted for approximately 3 weeks. Intruded teeth should be allowed to re-erupt. It is not possible to predict if the pulp will remain vital, although the prognosis is better when the apex is incompletely formed and the displacement is small. Consequently, it is important to re-examine the tooth at regular 6-month intervals to determine if endodontic treatment will be required. Occasionally, displaced teeth become ankylosed owing to damage of the periodontal ligament. Ankylosis becomes a problem for immature teeth as eruption is stopped, and, if that occurs, the crown may have to be lengthened by build-up of the incisal edge. However, if a completely intruded tooth becomes ankylosed, it will probably have to be extracted.

Avulsion. Teeth that are avulsed create an emergency situation; treatment must be performed immediately. The longer the tooth remains out of the mouth, the poorer is the prognosis. Teeth replanted in less than an hour after avulsion have a relatively good prognosis.

When the dentist is called for treatment, the parent should be advised to come immediately. If the root is not fractured and if the parent is able to do so, the tooth should be placed back into the socket with the child biting on a handkerchief for the trip to the dentist. If the tooth cannot be replaced, it should be kept moist in the child's expectorated saliva.

The child is examined to determine if other injuries are present, if the alveolus is fractured, and if the root is fractured. Rarely, a tooth is replaced a few minutes after injury with no endodontic treatment performed. However, if the tooth was not replaced, it is carefully washed with warm water with great care not to further damage the periodontal ligament. The clot in the socket is carefully curetted, and the tooth is replaced and splinted for 3 weeks. Local anesthesia is usually unnecessary if only a short time has elapsed since injury. One to 2 weeks following replantation, the pulp

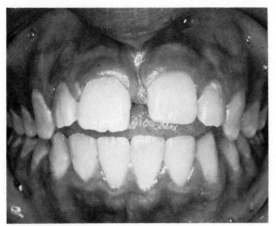

FIGURE 2–54 Replanted avulsed maxillary left central incisor that became ankylosed, preventing further eruption, while adjacent teeth continued to erupt.

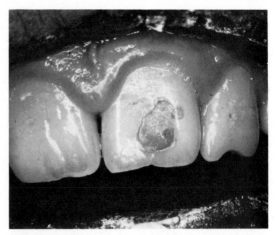

FIGURE 2–56 Enamel defect in permanent incisor caused by trauma to primary tooth.

chamber should be opened and endodontic treatment performed. If the apex is incompletely formed, apexification techniques are used. If the patient is not seen for many hours after avulsion, the pulpectomy can be performed and the canal sealed with a silver point prior to replantation. The prognosis is not good, and this procedure is performed only in the developing dentition in order to delay a prosthetic replacement.

Replanted teeth become reattached with a vital periodontal ligament or become ankylosed with no periodontal ligament (Fig. 2–

54). Anklosed teeth eventually experience external resorption (Fig. 2–55) and are lost within 1 to 2 years because of lack of sufficient root attachment. Occasionally, replaced teeth become infected soon after replacement and must be removed.

If the tooth was relatively dirty prior to replantation and if the child has not had a tetanus booster within 5 years, the child should be referred for a tetanus booster injection.

Treatment of Primary Teeth

Treatment of traumatized primary teeth is similar to treatment of permanent teeth. Major considerations are the age of the child, the length of time until normal exfoliation, and the underlying developing tooth (Fig. 2–56). Avulsed teeth are usually not replanted, and extremely mobile teeth might be extracted rather than retained. Teeth severely intruded with resulting impingement on the developing permanent tooth bud should be extracted.

Primary teeth that become ankylosed

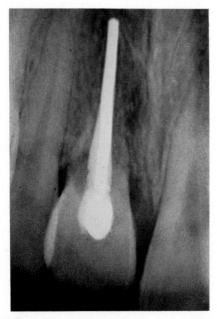

FIGURE 2–55 Radiograph of replanted tooth with external root resorption.

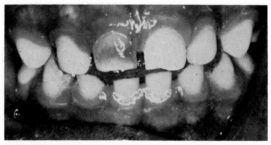

FIGURE 2–57 Discoloration of primary tooth due to trauma.

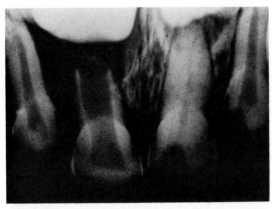

FIGURE 2–58 Radiograph of maxillary primary incisors following trauma. Left incisor—obliteration of pulp canal and chamber. Right incisor—wide pulp canal due to necrotic pulp preventing secondary dental formation; periapical involvement is seen.

should be extracted so that they will not interfere with the normal eruption of the permanent successor.

Concussed teeth usually undergo a change in color, becoming gray, dark brown, yellow, or pink (Fig. 2–57). The gray appearance often indicates a nonvital tooth that should be observed closely for any other signs or symptoms of necrosis (Fig. 2–58). A dark red or brown color usually develops following brief pulp hemorrhage with leakage of blood pigments into the pulp chamber. The pulp may or may not remain vital. A yellow color indicates that reparative dentin has filled the pulp chamber. Vitality is frequently maintained; however, if the pulp becomes nonvital, extraction is necessary. Occasionally, traumatized primary teeth become pink owing to internal resorption in the crown. If the resorption perforates the root, extraction is indicated.

Prevention

Children participating in active sports should be fitted with a custom-made mouthguard. The mouthguard is easily made with an Omnivac unit from a sheet of soft vinyl on a model of the patient's upper arch. In many sports leagues, mouthguards are mandatory. When they are not, dentists should encourage their use to prevent frequent dental injury.

TREATMENT OF THE HANDICAPPED

Perhaps the most neglected group requiring dental care in the population are the handicapped, in particular those individuals who because of severe physical or mental disability often appear and act differently; examples include the child with cerebral palsy who exhibits spastic, uncontrolled movements, the child with Down's syndrome facial features, and the retarded adult with the mental age of a child. Because of a lack of familiarity with them, many dentists will avoid or refuse to treat such persons. Also, because of the complexity of problems with which a handicapped person must deal, dental care tends to receive very low priority and consequently is neglected.

The handicapped sometimes present with physical and behavioral problems. Nevertheless, a practitioner with a caring attitude and a slightly modified approach will be able to treat most handicapped individuals and derive much satisfaction from doing so. The nature of the treatment will depend on the type of handicap; the actual dental care is little different from that performed for normal individuals. However, because dental care receives such a low priority, it is even more important to emphasize and practice preventive techniques. Some handicapped persons may require modification of routine medication, whereas others may require antibiotic premedication; consequently, it is advisable to consult with the patient's attending physician prior to the initiation of treatment. Most handicapped patients can be managed with patience and the tell, show, and do technique. This is particularly useful with the blind or the deaf patient. Nitrous oxide conscious sedation is very beneficial for the fearful, and oral premedication may also be advantageous. Some individuals may require treatment under general anesthesia, and these patients should be referred to the appropriate specialist.

QUESTIONS

1. What is the "tell, show, and do" technique?
2. Should the nose be covered in the hand over mouth exercise (HOME) to control child behavior?

3. What agents are used to premedicate a child for dental treatment? What dosages are recommended?

4. What radiographs should be taken at the first complete clinical examination of a child 5 years of age?

5. What recommendations should be made for toothbrushing in a 3-year-old child?

6. What technique is used to anesthetize the first permanent molar in a 10-year-old child?

7. How are palatal tissues anesthetized in a young, apprehensive child?

8. How many teeth should be isolated routinely when rubber dam is applied?

9. In a routine class II amalgam cavity preparation in a primary molar, what determines the extension of the proximal box buccolingually? gingivally? pulpally?

10. When a primary tooth is prepared for a stainless-steel crown, should all of the cervical bulge be reduced so that the crown could more easily fit the tooth?

11. What tooth preparation is performed when a fractured incisor is restored with the acid-etch technique?

12. What are the indications for indirect pulp treatment?

13. What treatment should be performed on a primary molar when a parulis is present?

14. Should a formocresol pulpotomy be performed in a primary molar with furcation involvement? Why (or why not)?

15. When and how is the apexification procedure performed?

16. In what direction should the forceps be moved when a primary tooth is loosened in its socket?

17. Of what significance is a negative response to the electric pulp test when a tooth was injured 1 month previously?

18. What treatment should be performed when a permanent (or primary) tooth is intruded beneath the gingiva?

19. How is a mobile tooth splinted?

20. What treatment should be performed when a primary incisor becomes yellowish after trauma?

See answers in Appendix.

REFERENCES

1. Andreason, J. O.: Traumatic Injuries to the Teeth. St. Louis, C. V. Mosby Co., 1972.
2. Braham, R. L., and Morris, M. E.: Textbook of Pediatric Dentistry. Baltimore, Williams & Wilkins Co., 1980.
3. Castaldi, C. R., and Brass, G. A.: Dentistry for the Adolescent. Philadelphia, W. B. Saunders Co., 1980.
4. Dixter, C., Langlais, R. P., and Lichty, S. G.: Exercises in Dental Radiology—Vol. 3: Pediatric Radiographic Interpretation. Philadelphia, W. B. Saunders Co., 1980.
5. Davis, J. M., Law, D. B., and Lewis, T. M.: An Atlas of Pedodontics, 2nd ed. Philadelphia, W. B. Saunders Co., 1981.
6. Finn, S. B.: Clinical Pedodontics, 4th ed. Philadelphia, W. B. Saunders Co., 1973.
7. Forrester, D. J., Wagner, M. L., and Fleming, J.: Pediatric Dental Medicine. Philadelphia, Lea & Febiger, 1981.
7a. Frankl S. N., Shiere, F. R., and Fogels, H. R.: Should the parent remain with the child in the dental operatory? J. Dent. Child. *29*:150–163, 1962.
8. McDonald, R. E., and Avery, D.: Dentistry for the Child and Adolescent, 3rd ed. St. Louis, C. V. Mosby Co., 1978.
9. Nowak, A. J.: Dentistry for the Handicapped Patient. St. Louis, C. V. Mosby Co., 1976.
10. Rapp, R., and Winter, G. G.: Color Atlas of Clinical Conditions in Pedodontics. Chicago, Year Book Medical Publishers, 1979.
11. Ripa, L. W., and Barenie, J. T.: Management of Dental Behavior in Children. Littleton, PSG Publishing Co., 1979.
12. Snawder, K. D.: Handbook of Clinical Pedodontics. St. Louis, C. V. Mosby Co., 1980.
13. Starkey, P.: Teaching manual for The Management of Child Behavior in the Dental Office (a teaching videotape). Indiana University, Indianapolis, Indiana, 1970 (mimeograph; 9 pp.).
14. Wright, S. B.: Behavior Management in Dentistry for Children. Philadelphia: W. B. Saunders Co., 1975.

ALVIN L. MORRIS

3

ORAL MEDICINE IN GENERAL PRACTICE

OBJECTIVES

The purpose of this chapter is to provide guidance for the practical application of the medical history in general dental practice. A further objective is to assist the practitioner in the management of dental patients with the following systemic illnesses: hypertension, cardiovascular disease, rheumatic and congenital heart disease, diabetes, hepatitis, and coagulation disorders.

This chapter will not increase the reader's basic knowledge of oral medicine; rather, it will provide guidelines for the practical application of that knowledge in the day-to-day management of patients receiving dental care. To achieve this, only the most commonly encountered oral medicine problems, given above, will be considered.

Increasing one's knowledge of the field of oral medicine should be a continuing goal of the general practitioner. Toward that end, many excellent books and articles are referenced at the end of this chapter. But frequently, it may be observed that dentists know a good deal more about oral medicine than is revealed in their practice behavior; therefore, the application of oral medicine knowledge in general practice must be increased. The more one knows about the fascinating and complex field of oral medicine, the more one recognizes that most questions related to human biology have complicated answers. But practitioners are forced, routinely, to make simplified "yes" or "no" decisions on behalf of their patients: "I will or will not refer this patient to a physician." This chapter will assist the practitioner in making such decisions by providing guidelines, but they must be applied with judg-

ment on the basis of knowledge gained from many sources.

MANAGEMENT OF THE ORAL MEDICINE PATIENT

The general practitioner who decides that the conscientious practice of dentistry requires the inclusion of an oral medicine component immediately asks himself or herself four questions:
1. What am I going to do about a medical history in my practice?
2. What am I going to do about a head and neck and oral soft tissue examination in my practice?
3. What am I going to do about referring patients to physicians?
4. What am I going to do about using clinical diagnostic laboratories?

The first question will be discussed as a separate section later in this chapter.

The Soft Tissue Examination

The conscientious practice of dentistry demands that patients receive a head and neck and oral soft tissue examination. This statement requires no defense or elaboration. How such an examination is performed is relatively unimportant. Every dentist was taught this procedure at some time, and several texts describe and illustrate excellent techniques. The important point is to develop one's own technique and then to follow it routinely in a systemized fashion. A perfectly adequate head and neck and oral soft tissue examination takes no more than

TABLE 3–1 Alternative Procedures Following Detection of a Lesion

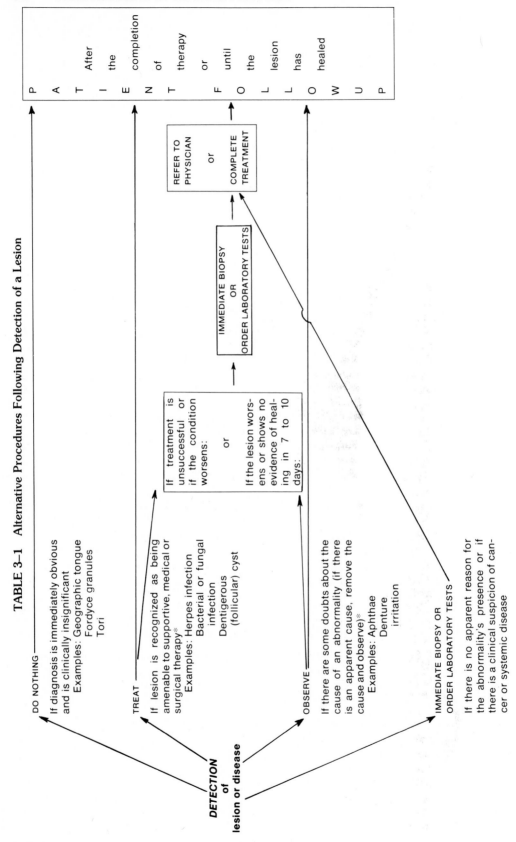

* A cytologic specimen should be considered at this point because a positive smear would lead to a diagnostic biopsy in less time than the usual 7 to 10 days allowed for treatment or observation and thus might result in earlier detection of malignant disease.

Patient's Name _____ Date _____

REGIONAL EXAMINATION

	WNL	Abnor-mality		WNL	Abnor-mality		WNL	Abnor-mality
1. Face	____	____	5. Floor of mouth	____	____	9. Gingiva	____	____
2. Lips	____	____	6. Palate—Hard	____	____	10. TMJ	____	____
3. Buccal Mucosa	____	____	7. Palate—Soft	____	____	11. Lymph nodes	____	____
4. Tongue	____	____	8. Pharynx	____	____	Blood Pressure	____	____

WNL = *Within Normal Limits.* **All abnormalities must be explained on reverse side.**

FIGURE 3–1 Sample form for recording initial soft tissue examination.

2 minutes in the absence of pathologic findings.

Most dentists will point out that they do perform a soft tissue examination as part of the initial patient work-up. Many will admit that they rarely perform such an examination thereafter. The following guidelines for the soft tissue examination are suggested:

1. A record of a completed examination should be part of the formal patient record initiated at the first appointment. It is important for medicolegal considerations, is good patient management, and is appreciated by patients. A simple, brief record is adequate (Fig. 3–1).

2. A record of a soft tissue examination should be made in the patient's chart when the patient is seen on recall or at least at yearly intervals. This, too, is important for medicolegal considerations. An example of the interim examination form will be presented later with the interim history form.

3. A soft tissue examination should be performed routinely as the initial step in every patient seen. It takes less than 2 minutes, and patients appreciate it and are impressed by it. The examination prevents unnecessary trauma to painful lesions, e.g., aphthous ulcers, and provides reassurance at the end of the day that no patient treated has a carcinoma under the tongue. How many dentists can make that statement with assurance?

References to oral soft tissue changes that are significant to the consideration of systemic disease will be made later. A more frequent finding, as a result of soft tissue examination, will be oral lesions. A detailed consideration of clinical oral pathology is beyond the scope of this chapter. A guide for the management of oral lesions, developed by Rovin, is presented in Table 3–1.

Referral to Physicians

With a common interest in the physical, emotional, and social well-being of their patients, it is inevitable that the practices of physicians and dentists will interrelate. It must be realized that information on dentistry is one of the voids in the education of physicians. Accordingly, the dentist must assume the responsibility for helping physicians gain an understanding of present-day dentistry. If a good relationship based on mutual respect is to exist, dentists must not be overly dependent on the physician but must bring their own training and experience to bear. To turn indiscriminately to the physician for information on the significance of every systemic problem reported by the patient is neither appropriate nor professional. On the other hand, the dentist should feel no reluctance to consult with the physician when the best interests of the patient are at stake.

When a patient has a physician of record, any referral should be to that physician. Patients who have no established pattern for pursuing their medical care needs may be referred to a physician of the dentist's choice. In selecting a physician who will be a primary referral resource, the dentist should contact the physician personally in order to discuss the nature of their professional needs and to learn the organizational and operational pattern of the physician's practice.

It is common for patients to deny having a physician of record but to indicate a group practice, Health Maintenance Organization, or hospital clinic as their source of medical care. The dentist should not refer a patient to a faceless institution; such a referral is not a satisfactory approach to patient management. A visit to an institution that the dentist must frequently contact is in order, both to understand the nature of the organization and to establish which staff members to contact.

All referrals should be made in writing, and the wise dentist keeps a copy of any communication leaving his office. Occasionally, however, a consultation with a physician by telephone about a patient with a medical problem who requires immediate dental treatment is necessary. It is impractical to request that the busy physician record in writing advice given over the telephone. The dentist, however, should file a written and dated record of the call in the patient's chart. The telephone consultation described should always involve a physician who is familiar with the patient. It is not appropriate to request advice regarding a patient whom the physician has not seen and about whom the questions are hypothetical.

Referral for Treatment. It is not uncommon for the dentist to suspect diabetes, hypertension, or other systemic conditions that have been undetected or have worsened significantly since the patient's last contact with a physician. A referral for treatment involves the transfer of patients so that they may benefit from the particular expertise of another health practitioner. In contrast to the referral for consultation, referral for treatment implies that the primary responsibility for a patient, or for a particular aspect of treatment, is being passed to another. Accordingly, the practitioner accepting the referral is at liberty to proceed independently. Although dentists who make referrals usually pass along information of value, they may not dictate the future course of the patient's care, nor should they tell the patient what to expect.

It is good patient management and good professional ethics to make all referrals in writing. When a dentist refers a patient to a physician for treatment, a letter should be submitted in which the purpose of referral is described in detail. Comments should be included concerning the patient's oral condition along with additional pertinent information. The dentist should state the tentative diagnosis of the patient's medical problem and the reasons for this diagnosis.

Referral of a patient to a physician without any accompanying information may be detrimental to the patient. If a patient is referred with a vague request such as "The blood should be checked," the physician may face a dilemma. There may be no obvious reason to "check the blood," but in order to save face for the dentist and to meet the patient's expectations, a battery of expensive but unnecessary laboratory tests may be requested. A similar problem may result following a vague request that the patient's endocrine status be checked or that the patient be checked for nutritional deficiency. No one's interests are served when unreasonable and unfounded requests are made of the physician.

Referral for Consultation. A consultation is a deliberation between two professional individuals concerning the diagnosis or proper method of treatment of a patient. When a dentist consults with a physician, the basic responsibility for the patient resides with the individual initiating the consultation—the dentist. The dentist should correlate the information received from the physician with all other data obtained during clinical examination and from the patient's history. The ultimate decision regarding the dentist's course of action must be made by the dentist, who is thereafter responsible for that decision. It is neither appropriate nor legally defensible to ask or to expect the physician to assume responsibility for care received by the patient in the dentist's office. By the same token, physicians should not be led to believe that they can or should dictate the course of dental treatment.

In referring patients for consultation, dentists frequently ask whether the patient's medical problems contraindicate anticipated dental treatment. Such a question is often indicated and in some cases is crucial. Equally important is information on how the patient may be better managed in the dental office. It is not justifiable for dentists to shift responsibility for a patient's well-being to physicians so that they may proceed uninhibited in providing routine dental treatment. The time and expense related to any referral to a physician should be justified on the basis of what is in the best interest of the patient, not the dentist. Referral must not represent an extravagant use of someone else's money to purchase peace of mind for a nondiscriminating dentist.

Clinical Diagnostic Laboratories

Although a marked departure from the traditional teaching of oral medicine, it is recommended that the conscientious general practitioner *not* be concerned with the use of clinical diagnostic laboratories in the day-to-day practice of dentistry. Certainly, knowledge of laboratory tests and the significance of their results is essential. Although it is necessary to understand the application of clinical laboratory testing to the diagnosis of the patient's problem and to the management of patients, it is not necessary that the general dental practitioner use clinical laboratory services directly.

It is recommended by some that the dentist who suspects systemic illness refer patients to a physician only after the suspicion has been confirmed through laboratory tests. The problem with this approach is that the physician will immediately repeat the tests. Thus, time has been lost, and money has been wasted. It is possible to make a discriminating referral for treatment on the basis of the medical history and clinical examination.

There are many patients whose treatment for perplexing soft tissue lesions, pain, or infection can be pursued intelligently only on the basis of data derived from laboratory tests. These patients are candidates for referral to dental specialists, not physicians. It is important that the general practitioner have the ability to identify such patients. Such ability assures superior care for patients and provides satisfaction for the dentist. Neither care nor satisfaction is compromised when the dentist leaves the direct interaction with clinical diagnostic laboratories to others.

THE MEDICAL HISTORY IN DENTAL PRACTICE

Purpose of the Medical History

Taking a medical history, once viewed as a procedure applied to the management of special patients, is now recognized as an essential element of routine patient care. There are four major reasons why the dentist takes such a history: (1) to be certain that the rendering of dental care will not be detrimental to the systemic health and well-being of the patient; (2) to ascertain whether the presence of some systemic illness or drugs being used in its treatment will interfere with or compromise the ability of the dentist to accomplish treatment objectives; (3) to detect unrecognized systemic illness that may require referral of the patient; and (4) to have

a written record in the event of unwarranted malpractice litigation.

The Health Questionnaire

There are several valid and appropriate approaches to history-taking. Some dentists prefer to record information on a blank sheet of paper, whereas others follow a form that guides the process of information seeking. A practical and popular method is the use of a health questionnaire. Since a number of dental schools use a health questionnaire in their clinics, many dentists are familiar with its use. The one presented here (Fig. 3–2) is based on the questionnaire compiled from forms used at four dental schools and which appeared in Accepted Dental Therapeutics, the publication of the Council on Dental Therapeutics of the American Dental Association. Every effort has been made to develop a questionnaire that is sufficiently complete and yet concise enough to have practical application in daily practice.

It should be noted that a questionnaire serves as a useful tool in seeking health information and, in this context, is not intended to be a substitute for the detailed medical history that may be required in some instances.

Significance of Positive Responses

A potential conflict concerning the material that follows must be acknowledged. How does one present enough information to be meaningful without developing an inordinately long and cumbersome discussion? Chapters in books on pathology and internal medicine have been written on the subject of each item of the questionnaire. An attempt has been made in this section to present a practical interpretation of the questionnaire rather than an academic analysis covering all possible implications of the questions. The dentist must refer to other sources in seeking to improve the wisdom with which the medical history is employed in practice. A more detailed consideration of systemic diseases of particular significance to the dentist is presented later in this chapter.

Chief Mouth Complaint

The *Chief Mouth Complaint* is, in fact, a brief explanation of why patients come to the dentist's office. The answer will provide immediate insight into the patients' interpretation of their oral or dental problems as

HEALTH QUESTIONNAIRE

Name_____Sex_____Age_____

Address_____

Telephone _____Occupation_____Marital Status_____

Name and Address of my Physician_____

What is your CHIEF MOUTH COMPLAINT (in a FEW words)?_____

_____

DIRECTIONS

If your answer to the question is YES put a circle around "YES."
If your answer to the question is NO put a circle around "NO."
Answer all questions and fill in blank spaces when indicated.

Answers to the following questions are for our records only and will be considered confidential.

1. Do you have a health problem.....................................YES   NO
   a. Has there been any change in your general health within the
      past year.. YES   NO

2. My last physical examination was on_____

3. Are you now under the care of a physician........................... YES   NO
   a. If so, what is the condition being treated_____

4. Have you had any serious illness or operation........................ YES   NO
   a. If so, what was the illness or operation_____

5. Have you been hospitalized or had a serious illness within the past
   five (5) years... YES   NO
   a. If so, what was the problem_____

6. Do you have or have you had any of the following diseases or problems.
   a. Rheumatic fever or rheumatic heart disease..................... YES   NO
   b. Congenital heart lesions or a heart murmur..................... YES   NO
   c. Cardiovascular disease (heart trouble, heart attack, coronary
      insufficiency, coronary occlusion, high blood pressure,
      arteriosclerosis, stroke)...................................... YES   NO
      1) Do you have pain in chest upon exertion..................... YES   NO
      2) Are you ever short of breath after mild exercise............ YES   NO
      3) Do your ankles swell.. YES   NO
      4) Do you get short of breath when you lie down, or do you require
         extra pillows when you sleep................................ YES   NO
   d. Allergy.. YES   NO
   e. Asthma or hay fever.. YES   NO
   f. Hives or a skin rash... YES   NO
   g. Fainting spells or seizures.................................... YES   NO
   h. Diabetes... YES   NO
      1) Do you have to urinate (pass water) more than six times a day... YES   NO
      2) Are you thirsty much of the time........................... YES   NO
      3) Does your mouth frequently become dry...................... YES   NO
   i. Hepatitis, jaundice or liver disease........................... YES   NO
   j. Arthritis... YES   NO
   k. Inflammatory rheumatism (painful swollen joints).............. YES   NO
   l. Stomach ulcers.. YES   NO
   m. Kidney trouble.. YES   NO
   n. Tuberculosis.. YES   NO
   o. Do you have a persistent cough or cough up blood.............. YES   NO
   p. Low blood pressure.. YES   NO
   q. Venereal disease.. YES   NO
   r. Other_____

7. Have you had abnormal bleeding associated with previous extractions,
   surgery, or trauma... YES   NO
   a. Do you bruise easily.. YES   NO
   b. Have you ever required a blood transfusion.................... YES   NO
      If so, explain the circumstances_____

FIGURE 3–2   Sample health questionnaire for recording patient's medical history.

Illustration continued on opposite page

8.   Do you have any blood disorder such as anemia........................ YES   NO

9.   Have you had surgery or x-ray treatment for a tumor, growth, or other
     condition of your mouth or lips.................................... YES   NO

10. Are you taking any drug or medicine............................... YES   NO
     If so, what_____

11. Are you taking any of the following:
     a. Antibiotics or sulfa drugs..................................... YES   NO
     b. Anticoagulants (blood thinners)................................ YES   NO
     c. Medicine for high blood pressure............................... YES   NO
     d. Cortisone (steroids).. YES   NO
     e. Tranquilizers...YES   NO
     f. Aspirin... YES   NO
     g. Insulin, tolbutamide (Orinase) or similar drug................... YES   NO
     h. Digitalis or drugs for heart trouble............................ YES   NO
     i. Nitroglycerin... YES   NO
     j. Other_____

12. Are you allergic or have you reacted adversely to:
     a. Local anesthetics.. YES   NO
     b. Penicillin or other antibiotics................................. YES   NO
     c. Sulfa drugs... YES   NO
     d. Barbiturates, sedatives, or sleeping pills....................... YES   NO
     e. Aspirin... YES   NO
     f. Iodine..YES   NO
     g. Other_____

13. Do you have any disease, condition, or problem not listed above that
     you think I should know about..................................... YES   NO
     If so, please explain_____
     _____

14. Do you have pain in your mouth.................................... YES   NO

15. Do your gums bleed... YES   NO

16. When were you last seen by a dentist_____

17. What did the dentist do for you at that time_____

18. Have you had any serious trouble associated with any previous dental
     treatment.. YES   NO
     If so, explain_____
     _____

WOMEN

19. Are you pregnant... YES   NO

20. Do you have any problems associated with your menstrual period....... YES   NO

Remarks:_____
_____
_____
_____
_____
_____
_____
_____

                                        _____
                                        Signature of Patient

Date_____

                                        _____
                                        Signature of Dentist

FIGURE 3–2 *Continued*

well as reveal the level of their expectations. In some instances the oral complaint itself will be strongly suggestive of a systemic health problem, e.g., bleeding or sores that do not heal.

The dentist should review the entire questionnaire briefly, noting particularly any positive answers, before beginning to question the patient for more detailed information. A general impression of the patient's health and some insight into how to proceed with the medical history is gained in this manner. If there are multiple positive responses, the dentist should avoid spending too much time pursuing answers to the first five questions, which are general in nature.

Because of the occasional low level of understanding or unusual attitudes toward health and disease found among patients, conflicting and confusing responses can be expected. The dentist should calmly and quietly elaborate on misunderstood questions; this will lead to clarification of any problems.

1. *Do you have a health problem?*

Patients answering in the affirmative should be questioned further regarding their health problems. At this time, intelligent, informed patients will provide most of the necessary significant information. Although listening to patients relate their illness and their reaction to it may be useful, it can result in wasted time. Once the nature of the illness is ascertained, it is wise to pass on to other parts of the questionnaire from which more specific information will probably be obtained. The chief medical complaint of patients, in their own words, should be recorded under *Remarks.*

1a. *Has there been any change in your general health within the past year?*

A "yes" answer may be given by a patient who has claimed good health in the previous response. Thus, a more subtle opportunity to gain an impression of the patient's overall health status is provided. Questions 2 and 3 also serve as a check on patients' assessment of their own health status.

4. *Have you had any serious illness or operation?*
4a. *If so, what was the illness or operation?*
5. *Have you been hosptialized or had a serious illness within the past five years?*
5a. *If so, what was the problem?*

These questions also offer insight into the patient's general health status; however, their focus is on the past. A "yes" answer often requires a searching follow-up. It is not unusual for a patient to answer positively at this point but negatively throughout the rest of the questionnaire. Thus, the answer may be the only lead to the patient's health problem. The patient's recollection of the past may be too vague to permit a positive response to the questions that follow. In such instances it may be necessary to inquire into the symptoms and sequelae associated with the past episode.

6. *Do you have or have you had any of the following diseases or problems?*
6a. *Rheumatic fever or rheumatic heart disease.*

Damage to heart valves is frequently associated with this disease. Patients who give a positive answer must receive prophylactic antibiotic medication before tooth extraction or other manipulative procedures involving soft tissue or bone can be performed. (See the section on rheumatic fever later in this chapter.)

6b. *Congenital heart lesions.*

Such patients also require the protection described under 6a. If further questioning reveals that the congenital defect has interfered with the patient's life by altering work or play habits, consultation with a physician is indicated. Special precautions may be necessary in the management of such patients.

6c. *Cardiovascular disease (heart trouble, heart attack, coronary insufficiency, coronary occlusion, high blood pressure, arteriosclerosis, stroke).*
6c. *(1). Do you have pain in chest upon exertion?*

Such pain, frequently indicating angina pectoris, results when the musculature of the heart is insufficiently oxygenated because of restricted blood flow. The symptom indicates atherosclerotic changes in the coronary vessels; a decrease in their diameter prevents the flow of blood required by exercise.

6c (2).) *Are you ever short of breath after mild exercise?*

This symptom indicates valvular heart disease that interferes with efficient flow of blood through the heart. When the mitral valve (the valve between the left atrium and left ventricle) is altered by atherosclerotic changes, blood regurgitates into the atrium when the ventricle contracts. Extra blood must be accommodated by the atrium and, in turn, by the pulmonary veins and, finally, by the vasculature of the lungs. This increased pressure results in accumulation of fluid within the lungs and thus in a shortness of breath. Shortness of breath may also indicate some chronic respiratory disease.

6c (3). *Do your ankles swell?*

This finding is frequently a symptom of congestive heart failure, which results when there has been a prolonged impairment of the ability of the heart to maintain an adequate flow of blood to the tissues. The passive engorgement of the venous system results in edema of the legs.

6c (4). *Do you get short of breath when you lie down, or do you require extra pillows when you sleep?*

Orthopnea (shortness of breath when supine) is a further indication of heart failure, particularly left ventricular failure. It is an extension of the problem described in 6c (2).

Patients answering "yes" to any of the questions under 6c require extra care and judgment on the part of the dentist. The welfare of these patients often depends on effective communication between physician and dentist (see section on cardiovascular disease later in the chapter).

6d. *Allergy.*

6e. *Asthma or hay fever.*

6f. *Hives or skin rash.*

All three of these questions seek to determine whether the patient has an allergic diathesis. In responding to 6d, the patient may identify the allergen to be avoided. A "no" answer to 6d but a positive response to 6e or 6f should make the dentist suspicious. Of particular concern are possible allergic responses to agents commonly used by the dentist, such as local and topical anesthetics, barbiturates, iodine, antibiotics, aspirin, and codeine (see 12). The dentist must always be alert to the possibility of an abnormal reaction to any of the drugs or chemicals used in treatment.

6g. *Fainting spells or seizures.*

It is important that the dentist know if a patient has epilepsy. Precipitation of a seizure during treatment can be avoided by careful management or sedation of the excitable patient. Also, a history of epilepsy may help to explain oral findings such as gingival enlargement associated with phenytoin (Dilantin) therapy or lingual lacerations or scars.

If the patient reports fainting related to dental treatment, especially during the administration of an anesthetic, the dentist can adjust the management of the patient

accordingly. If there is a history of recent or unexplained lapses in consciousness, then the patient should be referred to a physician for a suspected central nervous system disorder or lesion.

6h. *Diabetes.*

(1). *Do you have to urinate (pass water) more than six times a day?*

(2). *Are you thirsty much of the time?*

(3). *Does your mouth frequently become dry?*

A "yes" answer to any or all of these specific questions under 6h is strongly suggestive of diabetes mellitus. Although a positive history of controlled diabetes does not contraindicate routine dental care, it does require modification in patient management (see section on diabetes later in the chapter).

6i. *Hepatitis, jaundice, or liver disease.*

(See the section on hepatitis later in the chapter).

6j. *Arthritis.*

The dental significance of osteoarthritis is limited to its possible involvement of the temporomandibular joint, in which case joint pain or reduced mobility may be present. Some patients with arthritis take large amounts of aspirin (see 11f). The dentist must be sure that the patient is not referring to 6k in answering this question.

6k. *Inflammatory rheumatism (painful swollen joints).*

A "yes" answer should prompt careful questioning of the patient, and perhaps the physician, to determine if the painful joints are related to rheumatic fever or Sydenham's chorea. Both conditions frequently result in lesions of the heart valves (see 6a). In giving a positive answer to 6k, the patient may be indicating the presence of rheumatoid arthritis, which is frequently treated with steroids or aspirin (see 11d and 11f).

6l. *Stomach ulcers.*

The patient placed on a chronically restricted diet because of ulcers may manifest oral signs and symptoms of nutritional deficiencies. The absence of a detergent diet may also have oral hygiene implications or be responsible for an abnormal tongue coating. Drugs commonly used in the management of the patient with an ulcer frequently produce dryness of the mouth. The dentist must not prescribe steroids for the patient with an ulcer because of possible interference with connective tissue repair.

6m. *Kidney trouble.*

The clinical observation that acute glomerulonephritis occasionally develops after oral or pharyngeal infections emphasizes the need to eliminate oral infection in the patient with kidney disease. Surgical procedures, however, should not be carried out in patients with active or acute nephritis. If an emergency makes tooth extraction necessary, it should be performed only after administration of antibiotics.

Oral signs and symptoms of anemia or nutritional deficiencies may be observed in patients experiencing proteinuria resulting from chronic kidney disease. The stomatitis associated with uremia is usually a late symptom in the very ill patient.

6n. *Tuberculosis.*

Dentists should use a face mask and take other precautions to prevent their own exposure when working on a patient with diagnosed tuberculosis. Through infrequent, tuberculosis lesions sometimes may be found in the oral cavity.

6o. *Do you have a persistent cough or cough up blood?*

In asking this question, dentists are emphasizing their role as medical "case-finders." A positive response may indicate tuberculosis, lung carcinoma, or other chronic pulmonary diseases. The patient should be referred to a physician before any dental treatment, other than emergency care, is provided.

6p. *Low blood pressure.*

In most instances, chronic hypotension, even a systolic pressure of 100 mm Hg, can be regarded as a favorable health finding. Frequently, a patient who claims to have "low blood" is referring to anemia.

6q. *Venereal disease.*

Syphilis is the disease with which this question is primarily concerned. Although it is the rare patient who will admit to a history of venereal disease, when a positive response is given, a serologic test for syphilis should be obtained to rule out active disease.

6r. *Other.*

Patients should be encouraged to list any condition that may reveal the status of their health.

7. *Have you had abnormal bleeding associated with previous extractions or trauma?*

(See the section on bleeding problems later in the chapter).

7a. *Do you bruise easily?*

This question is often misinterpreted, and many women will answer "yes." The dentist should look for evidence of purpura. A frankly abnormal tendency to bruise should make one suspicious of thrombocytopenic purpura, but it may also be a symptom of leukemia or advanced vitamin C deficiency. Referral of such a patient to a physician is indicated.

7b. *Have you ever required a blood transfusion?*

This question offers another attempt to identify a bleeding tendency. Of course, it may lead to evidence of another blood dyscrasia or an elboration on another past medical event.

8. *Do you have any blood disorder such as anemia?*

It is common for patients to report having anemia or that "the doctor is building up my blood." Since physicians often given this explanation as part of their management of real or imagined diseases, one must not overreact to a "yes" answer. If it becomes clear that the patient is receiving medication for a blood problem or if clinical examination suggests anemia, the physician should be contacted.

9. *Have you had surgery or x-ray treatment for a tumor, growth, or other condition of your mouth or lips?*

If surgery has been performed, it is important that the dentist be informed in order to better interpret oral findings. It is most important, however, to know whether the facial bones have been subjected to irradiation. If so, no surgery involving bone should be performed since the diminished blood supply may result in osteoradionecrosis. The physician must be contacted for details concerning treatment. Any patient with a history of an oral neoplasm must be examined with special care for any evidence of recurrence.

10. *Are you taking any drugs or medicine?*

Although the drugs covered under the next question are of special interest, it is important to learn of *any* medication being used by the patient. The dentist should point out that the question refers to any medication, including nonprescription items purchased at the drugstore. This question may be the only one on the questionnaire that leads to information about a health problem.

11. *Are you taking any of the following:*

11a. *Antibiotics or sulfa drugs.*

A positive answer requires that the prescribing physician be contacted for further information. The dentist should not rely on the patient's explanation of why the drug is being taken.

11b. *Anticoagulants (blood thinners).*

A "yes" answer indicates the patient has experienced a heart attack or has peripheral vascular disease. The physician must be contacted. Elective dental treatment should be delayed for a minimum of 6 months after the attack. The patient on anticoagulants requires special planning when surgery is contemplated.

11c. *Medicine for high blood pressure. (See 6c.)*

11d. *Cortisone (steroids).*

The physician of the patient taking steroids must be contacted for further information. Since the inflammatory reaction may be suppressed, the usual signs and symptoms by which the dentist recognizes severe infection may be masked. The patient taking steroids may have a suppression of adrenal cortex function with a diminished systemic capacity to withstand the stress of emergency procedures or tooth extraction.

11e. *Tranquilizers.*

Since these drugs are in common use, the dentist must be alert to the side reactions that occur with relative frequency. Patients taking major tranquilizers, such as the phenothiazines, may faint easily and may be more difficult that usual to revive. The phenothiazine derivatives are known to potentiate the actions of sedative drugs such as the barbiturates. Orthostatic hypotension is seen in patients taking chlorpromazine and related drugs. These patients may go into syncope on being suddenly placed in the upright position and released from the dental chair. Nasal congestion, reduced salivary flow, and spasms of facial musculature are not uncommon in patients after prolonged administration of tranquilizers.

11f. *Aspirin.*

Bleeding complications may be seen in patients with arthritis who take large amounts of aspirin regularly.

11g. *Insulin, tolbutamide (Orinase) or similar drug. (See 6h.)*

11h. *Digitalis or drugs for heart trouble.*

11i. *Nitroglycerin. (See 6c).*

12. *Are you allergic or have you reacted adversely to:*

12a. *Local anesthetics.*

True allergic reactions to the anesthetic agents frequently used today are extremely rare, although a "yes" answer to this question is common. The patient is usually referring to an episode of fainting associated with the administration of an anesthetic on a previous occasion (see Chapter 10, Oral Surgery in General Practice).

The patient may identify the local anesthetic agent as Novocain (actually a brand name for procaine) when in fact the local anesthetic used may have been an agent other than procaine. If, after careful questioning, it is possible to identify the specific agent, the dentist should use a local anesthetic of another type. Local anesthetics may be divided into at least four types: (1) para-amino-benzoates, as represented by procaine (Novocain), butethamine (monocaine), tetracaine (Pontocaine), and butacaine (Butyn); (2) meta-amino-benzoates, as represented by metabutethamine (Unacaine) and metabutoxycaine (Primacaine); (3) benzoates with no aromatic amino group, as represented by meprylcaine (Oracaine) and isobucaine (Kincaine); and (4) amide types, as represented by lidocaine (Xylocaine, Lidothesin, Octocaine), mepivacaine (Carbocaine), and pyrrocaine (Dynacaine). If the allergic reaction appears to have been serious and if there is doubt as to the specific agent, referral to an allergist is indicated.

12b. *Penicillin or other antibiotics.*

As with any allergy, a positive answer to this question should be prominently recorded on the front of the patient's record. Erythromycin is the preferred antibiotic for the penicillin-sensitive patient.

12c. *Sulfa drugs.*

These drugs are rarely required in the management of the dental patient and should be avoided when sensitivity is reported.

12d. *Barbiturates, sedatives, or sleeping pills.*

The exact agent involved should be identified if the patient responds "yes." If sedation is necessary, a substitute drug may be used, such as meperidine hydrochloride (Demerol), promethazine hydrochloride (Phenergan), or ethinamate (Valmid).

12e. *Aspirin.*

Allergic responses to aspirin are not common; however, abnormal reactions, particularly gastritis, are frequently seen. Acetaminophen or codeine may be substituted as required.

12f. *Iodine.*

12g. *Other.*

If the patient indicates an abnormal reaction to iodine *or any other agent* used in the dental office, such reaction should be prominently recorded on the front of the patient's record.

13. *Do you have any disease, condition, or problem not listed above that you think I should know about?*

Patients should be asked to give this question careful thought, even though they may have answered "no." This request convinces them of the dentist's interest in their health and well-being. It also provides the opportunity to pursue any aspect of the medical history in greater depth.

14. *Do you have pain in your mouth?*
15. *Do your gums bleed?*

Positive answers may have medical significance, but the questions are chiefly of value in providing insight into the dental problems to be anticipated. These questions, with the three that follow, constitute the dental history portion of the health questionnaire.

16. *When were you last seen by a dentist?*
17. *What did the dentist do for you at that time?*
18. *Have you had any serious trouble associated with any previous dental treatment?*

Answers to these questions reveal the emphasis that the patients have placed on their oral health in the past and also give some indication of their dental "I.Q." Although the last question may or may not have medical significance, the answers obtained may be helpful as plans are made for the overall management of the patient.

19. *Are you pregnant?*

The patient may suspect that she is pregnant but may not have contacted her physician. Although routine dental treatment is not contraindicated in an uncomplicated pregnancy, special considerations are appreciated and often necessary. Draping with a lead apron when taking radiographs is indicated for all patients but should be done with special care with pregnant patients. Any medical problem, such as heart or kidney disease, may be compounded during pregnancy. When any drug is to be administered, the dentist must be certain that its use is not contraindicated in the pregnant patient. It is wise to contact the physician of any pregnant patient before dental treatment is begun.

20. *Do you have any problems associated with your menstrual period?*

In addition to serve as a "case-finding" clue, a "yes" answer may be important to the interpretation of a subsequent oral finding.

Medical History for the Child Patient

Taking a medical history is equally as important in the management of the child patient as it is in the adult. The health questionnaire presented here is longer than is required for a child and may prove confusing. For this reason, an abbreviated questionnaire for children is recommended for every general practitioner's office (see Chapter 2, Pedodontics in General Practice).

Interim History

There is a tendency to assume that once a medical history is taken and filed, one has discharged all professional and legal respon-

---

Name _____   Date_____

INTERIM HISTORY *(Please comment on any answer other than "No")*

1. Have you been seen by a physician since you last visited my office?   No _____
2. Are you aware of any change in your health since I last treated you?   No _____
3. Are you taking any drugs or medicine at the present time?   No _____
4. Has there been any change in your mouth or teeth?   No _____

BLOOD PRESSURE _____

INTERIM SOFT TISSUE EXAMINATION	Normal	See Comments
1. Lymph Nodes	_____	_____
2. Vermilion—Labial and Buccal Mucosa	_____	_____
3. Tongue	_____	_____
4. Palate	_____	_____
5. Pharynx	_____	_____

COMMENTS

FIGURE 3–3   Sample form for recording interim medical history.

sibility. The importance of taking an interim medical history when the patient is recalled must be emphasized. Medically speaking, the patient may be an entirely different individual 6 months after the original history was taken, although there may be no clinical manifestation of this difference. The records of each office should include an abbreviated medical history form similar to the one shown in Figure 3–3. Note that this form also provides for an interim soft tissue examination.

Summary

In the health fields, there are many instances when the art of practice is as important as the science. Such is the case in taking a medical history. The art of listening is a necessary attribute of the dentist who would diagnose and treat with wisdom and skill. It must be remembered that the patient is telling something of importance, even if it is misinformation.

When all the data have been collected in questionnaire form, the dentist must interpret their quantity, quality, and significance. The importance of a given positive answer will vary, depending on the individual giving it and on how the question is interpreted. The dentist who overreacts to every "yes" answer is practicing with no more skill than the one who takes an inadequate history.

If one's goal is to treat patients rather than teeth or disease, the value of taking a complete health history cannot be overemphasized. It is through this procedure that vital information is obtained, that patients begin to gain confidence in their choice of practitioner, and that dentists demonstrate their concern for the patient's well-being. The history serves as an excellent vehicle for the establishment of rapport with the patient.

THE DENTAL PATIENT WITH COMMON SYSTEMIC ILLNESSES

In keeping with the objectives of this chapter and book, only the more common systemic conditions are discussed in this section. Common, as used here, refers to illnesses that occur with such frequency in our population that they are inevitably encountered on a routine basis in general dental practice.

The material that follows is organized from a patient management perspective. It is based on predictable scenarios of patients who reveal systemic illness either from their medical history or from clinical findings. An effort is made to assist dentists with their "now what" questions ("So I've identified systemic illness, now what?"). The point is made that the answer does not lie simply in the referral of the patient to a physician. Rather, it is emphasized that the general dentist who includes oral medicine as a component of dental practice seeks information on systemic illnesses for one or more of the following purposes:

1. Identification. In some cases, all the dentist wants or needs to know is that some systemic illness has occurred or does exist. In order to understand the patient better and to prepare for assuming responsibility for one segment of the patient's overall health, the dentist wishes to identify *in the patient's record* the history or presence of a systemic disease. In some cases, no response other than identification is necessary or appropriate.

2. Monitoring. In some cases, having identified a systemic illness, the dentist will merely wish to monitor the status of the disease on a regular basis. Frequently, no other response is required.

3. Referral for Follow-up. In some cases, information obtained through the history, monitoring of the patient, or clinical observations will suggest to the dentist that the patient needs to be referred to the physician in order to follow up on the management of the patient's illness. Such referral is made in the overall interest of the patient and does not imply delay, interruption, or modification of dental treatment.

4. Referral for Assessment. In some cases, information received from the patient or through clinical observations or both makes the dentist suspicious that some as yet unidentified systemic illness may exist. In execution of the important case-finding role of dentistry, the patient is referred to a physician for assessment. Such referral may or may not have implications for the dental management of the patient.

5. Referral for Clearance. In some cases, the patient's history or clinical observations related to known or as yet unidentified systemic illness raise the question of whether routine dental care might complicate or jeopardize the systemic status of the patient. Referral is therefore made for assessment, but an additional specific purpose is to receive clearance from a physician that dental care is not contraindicated.

6. Referral for Treatment. In some cases, the history or clinical observations reveal overt evidence of significant, new, or uncontrolled disease that demands immediate attention. Referral to a physician takes precedence over any effort to provide dental treatment.

7. Consultation. In some cases, patients will report having a systemic condition that has significance in terms of patient management. If the patient has a physician of record, the dentist may wish to contact the physician for a consultation on the status of the patient and strategy for management. Referral of the patient is not necessary to accomplish this goal. If the patient has no physician of record, referral to a physician for assessment is required.

In consideration of the systemic illnesses that follow, reference is made to the aforementioned purposes of identifying the disease. In each case, implications for the dental management of the patient are discussed.

For every disease there is only one correct diagnosis, whereas there may be multiple approaches to treatment and patient management. Accordingly, sensitivity to the importance of systemic considerations in dentistry (an oral medicine philosophy of practice) and the ability to identify illness are viewed as more important than knowledge of how to treat or manage systemic disease. The dentist cannot respond to systemic illness unless or until it is identified. Drug therapy and other approaches to managing diseases are continually changing. Guidelines related to the management of patients must be viewed in that light, and dentists must be willing to continue to update their knowledge through many sources.

No guidelines for responding to the needs of patients can be applied comfortably to every case. There are always those patients who, for a variety of reasons, defy simple categorization. Accordingly, guidelines do not relieve the dentist of the necessity of exercising professional judgment.

HYPERTENSION

Hypertension is the systemic disease that provides dentists with the most frequent opportunity to perform their case-finding role, i.e., their role in identification of undetected illness. Although the medical history may contribute to that process, ultimately it is the level of the patient's blood pressure, as recorded in the dental office, that alerts the dentist to the presence of hypertension. For every undetected hypertensive patient identified in the dental office, there will be many patients reporting a history of the disease. Here again, the dentist's response to this information will be determined by the patient's blood pressure reading in the office. The point is, *the dentist cannot practice oral medicine responsibly in general practice without routinely taking blood pressures.* There is little excuse for not doing so, since any member of the dentist's staff can, with little difficulty, learn to use the sphygmomanometer with reliable results.

Identification. The average American adult's blood pressure is 120/80 mm Hg, but it varies with age and weight. Blood pressure ranges from 90/60 to 140/90 mm Hg are considered normal. Until recently, the diagnosis of hypertension was not made unless the systolic pressure was over 150 mm Hg and the diastolic pressure over 100 mm Hg. The diastolic pressure is the more significant reading. Whereas patients with a reading in the 90 to 95 mm Hg range were previously categorized as prehypertensive or borderline hypertensive, they are now diagnosed as definitely hypertensive and are considered candidates for treatment.

For the first 10 or 20 years after onset, hypertension is asymptomatic, but slowly and surely it strains the heart and damages the arteries supplying vital organs. Only if blood pressure readings are taken frequently will the disease be recognized before irreversible vascular damage is done. With proof that even the mildest cases of hypertension benefit from treatment, the dentist has an increasingly beneficial role to play in identifying the 20 to 30 million undiagnosed hypertensive individuals in the United States.

One blood pressure reading of over 140/90 mm Hg taken in the dental office does not justify a diagnosis of hypertension. Certainly, a dental visit and the environment of the dental office are stressful to many patients, thereby producing the normal response of blood pressure elevation. At an initial visit, before a relationship of trust and rapport has been established, suspicion of frank hypertension is elicited by two blood pressure readings in excess of 160/100 mm Hg, taken at a 30-minute interval. Readings in the range of 140/90 to 160/100 mm Hg must be confirmed consistently at two subsequent visits to justify further action by the dentist.

The Dentist's Response. The response of the dentist who identifies *undetected* hypertension will depend upon the severity of the blood pressure elevation. The patient with exceedingly high blood pressure, in the range of 200/115 mm Hg, or with frank symptoms of severe headaches, nosebleeds, ringing in the ears, dizziness, and fainting should be referred to a physician for treatment immediately. Routine dental care should be postponed until the patient's disease is controlled.

Asymptomatic patients with blood pressure in the range of 160/100 mm Hg should likewise be referred for treatment, but the dentist can begin the early stages of the patient's treatment plan, e.g., prophylaxis, x-rays, impressions, and pain control. Patients with blood pressures between 140/90 and 160/100 mm Hg should be referred to the physician for assessment, but routine dental care can be pursued.

Patients who report having hypertension and are *under a physician's care but have normal blood pressure* readings in the dental office are *not* candidates for automatic referral to the physician. Such patients can usually provide explicit details of how they are being treated. They can receive routine dental care but should be told to notify their physician at their next visit that dental work is being done.

Hypertensive patients *under a physician's care but with abnormal blood pressure* readings in the dental office should be managed using the guidelines suggested for patients with undetected disease.

Office Management of the Hypertensive Patient. Normotensive patients should have their blood pressure checked on an annual basis in the dentist's office, but identified hypertensive patients should be monitored at least once every 6 months. Patients who have been referred for treatment should have their blood pressure taken at each dental appointment until their disease is under control. Patients whose blood pressure is in the 140/90 to 160/100 mm Hg range must have their pressure taken at each visit until hypertension is confirmed or shown not to exist.

A predominant objective in the management of hypertensive patients in the dental office is the control of stress. Drugs should be used only to achieve a level of stress reduction not possible through careful and compassionate interaction with the patient. Patients who trust that the dentist and staff are sincerely concerned with their well-being, who are treated with kindness, and who are given special considerations such as short appointments scheduled in the morning, for which they are not kept waiting, frequently do not require drugs to control their stress. The dentist must determine those patients for whom premedication is required. Of paramount importance for all patients is adequate control of pain during treatment.

Consideration of the hypotensive therapy being administered by the physician is the other major requirement in managing hypertensive patients in the dental office. Treatment is often prescribed in a sequential manner as the goal of normal blood pressure is pursued. Some patients achieve that goal through nondrug interventions such as reducing weight, restricting sodium in their diets, exercising, and reducing stress. If drugs are required, a diuretic alone will reduce the diastolic pressure to 90 mm Hg in about half of the hypertensive individuals. For the remaining patients, a drug that blocks the sympathetic nervous system is added to their regimen. There is no particular best drug, and several may be tried until the best result for a particular patient is found. The dentist must be aware of what drug or drugs are being used for a given patient. Common side effects of these drugs are xerostomia and postural hypotension. Some agents also potentiate the effect of barbiturates.

A special management problem is encountered when a patient with severely elevated blood pressure requires emergency dental care. If the nature of emergency is such that it can be handled through the use of pain-control agents and treatment of infection, then such an approach is advised. If the control of the patient's acute pain cannot be achieved without surgical or operative intervention, then such intervention must not be denied. Withholding emergency treatment for severe pain because treatment might further elevate blood pressure and precipitate a medical emergency is not justified. In such patients, it is likely the pain and distress of their dental problem is contributing to elevated blood pressure, probably in excess of the elevation that would be associated with pain-relieving procedures. The general practitioner should not hesitate to refer such a patient to a dental specialist or for treatment in a hospital environment, if the benefits of referral are immediately available to the patient. In any event, for humane reasons and in the best interests of the patient's systemic problem, relief must be given promptly.

CARDIOVASCULAR DISEASE

In this section, consideration is given only to angina pectoris, myocardial infarction, and congestive heart failure, i.e., those cardiac-related conditions most frequently encountered in the dental office. The following section includes reference to cardiac conditions that are relevant to a consideration of bacterial endocarditis.

Cardiovascular disease is the leading cause of death in our population and, accordingly, is present in a high proportion of dental patients who have reached or passed middle age. The question is not whether dentists will encounter cardiovascular disease in their patients but what will be the reaction to this inevitability. It is not a question of whether dentists will have an oral medicine component to their practice but whether oral medicine will be practiced well or poorly. To practice comfortably and responsibly, general dental practitioners must have confidence in their knowledge of cardiovascular disease. Information contributing to such knowledge can be found in the references at the end of this chapter.

Identification. Most patients with cardiovascular disease being treated in the dental office will be aware of their condition and will be under the care of a physician. There is little worry that they will fail to reveal the history of a heart attack or a previous diagnosis of chronic heart disease, since few such patients fail to grasp the significance of their illness, and many are preoccupied with its status. Adherence to a drug regimen is often a dominant element in their daily lives. Encouraging these patients to discuss their illness and its treatment is not difficult and is highly productive for the dentist. Such discussion will provide needed information regarding response to treatment and the extent to which patients are compromised by their illness both physically and emotionally.

Since many people visit a dentist regularly but avoid physicians unless frankly ill, patients with undetected cardiovascular disease are frequently encountered by the general practitioner. Carefully questioning the patient about the responses made on the health questionnaire permits ready identification of the characteristic pain of *angina pectoris*, i.e., crushing, heavy, squeezing pain (in an area of the midchest and about the size of a fist) that may radiate to the left arm, the neck, or the jaw. The pain is most commonly precipitated by physical exertion, excitement, or emotional tension and seldom lasts longer than a few seconds or minutes. It is important to learn the frequency of such episodes.

Congestive heart failure is a symptom rather than a disease, indicating that cardiac reserve has been exceeded and that the heart is unable to maintain adequate circulation. An early symptom is increasing breathlessness due to the accumulation of fluid in the lungs following moderate exertion. Pulmonary edema may produce chronic coughing and cyanosis of fingers and lips as pulmonary circulation is compromised. Advanced symptoms include pitting edema of the legs, congestion of large neck veins, and orthopnea. It should be noted that congestive heart failure is not a symptom of acute disease but reflects a prolonged period of compromised cardiac output.

The Dentist's Response. If *undetected* heart disease is suspected, referral to a physician for assessment must be accomplished at the first dental visit with an expectation that future visits may be delayed. The dentist must use judgment, however, and not alarm the patient by overreacting. If the patient's symptoms are so severe that abandonment of all dental considerations is indicated, it is unlikely the patient would be in the dental office. Usually, procedures typical of the first appointment can be accomplished. The dentist must be judicious in explaining the reason for referral and should not alarm the patient by announcing a diagnosis of heart disease.

Again, judgment is required in how the dentist reacts to the presence of heart disease revealed through the medical history. As a rule of thumb, patients who are fully ambulatory and are free of cardiac symptoms can receive dental care, and routine first-appointment procedures can be accomplished. An exception is the post–myocardial infarction patient whose heart attack occurred less than 6 months previously or whose therapeutic regimen is unknown. Dental prophylaxis should not be performed until information concerning anticoagulant drug therapy has been obtained from the physician.

Although symptom-free cardiac patients can be treated as dental outpatients, their management may require modification. Referral of such patients for assessment is not usually indicated; however, consultation with the physician is required. The status of the patient's systemic condition and the drugs being employed in therapy must be known. In the process of this consultation, the dentist will learn whether cardiac surgery for valve reconstruction or the placement of prostheses or pacemakers has been performed. It is also appropriate to inquire whether there are contraindications to dental treatment. It is important to inform the physician whether oral surgical procedures are anticipated.

If the medical history reveals the presence of cardiovascular disease and if, on questioning, it is learned that the patient is *not* free of signs and symptoms, referral to the physician for assessment is indicated before the dentist embarks on a plan of treatment. Such referral does not pertain to the angina patient who reports only an occasional episode requiring the use of nitroglycerin.

Office Management of the Patient With Cardiovascular Disease. Although angina pectoris, myocardial infarction, and congestive heart failure are discussed separately, it is not to be implied that they are mutually exclusive and do not commonly coexist. The three conditions have in common a tendency for exacerbation of symptoms in response to stress and tension. Accordingly, for all conditions, sedative premedication before the administration of a local anesthetic or the performance of dental operative procedures is often indicated. Other generalizations applicable to all these conditions can be made:

1. Local anesthetics containing epinephrine in the concentration of 1:100,000 can be used safely if aspiration procedures are followed.
2. Usually no more than three anesthetic Carpules should be administered during a single appointment.
3. Vasopressor-containing solutions should not be used in gingival packing materials.
4. Any cardiovascular patient who is demonstrating distressed breathing should be placed in an upright sitting position.
5. The dental procedure should be terminated for any patient who develops chest pain, shortness of breath, profuse sweating, pallor, or a rapid or irregular pulse.
6. The administration of general anesthesia in the general practitioner's office to patients with known cardiovascular disease is not recommended.
7. Cardiovascular patients who are *not* symptom-free and who require surgical procedures should be referred to a hospital environment for treatment.

Post–myocardial infarction patients should not be scheduled for elective dental treatment for 6 months following their heart attack. Ultimately, these patients may resume a robust normal life, but neither the patients nor the dentist can ignore the probable existence of systemic conditions predisposing to another infarction. Although the use of anticoagulants is decreasing, many patients who have suffered a heart attack are kept on such therapy indefinitely. It is recommended that the general practitioner refer any patient on anticoagulants to an oral surgeon for extractions and to a hospital-based dental clinic for deep scaling or periodontal surgery. Emergency dental care for a patient with a history of recent myocardial infarction (within 6 months) should be as conservative as possible. Following the 6-month period, the patient not on anticoagulant therapy can receive any dental treatment indicated.

The patient with *angina pectoris* who experiences an anginal attack while in the dental chair should have a nitroglycerin tablet placed under his tongue immediately. Use of the patient's own tablets, which are invariably available, is recommended. If the patient is totally pain-free in 2 to 3 minutes, completion of necessary dental procedures to bring the appointment to an end can be considered. Such an episode should prompt reconsideration of administering premedication at the next visit. An anginal pain that persists for more than 3 minutes after nitroglycerin administration suggests the possibility of a *myocardial infarction* and emergency procedures should be instigated. An anginal attack lasting longer than 20 minutes is considered, by definition, to be an infarction.

Once patients with *congestive heart failure*

have been identified and referred and are under good medical management, they can receive any indicated dental treatment when given the benefit of the special dental management considerations listed earlier. Even patients considered to be under good medical management may have some pulmonary edema and should be treated sitting upright if more comfortable in that position. These patients are often on digitalis therapy, which may make them more prone to develop nausea. Careful attention should be given to those dental procedures or manipulations that tend to trigger gagging.

The office management of patients whose medical treatment included cardiac surgery for any purpose is considered in the following section. It should be stressed that rarely can the dentist discharge his responsibilities to a patient with cardiovascular disease merely through a single referral or consultation with the physician. Continuing consultation and cooperation between dentist and physician are usually required.

RHEUMATIC AND CONGENITAL HEART DISEASE

The emphasis in this section is on those systemic conditions that place the patient at risk of developing bacterial endocarditis following dental procedures. Traditionally such risk has been associated primarily with rheumatic and congenital heart disease. Advances in recent years in the surgical management of cardiovascular disease have resulted in a growing number of high-risk patients, e.g., those requiring placement of prosthetic heart valves or those needing prosthetic intravascular or intracardiac materials. To this group can be added the relatively few patients, at the present time, who have received renal transplants.

This section will help the dentist make appropriate decisions concerning patients with the aforementioned conditions. Details on specific antibiotic regimens to achieve prophylaxis are readily available and so are not included here. The textbook by Little and Falace (see references) includes an excellent chapter on this subject.

Identification.   The dentist cannot be expected to identify undetected rheumatic and congenital heart disease. Gross signs and symptoms such as dyspnea and cyanosis, which reflect congestive heart failure, do not develop until later stages of these diseases. Therefore, the dentist must depend on the medical history to identify patients with known disease. *Failure to identify existing systemic conditions requiring antibiotic prophylaxis places both the patient and the dentist in a particularly vulnerable position.*

The Dentist's Response.   Judgment is required in deciding how to respond to patients who indicate on the health questionnaire that they have had rheumatic fever or a heart murmur. What must be decided is whether the patient's rheumatic fever resulted in rheumatic heart disease, which probably occurs in over half of the cases. If rheumatic fever occurred as an isolated medical incident *over* 10 years ago, *and* if the patient denies any follow-up treatment for heart disease after recovery, *and* if the patient has been living a normal life with *no* restriction of physical activities, then no response on the part of the dentist is indicated. Similar scrutiny of the medical history is required of patients who report a heart murmur as an isolated incident. If the reported condition occurred *less* than 10 years ago, *or* if the history of the patient's health over the past 10 years is vague or confusing, *or* if the patient has been under the care of a physician, *or* if the patient has restricted physical activities in day-to-day living, the dentist must request a referral for follow-up.

Patients who report having rheumatic or congenital heart disease, patients under 40 years of age who are being followed by their physician for an unidentified heart condition, and all patients who have had heart surgery must be the subjects of consultation with the physician. Referral of the patient is not usually required if the patient has a physician of record, but *no* dental procedures should be performed until the dentist has conferred with the physician. How the dentist responds from that point depends on the results of that conference.

Office Management of Patients With Rheumatic and Congenital Heart Disease.   No dental procedures should be performed on a patient suspected of needing antibiotic prophylactic coverage until the need has been confirmed or denied through consultation with the physician. How to manage those who do require prophylactic antibiotics cannot be neatly categorized, and the regimen to be followed should be agreed upon with the patient's physician on a patient-by-patient basis.

The decision as to what dental procedures require antibiotic prophylactic coverage must be made by the dentist. The physician is not qualified to make that judgment. Although this subject has been widely discussed, the view of the American Heart Association has grown increasingly conservative. It is recommended that the dentist conform, without equivocation, to the current view of that association and provide antibiotic prophylaxis for *all* dental procedures (including routine dental prophylaxis) that are likely to cause gingival bleeding. The dentist must decide in advance what procedures are likely to be associated with gingival bleeding.

It is imperative that both the dentist and the patient give scrupulous attention to the establishment and maintenance of optimal oral hygiene when the risk of bacterial endocarditis exists. Dental floss and devices using water under pressure should be used with much caution, and they are not recommended if the condition of the gingivae predisposes the patient to easy bleeding.

According to the American Heart Association, patients requiring antibiotic prophylaxis and for whom the foregoing management considerations pertain include the following:

1. patients with congenital heart disease, excluding simple atrial septal defects;
2. patients with valvular heart disease, either congenital or acquired;
3. patients with previously documented bacterial endocarditis;
4. patients with mitral or tricuspid valve prolapse;
5. patients with an artificial heart valve or any form of valvular reconstruction; and
6. patients with a foreign body implanted within their hearts.

Antibiotic prophylaxis *may* be indicated for:

1. patients with prosthetic grafts implanted within the arterial or venous system and patients with left ventricular aneurysm repair;
2. patients with permanently implanted transvenous pacemakers;
3. patients with ventriculoatrial shunts;
4. renal dialysis patients with arteriovenous shunts; and
5. patients with idiopathic hypertrophic subaortic stenosis.

Certain species of microorganisms cause the majority of cases of infective endocarditis, and their antimicrobial sensitivity patterns have been used to develop the formal recommendations for prophylaxis. Since recommendations for all possible clinical situations are impossible to develop, practitioners must use their clinical judgment when special circumstances exist. Despite antibiotic prophylaxis, dentists should be alert to unusual clinical events when providing care for patients at risk.

DIABETES

It is estimated that there are between four and five million people in the United States who have diabetes mellitus, but only half of them are aware of their condition. Almost one out of ten patients over 65 years of age can be expected to have the disease. A general practitioner with a patient load of 2000 can expect about 40 of them to be diabetics. The complications of diabetes seriously compromise the quality of life and contribute to early death, but both morbidity and mortality can be influenced by early diagnosis and subsequent control of the disease. Uncontrolled diabetic patients have increased susceptibility to develop infection, exaggerated response to existing infection, and delayed healing of surgical wounds, all of which are relevant to dental practice. In addition, controlled diabetics can easily lose their controlled status through actions of the dentist. One manifestation of such loss may be acute episodes occurring in the dental office. Thus, general practitioners have ample motivation to prepare themselves to deal with diabetes in daily practice.

Identification. The patient who denies knowledge of diabetes on the health questionnaire but has the cardinal symptoms of diabetes (increased thirst and urination, increased eating—often with weight loss) should be assumed to be diabetic. Patients with milder forms of undetected disease require more discriminating judgment. The decision that diabetes may exist will depend upon the severity or the number of the following factors that are present: 1. repeated skin infection, especially difficulty with frequent boils; 2. blurred vision; 3. marked irritability; 4. paresthesias; 5. headache; 6. increased drinking, urinating, and eating; 7. age over

40; 8. obesity; and 9. a history of relatives with diabetes.

Dentists will wish to explore these items carefully, especially if their index of suspicion of diabetes is increased owing to the presence of some or all of the following oral findings: 1. generalized periodontal disease that appears more advanced than expected in a patient of that age or that suggests an exaggerated soft tissue response to the level of oral hygiene observed; 2. multiple periodontal abscesses; 3. burning tongue; and 4. dry mouth.

The Dentist's Response. Patients with frank signs and symptoms of diabetes should be referred, without delay, to a physician for assessment and treatment. All of the comments related to identification should be considered when the dentist decides whether a patient being treated for known diabetes should be referred to a physician for follow-up.

Having identified known diabetes, the primary interest of the dentist is in learning the extent to which the disease is controlled and the stability of that control. Toward that end, the following information is pertinent:

1. Is the diabetes being treated through diet control or with drugs?
2. Is insulin required more than once a day?
3. Have there been recent changes in the level of insulin or the amount of oral drugs prescribed?
4. Have there been episodes of unconsciousness (insulin shock) during the past year?

Information on stability is important to consider as the dental management of the patient is planned. Patients who appear to be poorly controlled, who are no longer symptom-free, or who have not seen their physician for an extended period of time should be referred to a physician for follow-up.

Diabetes that occurs in young people (frequently under the age of 25) has a sudden onset, is more acute in its clinical course, and is characteristically brittle, i.e, there is great difficulty in maintaining a controlled blood glucose level through drug therapy. When patients with this form of the disease are identified, even if symptom-free, the dentist should consult with the physician before embarking on a course of treatment. Patients with the adult-onset type of diabetes who are under good medical control and who are free of symptoms can proceed with their dental treatment.

Office Management of the Diabetic Patient. Known diabetics are engaged in a battle to control the level of their blood glucose every day of their lives. Dental disease and dental treatment represent a significant threat. The primary goal of the dentist in managing the diabetic patient is to minimize that threat.

The daily level of a diabetic patient's blood glucose is controlled through achieving a balance between caloric intake, exercise, and drug therapy. The dentist is in a position to influence significantly two of these factors. Consider the scenario of diabetic patients who arise in nervous anticipation of a midmorning dental appointment. They religiously take their insulin but, because of nervousness or discomfort, fail to eat a usual breakfast. After a 45-minute wait in the dental office, it can be reliably predicted that they are in glucose imbalance. If their hypoglycemia is severe enough, they may experience anxiety, sweating, headache, disorientation, or motor disturbances while in the dental chair. Their symptoms may proceed to mild convulsions, and they may go into insulin shock. Let us assume that such patients and their dentists recognize the symptoms of an insulin reaction, and orange juice or any available sugar-containing drink is consumed to ward off the reaction. The patients recover sufficiently to complete an abbreviated dental procedure and are told to go home and rest. Because of residual local anesthesia, they find it difficult to eat at lunch time. After resting throughout the afternoon they eat a very light dinner because of soreness in their mouths, further contributing to a glucose imbalance that has existed most of the day.

Obviously, this hypothetical scenario should be avoided. Although routine elective dentistry should be delayed in the diabetic known to be uncontrolled, patients whose glucose intake is balanced can comfortably receive routine care if managed properly. It should be emphasized that they must take both their insulin and a normal level of calories at breakfast. The dentist should confirm that both were achieved. Their appointments should be scheduled 1 to 2 hours after breakfast. If the procedure is one that can be expected to interfere with eating, patients must be counseled regarding their diets. As the length and complexity of the dentistry being performed increases, the attention given to these management procedures must intensify.

If a diabetic whose control is known to be highly unstable requires surgery, it is recommended that the general practitioner refer the patient to an oral surgeon who can decide whether the procedure should be performed in the hospital. A similar recommendation applies to any diabetic who requires treatment for a severe infection of dental origin.

HEPATITIS

This section deals exclusively with hepatitis resulting from exposure to the hepatitis B virus, the form of the disease that is most common and by far the most significant to the general practitioner. During the decade ending in 1976, there was a 1000 per cent increase in reported cases of hepatitis B. The number of cases reported during 1977 was twice that recorded during 1973. During the 1972 annual session of the American Dental Association, 13.6 per cent of 1200 dentists who volunteered for screening presented evidence of prior infection as shown by B virus serum antibodies. Positive tests for antibodies were four times greater in dentists than among a comparable sample of first-time volunteer blood donors. It is estimated that up to 10 per cent of individuals infected become chronic carriers of the hepatitis B surface antigen (HB_sAg) with variable degrees of infectivity. In one study, 1 per cent of dentists and 2.3 per cent of oral surgeons were identified as carriers.

Transmission of the disease is primarily by parenteral inoculation with contaminated blood. As little as 0.00001 to 0.0000001 ml of infectious blood may transmit the disease. Dental personnel with the inevitable minute nicks or cuts on the hands are clearly at risk. The role of saliva in transmission is less well defined, and contagiousness by this route is probably low. It is nonetheless significant that over half of patients with antigen-positive serum also reveal antigen in their saliva.

General dental practitioners have a twofold interest in hepatitis: first, to be certain that their offices are not a source of transmission of the disease from one patient to another; and second, to minimize the risk of exposing personnel in the dental office to the disease. Strict attention to these interests must dominate the approach taken in managing all patients, a small percentage of whom will surely have a history of hepatitis.

General practitioners cannot isolate themselves from the problem of dealing with this disease.

The increase in hepatitis in the population has been accompanied by an increase in clinical and laboratory research related to the disease and its management. This is a dynamic field with new and clinically significant literature appearing on an almost monthly basis. General practitioners who do not keep abreast of the current literature, through reading or attending scientific meetings, will quickly find their approach to hepatitis in day-to-day practice outdated.

Identification. It is unlikely that the dentist will be the first to identify undetected hepatitis. Patients with jaundice (first detectable in the sclera) are obviously suspect. Jaundice, however, is preceded by several weeks of a prodromal phase of flulike symptoms that may include nausea, vomiting, malaise, and fever. If the prodromal phase is mild, it will probably not be identified by the dentist. Frequently, it is sufficiently severe to prompt a visit to the physician.

Approximately 5 per cent of patients with acute hepatitis develop a chronic active hepatitis that may persist for a prolonged period, with signs and symptoms of chronic liver disease. The dentist must be alert for such patients.

From a practical viewpoint, the dentist will probably identify hepatitis through the medical history. It should be noted that most patients will readily report a history of hepatitis, but some, whose candor in the past has resulted in their being denied dental treatment, will intentionally fail to report having had the disease. For such patients, questions on the health questionnaire regarding past hospitalizations and recent care by a physician become particularly relevant.

The Dentist's Response. Any jaundiced patient should be referred to a physician for assessment immediately.

The response of the dentist to patients with a recent (within 10 years) history of hepatitis may change within the next few years because of advances in the field, but at the present time the only responsible reaction is to establish at once that their serum is hepatitis B surface antigen–negative. Even if the hepatitis occurred 5 to 10 years ago and if such patients have been free of any symptoms in the interim, it is in the best interest of the patients and the dentist to establish that they are serum-negative. Frequently, the answer is readily available through consultation, perhaps by phone, with the physician or health facility used by the patients. If the status of their serum is not a matter of record, then these patients must be referred for a radioimmunoassay (RIA) test. Such referral can, of course, be made to a physician, but as an exception to an earlier recommendation, this is a circumstance in which it is logical for the referral to be made directly to a commercial laboratory.

If such patients are serum-negative, usually reported as "negative for hepatitis," they can be treated as normal patients. If their serum is positive, they must be questioned carefully to establish that there are no signs and symptoms indicative of chronic active hepatitis. In the absence of any indication of disease, these patients are thereafter designated as heptatis B carriers.

Although there have been reports of patients remaining hepatitis B surface antigen–positive for many years without symptoms of liver disease, such cases are rare, and there is little justification for demanding laboratory tests on a patient whose episode of hepatitis occurred more than 15 years ago and who has been free of recurrent episodes or symptoms such as cirrhosis since that time.

Office Management of the Patient With Hepatitis.   The patient who has had hepatitis in the past and is not a carrier can be treated in a routine manner in the dental office. The patient with active hepatitis should receive emergency care only. If the emergency cannot be handled conservatively through drugs to control pain and infection, the patient should be referred to an oral surgeon or to a hospital dental service.

The special challenge for the general practitioner is in the management of the hepatitis carrier. The simplest way is to refuse to treat the patient. Such an approach may have legal implications but, more importantly, hepatitis carriers cannot be abandoned by the dental profession. In some cities there are hospital-based dental clinics where arrangements have been made for managing routine dental care for carriers. Some dental societies have identified dentists who have recovered from hepatitis and have permanent immunity as evidenced by serum levels of antibodies (anti-HB$_s$).

If the hepatitis carrier cannot be responsibly referred, the dentist should provide treatment while taking the following special precautions: The dentist and the assistant must wear face masks and gloves and have their eyes protected; a rubber dam should be used if possible; aseptic technique should be employed; and the air syringe should be used judiciously. Consideration should be given to use of the slow-speed handpiece. Following the appointment, special attention must be directed to cleaning and sterilizing instruments and handpieces as well as the light handle and other contaminated surfaces.

The special dilemma that hepatitis provides for the dentist has not yet been mentioned. Great emphasis is placed upon the carrier even with the knowledge that less than 10 per cent of hepatitis patients end up as carriers and that, by and large, carriers are not highly infectious. Antigen-positive serum in active disease is much more contagious. The dilemma stems from the fact that the incubation period for hepatitis is 2 to 6 months and that *the antigen appears in the serum up to 2 months before the onset of any clinical symptoms.* This fact is used by many to support their opinion that dentists should wear masks and gloves routinely. Regardless of how the practitioner reacts to that suggestion, there is strong motivation for every practitioner to scrutinize critically the sterilization and aseptic techniques that are employed routinely in the office. There should be no difference in those routine techniques and those employed in dealing with the hepatitis carrier.

Dentists or office personnel may experience an acute exposure to hepatitis B, e.g., an accidental cut or needle stick while working on a patient who has active hepatitis or who is a known carrier. In the event of acute exposure, it is recommended that hepatitis B immune globulin be administered as soon as possible (at least within 2 to 3 days) followed by a booster shot 1 month later.

A vaccine said to be highly effective against hepatitis B has been developed and is available for general use. It holds excellent promise for dealing with postexposure prevention of the disease. There is reason for optimism that a vaccine will be developed that can be administered prophylactically to all dental personnel, thereby conferring permanent immunity. Until that time, dealing with hepatitis remains a challenge for the general practitioner.

COAGULATION DISORDERS

An abnormal tendency for the patient to bleed excessively is obviously an important problem. The systemic conditions that can contribute to bleeding disorders are many, and the mechanisms that affect coagulation adversely are complex. Although not common, these problems are of such significance that some comment is warranted. The conditions under consideration are not those systemic conditions that predispose to easy or spontaneous hemorrhage (the thrombocytopenic and nonthrombocytopenic purpuras), but rather those associated with disorders in the mechanisms by which bleeding is controlled.

Identification. There is no question about whether general dentists will identify a coagulation disorder. The only question is whether they will make the identification by way of the patient's history of by way of an unpleasant clinical experience. By and large, the choice is up to the dentist. It is possible that an acquired disorder may develop and be undetected until difficulties are encountered during dental treatment. Most disorders, however, are inherited or are chronic in their onset, so that the existence of a problem has been recognized by the patient.

The patient who reports abnormal bleeding associated with previous extractions must be questioned carefully. Such a response is common and most frequently reveals an exaggerated response to an unpleasant experience or postoperative trauma to the extraction site. Significant abnormal bleeding is that which continues for many hours following any laceration, often requiring special procedures for its control. A history of blood transfusions may be the most important indicator that a bleeding disorder exists.

The Dentist's Response. If upon taking the medical history the dentist identifies a bleeding disorder, a consultation with a physician for additional information is warranted. If the disorder is confirmed, the general dental practitioner should refer the patient to an oral surgeon or other specialist for any surgical procedure. If deep periodontal scaling or periodontal surgery is required, it should be performed in a hospital environment.

Office Management of Patients with Bleeding Disorders. Although special care must be exercised, all nonsurgical procedures can be handled routinely. Special attention must be directed to a treatment plan that assures preservation of the teeth in order that extractions may be avoided. Elective surgery, e.g., third molar extractions, is contraindicated. Should an undetected coagulation disorder result in an abnormal bleeding episode, referral to an oral surgeon for control of the hemorrhage is indicated.

QUESTIONS

1. Any patient who reports having had hypertension, heart disease, or diabetes should be referred to a physician for medical clearance before dental treatment is begun. True or false?

2. The clinical observation of signs and symptoms is more important than the medical history in identifying systemic illness in dental patients. True or false?

3. What are the highest systolic and diastolic blood pressure readings that can be accepted as being in the normal range?

4. What is the predominant objective in the management of hypertensive patients in the dental office?

5. The dentist should be suspicious of what systemic condition when a patient enters the office out of breath? What is the cause of the dyspnea?

6. What is the difference between postural hypotension and orthopnea?

7. What drugs used in treating what disease can create difficulties with postural hypotension in dental patients?

8. Local anesthetics containing epinephrine should be used in patients with cardiovascular disease. True or false?

9. How long following a heart attack should the dentist wait before providing routine dental care?

10. The patient suffering an anginal attack in the dentist's office should be suspected of hav-

ing a heart attack if his pain persists for how long following administration of nitroglycerin?

11. A routine prophylaxis, if carefully performed, does not require antibiotic prophylaxis in patients with rheumatic heart disease. True or false?

12. What is the predominant objective in the management of diabetic patients in the dental office?

13. Diabetes occurring in older people can be expected to present fewer management problems for the dentist than that occurring in young people. True or false?

14. In dealing with diabetics whose blood glucose levels are difficult to control, is it too much or too little insulin that is likely to create greater problems for the dentist?

15. What is the predominant objective in dealing with hepatitis in the dental office?

16. Any patient with hepatitis B surface antigen in his or her blood is a hepatitis carrier. True or false?

17. There is no reason for dentists to be concerned about patients who have no history of hepatitis and are totally free of any symptoms of the disease. True or false?

18. Which three of the following diseases are most likely to be undetected when they exist in patients coming to the dental office: hepatitis, hypertension, rheumatic fever, diabetes, heart disease, coagulation disorders?

19. The drugs used in the treatment of which three of the following diseases are of the most significance in dental management: hepatitis, hypertension, rheumatic fever, diabetes, coagulation disorders, myocardial infarction, angina pectoris?

20. Under no circumstances should dental treatment be provided for patients whose systolic blood pressure is over 190. True or false?

See answers in Appendix.

REFERENCES

1. Lynch, M. A.: Oral Medicine, Diagnosis and Treatment, 7th ed. Philadelphia, J. B. Lippincott Co., 1977.
2. Little, J. W., and Falace, D. A.: Dental Management of the Medically Compromised Patient. St. Louis, C. V. Mosby Co., 1980.
3. Bodak-Gyovai, L. Z., and Manzione, J. V.: Oral Medicine, Patient Evaluation and Management. Baltimore, Williams & Wilkins, 1980.
4. Accepted Dental Therapeutics, 38th ed. Chicago, Council on Dental Therapeutics, American Dental Association, 1979.
5. Physician's Desk Reference, 36th ed. Oradell, N.J., Medical Economics Company, Inc., 1982.
6. National High Blood Pressure Education Program. Report of the Joint National Committee on Detection, Evaluation and Treatment of High Blood Pressure. Bethesda, Md., National Institutes of Health, Publication No. 81–1088, 1980.
7. Hypertension. J. Prev. Dent., 68:162–193, 1980.
8. Kaplan, N. K.: The control of hypertension: A therapeutic breakthrough. Am. Sci., 68:537–545, 1980.
9. Kaplan, E. L.: Prevention of bacterial endocarditis. Circulation, 56:139A–143A, 1977.
10. Rothstein, S. S., Goldman, H. S., and Arcomano, A. S.: Hepatitis B virus: An overview for dentists, J. Am. Dent. Assoc. 102:173–176, 1981.
11. Sachs, H. L.: Dentistry and hepatitis B: The legal risks. J. Am. Dent. Assoc. 102:177–179, 1981.
12. Shields, W. B.: Dentistry and the issue of hepatitis B. J. Am. Dent. Assoc. 102:180–182, 1981.
13. Alexander, R. E.: Hepatitis risk: A clinical perspective, J. Am. Dent. Assoc. 102:182–185, 1981.
14. Rothstein, S. S., and Goldman, H. S.: Sterilizing and disinfecting for hepatitis B virus in the dental operatory. Clin. Prev. Dent., 2:9–14, 1980.

DANIEL P. CASULLO

4

DIAGNOSIS AND TREATMENT PLANNING IN GENERAL PRACTICE

The practice of general dentistry will become increasingly demanding from the standpoints of diagnosis, treatment planning, ensuring high-quality care, and assuming the responsibility for the overall management of patient care. While the vast majority of dental care will continue to be provided by the general practitioner, much will be provided in conjunction with the dental specialist. The diagnosis and treatment planning skills of the general dentist are of great import, since he is coordinator of total patient care.

The gathering, deciphering, and organizing of data to make accurate diagnoses, to formulate integrated treatment plans, and to recognize problems that would be best treated by the specialist make diagnosis and treatment planning a challenging procedure. Treatment planning cannot be dictated by a prescribed set of rules; it is a highly individualized process. Every patient has unique desires, complaints, and financial resources while exhibiting varying degrees of disease, deformity, and abnormality. Every dentist has a unique perspective on patient care, a specific range of technical skills and a particular personal demeanor. Nevertheless, a treatment plan must evolve that will recognize health, identify disease, assess patient needs, and then coordinate and make treatment procedures sequential to ensure a functionally healthy dentition. Use of guidelines and devices, along with the exercise of sound clinical judgment, should result in a viable, rational, and effective treatment plan designed to satisfy the requirements of both patient and doctor.

GOALS

The purpose of this chapter is to present fundamental principles and organizational devices that may be applied to the development of any dental treatment plan. This will include (1) a discussion of a philosophy of treatment based upon disease versus health and patient complaints, (2) an interdisciplinary (organizational) treatment planning worksheet, (3) a procedure for planning the sequence of therapy, and (4) presentation and illustration of these basic principles.

FORMULATING A TREATMENT PLAN

Interdisciplinary Treatment Planning Worksheet

An interdisciplinary treatment planning worksheet is a useful heuristic device that allows the clinician to organize patient data in a clear, concise fashion (Fig. 4–1). It aids in the systematic assessment of individual problems as they relate to the development of appropriate treatment. The interdisciplinary worksheet organizes the significant medical and dental history, records patient complaints and desires, and records information exchanged between clinician and patient and clinician and specialist. This interdisciplinary worksheet is an adjunct to the routine use of radiographs, study models, and complete medical history. If the problems of the patient are dominated by one or more

105

specific entities such as periodontal disease, occlusal disease, temporomandibular joint pain and/or restorative dentistry, the clinician can record all data on a worksheet record designed for that specific entity.

The clinician would then transfer all significant findings on the interdisciplinary worksheet in order to organize and correlate data and to finalize the treatment plan. During the actual treatment session and re-evaluation phases of therapy, the clinician would refer to the detailed records designed for the specific area. However, when patient needs are relatively simple, there is no need to use specialty charts or worksheets (i.e., periodontal or occlusal chartings). Data can be recorded directly on the interdisciplinary worksheet.

Patient Name_____ DATE_____

SIGNIFICANT MEDICAL AND SYSTEMIC DISEASE OR CONDITION

_____

SIGNIFICANT DENTAL/SOCIAL HISTORY

Chief dental complaint and history_____

_____

Other complaints:

    Mastication_____ Aesthetics_____

    Comfort_____ Phonetics_____

Understanding of dental problem_____

_____

_____

Desires_____

Attitude_____

Age_____ Gender_____ Occupation_____Financial Resources_____

Other Considerations_____

CONSULTATIONS WITH DENTAL SPECIALISTS OR PHYSICIAN

_____

SIGNIFICANT SIGNS, SYMPTOMS AND ETIOLOGY OF DISEASE AND SIGNIFICANT MECHANICAL FACTORS

Caries

_____

Pulpal Disease

_____

Inflammatory
Periodontal Disease

_____

Occlusal
Traumatism

_____

Severe Wear

_____

Significant
Mechanical Factors

_____

TMJ Dysfunction
and Other Oral
Disease

FIGURE 4–1   Interdisciplinary Treatment Planning Worksheet. The interdisciplinary treatment planning worksheet is a simple device for organizing all patient data and for formulating an ideal treatment plan and any required alternative therapy.

Illustration continued on opposite page

IDEAL TREATMENT PLAN   Patient Name_____Date_____

ALTERNATIVE TREATMENT PLANS

RATIONALE FOR ACTUAL TREATMENT PLAN

FINANCIAL ARRANGEMENTS

FIGURE 4–1 *Continued*

Medical History

Past or present systemic disease can interfere with host resistance, thereby compromising the ability of the clinician to establish or maintain health, and can jeopardize the long-term survival of the dentition. Recognition of and appropriate attention to compromising medical disorders are fundamental to successful treatment planning. (The reader is referred to Chapter 3, Oral Medicine in General Practice, for discussion of the most prevalent medical conditions that influence treatment.)

Dental and Social History

The clinician must record the patient's priorities and complaints, and the reason for the visit as well as the past dental history. An important consideration, often overlooked by clinicians, is the patient's subjective esthetic and functional requirements. During the examination process, the dentist and staff members have the opportunity to observe and to interpret patient behavior and attitudes. Many patients have a great awareness of what dentistry can offer, whereas others are ignorant of what is required for good dental care. It is important to record impressions and speculations about the patient's fears, emotional stability, financial resources, and degree of dental awareness. This information can help the clinician determine whether a patient will make a serious commitment to treatment and maintenance care.

In the dental history, previous dental treatment that has altered natural structures and their self-protecting relationship has the potential to interfere with the adaptive capacity of the tissue and to compromise the future health of a dentition. Some of the more common undesirable results associated with dental treatment are (1) in restorative dentistry: masking of caries by cast restorations and interferences with oral hygiene (Fig. 4–2); (2) in periodontal surgery: exposure of the labial plate or bone, dehiscences and fenestrations, exposure of root surfaces, root caries, and sensitivity; (3) in orthodontics: blunted or shortened roots, gingival clefts, periodontal defects, relapse, and interference with oral hygiene (Figs. 4–3, 4–4); (4) in endodontics: overinstrumentation,

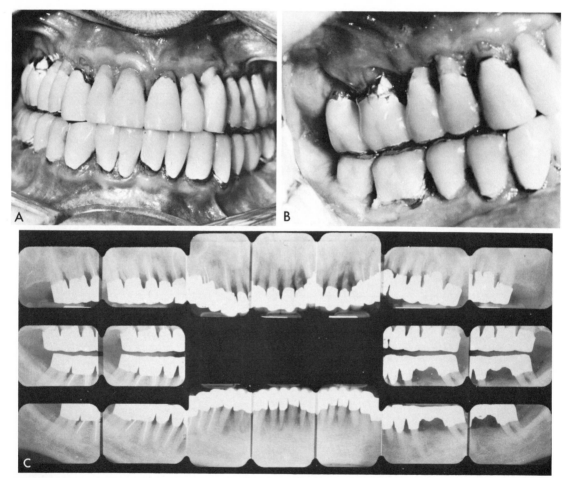

FIGURE 4–2 Complications Associated With Restorative Dentistry. *A,* The complex restorative dentistry rendered in the full mouth reconstruction of this 54-year-old patient failed after 4 years. *B,* Right buccal view. *C,* Extensive disease is evidenced by advanced bone loss, periapical radiolucencies, and severe root caries. Sophisticated restorative dentistry places an enormous burden on both patient and doctor to maintain the health of the dentition. The determination of the cause of failure is critical in an analysis of etiology and subsequent treatment.

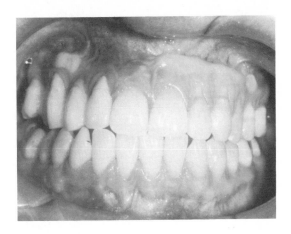

FIGURE 4–3 Loss of Periodontal Structures Associated With Orthodontics. Extended orthodontic treatment and periodontal surgery were completed in this 20-year-old patient with thin and friable gingival tissues. Advanced recession with root exposure resulted.

perforations, and root fractures; (5) in occlusal adjustment: induced occlusal awareness and tooth sensitivity.

Ideally, the goal of all dental practitioners is the prevention of disease and the preservation of the natural dentition. The goal of the treatment plan is to enhance the prognosis for long-term survival and function of both the natural dentition and artificial prostheses. Prevention, in general practice,

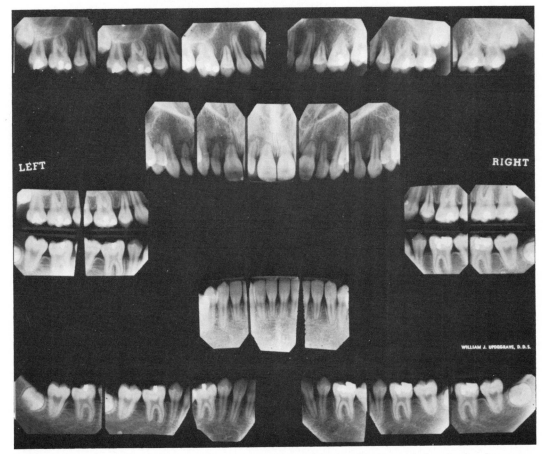

FIGURE 4–4 Loss of Root Structure Associated With Orthodontics. Extended orthodontic treatment in this 15-year-old patient resulted in blunted roots and a poor crown-to-root ratio.

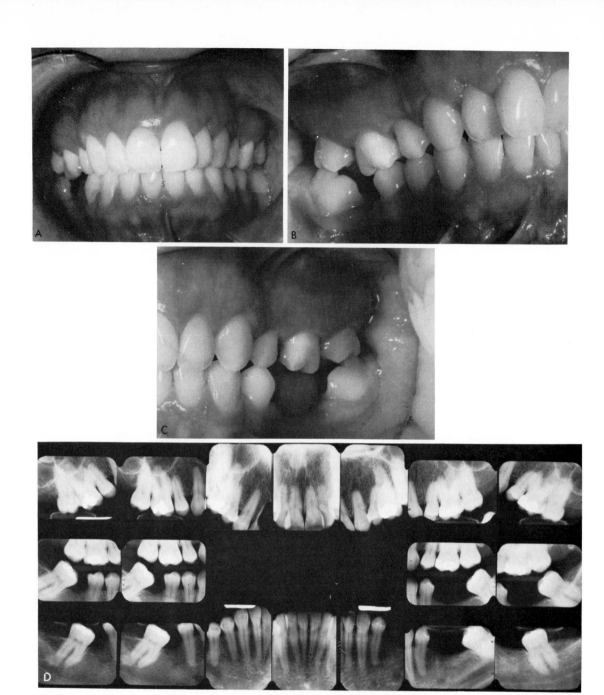

FIGURE 4–5 Physiologic Occlusion Associated With Multiple Missing Teeth and Occlusal Aberrations. *A,* This is a healthy dentition of a highly resistant 34-year-old patient. No signs or symptoms of disease or patient complaints were associated with this physiologic occlusion in spite of multiple missing teeth and occlusal deformities. *B,* The right buccal view shows the aberrations in form due to loss of molars. *C,* The lower left molars and premolars were lost at age 14; the maxillary second molars were extracted at age 20, when orthodontic treatment was instituted to correct crowding of the maxillary anterior teeth. Posterior tooth loss and malpositioning has caused aberrations in occlusal morphology with consequent interferences in protrusive and lateral-protrusive movements. *D,* The radiographic picture, demonstrating a healthy attachment apparatus, confirms the absence of a clinical indication of disease. This physiologic occlusion requires maintenance therapy only.

is directed not only to avoid the onset of disease but also to avoid overzealous and unwarranted treatment. Past dental history must be studiously considered before any new diagnosis can be made.

Clinical Examination: Recognition of Signs and Symptoms of Disease

The dental examination includes an analysis of each component of the masticatory

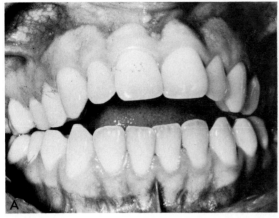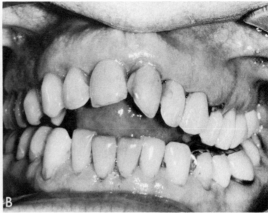

FIGURE 4–6   The Physiologic Class II, Division I Malocclusion. *A,* The occlusal relations and morphology that characterize the Class II, Division I malocclusion unquestionably create an environment that is not conducive to health. Nevertheless, if the occlusion is physiologic, there is no reason to intervene therapeutically. Treatment would be prophylactic and is contraindicated for this 34-year-old patient. *B,* This is the physiologic occlusion of a 77-year-old patient with a Class II, Division I malocclusion, demonstrating that with high resistance, severe occlusal aberrations do not preclude the possibility of the long-term survival of the dentition.

system. The physiologic occlusion or physiologic masticatory system (Fig. 4–5) is one that is surviving in health, although it may not conform to a preconceived idea of normal or ideal.[1] Therefore, when a patient exhibits healthy dentition, manifests no signs or symptoms of disease, and has no complaints or discomfort about appearance, phonetics, or mastication, treatment is contraindicated even though the masticatory system may not be ideal. Often, clinicians find aberrations in occlusal morphology or relationships in the adult patient. However, if those abnormalities have not caused or contributed to disease or dissatisfied the patient, then treating them prophylactically is unwarranted. For example, a patient may present with a skeletal-dental deformity such as the Class II, Division I malocclusion yet manifest no signs or symptoms of disease and have no complaints (Fig. 4–6). In such an instance, treatment is not indicated.

Examination analysis should eliminate all factors not associated with specific disease processes, and include all clinical signs and subjective symptoms that indicate the presence and severity of disease and influence the feasibility of treatment.

Diagnosis of Disease

Diagnosis is the process of defining a specific disease based on analysis of the host tissue response to etiologic factors. A specific diagnosis describes the extent and location of the tissue injury in relation to the etiologic factors identified. The verification of correct diagnoses and treatment is determined by the elimination of all etiologic factors and the alleviation and correction of the accompanying signs and symptoms of disease.

The dental diseases most often seen in general practice include caries, pulpal disease, plaque-induced periodontal disease, occlusal trauma, severe wear, and TMJ dysfunction. The extent and diagnosis of each disease entity and significant mechanical factors should be recorded as completely as possible. Table 4–1 lists some of the most common signs and symptoms of disease and significant mechanical factors, which can be recorded on the interdisciplinary treatment-planning worksheet.

Identification of Mechanical Factors

To ignore or dismiss the mechanical factors of occlusion and their influence on the correction of disease can lead to frustrating and disastrous results. In planning treatment of the mechanical phase of therapy, one should give primary consideration to the health of the remaining teeth and their periodontal support. The presence of a severe malocclusion as well as the quality and quantity of the remaining attachment is extremely important, since the correlation of severe malocclusion to advanced disease and required tooth replacement devices has made treatment quite complex (see Chapter 8, Oc-

TABLE 4–1   Examples of Common Significant Findings To Be Recorded on the Interdisciplinary Treatment-Planning Worksheet

Periodontal Disease	Caries	Pulpal Disease	Occlusal Traumatism	Wear	TMJ Dysfunction	Mechanical Factors
Diagnosis	Caries	Pain	Diagnosis	Flattened occlusal surfaces or incisal edges	Head and neck pain	Malocclusions
Plaque and calculus deposits	Sensitivity	Sensitivity to hot and cold	Mobility and fremitus patterns			Malposed teeth
Inflammation	Poor home care	Sensitivity to percussion	Parafunctional habits	Cosmetic complaint	Clicking	Missing teeth
Bleeding	Questionable restorations	Fractured roots	Interferences	Crown fracture	Crepitus	Posterior landmark relations
Suppuration	Nutritional factors	Radiographic radiolucency	Sensitivity	Interferences	Limited mandibular opening	
Edema		Broken instruments or posts	Widened PDL space	Parafunctional habits	Mandibular deviation	Anterior tooth guidance relations
Soft tissue deformities		Fistulas	Loss of definition and continuity of the lamina dura	Sensitivity or pain	Parafunctional habits	Inadequate restorations
Pocket depths		Sinus tract	Root resorption	Exposed dentin	Interferences	Abutment teeth; strategic location and periodontal support
Recession		Interferences	Root fractures		Negative radiographic signs	
Furcation involvements		Parafunctional habits				Deficient edentulous ridges
Mobility and fremitus patterns		Resorption (internal and external)				Abnormal plane of occlusion
Poor home care						Aberrant curves of occlusion
Inadequate nutrition						
Loss of definition and continuity of the alveolar bone						

clusion in General Practice). Tooth replacement devices must be utilized very judiciously. The main criteria for replacing missing teeth are to treat disease and to treat patient complaints about appearance, phonetics, and mastication.

The Ideal Treatment Plan

The final stages of treatment planning require the interpretation of all data gathered during the examination and communication process. The interdisciplinary treatment-

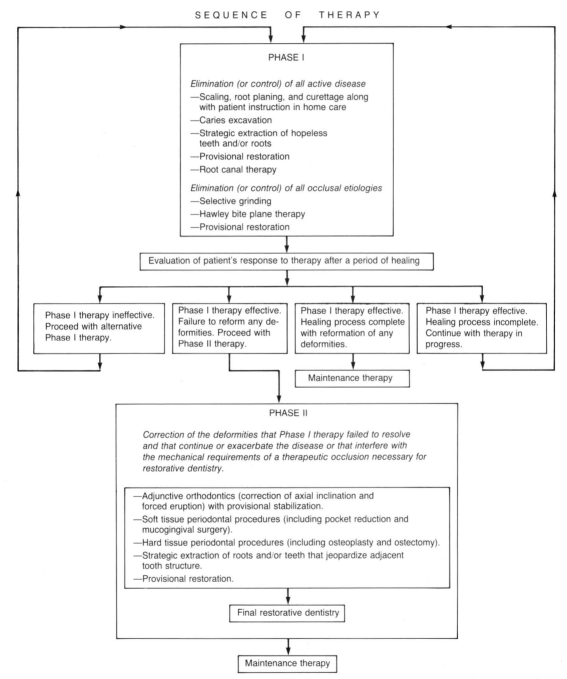

SEQUENCE OF THERAPY

PHASE I

Elimination (or control) of all active disease
—Scaling, root planing, and curettage along with patient instruction in home care
—Caries excavation
—Strategic extraction of hopeless teeth and/or roots
—Provisional restoration
—Root canal therapy

Elimination (or control) of all occlusal etiologies
—Selective grinding
—Hawley bite plane therapy
—Provisional restoration

Evaluation of patient's response to therapy after a period of healing

| Phase I therapy ineffective. Proceed with alternative Phase I therapy. | Phase I therapy effective. Failure to reform any deformities. Proceed with Phase II therapy. | Phase I therapy effective. Healing process complete with reformation of any deformities. | Phase I therapy effective. Healing process incomplete. Continue with therapy in progress. |

Maintenance therapy

PHASE II

Correction of the deformities that Phase I therapy failed to resolve and that continue or exacerbate the disease or that interfere with the mechanical requirements of a therapeutic occlusion necessary for restorative dentistry.

—Adjunctive orthodontics (correction of axial inclination and forced eruption) with provisional stabilization.
—Soft tissue periodontal procedures (including pocket reduction and mucogingival surgery).
—Hard tissue periodontal procedures (including osteoplasty and ostectomy).
—Strategic extraction of roots and/or teeth that jeopardize adjacent tooth structure.
—Provisional restoration.

Final restorative dentistry

Maintenance therapy

FIGURE 4–7 Sequence of Therapy. The sequence of therapy is an organized representation of the basic principles of therapy. It is a guide for the formulation of the patient treatment plan, requiring the integration of the various dental disciplines.

planning worksheet is studied in conjunction with other diagnostic materials such as study models, photographs, radiographs, and consultation records in order to formulate the ideal treatment plan. The formulation and sequencing of treatment should be directed toward the ideal treatment plan, that unique combination of treatment modalities and the sequence of therapy that will prevent, eliminate, and control disease most effectively and maximize the healing, regeneration, and preservation of all tissues. The ideal treatment plan provides the basis for alternative treatment plans. In many situations, a treatment plan may be formulated and accepted at one visit; in more complex situations, it is best to gather all data, exchange information with the patient and consulting specialists, and then schedule an appointment to discuss a proposed ideal treatment plan as well as any appropriate alternative plan.

The Alternative Treatment Plan

Alternative treatment plans are more difficult to formulate because of the restraints put on the clinician and what he feels is best for the long-term survival of the patient's dentition. If finances are the primary restraint, materials and methods of tooth replacement and the extent of any prostheses can be changed. If other complicating factors such as time, health, or patient attitude necessitate the use of an alternative plan, other aspects of treatment can be amended.

The alternative treatment plan should be based on the fundamentals presented in the sequence of therapy (Fig. 4–7). The first phase of therapy prevents the further breakdown of tissues, regains patient function and comfort, and maintains the dentition in a condition optimal for the second phase of therapy. At the very least, all alternative treatment plans should include Phase I therapy and rigorous maintenance therapy.

SEQUENCE OF THERAPY

The sequence of therapy is divided into three phases. The first phase includes communication between the doctor and the patient, treatment planning, and the elimination or control of all active disease. The second phase of therapy is implemented to correct any remaining deformities that cause or contribute to the perpetuation of disease. The third phase concerns the ongoing maintenance of dental health. Inadequate maintenance can lead to the recurrence of disease, resulting in extensive loss of teeth and supporting structures. Subsequent treatment becomes difficult to execute as poor maintenance jeopardizes the long-term survival of the entire dentition. Therefore, all treatment planning and treatment must incorporate the continuous maintenance of health for the prevention of disease and for the preservation of the natural dentition and of prosthetic devices.

The principles of establishing the optimal sequence of therapy are fundamental, logical, and consistently applicable. Naturally, emergencies involving acute pain or tooth avulsion are treated first. Lesions of suspicious origin, salivary gland or duct abnormality, swelling, and head or neck pain are also managed immediately by the dentist, and, if necessary, the patient is referred to an appropriate specialist for diagnostic tests before any treatment is initiated.

Phase I Therapy

After all emergency procedures are performed, it is time to evaluate the patient's desires, complaints, and ability to overcome any fear of dental treatment. Philosophically, Phase I therapy represents procedures that are necessary for the patient's well-being and dental health. In practice, Phase I takes into account the attitude of the patient while using conservative measures to promote maximal healing, regeneration, and preservation of the natural dentition and its supporting structures. Phase I therapy saves teeth with a questionable prognosis and often eliminates the need for advanced periodontal surgical procedures as well as minimizing the need for extractions and complex restorative therapy.

Throughout Phase I therapy, frequent reevaluations are scheduled at appropriate intervals to assess the patient's response to treatment and to revise the planned sequence of therapy. For example, as Phase I progresses, rapidly healing tissue may dramatically eliminate the need for a particular procedure, while tissue that fails to heal will necessitate additional Phase I or Phase II therapy.

After attending emergency situations, Phase I therapy begins with patient instruction in oral hygiene and general dental health education. Following successful patient education, scaling, root planing, soft tissue curettage, and open-flap curettage (if needed) are instituted to control inflammatory periodontal disease. Caries control, strategic tooth extraction, and root canal therapy are also carried out. Occlusal adjustment via selective grinding and Hawley bite plane and nightguard therapy is used to control excessive forces associated with severe wear, occlusal traumatism, and myofacial pain dysfunction syndrome. Temporary stabilization or provisional crowns during Phase I therapy should be used only when absolutely necessary to control disease.

If therapy is terminated at this stage, soft tissue deformities and osseous craters may remain, missing teeth have not yet been replaced (although the Hawley bite plane with tooth replacements may suffice), and contributing malocclusions have not yet been corrected. However, there has been the control or elimination of active disease during this phase. It is critical that Phase I treatment be completed before the more advanced Phase II treatment is begun. Also critical is the constant monitoring of treatment, since diagnosis and prognosis are tentative until the patient's response to therapy can be observed. If patient desire for, or commitment to, further therapy changes, a disease-free dentition can be maintained indefinitely, and no complex, irreversible procedures will have been initiated.

Phase II Therapy

Phase II therapy, predicated on successful Phase I therapy,* corrects any remaining deformities that may cause or contribute to the perpetuation of disease. Phase II generally involves advanced periodontal procedures, orthodontics, and advanced restorative procedures or all three. Patient commitment should be reascertained prior to the initiation of extensive Phase II treatment.

Adjunctive orthodontics with Hawley bite plane therapy, provisional restorations, soft tissue periodontal therapy including pocket

---

*Phase II therapy should not be executed in the presence of active disease.

reduction and mucogingival surgery, hard tissue periodontal therapy such as osteoplasty and ostectomy, and final restorative dentistry are all Phase II treatment modalities. All final restorative therapy must be planned prior to adjunctive orthodontics and periodontal surgery. If orthodontic treatment is planned, it should be completed prior to Phase II periodontal surgery since orthodontic treatment can ameliorate periodontal defects and soft tissue deformities, reducing the amount of resective periodontal procedures required in the future. Moreover, the need for periodontal surgery should not be assessed until the attachment apparatus has been allowed a period of healing following orthodontic tooth correction. Final restorative therapy is implemented after total re-evaluation of all previous therapy. If any residual problems remain, they must be corrected prior to the final restorative phase of treatment. Provisional restorations must be functioning in a healthy environment prior to the placement of final restorations to ensure success of the final prosthesis and all previous therapy.

Considerations for Establishing a Prognosis

A prognosis is a prediction of the likelihood of recovery from disease and the ability to maintain the corrected environment. The extent and duration of etiologic factors, the amount of disease present, the extent of the deformity created by the disease, the qualitative aspects of dentition (excessive forces, alveolar bone and mobility, root length and form), arch integrity and the number and distribution of the remaining teeth in the occlusal scheme, any influential systemic factors, and the patient's age, manual dexterity, and attitude are all factors that one must consider when establishing a prognosis.

Certain variables can be correlated in developing the prognosis of a single tooth or the entire dentition. Some clinical guidelines should be stated: (1) An older patient with many etiologic factors and advanced disease has a better prognosis than a younger patient with comparable disease and no discernible etiology; (2) the control of any emotional or systemic factors can be very influential in a prognosis; (3) the better the patient's understanding and cooperation, the better the prognosis; (4) as the amount of deformity created by the disease increases, the prognosis worsens; (5) as inflammation, bleeding, and suppuration increase, the more influential the destructive capabilities of excessive forces, interferences, and malocclusion become.[1]

Generally, the prognosis is better in the older of two patients with equal levels of disease and deformity, despite an increased healing time in an older patient. The younger patient is considered more susceptible to disease and, because of the progressive nature of periodontal disease, occlusal disease, and dental caries, will be more likely to experience further breakdown of the involved structures, thus warranting a more guarded prognosis.

PRESENTING THE TREATMENT PLAN TO THE PATIENT

When the treatment plan is presented, the clinician must inform the patient of the following:
1. the current status of the patient's dentition;
2. the prognosis for individual teeth, the entire dentition, and any necessary restorations as well as how the loss of strategically located teeth with questionable prognosis would alter the treatment plan;
3. the rationale for the treatment plan and the planned sequence of therapy;
4. the immediate and long-term benefits of the proposed treatment;
5. the projected duration of treatment; and
6. the estimated cost.

When presenting the ideal treatment plan, the clinician should make certain that the patient fully understands the nature and extent of the problem and the therapy proposed to resolve the problem. It must be made clear that this treatment is what the clinician feels is best for the patient. The patient should be encouraged to voice any concerns or desires and to ask questions. The clinician should then clarify any misconceptions or unrealistic expectations.

With proper education and presentation of data, the patient can better understand his problems and the planned corrective treatment. Patient cooperation and willingness improve the overall prognosis, and, if an alternative treatment plan is tentatively chosen, the educated, informed patient may very well proceed to Phase II therapy in the future.

Rationale for the Actual Treatment Plan

The rationale for a treatment plan consists of a precise explanation of the factors that dictated the choice of that particular plan. The explanation includes the reasons for modification of ideal therapy, among them consideration of modifying influences such as the patient's cooperation, systemic problems, and finances and the judgments made by the clinician regarding individual teeth or dental arches with a questionable prognosis. The rationale for therapy also provides contingency plans to be implemented if teeth with a questionable prognosis are lost. Furthermore, it explains the goals of Phase I therapy and the need for re-evaluation prior to Phase II therapy as well as any instances in which the clinician should not proceed with Phase II therapy.

ILLUSTRATED TECHNIQUES

An illustration of patient care is presented to demonstrate the application of an interdisciplinary treatment-planning worksheet, the basic principles of treatment planning, the sequence of therapy, and the actual treatment. The fundamental principles of patient care are to prevent, eliminate, or control disease and to maintain healthy dentition within the confines of limiting factors. Other considerations in patient care that have a profound effect on treatment planning are establishing a prognosis (especially on questionable teeth), evaluating mechanical factors of occlusion, and choosing the proper restorative therapy (tooth replacement procedures) to enhance the long-term survival of the patient's dentition.

The goal of this section is not to present a myriad of treatment plans but to demonstrate a consistent, logical, and well-organized approach in formulating both the ideal and the alternative treatment plan. It is important to try to visualize the final result and all contingencies of treatment prior to beginning therapy. If the final result cannot be visualized, the alternatives available must be understood and accepted by the clinician and patient. The complexity of the individual patient's problems determines the clinician's ability to visualize and to control the final result. The alternative treatment plan is often the most difficult to formulate owing to all the encumbrances and limitations that are by this point placed on the clinician. In any case, the clinician must conclude therapy in a manner that will ensure a successful maintenance program.

Presentation of Patient Treatment Plans and Treatment

The treatment plans and treatment of six patients are presented. Each presentation demonstrates diverse problems in treatment planning due to a number of complicating variables. The comprehensive treatment-planning worksheet is presented for five of the six patients who presented with extensive problems. The ideal and alternative treatment plans and the rationale for the actual treatment plan have been recorded.

All alternative therapy must eliminate or control disease, dispel patient discomfort, and prevent further deterioration of the dentition via controlled maintenance. The sequence of therapy is based on the treatment plan agreed upon to achieve a result satisfactory to both clinician and patient. The patient care exhibited includes:

1. Management of a patient's dentition with Phase I therapy only.
2. Management of a patient's dentition with Phase I therapy and minimal Phase II therapy.
3. Management of a patient's dentition with Phase I therapy followed by Phase II therapy.
4. Management of a patient's dentition with combined Phase I and Phase II therapy.
5. Management of a severely broken-down tooth and its associated quadrant with Phase II therapy.
6. Management of a patient's dentition in which advanced disease exists with Phase I and Phase II therapy.

Case 1. Management of a Patient's Dentition With Phase I Therapy Only

This patient's care is an example of the diagnosis, treatment planning, and manage-ment of disease using Phase I therapy. Although the ideal treatment plan included Phase II therapy, the actual treatment plan was chosen to accommodate the patient's personal needs as well as the basic principles of therapy.

During routine diagnostic evaluation, the patient expressed unwillingness to undergo anything but rudimentary care, requesting that all remaining teeth be extracted and a full denture be fitted. The most important step in treatment was patient education and awareness.

Past dental history revealed that this 54-year-old patient had worn a maxillary partial denture all his adult life. The central incisors were lost at age 16, and, as other teeth were lost, they were either added to the old removable partial denture or a new removable partial denture was made to include them. The patient had no experience of regular care, and his infrequent visits had been on an emergency basis only.

The first visit required emergency treatment to alleviate pain. Root tips were extracted and a pulpotomy was done on the left lateral incisor. This tooth was eventually extracted because of the patient's financial situation. The patient returned 7 days later and was comfortable and willing to undergo a full set of intraoral radiographs and study models. The following office visits were aimed at motivating and educating the patient. The previous request for a denture was thereby revised and alternatives were sought.

Using the interdisciplinary worksheet (Case 1 Worksheet), an ideal treatment plan was formulated to include endodontics, orthodontics, and possible periodontal treatment as well as extensive restorative therapy. Because of the patient's financial limitations and unwillingness to undergo extensive procedures, an alternative treatment plan using Phase I therapy only was agreed upon. Although compromised, the actual treatment plan proved acceptable to both doctor and patient.

The sequence of treatment included scaling, root planing, caries control, hygiene instruction, and extractions (Fig. 4–8). A new maxillary removable partial denture was fabricated and inserted. The success of initial treatment and the continued maintenance therapy at 4-month intervals during the last 3 years has helped increase patient trust and

Text continued on page 122

INTERDISCIPLINARY TREATMENT PLANNING WORKSHEET

Patient Name___Anthony_____ DATE___9-21-78_____

SIGNIFICANT MEDICAL AND SYSTEMIC DISEASE OR CONDITION
         None

SIFNIFICANT DENTAL/SOCIAL HISTORY

Chief dental complaint and history_"Pain in upper left side of my mouth"   Patient has_
 not been to a dentist in 3 years; wears a maxillary partial denture.

Other complaints:
    Mastication___Not a problem_____ Aesthetics__Wants full dentures___
    Comfort__Pain in maxillary left quadrant_____ Phonetics___Not concerned____
Understanding of dental problem__Patient thinks he will have to lose all his teeth;_
 he has never been taught preventive dentistry.

Desires__Maxillary full denture. He would like all his maxillary teeth extracted._
Attitude_Good, but must be educated and motivated.
Age___54__ Gender__M__ Occupation__Clerk_____ Financial Resources_Limited_
Other Considerations__Patient wants short dental visits and work done quickly.__

CONSULTATIONS WITH DENTAL SPECIALISTS OR PHYSICIAN
         None

SIGNIFICANT SIGNS, SYMPTOMS AND ETIOLOGY OF DISEASE AND SIGNIFICANT MECHANCIAL FACTORS

Caries	#2-MFL #10-MFL #31-D (injury from scaling) 5-MDFLO 16-All
Pulpal Disease	#10 - necrotic pulp, periodontal lesion

Inflammatory
Periodontal Disease
	Dx-generalized moderate periodontitis, more severe around all
	  lower molars and #2, 15.
	Gen 3-5 mm pocket depths; greater depths are on periodontal
	  charting - teeth #2,18,19,30,31 and lower anteriors
	Heavy plaque and calculus, bleeding on probing

Occlusal Traumatism	Generalized one degree mobility with three degree mobility on teeth #2,10,15
Severe Wear	None

Significant
Mechanical Factors
	Maxilla-multiple missing teeth (all molars #5,8,9,11,13)
	  #11 strategic tooth loss
	Mandible-#19 & #30 missing-posterior molars are severely inclined
	  aberrant plane of occlusion and Curve of Spee

TMJ Dysfunction and Other Oral Disease	None

CASE 1 WORKSHEET Management of a patient's dentition with Phase I therapy only.

Worksheet continued on opposite page

IDEAL TREATMENT PLAN   Patient Name   Anthony   Date   9-21-78

1   Emergency care for pain
2   Patient education and motivation
3   Scaling, root planing
4   Caries control
5   Extraction #5, 16
6   RCT #10, post and provisional restoration
7   Ligate lower anteriors
8   Hawley bite plane and occlusal adjustment
9   Reevaluation
10   Upright mandibular molars with continuous scaling and root planing
11   Reevaluation for Phase II periodontal therapy
12   Periodontal surgery when required (possible mandibular molars and #2)
13   Reevaluation
14   Tentative restorative therapy — maxillary fixed prosthesis, 12 units of crown and
     bridge; mandibular posterior fixed bridges-6 units
15   Maintenance at 3 month intervals

ALTERNATIVE TREATMENT PLANS   I

1   Emergency care for pain
2   Patient education and motivation
3   Scaling, root planing
4   Caries control
5   Extraction #5, 16
6   RCT #10, post and provisional restoration
7   Ligate lower anteriors
8   Hawley bite plane and occ. adjustment
9   Reevaluation
10   Upright mand. molars with continuous
     scaling and root planing
11   Reevaluation for Phase II perio. therapy

12   Alternative restorative therapy:
A(1)   Maxillary 6 unit anterior bridge and
     removable partial denture
 (2)   Maxillary removable partial denture
     without fixed anterior section
B   Mandibular 6 unit bridges

RATIONALE FOR ACTUAL TREATMENT PLAN

The actual treatment plan was Alternative III and was dictated by patient's
willingness to go though extensive procedures and by financial limitations.

FINANCIAL ARRANGEMENTS

Payments made on a monthly basis.

CASE 1 WORKSHEET *Continued*

Patient Name ___Anthony___   Date _9-21-78_

ALTERNATIVE TREATMENT PLANS   II

1	Emergency care for pain
2	Patient education and motivation
3	Scaling, root planing
4	Caries control
5	Extract #2,5,16
6	Root canal therapy #10
7	Ligate lower anteriors
8	Hawley bite plane and occ. adjustment
9	Reevaluation
10	Restorative therapy: Maxillary fixed bridge #6 to 12, posterior removable partial denture

11 Maintenance 3 to 4 month intervals to
   include topical fluoride to prevent
   root caries (#31)

                                III

1	Emergency care for pain
2	Patient education and motivation
3	Scaling, root planing
4	Caries control
5	Extract #2,5,10,16
6	Hawley bite plane for noct. parafunction
7	Reevaluation
8	Maxillary removable partial denture
9	Maintenance 3 to 4 month intervals to include topical fluoride

CASE 1 WORKSHEET   *Continued*

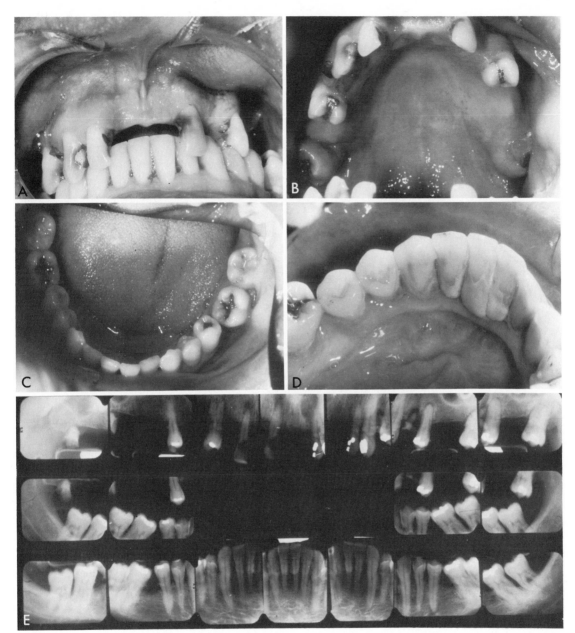

FIGURE 4–8 **Management of a Patient's Dentition With Phase I Therapy Only. A,** A 54-year-old patient complaining of pain in the maxillary left posterior quadrant. The maxillary left lateral incisor had a draining fistula. The maxillary left molar root (No. 16) was extracted and root canal therapy was started on the maxillary left incisor. **B,** The occlusal view of the maxillary arch demonstrates multiple missing teeth as well as severe periodontal destruction of the right molar. **C,** The occlusal view of the mandibular arch shows the severe inclination of the mandibular second and third molars. **D,** This lingual view of the mandibular anterior and premolar areas demonstrates heavy calculus deposits and soft tissue inflammation. **E,** The preoperative radiographs demonstrate the patient's neglect of and lack of concern for his oral health. Note the heavy calculus deposits, advanced periodontal disease, severe caries, poor tooth position, and distribution of abutment teeth in the maxillae.

Illustration continued on following page

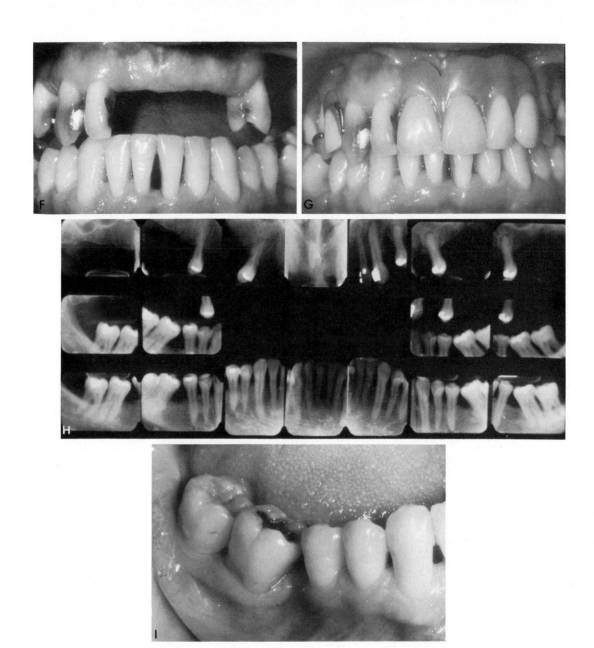

FIGURE 4–8 *Continued F,* After Phase I treatment all disease was eliminated. The patient was comfortable and satisfied. Note the shrinkage of the soft tissue as well as the change in color and texture. *G,* The final restorative therapy consisted of a maxillary removable partial denture. Maintenance therapy included periodic scaling, root planing, occlusal adjustment, and fluoride treatment. *H,* Postoperative radiographs demonstrate the results of Phase I therapy. *I,* The patient was placed on a 3-month maintenance therapy. Note exemplary oral hygiene as seen on the postoperative radiograph *(H)* and this view of the mandibular right quadrant at the time of maintenance therapy.

awareness so that advanced therapy to save the maxillary teeth will be an acceptable procedure if needed in the future. Using a formula of accommodation of the patient's needs, alleviation of pain, and education of the patient, the practitioner was able to bring the patient's goals for dental care closer to his own, thus ensuring a brighter prognosis for continued dental health and treatment. The purpose of this case is to demonstrate simple patient care and management of dental disease with conservative and alternative treatment.

Case 2. Management of a Patient's Dentition With Phase I Therapy and Minimal Phase II Therapy

This 41-year-old patient presented with a multitude of symptoms of advanced disease. They included extensive caries, plaque and calculus, poor tooth position, open contacts, and acquired tongue thrust in addition to inadequate oral hygiene.

The dental caries were recorded by quadrant on the interdisciplinary worksheet (Case 2 Worksheet). The periodontal and occlusal deformities were so extensive that they required individual specific chartings. Significant findings were then entered on the interdisciplinary worksheet to be integrated

---

INTERDISCIPLINARY TREATMENT PLANNING WORKSHEET

Patient Name   Frances   Date   9-12-72

SIGNIFICANT MEDICAL AND SYSTEMIC DISEASE OR CONDITION
          Rheumatic fever

SIGNIFICANT DENTAL/SOCIAL HISTORY
Chief dental complaint and history "I don't like the black fillings on my front teeth."
      Amalgam fillings placed 15 years ago because of high caries rate.

Other complaints:
    Mastication   Negative   Aesthetics   Chief complaint
    Comfort   Negative   Phonetics   Negative
Understanding of dental problem   Patient unaware of disease in her mouth.

Desires   Patient wants to know what has to be done and consider options.

Attitude   Good
Age   41   Gender   F   Occupation   Housewife   Financial Resources   Limited
Other considerations   Patient has no pain, but advanced disease.

CONSULTATIONS WITH DENTAL SPECIALISTS OR PHYSICIAN
      Physician contacted by letter; patient is on long-term antibiotics.

SIGNIFICANT SIGNS, SYMPTOMS AND ETIOLOGY OF DISEASE AND SIGNIFICANT MECHANICAL FACTORS

Caries	#3 - MOD	#9 - ML & DL	#19 - MODL	#29 - DO
	#5 - MOD	#10 - ML & DL		#30 - MODL
	#7 - ML & DL	#13 - MOD		
	#8 - ML & DL	#14 - MOD		

Pulpal Disease   #3 & #14 may need RCT for D-B root resection

Inflammatory Periodontal Disease	Gen. heavy plaque and calculus accumulation, edema, bleeding, soft-tissue deformity, poor home care.
	Pocket depths - mand. - generalized 5-7 mm, Greater depths - 9 mm tooth #3-D
	             max. - generalized 4-6 mm, Greater depths - tooth #5-M
	   Tooth #3 & #14 Distal Cl. III furcation involvements. tooth #19-M
	   Dx - Gen. periodontitis with primary occ. traum. 7 mm tooth #22-M

Occlusal Traumatism	Gen. primary occlusal traumatism Fremitus #6,7,8,9,10,11 Gen. mobility at widened PDL spaces
Severe Wear	Minimal - canines
Significant Mechanical Factors	Missing teeth - #1,2,15,16,17,22 Worn, broken down restorations Flared anterior teeth (max and mand) Poor marginal ridge relations; poor posterior occlusal contacts.
TMJ Dysfunction and Other Oral Disease	Acquired tongue thrust associated with spaces.

CASE 2 WORKSHEET. Management of a patient's dentition with Phase I therapy and minimal Phase II therapy.

Worksheet continued on following page

IDEAL TREATMENT PLAN   Pt. Name Frances   Date 9-12-72
   Premedicate with Penicillin for all treatment.
   Scaling and root planing, curettage and home care instruction.
   Retract and ligate lower anteriors and place Hawley bite plane.
   Operative dentistry and occlusal adjustment.
   Anterior space closure with elastics.
   Stabilization with A-splint
   Re-evaluation of periodontal and occlusal therapy; evaluate #3 & #14 for
      D-B root amputation.
   Root canal therapy and root amputation.
   Continued scaling and root planing.
   Perio surgery if required.
   Re-evaluation and maintenance. (3 month intervals)
   Patient may require advanced restorative therapy.

ALTERNATIVE TREATMENT PLANS

   Scaling, root planing and curettage, HCI
   Operative dentistry and occ. adjustment
   Nightguard.
   Constant maintenance 3 months.

RATIONALE FOR ACTUAL TREATMENT PLAN

   Ideal treatment plan was possible. Patient is extremely cooperative, but
   limited by finances. Arch integrity allows us to avoid advanced restorative
   therapy, yet it may be required in the future. Periodontal health must be
   established. Occlusal adjustment must be in concert with operative dentistry.
   Phase II periodontal therapy must be modified because of financial constraints upon
   advanced restorative therapy.
   All stabilization of teeth that are moved must be executed with A-splints. Any
   open embrasure spaces can be controlled with A-splints.

FINANCIAL ARRANGEMENTS

   12 months of treatment. Financial arrangements were made on installments.

CASE 2 WORKSHEET *Continued*

into the development of an ideal treatment plan. Long-standing periodontal disease had severely compromised the gingival architecture; pocket depths and recession were extreme. Extensive loss of attachment apparatus along with the parafunctional force associated with tongue thrust had resulted in the mesial drifting of teeth, generalized tooth mobility (secondary occlusal traumatism), and spacing and flaring of the anterior teeth. The existing maxillary incisor restorations were defective and esthetically unacceptable.

Treatment planning required Phase I

therapy to control disease through instruction in proper oral hygiene and the administration of scaling, root planing, and curettage (Fig. 4–9). After retraction and ligation of the lower incisors, occlusal adjustment and Hawley bite plane were planned and then executed along with the operative dentistry and caries control to eliminate all interferences associated with deformed tooth relations. Adjunctive orthodontic treatment was also utilized to retract the maxillary anterior teeth. Since financial considerations precluded advanced restorative treatment as a viable procedure, only minimal Phase II periodontal therapy was executed. A healthy dentition was nevertheless achieved, but a long-term favorable prognosis would depend on the strict observance of careful

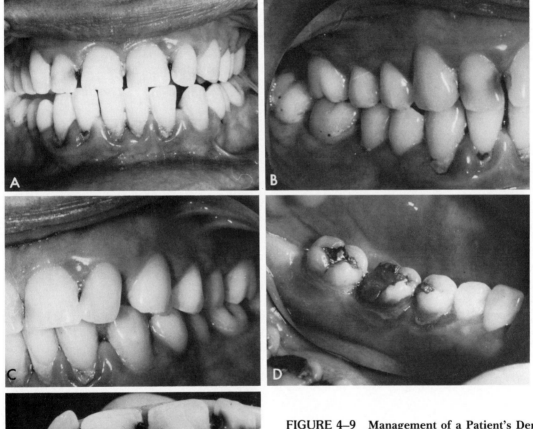

FIGURE 4–9 Management of a Patient's Dentition With Phase I Therapy and Minimal Phase II Therapy. A, This labial view demonstrates the etiology and deformity present. Extrusion of the unopposed mandibular second molar (also a problem on the right side) has resulted in posterior interferences in protrusive and lateral-protrusive movements. **B,** Right buccal view demonstrating intact dentition from first molar to first molar, unopposed and inclined second molar, and severe soft tissue deformity due to long-standing plaque and calculus. **C,** Left buccal view. **D,** Inadequate home care of the lingual surfaces of the teeth has led to excessive plaque accumulation and calculus formation. A severe inflammatory response has resulted, causing soft tissue deformities. Note inadequate restorative dentistry and poor proximal relations. **E,** Poor anterior tooth relations and soft tissue response are seen on this palatal view of the maxillary incisor. The mesially inclined lateral incisors have compromised the embrasure spaces.

Illustration continued on following page

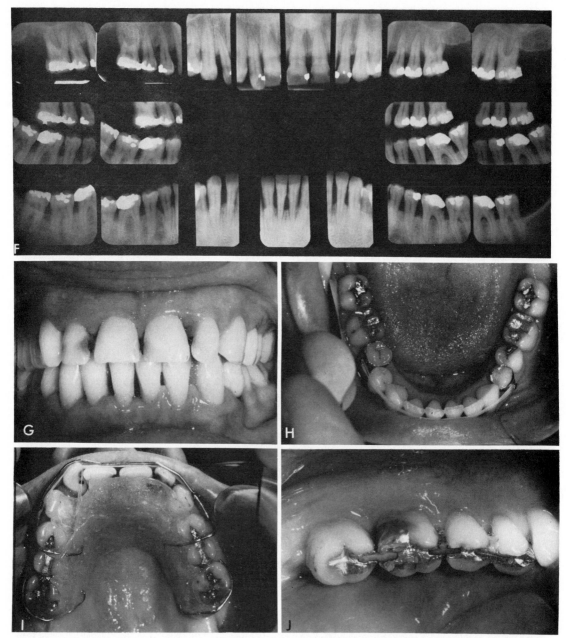

FIGURE 4–9 *Continued* **F,** The preoperative radiographs demonstrate recurrent caries associated with worn and fractured restorations, which have resulted in the breakdown of the mandibular molars, and advanced periodontal disease, which has resulted in widespread bone loss, especially around the maxillary first molar. **G,** Favorable soft tissue changes occurred within 2 weeks after the patient was instructed in proper oral hygiene, and scaling and root planing were initiated. Caries control was executed. Tooth movement procedures could then be employed safely, along with continuous scaling and root planing. **H,** After only 2 weeks of adjunctive orthodontic treatment, the mandibular incisor teeth were retracted. The teeth are ligated to retain proper alignment and to stabilize occlusal relations for subsequent therapy and placement of the Hawley bite plane. **I,** The Hawley bite plane was used for the orthodontic correction of the maxillary anterior teeth. (The bite plane also facilitated occlusal adjustment.) **J,** While adjunctive orthodontics was in progress, the posterior occlusion was treated: Selective grinding was implemented to shorten the extruded mandibular second molars and eliminate the interferences. Amalgam fillings and A-splints were placed to restore the broken-down carious teeth, to prevent the extrusion of the still unopposed mandibular second molars, and to stabilize occlusal relations. Note the soft tissue response.

Illustration continued on following page

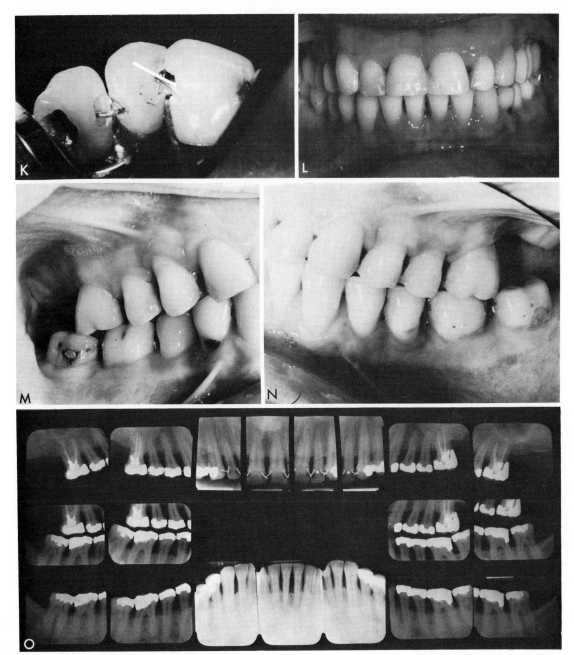

FIGURE 4–9 *Continued* ***K,*** The defective restorations in the maxillary anterior teeth were replaced with composite resins using TMS pins to maximize stabilization for cosmetic reasons. Currently, extracoronal acid etch ligation would be recommended. A nightguard was placed, and active treatment ended here. Maintenance therapy was started. ***L,*** Management of the posterior dentition and orthodontic repositioning of the maxillary anterior teeth were completed after 6 weeks. Soft tissue health and adequate embrasure spaces were reestablished. ***M,*** The right buccal view 2 years after the start of treatment. The isolated periodontal defects associated with the distobuccal roots of the maxillary first molars have not responded to treatment. Because the deformities jeopardized the integrity of the osseous structures of adjacent roots of the same teeth, the roots were removed in an effort to gain optimal quantity of the attachment apparatus. ***N,*** The left buccal view. ***O,*** Eight-year postoperative radiographs demonstrate the maintenance of the periodontal tissues. The area of greatest concern is maintenance of tooth position and occlusal relations, because of the instability of the methods of stabilization. Proximal contacts and embrasure spaces were controlled with A-splints.

maintenance therapy. The maintenance phase of therapy became a critical part of the treatment plan. It was the sole remaining source of re-evaluation in a case with potential for further deterioration. Maintenance visits every 3 months provided an opportunity to closely monitor A-splint wear and fracture, continuing periodontal health and occlusal stability, and the patient's oral hygiene.

Since there was successful maintenance of arch integrity in both quadrants, no extensive tooth replacement prostheses were required. Occlusal stability, orthodontic stabilization, and periodontal health were achieved with operative dentistry. This was a tenuous and compromised mode of therapy. As stated, maintenance of the restorative dentistry is critical and an encumbrance to long-term periodontal health.

Case 3. Management of a Patient's Dentition With Phase I Therapy Followed By Phase II Therapy

This 58-year-old patient had swelling and severe pain in her lower jaw. She complained about the appearance of her dental prostheses and the difficulty of oral hygiene and was generally discouraged with dentistry. An office examination revealed extensive caries under many existing crowns, generalized periodontal disease, occlusal traumatism, severe wear, and numerous missing teeth. The left mandibular lateral incisor presented a special problem because of its strategic location and the severity of the disease process.

This patient's care is an example of the diagnosis and treatment planning used to establish a prognosis for a single tooth in Phase I therapy (Fig. 4–10; Case 3 Worksheet). The patient's attitude and financial resources precluded any discussion about saving the maxillary anterior teeth. Since the best option for the long-term retention of the patient's lower dentition was to save the left mandibular lateral incisor (No. 23), an ideal treatment plan was developed on that basis. The goals of ideal treatment were to restore the health of the entire masticatory system and, specifically, to maintain the integrity of the lower arch by saving tooth No. 23 and then to replace the mandibular right

bridge. Plans were made for extraction of the maxillary teeth, to be replaced immediately by a maxillary full denture. Also anticipated by both patient and practitioner was the goal of the simple maintenance of optimal hygiene.

Alternative treatment plans are usually devised to suit the patient's special demands and financial or time limitations (see Case Illustration 1). In this instance, optional plans were based on special dental demands and limitations and were discussed even prior to the administration of emergency treatment. The probability, however marginal, that tooth No. 23 could be saved was worth any effort, since failure to save it would result in a less acceptable and completely different treatment plan, sequence of treatment, and final result.

If the left mandibular lateral incisor were extracted, the options available for treatment would dramatically increase the cost and duration of therapy and involve the preparation and alteration of previously unrestored and healthy dentition. An extracoronal fixed bridge for teeth Nos. 21 to 27 (etched cast metal resin-bonded restoration) or a full mandibular fixed prosthesis was considered as a viable alternative if it became necessary. The poor distribution of the remaining teeth and the anterior edentulous space would place an extreme burden on the remaining dentition, so the use of a removable partial denture was considered unacceptable by the clinician. All the treatment required for a maxillary fixed bridge with precision attachments was considered unacceptable by the patient. It was mutually agreed upon to expend all energy and finances to maintain mandibular arch integrity. The patient was aware of all alternative treatment if tooth No. 23 was lost.

The ideal and the alternative treatment plans recorded on the interdisciplinary worksheet involve specialized treatment in endodontics and periodontics. To relieve severe pain on the first visit, the lower anterior teeth were ligated with wire, and tooth No. 23 was treated endodontically and scaled and root planed. Eight weeks after root canal therapy was completed, suppuration continued. A periodontal surgical procedure was done to remove inaccessible calculus and to completely clean out tooth No. 23's periodontal defect. The interdisciplinary worksheet provided a convenient vehicle for the planning, explanation, and documentation of the development of a prognosis of this tooth and the patient's dentition.

The worksheet's treatment plans also reflect the practitioner's careful inclusion of frequently scheduled re-evaluations to monitor every step in the sequence of treatment.

The completion of each sequence of treatment, in this particular case, predicated the choice of any subsequent stages of treatment. The anticipation by the clinician of all the various degrees of therapeutic success and their resultant effect on later procedures facilitated uninterrupted therapy and

Text continued on page 134

INTERDISCIPLINARY TREATMENT PLANNING WORKSHEET

Patient Name___Helen_____ DATE___1-12-80_____

SIGNIFICANT MEDICAL AND SYSTEMIC DISEASE OR CONDITION
___None_____

SIFNIFICANT DENTAL/SOCIAL HISTORY
Chief dental complaint and history__"I have pain in the front of my mouth." Patient had_
_swelling for the past 4 months and pain is severe now._____

Other complaints:
     Mastication__Can't chew because of pain_____ Aesthetics_Unhappy with looks of teeth_
     Comfort_Uncomfortable when chewing_____ Phonetics__Negative_____
Understanding of dental problem___Patient feels she has been taking care of her teeth____
_and can't understand why she has problems._____

Desires__Patient wants to look better and wants to be comfortable._____
Attitude_Impatient_____
Age___58__ Gender__F___ Occupation_Seamstress_____Financial Resources__Limited__
Other Considerations___Patient unhappy with past dentistry._____

CONSULTATIONS WITH DENTAL SPECIALISTS OR PHYSICIAN
___None_____

SIGNIFICANT SIGNS, SYMPTOMS AND ETIOLOGY OF DISEASE AND SIGNIFICANT MECHANCIAL FACTORS

Caries	#8-under crown # 9-under crown #28-under crown #10-under crown #31-under crown #11-under crown
Pulpal Disease	#23 non-vital; endo-perio lesion
Inflammatory Periodontal Disease	Gen. periodontitis with secondary occlusal traumatism on #23; #31 Class II furcation Gen. plaque and calculus, bleeding on probing; suppuration in area of #23 (Endo-perio lesion)
Pocket Depths:	Maxilla - Generalized 5-8 mm Mandible - Gen. 3-4 mm except #23,24 - 10 mm on labial and proximal
Occlusal Traumatism	Secondary occlusal traumatism #23 Maxillary splint is very loose
Severe Wear	#24, 25 - may be associated with holding a needle between her teeth
Significant Mechanical Factors	Multiple missing teeth - especially maxillas If #23 is lost, must fabricate lower fixed anterior bridge Poor force deliverance and distribution to all occluding teeth (anteriors)
TMJ Dysfunction and Other Oral Disease	None

CASE 3 WORKSHEET Management of a patient's dentition with Phase I therapy followed by Phase II therapy.

Worksheet continued on following page

IDEAL TREATMENT PLAN   Patient Name___Helen_____   Date_1-12-80_

1   Emergency treatment #23 inclined
     (a) stabilization   (b) scaling   (c) root canal therapy
2   Stabilize lower anteriors with wire and acrylic
3   Scaling, root planing and curettage
4   #23 complete root canal
5   Remove fixed bridge from #29-32 and place provisional restoration
6   Reevaluation – #23 may completely heal with root canal therapy and minimal scaling
     and root planing. It it does not, then do open flap exploratory procedure to
     clean out inaccessible calculus.
7   Set up lower plane of occlusion optimally for maxillary denture.
8   Extraction of #8,9,10,11; immediate insertion of maxillary full denture
9   Reevaluate entire lower arch for strategic extraction of #23 or keep it and
     avoid fixed bridge; or evaluate need for periodontal surgery of lower anteriors
10   Convert ligation to NUVA-seal – NUVA-fill
11   Complete fixed bridge #29-31
12   Rebase maxillary denture
13   Maintenance – 4 month intervals

ALTERNATIVE TREATMENT PLANS   I

1   Emerg. tx. #23 inclined (a) stabilization   10   Complete fixed bridge 29-31
     (b) scaling (c) root canal therapy   11   Rebase maxillary denture
2   Stabilize lower ant. with wire & acrylic   12   Maintenance at 4 month intervals
3   Scaling, root planing and curettage
4   #23 complete root canal
5   Remove fixed br. 29-32, place prov. rest.
6   Ext. #23; place cast ling. extracoronal
     br. with pontic (Maryland bridge)
7   Ext. #8,9,10,11; incert imm. max. denture
8   Reevaluate (a) stability of ant. splint
     (b) periodontal need, especially #31
9   Maintain lower fixed extracoronal bridge

RATIONALE FOR ACTUAL TREATMENT PLAN

The actual treatment plan will be determined during therapy. The prognosis of #23
must be established. If all goes well, the lower cast fixed restoration can be kept
to #29-32. Maxillary fixed bridge with precision attachments was considered, but
patient's attitude completely precluded a discussion about such treatment. If #23
is lost, part of fee may have to be absorbed by clinician.

FINANCIAL ARRANGEMENTS

Monthly payments; fill out insurance forms.

CASE 3 WORKSHEET   *Continued*

Worksheet continued on opposite page

Patient Name Helen   Date 1-12-80

ALTERNATIVE TREATMENT PLANS   II

1 Emerg. tx. #23 inclined (a) stabilization
     (b) scaling (c) root canal therapy
2 Stabilize lower ant. with wire & acrylic
3 Scaling, root planing and curettage
4 #23 complete root canal
5 Remove fixed br. 29-32, place prov. rest.
6 Ext. #23 and place mand. fixed prov. rest.
7 Ext. #8,9,10,11; insert imm. full dent.
8 Reevaluation for periodontal needs
9 Complete mandibular fixed restoration:
     #21 to #27
     #28 to #31 with interlock between #27-28

10 Rebase maxillary full denture
11 Maintenance at 4 month intervals

CASE 3 WORKSHEET *Continued*

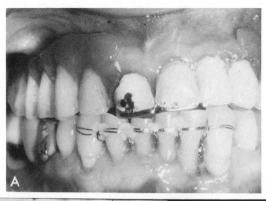

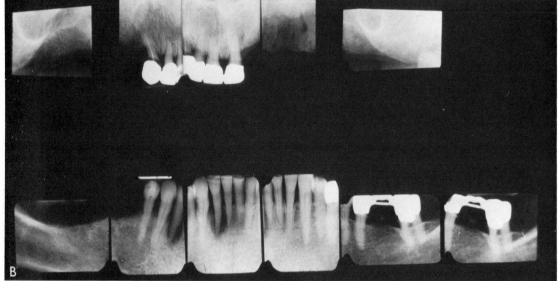

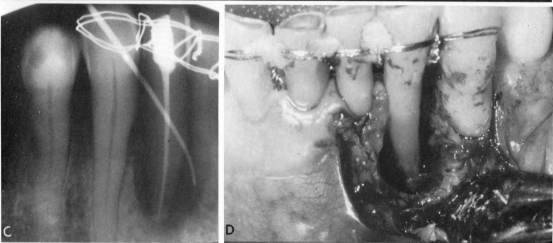

FIGURE 4–10 Management of a Patient's Dentition With Phase I Therapy Followed by Phase II Therapy. *A,* This 58-year-old patient presented with the chief complaint of pain on the lower left lateral incisor, inability to chew, and difficulty with cleaning her teeth. Only four anterior teeth remain in the maxilla. The patient was wearing a removable maxillary appliance and no mandibular tooth replacement device. *B,* The full set of radiographs demonstrates extensive caries under the fixed prosthesis, generalized heavy calculus deposits, and severe bone loss around the lower left lateral incisor. *C,* Eight weeks after the completion of root canal therapy, suppuration continued around tooth No. 23. This radiograph shows gutta percha in the periodontal pocket extending close to the apex of the adjacent incisor. A decision was made to perform a periodontal exploratory procedure.

Illustration continued on opposite page

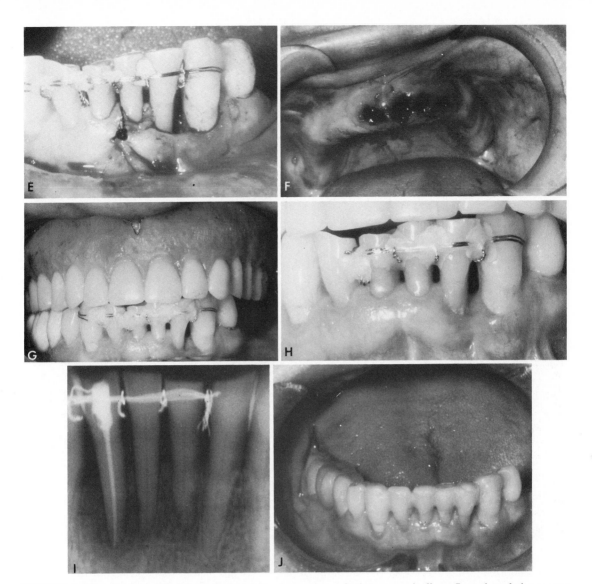

FIGURE 4–10 *Continued D,* This photograph shows the soft tissue surgically reflected and the severe periodontal defect completely cleaned out. The periodontal defect was not corrected by osseous surgery because it might have jeopardized the adjacent teeth. Strategic extraction, however, was a consideration. *E,* The soft tissue was repositioned to cover the adjacent osseous crest and the defects around tooth No. 23. Owing to the osseous topography of the defect and the extensive restoration required to replace this tooth, it was decided to evaluate the results of this procedure at 3-month intervals. *F,* The maxillary teeth were removed. *G,* The maxillary denture was inserted immediately after extraction, five months after initial treatment began. The lower plane of occlusion was corrected by means of selective grinding and a provisional three-unit restoration on the lower right. *H,* Eight months after the surgical procedure, the soft tissue had adequately healed, but there was some supragingival build-up of calculus. Oral hygiene procedures were reinforced and monitored carefully; the patient was seen every 4 weeks for scaling and root planing. *I,* The eight-month postoperative radiograph shows healing and re-formation of the attachment apparatus. It was now evident at this time that there could be a positive prognosis for tooth No. 23. *J,* The final restoration involved the rebuilding of lower anteriors with light-cured resin. The final fixed bridge on the lower right was in place 14 months after therapy began.

Illustration continued on following page

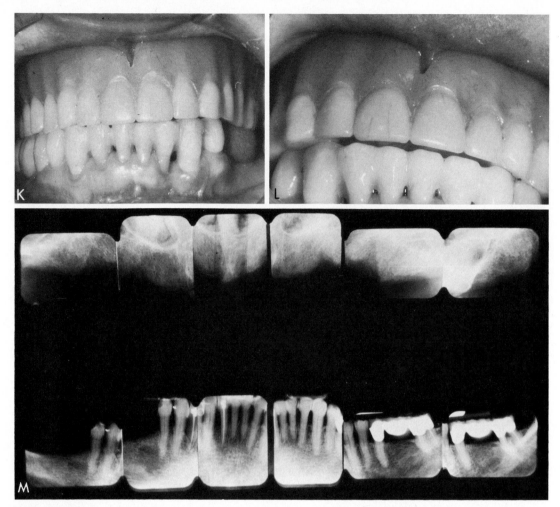

FIGURE 4–10 *Continued K,* A labial view of the final restoration, which did not include a mandibular partial denture. *L,* The occlusion of the denture is now balanced and includes canine support (see Chapter 8, Occlusion in General Practice). *M,* Final radiographs of the mandibular arch 14 months after initial treatment.

the understanding and acceptance by the patient of any future variation in treatment.

The efficacy of any logical and organized diagnosis and treatment plan is not measured only by the eventual attainment of the goals of dental health but also by the plan itself. This plan for example, was so well designed and far-reaching that both the practitioner and the patient were fully prepared to readily assume any necessary alternative therapy.

In the course of the diagnosis of, treatment planning for, and management of this patient, Phase I therapy was especially formulated to save a single tooth that threatened the entire sequence and goal of therapy. As the solitary tooth progressed from a questionable prognosis to a positive prognosis, the dental health of the masticatory system changed from an unpredictable situation that might require expensive, extensive, and highly involved Phase I and Phase II therapy to a relatively uncomplicated Phase I and minimal Phase II situation that could be treated in a reasonable brief period of time.

Case 4. Management of a Patient's Dentition With Combined Phase I and Phase II Therapy

A treatment plan using routine Phase I and Phase II therapy was developed for this 24-year-old patient who presented with ad-

INTERDISCIPLINARY TREATMENT PLANNING WORKSHEET

Patient Name ___Helene_____   Date ___9-24-72_____

SIGNIFICANT MEDICAL AND SYSTEMIC DISEASE OR CONDITION
_____Negative_____

SIGNIFICANT DENTAL/SOCIAL HISTORY
Chief dental complaint and history __Patient "did not like empty spaces in her mouth".__
___She lost her teeth at age 14-16 due to caries._____

Other complaints:
   Mastication __Inadequate_____   Aesthetics __Unhappy with spaces_____
   Comfort __TMJ pain, occlusal awareness__ Phonetics __Negative_____
Understanding of dental problem __Patient feels her discomfort and inability to____
___chew is related to the missing teeth._____

Desires ___Tooth replacement and anterior space closure._____
Attitude __Good, yet pt. missed 1st consultation appointment and was late for 2nd.__
Age __24__ Gender ___F___ Occupation _Secretary_____ Financial Resources _Adequate___
Other considerations _____

CONSULTATIONS WITH DENTAL SPECIALISTS OR PHYSICIAN
_____None_____

SIGNIFICANT SIGNS, SYMPTOMS AND ETIOLOGY OF DISEASE AND SIGNIFICANT MECHANICAL FACTORS

Caries	Negative at this time. Patient tooth loss was due to dental caries.
Pulpal Disease	#26 necrotic pulp (periapical lesion)
Inflammatory Periodontal Disease	Gen. plaque and calculus accum. esp. on ling. of lower anteriors. Soft tissue is thin, friable and bleeds on probing. Gen. 3-4mm pocket depths, 6mm at mesial of all molars. 3mm recession around lower anteriors, exposed roots and inadequate attached gingiva around the lower anteriors and lower left quadrant. Dx - periodontitis with more severe around lower anteriors. primary occlusal traumatism
Occlusal Traumatism	Primary occ. traum. associated with protrusive habit and nocturnal bruxing. Interferences between #2 & 31,#15 & 18. Heavy protrusive contact on #7 &26. Gen. mobility more severe around lower incisors especially #26.
Severe Wear	Negative
Significant Mechanical Factors	Posterior bite collapse - mesially inclined molars, distal drift of the bicuspids, flaring of the max. and mand. anterior teeth; inadequate support of OVD by posterior teeth. Lack of arch rhythmicity and continuity. Missing teeth #
TMJ Dysfunction and Other Oral Disease	Dull pain on both sides. Patient is more aware of pain upon waking in A.M. Dx: Myofascial pain dysfunction syndrome.

CASE 4 WORKSHEET.   Management of a patient's dentition with combined Phase I and Phase II therapy.

Worksheet continued on following page

IDEAL TREATMENT PLAN   Pt. Name Helene   Date   9-24-72

Scaling and root planing, curettage, home care instruction.
Root canal #26
Ligate the lower anterior teeth with wire.
Hawley bite plane for TMJ symptoms.
Re-evaluation.
Upright lower molar and #2.
Occlusal adjustment by selective grinding.
Stabilization of posterior teeth and establish occlusion with provisional restorations.
Re-evaluation.
Periodontal surgery (to correct mucogingival problems)
Final restorative therapy: A. Minimal max. and mand. posterior reconstruction —
    porcelain to gold; or
                        B. Possibly maxillary posterior reconstruction. Full
    lower reconstruction (lower anterior teeth may have to be included for stability).
Maintenance therapy.

ALTERNATIVE TREATMENT PLANS   I   II

Scaling, rt. planing, curettage, HCI.   Scaling, rt. planing, curettage, HCI.
Root canal #26   Root canal #26
Ligate lower ant. teeth with wire.   Ligate lower ant. teeth with wire.
Hawley bite plane for TMJ symptoms.   Hawley bite plane for TMJ symptoms.
Re-evaluation.   Re-evaluation
Occlusal adjustment   Free gingival graft lower ant. and left
Nightguard.   bicuspids.
Maintenance.   Nightguard and possible occl. adjustment.
                                               Maintenance.

RATIONALE FOR ACTUAL TREATMENT PLAN

Ideal treatment plan was agreed to and the lower anteriors may have to be
included in the fixed restorations if they prove to be unsatable. The
alternative treatment plans can be executed if patient proves unreliable.
Posterior occlusion must be reestablished to support occlusal verticle dimension.
This requires repositioning the malposed posterior teeth, fixed restorations.
If ideal restorative treatment cannot be executed, the occlusal problem should be
managed as best as possible with the Hawley bite plane, occlusal adjustment, and
nightguard therapy.

FINANCIAL ARRANGEMENTS

Monthly payments.

CASE 4 WORKSHEET *Continued*

vanced periodontal disease, occlusal trauma, extensive posterior tooth loss, loss of support for the occlusal vertical dimension, and poor spacing of the anterior teeth. All data were recorded on appropriate periodontal and occlusal examination charts, and significant findings were transferred to the inter-disciplinary worksheet for consideration in the development of a treatment plan (Case 4 Worksheet). The individual periodontal and occlusal chartings proved useful initially and also later during the actual treatment and re-evaluation stages of therapy. As part of the occlusal examination, study models were mounted on an articulator and the final proposed orthodontic, occlusal, and restorative therapy was planned and visualized (Fig. 4–11).

The excessive number and combination of etiologic factors present were correlated to the patient's age, the extent of the disease present, and the deformity created by the

Text continued on page 142

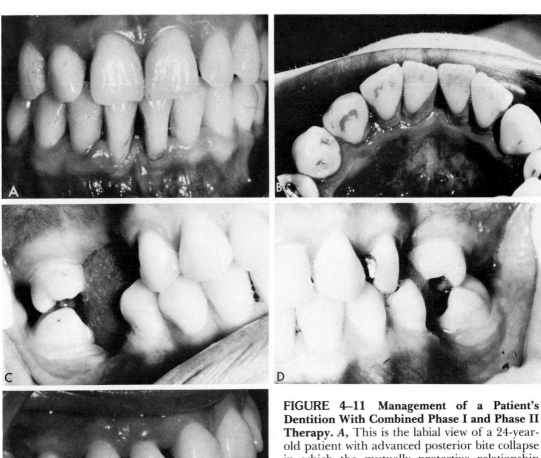

FIGURE 4–11 Management of a Patient's Dentition With Combined Phase I and Phase II Therapy. *A*, This is the labial view of a 24-year-old patient with advanced posterior bite collapse in which the mutually protective relationship between the anterior and posterior teeth has been destroyed. Loss of the support for occlusal vertical dimension by the posterior teeth has resulted in excessive off-axis force application to the anterior teeth. Notice the resultant flaring and spacing of the anterior teeth. In addition to the destructive force associated with the primary occlusal trauma, parafunctional activity engaged in by the patient increased both the magnitude and the duration of force. The constant, excessive, horizontal occlusal forces caused pulpal necrosis of the mandibular right lateral incisor, as well as generalized tooth sensitivity and TMJ pain. *B*, The lingual view demonstrates the thin, friable periodontium and inadequate masticatory mucosa along with poor oral hygiene and extensive plaque and calculus accumulation. The clinical signs include gingival edema, enlargement, and recession; severe mucogingival deformities in the mandibular arch; and mobility and fremitus of the anterior teeth. *C*, Throughout the patient's adolescence, posterior teeth were extracted as a result of extensive caries. This right buccal view shows the consequent mesial drifting of the molars that has led to soft tissue bunching, interferences in protrusive and lateral-protrusive movements, and a functional increase in cuspal height. *D*, The left side of the mouth is characterized by extensive tooth loss and manifests occlusal and periodontal deformities similar to the right side. *E*, Note the anterior tooth spacing and amount of overbite-overjet at the retruded contact position. The occlusal vertical dimension at the contact position is 1 mm greater than at the maximum intercuspal position. This is sometimes referred to as a "1-millimeter IC-RC discrepancy."

Illustration continued on following page

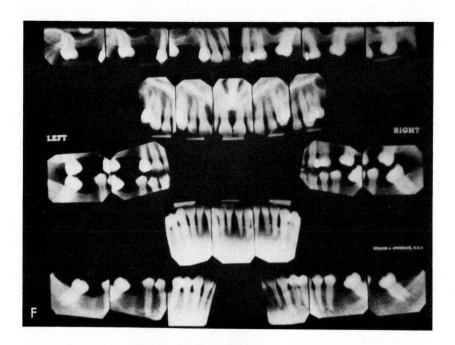

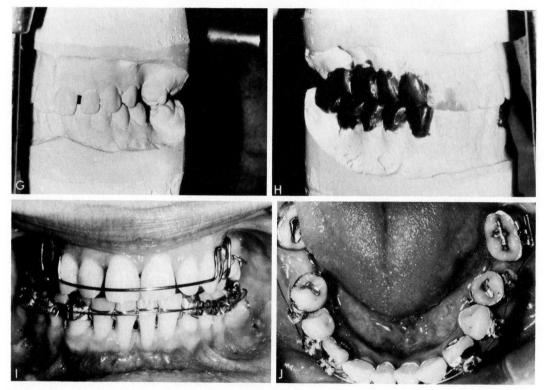

FIGURE 4–11 *Continued F,* Periodontal disease evidenced by advanced bone loss, especially around the mandibular anterior teeth, and by widening of the periodontal ligament. Pulpal necrosis of the mandibular right lateral incisor is manifested by the periapical radiolucency. *G,* A diagnostic mounting was indicated. Study models were mounted to the retruded contact position. *H,* For the fabrication of the provisional restoration, selective grinding was done and a wax-up of the proposed final restoration was made, estimating postorthodontic tooth positions and relations. *I,* Scaling, root planing, and oral hygiene instruction controlled soft tissue inflammation after 8 weeks. The mandibular right lateral incisor was treated endodontically and the periodontally weak anterior teeth were ligated to provide stabilization for Hawley bite-plane therapy, which was used diagnostically to confirm an occlusal etiology of TMJ symptoms. After 8 weeks, the pain was alleviated and a definitive diagnosis was established calling

138

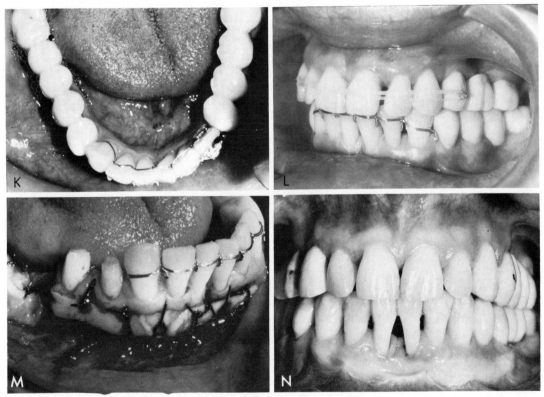

for Phase II adjunctive orthodontic therapy. *J,* Orthodontic appliances were used to upright the mandibular molars. *K,* After 6 months of orthodontic treatment, repositioning of the molars was achieved, eliminating the interferences and promoting re-formation of deformed soft tissues. Gold band and acrylic provisional restorations were placed immediately to retain corrected tooth positions, to help establish and stabilize arch rhythmicity, and to support the occlusal vertical dimension. *L,* With the function of the posterior teeth restored (and inflammation controlled), it was then possible to retract the maxillary anterior teeth. Cleats were incorporated into the provisionals to accomplish tooth movement, which took 2 weeks. *M,* During the clinical reevaluation, the mucogingival deformities in the mandibular arch had not responded to Phase I therapy. This was not surprising, because of the limited quantity of masticatory mucosa and the extensive nature of the defect. Periodontal surgery involving placement of free gingival grafts was effective in managing the mucogingival problem. *N,* Two months after surgery, the status of soft tissues was healthy. No further Phase II periodontal therapy was needed; occlusal function had been maintained, and corrected tooth positions had been retained. At this point in therapy, all provisional restorations were functioning in a healthy environment; therefore, fabrication of the final restorations was indicated.

Illustration continued on following page

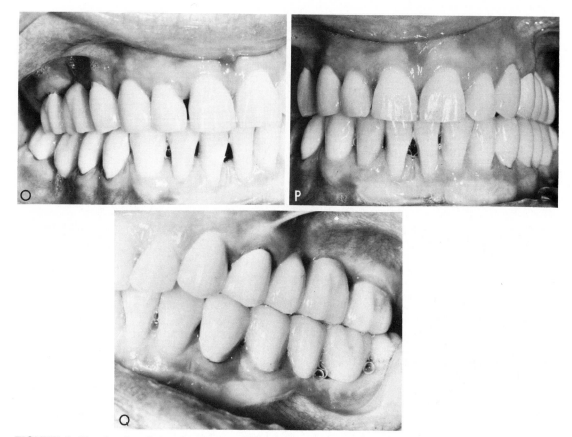

FIGURE 4–11   *Continued O,* After six months, the final fixed prosthesis was in place, as seen from a right buccal view, *(P)* from a frontal view, *(Q)* and from a left buccal view.

Illustration continued on opposite page

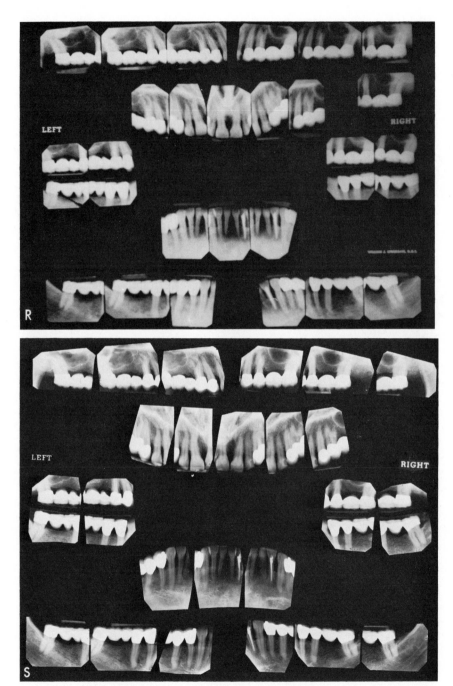

FIGURE 4–11   *Continued R,* These 4-year postoperative radiographs corroborate the clinical picture of health. During the maintenance phase of therapy, nightguard therapy was indicated to control nocturnal force generation. Continued assessment of the status of the mandibular incisors was of particular importance. These teeth had suffered the greatest amount of bone loss and were periodontally weak. Although stabilization via ligation has proved effective in the short run, these teeth may eventually require advanced restorative dentistry to enhance their long-term prognosis. *S,* Ten-year postoperative radiographs. A rigid maintenance program was followed.

active disease. The prognosis for the entire dentition was considered excellent. The patient was informed about the proposed treatment, the importance of her responsibility to this prodigious amount of therapy, and the favorable prognosis of the ideal treatment plan and sequence of therapy. The ideal treatment plan was accepted by the patient. All active inflammatory disease was eliminated, excessive occlusal forces were controlled, and temporomandibular joint pain was alleviated. Phase I therapy consisted of scaling, root planing, curettage, and home care instruction followed by root canal therapy, retraction and stabilization of the lower anterior teeth, and placement of a Hawley bite plane. After a re-evaluation of all therapy and patient complaints, Phase II therapy was started. Adjunctive orthodontic procedures were executed to correct tooth

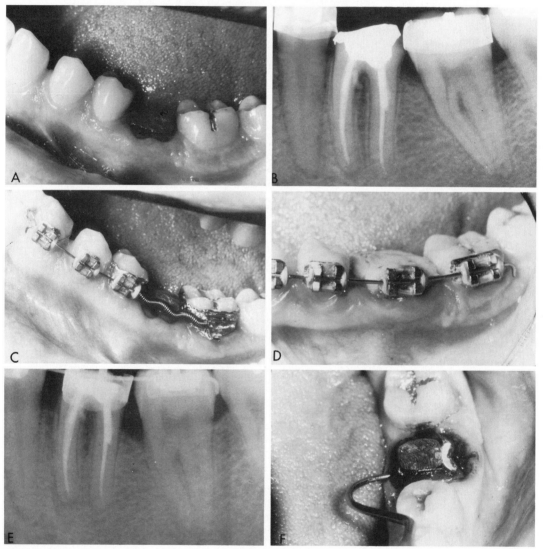

FIGURE 4–12 **Management of a Severely Broken Down Tooth and Its Associated Quadrant With Phase II Therapy. *A,*** Note the severe caries on the mandibular first molar. Owing to the loss of proximal tooth contacts, the mandibular second and third molars drifted mesially and the premolars distally. ***B,*** This preorthodontic radiograph shows the encroachment of the mandibular second molar and the second premolar on the first molar. In the furcation, there is a perforation on the distal aspect of the mesial root. ***C,*** An open coil-spring was used to move the premolars mesially and the molars distally. ***D,*** Once the embrasure space was adequate, the provisional restoration was cemented in place with zinc phosphate cement, the arch was rebanded, and the first molar was extruded. ***E,*** This radiograph was taken after the forced eruption of the first molar. Note the proximal angular crest created to avoid extensive osseous reduction from around the adjacent teeth. ***F,*** The Class III periodontal furcation involvement due to the root perforation was made more accessible by adjunctive orthodontics.

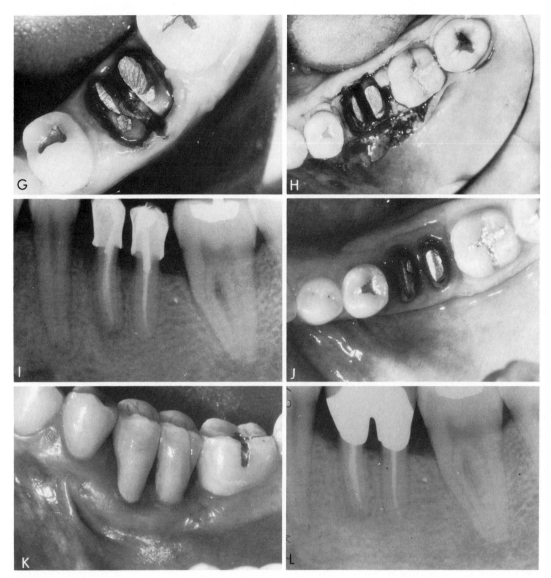

FIGURE 4–12 *Continued* **G,** The tooth was first hemisected and the extent of the perforation visualized. Note the gutta percha in furcation area. **H,** The roots were then completely prepared to open the embrasure space between the roots, to get below the perforation, and to fabricate a new provisional restoration. Since the perforation was inaccessible (below the osseous crest), buccal and lingual flaps were raised, osseous surgery executed, the provisional restoration cemented, and the flaps sutured in place. **I,** This radiograph was taken after cementation of the provisional restorations to check osseous contours, to determine the amount of sound tooth structure above the osseous crest, and to ensure that no cement was below the flaps. **J,** The teeth were reprepared 12 weeks after the surgical procedure. Final impressions were taken. Note the final root preparation, embrasure space, and soft tissue healing. **K,** The final restoration consisted of two splinted units. **L,** Final radiograph 6 months after surgical therapy, 18 months after the initial tooth movement. (In conjunction with Drs. Mark Lipkin and Carol Kirschenbaum.)

position and occlusal relations. Provisional restorations were then placed to maintain the corrected tooth position, to replace missing teeth, and to establish a therapeutic occlusion. After stabilization and an 8-week period of re-evaluation, Phase II periodontal procedures were executed.

Adherence to the planned sequence of treatment as devised in the treatment plan was important. This ensured that Phase I therapy would be completed and re-evaluated before Phase II therapy was attempted. Phase II periodontal treatment and advanced restorative dentistry were completed in the proper sequence, and a strict program of maintenance was instituted.

Case 5. Management of a Severely Broken-Down Tooth and Its Associated Quadrant With Phase II Therapy

This 18-year-old patient's care is an example of the extensive Phase II therapy required to correct a severe deformity created by dental caries and a mechanical perforation. The patient had periodontal health, yet extensive caries was present on the first molar. In an attempt to restore the lost tooth structure with amalgam and pins, a perforation occurred in the furcation area (the distal aspect of the mesial root) (Fig. 4–12).

The treatment plan used extensive Phase II therapy to manage the broken-down, perforated molar and its associated deformed posterior quadrant. Phase II therapy was directed toward two problems. The first problem was the collapse of the adjacent teeth into the area once occupied by the coronal aspect of the first molar. The second problem was the periodontal breakdown in the furcation area due to the mechanical perforation.

The treatment of these problems was complex. No Phase I therapy was administered after the initial examination and prevention and maintenance therapy. The treatment plan required a complete medical history, full-mouth radiographs, study casts, and the use of the interdisciplinary treatment planning worksheet. Adjunctive orthodontic procedures were used to create embrasure space for the placement of a provisional restoration, and then orthodontic extrusion was done to facilitate osseous surgery in the furcation area as well as hemisection and the placement of a final restoration.

Case 6. Management of a Patient's Dentition In Which Advanced Disease Exists With Phase I and Phase II Therapy

The management of a patient requiring Phase I and Phase II therapy to establish a positive prognosis for the entire dentition is exemplified in this patient's care. The patient, a 41-year-old male, complained of bleeding gums, bad breath, and general pain. He was very concerned about losing his few remaining teeth and requested that all efforts be made to save them. His willingness to undergo advanced therapy allowed the practitioner to pursue an ideal plan of treatment as well as to predict a more favorable prognosis. The prognosis for this patient's dentition is poor, yet his extreme desire to keep his teeth enhances the chances of success.

Significant symptoms of disease charted on the interdisciplinary worksheet were reflected in the extensive dental caries, generalized occlusal traumatism, advanced periodontitis, poor crown to root ratio, and poor distribution of remaining teeth (Case 6 Worksheet). The patient had lost an excessive number of teeth and an extraordinary amount of attachment apparatus. The immediate prognosis for the maxillary arch was questionable at best. Saving tooth No. 11, the maxillary left canine, was critical for the execution of a maxillary fixed prosthesis. In this case, a definite prognosis for the maxillary arch was established during Phase II therapy.

The extensive nature of the disease process and the severe deformity created by disease and associated with the many missing teeth required a complex sequence of therapy, which for this patient entailed simultaneous and continuous Phase I and Phase II therapy as well as strategically planned stages of re-evaluation.

The ideal treatment plan included Phase I scaling, root planning, hygiene instruction, curettage, caries control, fixed stabilization of the lower right and anterior teeth, and Hawley bite plane therapy (Fig. 4–13). Although general Phase I therapy was instituted first, followed by mandibular tooth movement and stabilization required for the maxillary Hawley bite plane placement, the treatment plan required that both phases of therapy then be administered simultaneously. Phase II therapy included adjunctive orthodontic and advanced periodontal procedures. The occlusal vertical dimension was established with the Hawley bite plane, and the malpositioned mandibular molars were uprighted and then stabilized. The maxillary anterior teeth were then retracted, and provisional restorations were put in place. After the therapy was re-evaluated clinically and radiographically, Phase II periodontal surgery was executed. The results of all therapy were once again evaluated, the need for and extent of the final prosthesis were confirmed, and the final prosthesis was executed.

Successful execution of simultaneous Phases

I and II of treatment enabled the clinician to retain the maxillary left canine, which was the key to this case. A questionable prognosis for the maxillary arch was overcome, and long-term retention of teeth became possible. A very complex and extensive amount of therapy is required to treat disease of this advanced nature. The poor distribution of abutments, the excessive off-axis forces, and the severe periodontal deformity created by all etiologic factors demands a combination of advanced periodontal, or-

Text continued on page 152

INTERDISCIPLINARY TREATMENT PLANNING WORKSHEET

Patient Name __Anthony P.__   DATE ___9-11-72___

SIGNIFICANT MEDICAL AND SYSTEMIC DISEASE OR CONDITION
   __Non-contributory__

SIFNIFICANT DENTAL/SOCIAL HISTORY
Chief dental complaint and history __"I can't chew." "My partial denture doesn't fit."__
 __Patient had progressive tooth loss and new partials made for the last 20 years.__

Other complaints:
   Mastication __Chief complaint__   Aesthetics __Patient unhappy__
   Comfort __Teeth hurt when patient chews__   Phonetics __Negative__
Understanding of dental problem __Patient understands advanced nature of his problem.__

Desires __"save his teeth" - new lower partial denture__

Attitude __Excellent__

Age __41__ Gender __M__ Occupation __Meat cutter__   Financial Resources __Pt. is able to pay over 2 yrs.__

Other Considerations _____

CONSULTATIONS WITH DENTAL SPECIALISTS OR PHYSICIAN
   __Blood sugar negative - CBC normal__

SIGNIFICANT SIGNS, SYMPTOMS AND ETIOLOGY OF DISEASE AND SIGNIFICANT MECHANCIAL FACTORS

	#3-DO	# 9-MLB	#18-MOD	#31-MOD
Caries	6-DL	11-MLF	19-MOD	
	6-ML	11-DLF	20-DO	22-DO
		15-MOD	21-DO	22-MF

Pulpal Disease (considerations)   #11 intentional extirpation

Inflammatory Periodontal Disease   Advanced periodontitis with secondary occlusal traumatism   See perio charting

Occlusal Traumatism   See occlusal charting. Generalized secondary occlusal traumatism

Severe Wear   Negative

Significant Mechanical Factors   Poor crown-root ratio Poor distribution of teeth, especially maxillary left Missing teeth #1,2,5,7,8,10,12,13,14,16 - #17,23,24,25,26,28,29,31,32

TMJ Dysfunction and Other Oral Disease   None

CASE 6 WORKSHEET. Management of a patient's dentition in which advanced disease exists with Phase I and Phase II therapy.

Worksheet continued on following page

IDEAL TREATMENT PLAN   Patient Name Anthony P.   Date 9-11-72

1 Consult physician for suspected systemic etiology
2 Scaling, root planing and curettage
3 Nutritional evaluation
4 Caries control
5 Retract lower canines
6 Stabilize lower canines to right molar and left premolars
7 Retract maxillary anteriors with modified Hawley bite plane
8 Upright mandibular left molars
9 Place provisional restorations
10 Reevaluation
11 Periodontal surgery – hemisect and extract distal root of #30
12 Reevaluation
13 Final restorative therapy:
   Maxillary fixed splint #3 to #11
   Maxillary removable partial denture for #12, 13, 14
   Mandibular fixed splint
   Telescope all teeth

ALTERNATIVE TREATMENT PLANS

1 Consult physician for suspected systemic etiology
2 Scaling, root planing and curettage   12 Periodontal surgery
3 Nutritional evaluation   13 Restorative therapy:
4 Extract teeth with poor prognosis-9,11,15   Mandibular fixed splint
5 RCT on 3,4,6 and copings for overdenture   Maxillary overdenture
6 Maxillary overdenture
7 Retract lower canines
8 Stabilize lower canines to rt. molar and
     left premolars
9 Upright mandibular left molars
10 Place prov. rest. on mandibular arch
11 Reevaluation

RATIONALE FOR ACTUAL TREATMENT PLAN

The ideal treatment plan will be started and probably take 2 years. The patient was
apprised of the questionable prognosis of key abutment teeth (#9,11) in the maxillary
arch. If these teeth prove to be a poor risk, then a maxillary overdenture will be
considered. The prognosis for the mandibular arch is excellent. The patient is
willing to go through with all the advanced therapy.

FINANCIAL ARRANGEMENTS

  Monthly installments.

CASE 6 WORKSHEET *Continued*

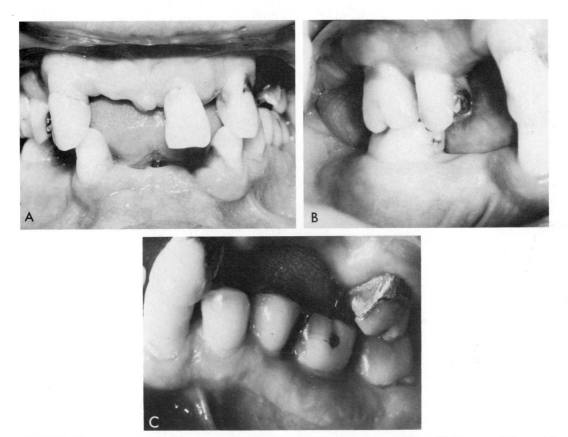

FIGURE 4–13 Management of a Patient's Dentition With Phase I and Phase II Therapy Where Advanced Disease Exists. *A,* This 41-year-old male's chief complaints were that he had a bad taste in his mouth, bleeding gums, and general discomfort. Finances, patient willingness to cooperate, and medical history were advantageous for optimal dental treatment. Note the flaring of the central incisor due to posterior bite collapse. *B,* This right buccal view demonstrates the multiple missing teeth, occlusal support on the two molars, and the flaring of the canine. *C,* On the left, the maxillary and mandibular second molars have drifted mesially, and the mandibular first molar and second premolar have overerupted.

Illustration continued on following page

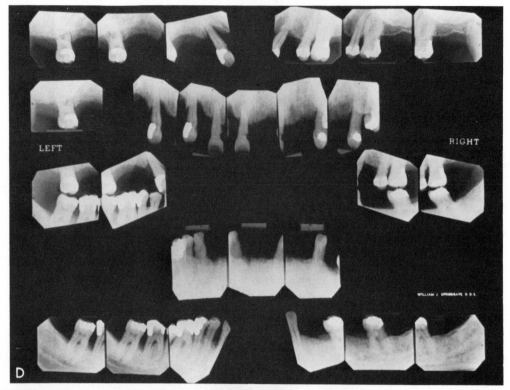

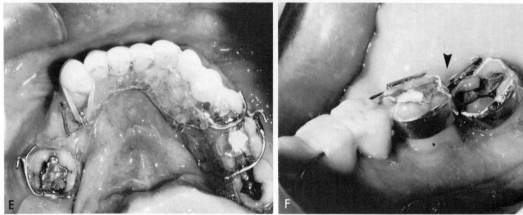

FIGURE 4–13 *Continued* **D,** The preoperative radiographs display the extensive destruction of the attachment apparatus. The radiographic picture is consistent with the clinical findings of 4- to 10-mm pocket depths and severe mobility patterns. The prognosis for the maxillary arch was poor. **E,** After initial scaling, root planing and curettage, caries control, and root canal therapy, Phase II therapy was started immediately, while Phase I therapy was continued. A mandibular removable appliance was used to reposition the canines. **F,** The mandibular molars, which were inclined mesially (arrow), were banded for uprighting. The provisional restoration on the anterior section served as anchorage and the Hawley bite plane disarticulated the molars, thus facilitating tooth movement.

Illustration continued on opposite page

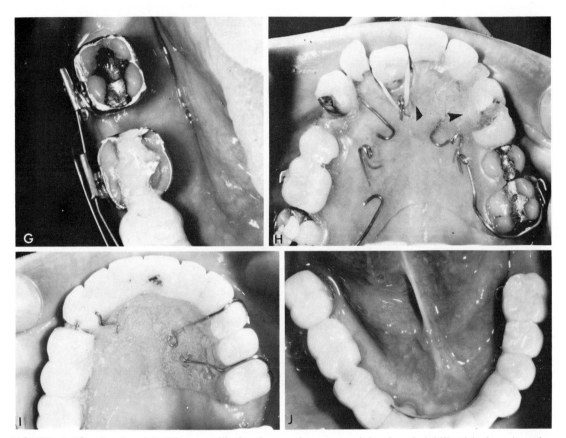

FIGURE 4–13 *Continued G,* The mandibular first molar was uprighted and stabilized in less time than the second molar. After 12 weeks, the second molar tooth movement was completed. *H,* The maxillary bite plane included palatal and buccal cleats to retract the maxillary canines and incisors. The arrows point to the final position of the left canine and the right central incisor, which had moved half the desired distance. Each anterior tooth was placed over basal bone and then stabilized with a fixed provisional restoration. *I,* The maxillary provisional restoration consisted of a combination of fixed and removable prostheses. The occlusal scheme, crown contours, and all requirements of the final restoration were established in the provisional restoration. *J,* The mandibular full-arch provisional restoration was placed.

Illustration continued on following page

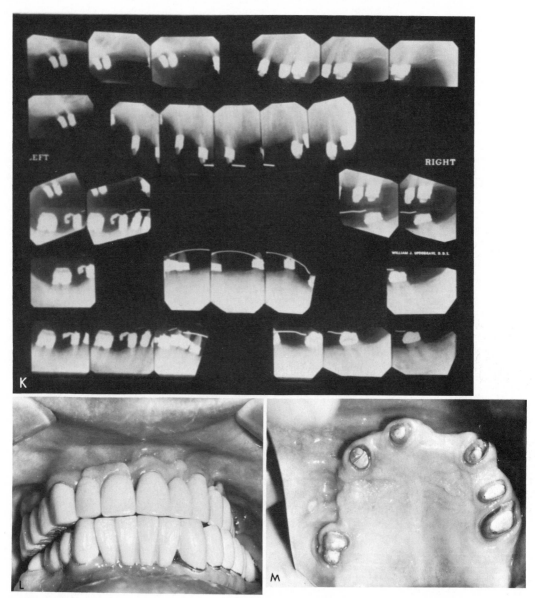

FIGURE 4–13 *Continued* **K,** After 6 months of stabilization and continuous scaling and root planing, a set of radiographs was taken and a clinical reevaluation was made of all periodontal, endodontic, orthodontic, occlusal, and restorative therapy. Advanced surgical procedures and pocket elimination were planned. After periodontal surgery, the provisional restorations were relined with new gold bands. **L,** The final restoration consisted of a maxillary fixed bridge from the first right molar to the left canine and a removable prosthesis in the left posterior section. The mandibular restoration was a bilateral fixed splint. **M,** Telescopes were utilized on both the maxilla and the mandible to protect the abutment teeth, provide parallelism, and allow future maintenance and conversion of the prosthesis.

Illustration continued on opposite page

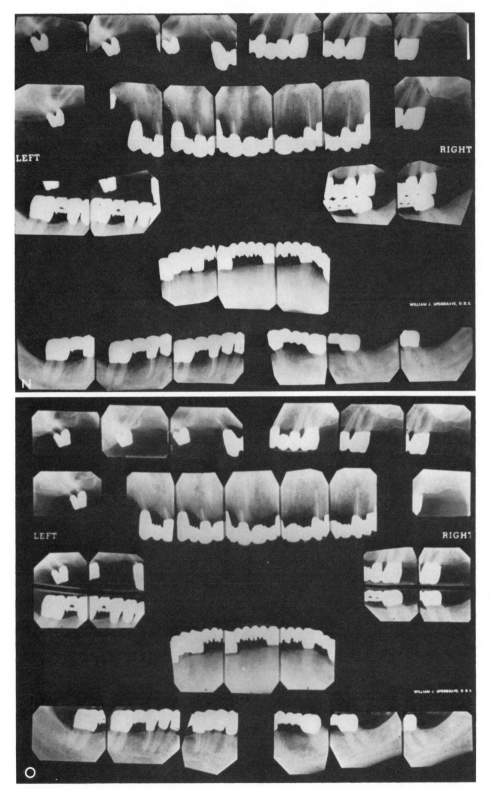

FIGURE 4–13 *Continued N,* Final radiographs, 1974. *O,* Postoperative radiographs, 1982. Note periapical radiolucency over maxillary left molar. The overcase was removed, and root canal therapy was done. (From Casullo, D. P., Matarazzo, F. S.: Occlusal considerations, Chapter 11. *In* Telescopic Prosthetic Therapy, Yalisove, I. and Dietz, J. (eds.). Stickley Press, Philadelphia, 1977.)

thodontic, endodontic, and restorative procedures.

The complex nature of this treatment requires fastidious attention to the basic principles of treatment planning and the sequence of therapy.

SUMMARY

Treatment planning is a unique and complex discipline usually addressed in an isolated manner by the various dental specialties. The purpose of this chapter was to present treatment planning as an interdisciplinary exercise based upon the fundamentals of the "Sequence of Therapy" (see Fig. 4–7). It is important that treatment planning be approached in the general practice setting in a systematic and standardized manner, that is, a routine set of sequenced steps. An interdisciplinary treatment planning worksheet has been provided as a tool for the organization of data gathered in both the dental examination and the communication phases of patient contact. It should offer an easy and consistently applicable method of presenting treatment plans to the patient as well as the rationale for the proposed therapy.

The basic and standardized mechanisms of treatment planning allow the clinician freedom of thought and expression based upon sound fundamental principles of therapy. There are no absolute rules, no unalterable courses, and no rigid thought processes. Instead, a philosophy of treatment and treatment planning will enhance the creativity of the individual clinician.

QUESTIONS

Please circle the correct answer(s). (There may be more than one correct answer.)

1. The sequence of therapy
    a. is significant only when planning for complex treatment
    b. is consistently divided into two phases and a maintenance phase
    c. is never modified or re-evaluated once Phase I therapy has begun
    d. for most cases never varies with the prognosis
    e. is a consistent and logical means of planning treatment

2. Phase I therapy includes
    a. elimination of active disease processes
    b. caries control
    c. communication with the patient
    d. treatment of emergencies
    e. verification of the diagnosis

3. An ideal treatment plan
    a. should be geared toward prevention
    b. should maximize survival of the prosthesis
    c. may require modifications and alterations during the course of treatment
    d. always involves extensive and complex therapy
    e. preserves the natural dentition using the most conservative means

4. An important objective of the clinician in treatment is
    a. to maintain patient health and to eliminate and control disease
    b. to ensure a result that is considered esthetically pleasing by the clinician
    c. to maximize patient comfort
    d. to replace missing teeth

5. Frequent evaluations of treatment
    a. are required during Phase I treatment to verify the diagnosis
    b. are important to assess the prognosis and patient's response to therapy
    c. may suggest that changes be made in the final treatment plan
    d. are important only when there is a questionable prognosis

6. Phase I therapy
   a. once initiated should not be modified regardless of the patient's response to treatment
   b. never includes occlusal therapy or appliances
   c. includes scaling, root planing, and other modalities to control inflammatory periodontal disease
   d. should never be started before the patient agrees to an ideal Phase II modality

7. The maintenance phase of therapy is
   a. highly important to ensure that therapy is successful and that there is no relapse or recurrence of disease
   b. unnecessary once the patient has demonstrated adequate home care
   c. never required more often than at 6-month intervals
   d. significant only when multiple teeth need replacement

8. A physiologic occlusion
   a. is a healthy occlusion
   b. manifests no signs or symptoms of disease
   c. meets the patient's requirements for comfort and appearance
   d. may contain aberrant morphology or aberrant occlusal relationships
   e. might not conform to the clinician's cosmetic ideals

9. The diagnosis of disease
   a. is not important for planning therapy and need not be verified
   b. is an analysis of the host's response to the etiologic factors
   c. may be difficult to determine if the patient shows few significant symptoms
   d. is important for both planning treatment and establishing the sequence of therapy

10. Communication with the patient is highly important to
    a. understand the patient's complaints
    b. ascertain the patient's level of understanding of dental needs and problems
    c. develop the patient's trust and motivation toward successful therapy
    d. avoid misunderstandings and answer any questions
    e. explain the doctor's philosophy of treatment and goals of therapy

11. A patient's own esthetic, phonetic, and functional requirements
    a. are not as significant as those of the clinician
    b. can never be modified by the clinician's views
    c. in a physiologic occlusion (healthy dentition) should not be influenced by the dentist's personal biases

12. Consultations with other specialists
    a. are rarely necessary
    b. must be received and recorded prior to planning treatment and establishing the sequence of therapy
    c. are usually an insignificant aspect for treatment planning
    d. are not as important as the opinion of the primary provider

13. Patient complaints
    a. are associated with mastication, esthetics, comfort, and phonetics
    b. may be totally subjective and unrelated to any pathology
    c. should always be treated regardless of cause or of the clinician's judgment
    d. are a secondary aspect of planning appropriate treatment

14. When using the interdisciplinary worksheets
    a. all significant data gathered from other sources should be recorded to help organize treatment plans
    b. the use of supplementary aids such as radiographs or study models is unnecessary
    c. it is not necessary to note the patient's needs or understanding of problems

15. In sequencing treatment
    a. all final restorative treatment must be planned prior to orthodontics and periodontal surgery

    b.   advanced periodontal osseous surgery is done prior to orthodontic therapy

    c.   final decisions as to strategic extractions of roots or teeth are always made before any treatment is initiated

    d.   the evaluation of prior treatment has little effect on Phase II therapy

16.   Unusual occlusal schemes in adult patients

    a.   should always be treated to make them closer to ideal

    b.   if representing a skeletal-dental deformity always require orthodontic treatment

    c.   when free of both disease and any patient complaints should not be treated

    d.   may warrant extensive treatment if esthetically unacceptable to the clinician

17.   At the termination of Phase I therapy

    a.   disease and excessive forces should be controlled

    b.   deformities, i.e., soft tissue and osseous craters, may remain

    c.   a re-evaluation before beginning Phase II is mandatory

    d.   therapy can stop here and be followed by maintenance only

    e.   patients may be dismissed until an emergency complaint arises

18.   In an extensive case, if Phase II advanced restorative treatment cannot be carried out

    a.   it is still mandatory that Phase II periodontal therapy (pocket elimination) be done

    b.   all patient treatment should be terminated at this time

    c.   the treatment plan could be modified to an alternative treatment plan for Phase II therapy

    d.   frequent maintenance can be done, and if advanced Phase II therapy is requested at some future time, it can then be implemented

19.   The rationale for the actual treatment plan

    a.   is important only for the clinician's records

    b.   should ideally be explained thoroughly to the patient

    c.   is an explanation of questionable prognosis and possible alternatives if problems develop

    d.   is never explained to the patient unless specifically requested

20.   Factors that may be considered in determining the prognosis are

    a.   patient's manual dexterity

    b.   age of patient and duration of disease

    c.   number of alternative treatment plans

    d.   systemic factors

    e.   amount of deformity created by the disease

21.   The prognosis may vary if

    a.   the dentist reaches a better understanding of the cause of the disease

    b.   the patient's financial status changes

    c.   the patient's understanding of the problem and attitude toward treatment improve

    d.   orthodontic treatment is instituted at an early point in therapy

22.   The formulation of the prognosis

    a.   is the process of evaluating the effects of the factors responsible for disease

    b.   involves an understanding of the multitude of dental disciplines involved in treatment

    c.   of a tooth or teeth is an ongoing process subject to modification based upon response to a treatment modality

    d.   of a tooth or teeth should be presented to the patient during the treatment planning visit

23.   An alternative treatment plan

    a.   is a poor substitute at best

    b.   rarely is used if the patient's finances allow for more extensive treatment

    c.   is an important and significant part of treatment planning

    d.   does not contradict the fundamentals presented in sequence of therapy

    e.   at the very least consists of Phase I therapy

24. The presentation of the treatment plan should include
    a. an explanation of the status of the patient's dentition and extent of disease
    b. prognosis insofar as it can be ascertained at this time
    c. immediate and long-term benefits of the proposed treatment plan
    d. duration and and cost of treatment
    e. presentation of alternative treatment plans as necessary

See answers in Appendix.

REFERENCES

1. Amsterdam, M.: Periodontal prosthesis—Twenty-five years in retrospect. *Alpha Omegan, 67*:8, 1974.
2. Amsterdam, N., and Abrams, L.: Periodontal prosthesis. *In* Goldman, H., and Cohen, D. W., (eds.): *Periodontal Therapy,* 5th ed., St. Louis, C. V. Mosby Co., 1973.
3. Casullo, D.: The integration of endodontics, periodontics and restorative dentistry in general practice. Part I. Diagnosis. Compend. Contin. Ed. Gen. Dent. *1* (2):137–147, 1980.
4. Casullo, D.: The integration of endodontics, periodontics and restorative dentistry in general practice. Part II. Sequence of therapy. Compend. Contin. Ed. Gen. Dent. *1* (4):268–281, 1980.

D. WALTER COHEN
NORMAN H. STOLLER

5

PERIODONTICS IN GENERAL PRACTICE

One of the most important aspects of general practice in the years ahead will be the inclusion of the advances in periodontics into everyday general dentistry. More attention to the recognition and treatment of periodontal diseases will become the responsibility of the general practitioner. The specialty of periodontics has contributed greatly to our understanding of the pathogenesis, etiology, and treatment of periodontopathies, and with more of our population living longer, greater effort by the general dental team will be required to incorporate these contributions into routine clinical practice. A study by Douglass and Day noted that about 3 per cent of a general practitioner's time is devoted to periodontics and orthodontics, and we can anticipate that this percentage will increase as the incidence of dental caries decreases and less effort is devoted to restorative dentistry.

There is a growing concern that the generalists of the 1980s and 1990s will have to assume more of the responsibility for recognizing and treating periodontal diseases than in the past. We may not have sufficient manpower to meet this challenge.

In the keynote address at the Eighth International Conference in Oral Biology (Tokyo, June 1980), devoted to the theme of the meeting, "Oral Disease Prevention," Chairman M. Skougaard made the following statement:

There has been a substantial increase in dental manpower during the last four to five decades. In some European countries the dentists/population ratio is approaching 1:1,000. If these facts are combined, the answer should be very simple; dental disease ought to be, if not eliminated, then at least drastically reduced. Unfortunately this is far from true. The situation with respect to periodontal disease is illustrated by a survey on the need for periodontal treatment conducted on a randomly-selected sample in Denmark. The results were extrapolated in order to obtain an estimate of the need for periodontal treatment in the entire adult population. On the basis of these calculations it was hypothesized that if every person in Denmark over the age of 25 were to receive periodontal treatment according to this professionally-assessed treatment need then every dentist in the country would have his full working capacity occupied carrying out oral hygiene instruction, scaling and pocket treatment. Similar estimates for other European countries have resulted in similar conclusions. It is unnecessary to discuss whether the estimations were too crude or the extrapolations too bold. The fact remains that periodontal disease is far from being eliminated. On the contrary the situation is so bad that traditional periodontal treatment of the adult population would be totally unrealistic.

Papers such as this make one question whether there is an oversupply of dentists in the United States. If all generalists recognized and began to treat the periodontopathies of their patients, would they still complain of voids in their appointment schedules? At a workshop held in Bethesda, Maryland, on May 13 and 14, 1981 under the auspices of the National Institute for Dental Research, the participants raised this issue, summarized as follows:

Chronic destructive periodontal disease is among the most prevalent human infectious diseases on this planet. Research has demonstrated that plaque-induced periodontal disease begins in the gingival tissues of young individuals, and if unrecognized and untreated such sites can be observed to advance with time to periodontitis. It is a major oral health problem that surpasses dental caries in its ravages in the human dentition, resulting in the loss of most permanent teeth in individual patients. It was the feeling of the Workshop that even if the dental profession could address the problem of recognition of disease, improve patient skills in plaque-control methods, and effect professional removal of hard and soft accumulations from the teeth and pocket treatment, there might not be sufficient trained manpower in the United States to accomplish the objective of meeting the periodontal needs of our society. It was the firm belief of the Workshop that the periodontal needs of the population must be identified and treated earlier, and if this goal is achieved, the cost-effectiveness of early treatment will save millions of hours for the United States work force and billions of dollars in future health care expenditures.

INTRODUCTION TO PERIODONTAL DISEASE

Epidemiology

The number of cases of untreated moderately advanced to advanced periodontitis that exist in the population of patients who regularly seek dental care is inexcusable. The reasons for this apparent neglect are numerous and complex. Historically, the emphasis of dental education was on the treatment of dental caries, despite the fact that periodontal disease accounts for perhaps 70 per cent of all tooth loss. Compounding this lack of education is the fact that although patients perceive themselves to be susceptible to dental caries, very few believe they are susceptible to periodontal disease. Even now that dental education has begun to place more emphasis on the management of periodontal disease, one still encounters many recent dental school graduates who fail to manage their patients' periodontal problems adequately.

In the United States, less than 3 per cent of the dental treatment of general practitioners is directed at periodontal disease. It is true that the treatment of periodontal pathology is often frustrating, since patient cooperation is such an integral part of the treatment process. Nevertheless, the disease can be controlled, and it is the dental team's obligation to do so. It is no longer acceptable to consider tooth mortality as a result of periodontal disease to be part of the aging process, nor is it acceptable to ignore gingivitis

in the adolescent or incipient periodontitis in the young adult. Numerous studies over the past few years have shown that the disease can be managed successfully, especially when treatment is instituted early in the disease process. The purpose of this section is to examine some of these studies.

For many years it was felt that periodontitis was a normal sequela of aging. Indeed, numerous epidemiologic studies performed in the 1950s and 1960s demonstrated quite clearly that the prevalence and severity of periodontitis increase with age. However, most of these same studies also show that periodontitis is related to oral uncleanliness, specifically, to the presence of microbial plaque. It has become increasingly clear that it is the oral hygiene status of the patient, not the age, that is responsible for the disease. The positive correlation seen between disease severity and age is the result of the disease being a chronic progressive disorder rather than a disease involving diminished host resistance.

Studies by Löe et al. have clearly demonstrated the effect of appropriate dental treatment on periodontal disease. Two diverse populations of patients were examined; one group consisted of Norwegian academicians, the other of Sri Lankan tea laborers. The Norwegians between the ages of 3 and 16 years were given free comprehensive dental care with a systematic preventive program. Free dental care was continued through age 21 years. The Sri Lankans received virtually no dental treatment and toothbrushing was unknown. By age 40, the average Norwegian in the study had lost 1.5 mm of attachment, and attachment loss was progressing at less than 0.1 mm per year. There were no cases of rapidly progressing adult or juvenile periodontitis in the group. In contrast, the Sri Lankans had lost 4.5 mm of bone by age 40 years. Attachment loss was progressing at an annual rate of 0.2 mm on the buccal surfaces and 0.3 mm in the interproximal areas. One per cent of 15-year-old Sri Lankans had localized loss of osseous support exceeding 10 mm. It would appear from the results of this study that if comprehensive dental care, including preventive care, is initiated early in life, the vast majority of periodontal breakdown can be prevented.

Another study carried out by Axelsson and Lindhe confirms the benefit of preventive dentistry and its effect on the periodontium. These investigators studied the effect of scaling, prophylaxis, and oral hygiene instructions delivered every 2 to 3 months to an adult population over the age of 35 years. The control population was seen once a year and received only symptomatic treatment. These subjects continued to manifest gingival inflammation and loss of periodontal support as well as new carious lesions. Attachment loss in the control population was progressing at the rate of 0.2 mm per year. The test population had almost no gingival inflammation, had no loss of attachment, and developed very little tooth decay over the 6-year study period.

A number of additional clinical trials performed over the past several years have demonstrated the efficacy of periodontal therapy in managing existing periodontal disease. Of particular note are those that follow their subjects for extended periods of time (at least 5 years). Ramfjord and his coworkers examined the effects of scaling, root planing, oral hygiene instructions, and the use of either apically positioned flaps or open flap curettage on periodontitis. Regardless of the surgical technique employed, the progression of the disease was essentially eliminated. Similar studies by Lindhe and Nyman yielded even more dramatic results. In the latter studies, more time was spent maintaining impeccable oral hygiene. Lindhe and Nyman showed that it is possible to arrest even advanced periodontitis with appropriate therapy when oral hygiene is maintained at nearly perfect levels with biweekly professional tooth cleaning. In a retrospective evaluation of the success of periodontal therapy provided in a private practice of periodontics, Hirschfeld and Wasserman analyzed tooth mortality in 600 patients who had been actively treated and then placed on periodontal maintenance at 4- to 6-month intervals for at least 15 years. Five hundred of the patients lost fewer than 3 teeth, and 300 lost no teeth at all. Seventy-six patients lost between 4 and 6 teeth, and 25 patients lost 10 to 23 teeth. Tooth loss tended to be bilaterally symmetric. It should be noted that many of the teeth lost during the period of this study had had extremely guarded prognoses prior to treatment.

A retrospective study by Becker et al. also demonstrated the progressive nature of periodontal disease. In that study, 29 patients who had refused periodontal therapy were examined 1 to 10 years after their initial examinations. All of the patients studied manifested increased loss of periodontal support. "Increases in the mean annual pocket depths per tooth per patient varied from 0.24 mm per year to 2.46 mm per year."

The epidemiologic data currently available regarding the prevention and control of periodontal disease are quite clear in their implications: (1) The disease can be prevented, (2) the management of existing disease can be effective, and (3) the prevention and control of the disease are primarily contingent on the ability of the patient and therapist to eliminate microbial plaque from the supra- and subgingival aspects of the periodontium.

The Soft Tissues of the Periodontium

The entire oral cavity is lined with mucosa. The keratinized surfaces of the mucosal lining, i.e., the palate, tongue, and gingiva, are referred to as masticatory mucosa, and the nonkeratinized surfaces are called the alveolar mucosa. The mucous membrane, which covers the alveolar process and makes contact with and actually attaches to the tooth, can be divided into two rather distinct zones, one keratinized, the other nonkeratinized. The keratinized tissue is the gingiva. Its most coronal aspect is referred to as the free gingival margin (FGM). In a healthy dentition it is 0.5 to 2 mm coronal to the cementoenamel junction. The junction of the gingiva with the nonkeratinized alveolar mucosa marks the most apical extent of the gingiva. This junction of gingiva with the alveolar mucosa is the mucogingival junction (MGJ). The distance from the FGM to the MGJ varies from tooth to tooth and from individual to individual. On the facial surfaces it varies in width from approximately 1 to 5 mm. It is usually narrowest on the buccal surface of the mandibular first premolar area and widest in the maxillary incisor region (Fig. 5–1). On the lingual aspect of the mandibular dentition, the width of the gingival tends to be narrowest in the central incisor region and widest in the second molar region. Its width is determined in part by the position of the tooth as it erupts into the dentition and in part by genetic predisposition. A tooth that erupts in facial ver-

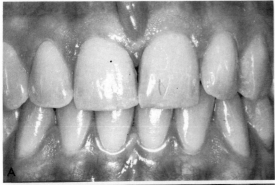

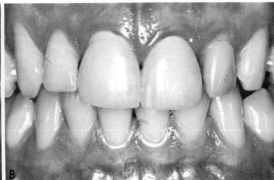

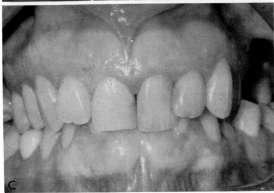

FIGURE 5–1 **Variation of Normal Gingival Width.** Typically, the gingival tissues are widest in the maxillary incisor region and are narrowest in the mandibular first premolar area. There are, however, great variations from one individual to another. For example, compare the mandibular anterior area in the patients shown in *A, B,* and *C*.

sion, for example, will tend to have a narrower band of gingiva on its facial aspect and a somewhat wider band on the lingual aspect.

The external surface of the gingiva is referred to as the oral epithelium. It is a keratinized or parakeratinized stratified squamous epithelium with rather distinct rete ridges. The underlying connective tissue is a dense vascular mass of nonelastic collagen fibers. The deeper fibers of the connective tissue are confluent with the periosteum of the alveolar process. Connective tissue fibers also insert into the portion of the root surface that is coronal to the crestal bone. These fibers, which fan out in all directions from the root surface, constitute the gingival fiber apparatus. Connective tissue fibers also pass from the cementum of one tooth to the cementum of the adjacent tooth in the interproximal area. These fibers are referred to as the transseptal fibers and are part connective tissue attachment.

Around the circumference of each tooth is the 0.5 to 2 mm deep gingival sulcus, where the sulcular epithelium of the gingiva contacts, but does not attach to, the tooth. This potential space between the gingiva and the

tooth is referred to as the gingival crevice or gingival sulcus. The sulcular epithelium is a relatively nonkeratinized stratified squamous epithelium that is confluent with the oral epithelium at the orifice of the sulcus. Apical to the sulcular epithelium is the junctional epithelium (JE). It forms an attachment between the connective tissue of the gingiva and the tooth surface. The JE is a nonkeratinized stratified squamous epithelium that is 15 to 30 cells thick at its most coronal aspect, where it meets the sulcular epithelium. It narrows to one cell at its most apical extent at, or just apical to, the cementoenamel junction. Hemidesmosomes attach the junctional epithelium to the dental cuticle. This attachment between the tooth and JE constitutes the epithelial attachment. The apicocoronal extent of the JE is from approximately 0.5 to 1 mm. The distance from the most coronal cell of the JE to the FGM is defined as the "histologic" sulcus (Fig. 5–2).

Classification of Periodontal Diseases

Periodontal diseases can be subdivided into those forms that are plaque-induced and the non–plaque-induced lesions (Table

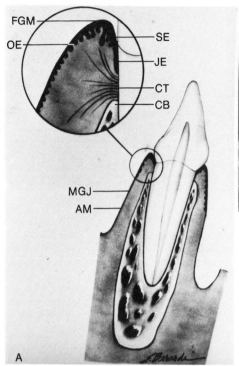

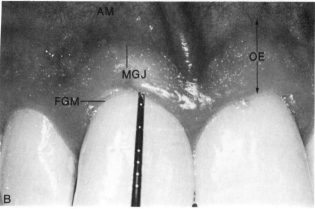

FIGURE 5–2 The Relationship of the Gingival Tissues. *A,* Free gingival margin (FGM), oral epithelium (OE), sulcular epithelium (SE), junctional epithelium (JE), connective tissue attachment (CT), crestal bone (CB), mucogingival junction (MGJ), and alveolar mucosa (AM). *B,* The periodontal probe is measuring the depth of the clinical sulcus (2 mm in this area).

5–1). The plaque-induced periodontopathies included gingivitis, acute necrotizing ulcerative gingivitis (ANUG), juvenile periodontitis, and periodontitis. The non–plaque-induced form is trauma from occlusion, or occlusal traumatism. Frequently trauma from occlusion is also coupled with periodontitis, and this combined form is called occlusal periodontitis as an abbreviation for occlusal traumatism and periodontitis. The plaque-induced forms of disease have their origin in the gingival unit, whereas non–plaque-induced pathology is seen initially in the attachment apparatus.

TABLE 5–1 Classification of Periodontal Diseases

Periodontium	
Gingival Unit	*Attachment Apparatus*
Free and attached gingiva	Alveolar bone
Alveolar mucosa	Periodontal ligament
	Cementum
Periodontal Diseases	
Plaque-Induced	*Non–Plaque-Induced*
Gingivitis	Trauma from
Acute necrotizing ulcerative gingivitis	occlusion
Juvenile periodontitis	
Periodontitis	
Occlusal Periodontitis	

EXAMINATION OF THE PERIODONTIUM

Clinical Examination

Prior to the initiation of an examination of the periodontium, a thorough health history should be taken and carefully evaluated. The examination of the periodontium begins with an inspection of the gingival tissues.

Gingival Tissues

The color of the healthy gingiva can vary from coral pink to black depending on the degree of pigmentation, the thickness of the tissues, and the underlying vasculature. The tissues should have a mat or stippled appearance. A marked reddening or a red-blue cyanotic color are indicative of underlying pathology and are therefore noteworthy. Likewise, changes in the gingival architecture from its normal knifelike appearance at the tooth–soft tissue interface are noteworthy. Perhaps the most subtle change in the gingival architecture is a slight swelling in the vicinity of the free gingival margin. This often leads to a slightly rolled gingival margin with a rather glossy appearance. The

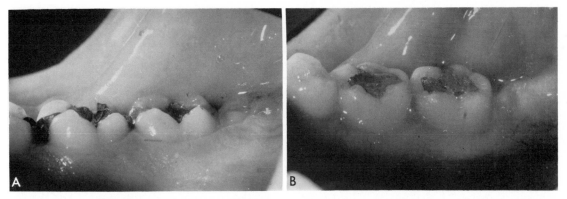

FIGURE 5–3 Variation of Normal Gingival Positions. The free gingival margin is often 3 to 5 mm coronal to the cementoenamel junction on the lingual aspect of the mandibular molars and on the palatal aspect of the maxillary molars. Note the coronal location of the gingival tissues in **A** and compare them with the gingiva in **B**. This variation may predispose to periodontal disease, since the sulci associated with the conditions tend to be somewhat deeper than normal.

consistency of the gingival tissues in health is rather firm and dense. In the diseased state they may feel boggy or spongy. The position of the free gingival margin (FGM) relative to the cementoenamel junction (CEJ) should be noted. It is not unusual to find the FGM in a considerably more coronal than normal position on the lingual surfaces of mandibular second and third molars (Fig. 5–3). This is an anatomic variation of normal, and although it may predispose to disease, it does not necessarily require treatment. This position of the free gingival margin should be documented either with careful measurements from the CEJ or, perhaps more practically, with a set of study models.

The width of the gingiva should also be noted. Of particular concern are areas where the FGM and MGJ are in close proximity to one another. The relationship of frenal attachments to the FGM is also noteworthy, especially when a gentle tug on the frenum results in movement of the FGM. There is a wide range of normal, which is particularly apparent when one observes the thickness or thinness of the periodontal tissues. At one extreme is a highly scalloped, very thin, delicate tissue with thin underlying alveolar bone. At the other extreme is the thick periodontium with a less scalloped, blunt-looking soft tissue (Fig. 5–4). The former is probably more prone to gingival recession as a result of either tissue trauma or periodontitis, whereas the latter is better able to withstand soft tissue trauma and does not recede as readily in the presence of periodontitis.

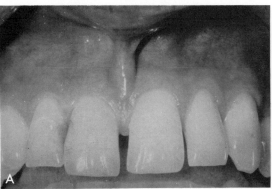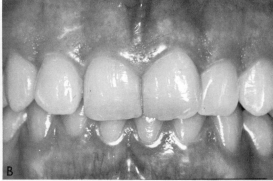

FIGURE 5–4 Variation of Normal Gingival Thickness. Variation of normal gingival thickness is reflected in **A** (thin architecture) and **B** (thick architecture). The gingival profile reflects the thickness of the underlying osseous tissues. Thin tissue is more prone to gingival recession than is thicker tissue.

Sulcular Epithelium

Attention should next be directed to the status of the sulcular epithelium. By gently inserting a calibrated periodontal probe just apical to the free gingival margin and by tracing the gingival crevice from mesial to distal, one can make a rapid determination of the health of the sulcular tissues. If the sulcular lining is intact and healthy, no bleeding will occur. If, however, the integrity of the sulcular epithelium is impaired, bleeding will almost certainly occur. The clinical pocket should then be carefully explored. The clinical pocket is defined as the distance from the free gingival margin to the most apical point that a calibrated periodontal probe reaches when it is gently inserted into the gingival crevice. In a healthy state, the clinical pocket and histologic pocket are nearly equal to one another. In a diseased state, however, when the integrity of the junctional and sulcular epithelia and their underlying connective tissue is impaired, the periodontal probe may not stop at the JE. Instead it may tear through these tissues and not stop until relatively healthy tissue is encountered (Fig. 5–5). The histologic pocket may differ from the clinical pocket by several millimeters. The presence of bleeding once again indicates underlying disease. Suppuration should also be noted when it occurs during the probing process.

Pocket Depth

In the absence of bone loss, an increase in the clinical pocket depth is the result of either a coronal movement of the free gingival margin or a loss of integrity of the JE, SE, and underlying connective tissue. Pockets of this type are called gingival pockets, or pseudopockets. When the tip of the periodontal probe passes more than 1 mm apical to the cementoenamel junction, one can assume that there has been an apical migration of the attachment apparatus. Pockets that are the result of attachment loss are termed periodontal pockets. By measurement of pocket depths in various areas around the circumference of the tooth, the topography of the attachment loss can be established. When the tip of the probe is apical

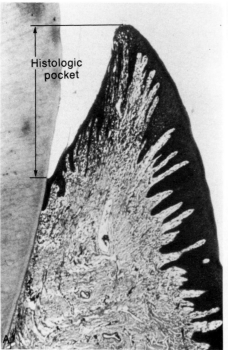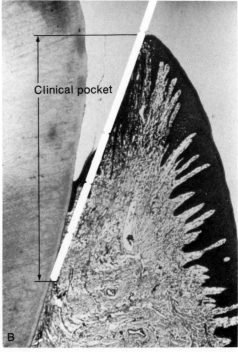

FIGURE 5–5   The Histologic and Clinical Pockets. *A,* The histologic pocket is defined as the distance from the free gingival margin to the most coronal cell of the junctional epithelium. *B,* The clinical pocket is defined by the distance a periodontal probe inserted into the gingival crevice will extend in an apical direction. Because the probe will easily penetrate inflamed tissues, the clinical pocket is deeper than the histologic pocket.

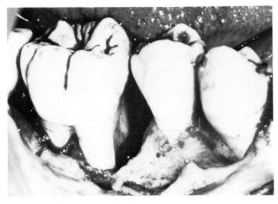

FIGURE 5–6   An Infrabony Pocket. This example is primarily that of a one-wall osseous defect, since the buccal, lingual, and mesial walls of the molar are missing. Only the distal wall of the premolar remains.

to the bone in surrounding areas, the periodontal pocket in that region is said to be an infrabony pocket. When the probe tip is coronal to the surrounding bone, the periodontal pocket is considered to be suprabony. Infrabony pockets are further classified according to the number of osseous walls remaining in the area probed (Fig. 5–6).

Accurate probing can be accomplished only if the tip of the probe is kept in contact with the tooth at all times. The long axis of the probe should be kept nearly parallel to the long axis of the tooth, except when one is probing the interdental area. In that area the contact between two adjacent teeth precludes probing the midinterproximal area without slightly tilting the probe off the long axis of the tooth. Utilizing the probe in this fashion will result in a slightly increased pocket depth. However, since the majority of osseous defects occur in the interproximal area, it is essential that it be fully explored (Fig. 5–7).

Furcations

All potential furcation areas should also be explored for the presence of attachment loss within the furcation. Either a specially designed Nabers probe or an appropriate curet can be used for this part of the examination. Furcation involvements are classified as being Class I (incipient) if the tip of the exploring device barely enters the furcation, Class II if the tip of the probe frankly enters the furcation, and Class III if the probe tip enters one furcation and exits at another, e.g., if the probe tip passes from the buccal furcation to the lingual furcation of a mandibular molar (Fig. 5–8). The findings obtained during the clinical examination should be carefully correlated with those of the radiographic examination. When incongruities seem to exist, they should be explored further. If, for example, a deep pocket is measured on the mesial aspect of a

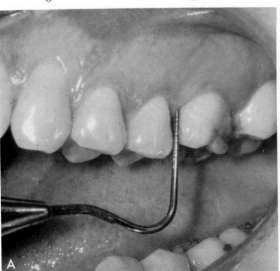
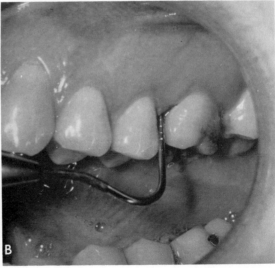

FIGURE 5–7   Probing the Interproximal Area. Since most osseous defects occur in the midinterproximal area, it is necessary to angle the periodontal probe in that direction. In **A,** the probe is placed too far in a buccal direction, missing the interproximal osseous defect, which becomes apparent in **B** when the probe is properly angled.

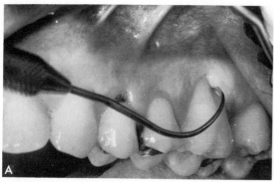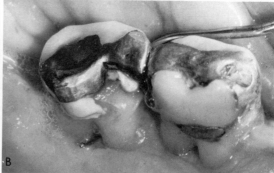

FIGURE 5–8   Exploring Furcations. Using a Nabers probe to explore an incipient Class II furcation *(A)* and a Class III furcation *(B)*.

tooth in which there is no apparent radiographic evidence of bone loss, it is appropriate that another radiograph be taken with the probe or other radiopaque object in place. Combined endodontic-periodontic lesions are often discovered in this manner. Similarly, when radiographic evidence of bone loss is apparent and when pocket depths seem minimal, the area should be reprobed. It is possible that a piece of calculus impeded the periodontal probe.

Mobility

The mobility of each tooth should be measured. There are a variety of ways to accomplish this; all are subject to error and lack of reproducibility. Perhaps the best technique available to the clinician is the one that requires the use of the ends of two mir-

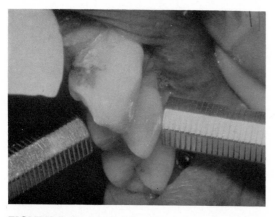

FIGURE 5–9   Measuring Horizontal Tooth Mobility. Two mirror handle ends are alternatively tapped on the facial and palatal aspect of the tooth. In addition to looking for movement, it is useful to feel the vibration of the instruments on the tooth and to listen to the sound of the percussion. A mobile tooth will elicit a dull sound.

ror handles (Fig. 5–9). By tapping the tooth in a buccolingual direction, one can see small displacements of the tooth as well as feel the vibration of the tooth as it hits one handle. In addition, it is useful to listen to the sound of the tooth as it is tapped. A loose tooth sounds duller.

Mobility can be classified in numerous ways. A clinically acceptable method is to score a tooth with no clinically perceptible mobility as 0. A tooth that barely moves but whose movement is just visible (a typical mandibular incisor, for example) is scored 1/2. Readily discernible mobility can be given a score of 1. Extreme mobility to the point at which function is impaired can be scored with a 3. A score of 2 can be utilized for mobilities between a 1 and a 3. This is a crude index, but it does have clinical applicability.

One should attempt to relate the mobility to the clinical situation. Horizontal tooth mobility is almost always the result of a combination of one or more of the following factors: inflammation of the periodontal tissues, loss of osseous support, excessive forces delivered to the tooth, and tooth anatomy. The 1/2 mobility typically seen in a mandibular incisor in an uninflamed periodontium is the result of root anatomy.

An additional measurement of the tooth mobility can be obtained by observing fremitus patterns. By placing one's finger on the tooth–soft tissue interface and then by having the patient articulate his teeth in all the various positions (intercuspal, protrusive, working, and so on), small movements of the tooth can be felt. These fremitus patterns should be correlated with mobility.

An integral part of the periodontal examination is evaluation of the patient's occlusion. One should routinely determine whether a particular occlusion is physiologic or pathologic.

Radiographic Aspects

When viewing the lamina dura and the periodontal ligament, the clinician must realize that only the proximal portions are visible. The buccal and lingual areas are not seen in the radiograph. Widening of the periodontal ligament space, however, is also diagnostic of what is happening in the buccal and lingual aspects. The interpretation then is based on the assumption that the entire periodontal ligament space has been recorded. Widening is diagnostic of heavy function or trauma, while narrowing is more often seen in minimal use. These findings, however, are correlated to those seen in the lamina dura and the alveolar housing. Widening of the periodontal ligament space and loss of lamina dura can be interpreted as resorption of the alveolar bone. Translucency observed in the supporting bone undermining the lamina dura is evidence of resorption of bone.

When viewing the crestal portion of the alveolar housing, the examiner looks for intact crestal bone, evidenced by the opaque nature of the lamina dura. Loss of this opacity (with evidence of translucency) is evidence of a resorptive lesion. The overall height of the interproximal septum in relation to the cementoenamel junction of the teeth offers evidence of whether loss of bone height has occurred. Thus, bone recession can be detected. The exact topography of osseous defects cannot be ascertained from the radiography; however, hemisepta can be recognized in this manner. Using the radiographs in combination with the clinical pocket depths is a valuable method for ascertaining the nature of the osseous defects.

Crestal Bone

This section is concerned with the radiology of the alveolus, which supports the teeth and centers on the crestal portion, the interproximal septum, and that area subjacent to the tooth roots, the periapical area. As previously stated, the topography of the crestal area is not recorded, and even in instances of craters the true crestal location cannot be discerned radiographically. For a long time, attempts have been made to insert opaque markers into the gingival detachments to vis-

ualize crestal contour. Hirschfeld points can be utilized to record pocket depth in relation to crestal bone.

The width of the interproximal septum is directly related to the proximity of the roots of the teeth. For example, the flaring and narrow interproximal bone found in the maxillary molar region is of much concern to the therapist. Once the marginal loss of tissue has occurred, the resultant change in local environment often makes it an impossible area for the patient to clean. Poor topography and continuation of disease result in tooth loss.

The examiner must be conscious of viewing the interradicular area of the molar teeth. Furca involvements associated with bone loss appear as translucencies in these anatomic areas. Associated with these furca involvements are crestal topography changes. These data must be considered together. For example, furca involvements of the maxillary molar teeth can occur from a buccal or a proximal entrance, but entrance to the mandibular molar teeth can occur only from the buccal or lingual aspects. The most difficult furca involvement to recognize in the radiograph is that of the maxillary first premolar, since entrance can be made only from the proximal side. Since the buccal aspect overshadows the lingual aspect, the interradicular bone may not be seen. Therefore, an impression of the involvement can be made only by topography of the bone crest after intentional mesiodistal distortion of the radiograph.

It must be stressed that incipient furca involvement is not recorded on the radiograph, since the loss of bone is too minimal to detect. Incipient lesions, therefore, must be found clinically.

Clinical Crown-to-Root Ratio

The determination of the clinical crown-to-root ratio is made on the basis of radiographic findings. The portion of the tooth embedded in bone is related to that which is not. When there is more tooth embedded in bone, the prognosis tends to be positive. When there is little of the tooth embedded in bone, the prognosis tends to be poorer. Although not definitive indicators of prognosis, these findings are indicative. However, the clinician must take into account possible regeneration of bone, possible gingival attachment at more coronal levels, and changes in clinical crown–clinical root relationship.

Darkfield Microscopy Examination

The subgingival flora at healthy and diseased sites in subjects with chronic periodontitis was studied by darkfield microscopy by Listgarten and Hellden in 1978. Their findings demonstrated clear-cut differences in the microbial composition of healthy and periodontally diseased areas in the same individuals. The proportion of motile rods and spirochetes was significantly higher at diseased sites than at healthy sites. In a subsequent report, Listgarten et al. indicated that mechanical débridement, with or without antibiotic therapy, altered the microbial flora of untreated periodontal lesions in patients with chronic periodontitis. Listgarten and Hellden described the technique of sampling by removing any detectable supragingival plaque with a Gracey curet. The cleaned curet tip is introduced below the gingival margin as far as the anatomy of the gingival sulcus will permit, and the removed subgingival debris is suspended in a solution of 0.85 sodium chloride containing 1 per cent gelatin. It may well prove to be efficacious to monitor the spirochete and motile rod populations of the subgingival flora to determine the optimal time periods for periodontal maintenance.

Arnim and others have advocated monitoring patient plaque-control methods by using phase-contrast microscopy to examine microbial plaque. This method is also used to motivate patients to perfect their personal oral hygiene methods.

Socransky and others have examined the aerobic and anaerobic flora from various forms of periodontal disease. The technique of removing and culturing anaerobic bacteria is sophisticated and has yielded a great deal of information in the specific flora related to different forms of human disease. These culturing techniques are not yet efficacious for routine clinical use.

ETIOLOGY OF PERIODONTAL DISEASE

Gingivitis and Periodontitis

The primary etiologic factor responsible for gingivitis and periodontitis is one or more of the bacterial components of microbial plaque. Plaque is a complex ecosystem consisting of a variety of bacteria and their carbohydrate and protein substrate. Plaque has the ability to adhere tenaciously to the tooth surface.

Plaque Microbiology

In excess of 180 different species of bacteria have been isolated from human dental plaque. It is not known at this time precisely how the bacteria found in plaque are transmitted from one mouth to another. As an individual matures, bacterial flora becomes progressively more complex. The particular organisms that an individual acquires in the course of a lifetime are probably determined by at least two factors: coming in contact with a given species in sufficient number and having an oral environment in which the species can survive.

Very little is known about the type of environment required for the various organisms, but it is known that most of the bacteria associated with periodontal disease are not present in an edentulous mouth. It has been speculated that the environment in the subgingival pocket created by gingivitis allows for the population of organisms that are associated with periodontitis. The relative proportions of organisms may vary dramatically from one area of the mouth to another. Plaque in a shallow, relatively healthy pocket on the facial surface of a tooth can vary greatly from the subgingival plaque obtained from an unhealthy pocket on the mesial aspect of the same tooth. Information gleaned from sophisticated culturing techniques has begun to show that flora associated with health, gingivitis, periodontitis, and juvenile periodontitis differ from one another (Table 5–2). It is still not known whether these differences result from selective bacterial growth, from the disease process, or from subsequent changes in the local environment, or whether the different flora actually caused the disease.

Plaque-Retentive Factors

A variety of factors influence the plaque-retentive nature of the tooth surface as well as the ability of the patient to mechanically remove plaque. Supragingival calculus, rough or poorly contoured restorations, unrestored caries in the gingival one third of the tooth, orthodontic appliances, and malposed

TABLE 5–2 Microbiota of Various Forms of Periodontal Disease

I. Periodontitis
   A. Predominant flora
      1. Chronic—several gram-positive organisms, esp. *Actinomyces* spp, other filamentous organisms, occasional streptococci, spirochetes, and other unidentified gram negative rods
      2. Rapid—primarily an asaccharolytic, anaerobic flora and mostly gram-negative rods (48–92% of total flora); some gram-positive
         a. *Bacteroides gingivalis*
         b. Other organisms
            1. Spirochetes
            2. *Eikenella corrodens*
            3. *Fusobacterium*
            4. *Campylobacter*
            5. *Selenomonas*
II. Juvenile Periodontitis (periodontosis)
   A. Predominant flora—saccharolytic, gram-negative, anaerobic rods
      1. *Actinobacillus actinomycetemcomitans*
      2. *Capnocytophaga* (surface gliders) (juvenile diabetics)
      3. Other gram negative-rods
         a. *Fusobacterium*
         b. Saccharolytic vibrios
         c. Unidentified
III. Marginal gingivitis
   A. Predominant flora:
      Actinomyces viscosus (A proportional increase in *A. viscosus* was significantly associated with development of marginal gingivitis.)
IV. Root surface caries
   A. Predominant flora:
      Type I ("*Streptococcus mutans* type")
         1. *A. viscosus* (47%)
         2. *S. mutans* (30%)
         3. Other streptococci (18%)
         4. *Veillonella* (4%)
      Type II (No *S. mutans*)
         1. *A. viscosus* (40%)
         2. *S. sanguis* (48%)
         3. Others including *Veillonella* (10%)
V. Acute necrotizing ulcerative gingivitis (ANUG)
   A. Predominant flora:
      Large spirochetes (±20 axial fibrils)
      B. melaninogenicus subsp *intermedius*

Courtesy of Professor Benjamin F. Hammond, Chairman, Department of Microbiology, School of Dental Medicine, University of Pennsylvania.

teeth can all act as impediments to the patient's attempts to remove plaque. The manual dexterity of the patient also influences plaque removal. This problem becomes most severe in mentally or physically impaired individuals.

Perhaps the most troublesome of the plaque-retentive features that contribute to the cause of the disease are those that occur as a direct result of the disease process. Among these factors are changes in the gingival architecture; increases in pocket depth either as a result of the coronal movement of the free gingival margin or as a result of the loss of periodontal attachment; the exposure of furcations and other concave surfaces on the roots; and the presence of subgingival calculus. Not only do these deformities make daily mechanical plaque removal difficult, if not impossible, but it is likely that they contribute to detrimental shifts in the relative proportions of various bacterial pathogens.

Anatomic and Environmental Factors

Mouth breathing, which has the effect of drying the gingival tissues, can exacerbate the effect of bacterial plaque. The mechanism is unknown. The effect of mouth breathing is usually most severe in the maxillary anterior sextant.

The quantity of attached gingiva has also been implicated as a modifying influence related to the progression of the inflammatory process. Studies by Lang and Löe imply that widths of attached gingiva less than 1 mm tend to be more inflamed than wider zones. However, conflicting results were reported in a similar study by Miyasato et al. They found no difference in the inflammatory response between wide and narrow bands of attached gingiva. Narrowed zones of gingiva may be more susceptible to mechanical trauma or frenal muscle pulls or both and, as a result, may manifest recession more readily.

Excessive forces delivered to the teeth may adversely affect the response of the periodontium to plaque in the presence of existing periodontitis. The precise mechanism for this interaction is not known, but the net result may be a more severe loss of periodontal support than in the case of periodontitis alone. In the absence of periodontitis, i.e., in either a periodontium that is uninflamed or one that is affected only by gingivitis, the effects of the force are limited to the periodontal ligament, the alveolar and supporting bone, and the cementum.

Host Factors

In addition to variations in the local environment, it is likely that there are a number of host-related factors that influence the susceptibility of the patient to periodontal disease. In particular, the immune, the reticuloendothelial, and the endocrine systems, as well as the nutritional status of the host, have been implicated in the etiology and pathogenesis of periodontal disease. There is no doubt that hormonal changes that occur during puberty and pregnancy influence the host response to plaque. Diabetes mellitus has been shown to adversely influence the severity of periodontitis. It has also been demonstrated that defects in neutrophil function are associated with juvenile periodontitis.

The drug phenytoin sodium (Dilantin) can also influence the response of the periodontium to plaque. In approximately 40 per cent of the individuals who take this drug, the gingival tissues become markedly hyperplastic. It has been shown that the hyperplastic response will not occur in the absence of plaque.

Numerous references to the impact of altered nutrition on the periodontium appear in the literature, and it is clear that healing of tissue can be affected by deficiencies in certain nutritional elements. The role that malnutrition plays in the cause of periodontal disease is probably related to an alteration of the tissue's ability to cope with bacterial plaque.

It must be emphasized that at this time only microbial plaque has been shown to be capable of initiating and perpetuating inflammatory periodontal disease. All other factors, both local and systemic, although important in the etiology of the disease, and even potentially necessary cofactors, have not been shown to initiate the disease in the absence of plaque.

Occlusal Trauma

The cause for the lesion of the attachment apparatus referred to as occlusal traumatism is excessive force. The type of force required to produce the lesion is dependent on the magnitude, direction, duration, and frequency of the force application as well as the quantitative status of the attachment apparatus. The quantitative state is a function of the individual tooth's root anatomy as well as of the quantity of periodontal support remaining around the tooth. It will take less force, for example, for the clinical manifestations of occlusal trauma to occur in a

short conically rooted premolar than in a long-rooted maxillary molar with divergent roots. If a tooth is periodontally compromised as the result of periodontitis, the forces that would be required to cause occlusal traumatism would presumably be less than if the periodontium were uncompromised.

The excessive forces the tooth receives can be categorized as belonging to one of three types: tooth-to-tooth, tooth-to–foreign object and tooth-to–soft tissue. Examples of tooth-to-tooth forces are those delivered during bruxism or clenching. They are felt to be most deleterious when they are exerted off the long axis of the tooth. Lip biting and tongue thrusting are examples of soft tissue–to-tooth habits. Pencil biting, eyeglass chewing, and nail biting all fall into the tooth-to–foreign object category. On occasion the forces required to cause damage to the attachment apparatus are so minimal that even those forces generated during normal function are excessive. This occurs only when the periodontium has been severely compromised as a result of periodontitis.

DIAGNOSIS AND PATHOGENESIS OF PERIODONTAL DISEASE

Gingivitis

Clinically, gingivitis is manifested by a change of the marginal gingiva (when not masked by pigmentation) to a redder than normal color. This color change is usually accompanied by a blunting of the gingival margin, so that the previously knifelike gingival margin becomes bulky and rolled. Occasionally the gingiva may become frankly hyperplastic, accounting for a substantial change in the position of the free gingival margin, particularly in the area of the papilla. The placement of a periodontal probe inserted into the pocket will reflect the depths from the free gingival margin to the point where the probe stops in the inflamed subsulcular connective tissue. In health, with the tip of the probe resting in the vicinity of the coronal part of junctional epithelium, this dimension is usually $\frac{1}{2}$ to 2 mm. The increase in depth noted in gingivitis reflects the coronal movement of the free gingival margin and the loss of soft tissue integrity of the sulcular and junctional epithelium as well as the underlying connective tissue, which allows the probe to pass apical to the soft tissue attachment. Because the probe passes through the epithelial tissue, it is not uncommon for bleeding to occur during probing. As a result of the underlying inflammation, a thin clear gingival fluid exudes out of the sulcus. Actually, the presence of gingival fluid precedes all of the other clinical changes and, at least for the researcher, is a useful tool for assessing early gingival inflammation. Purulent exudate may also be elicited from the gingival pocket during gingivitis. It is not a consistent finding, however.

Gingivitis does not manifest itself on radiographs, although in cases in which the gingiva has become grossly hyperplastic a more coronal than normal soft tissue shadow may be seen on the radiograph. The major contribution of radiographs is in ruling out the presence of bone loss.

The histopathologic changes that accompany an early gingivitis are characteristic of an acute inflammatory reaction. There is a loss of perivascular collagen, vasculitis, and an influx of lymphocytes and polymorphonuclear leukocytes into the connective tissues. The polymorphs actively migrate through the junctional and sulcular epithelium into the sulcus. After approximately 4 days, the inflammatory changes become more chronic in nature. Fibroblasts decrease in number, and the gingival fiber apparatus loses its integrity as collagen breakdown occurs. In 2 weeks' time the inflammatory infiltrate is predominantly made up of plasma cells. The junctional and sulcular epithelium lose their integrity as their intercellular spaces widen. In some areas the sulcular epithelium may be thin to the point of being ulcerated. It should be noted that although the junctional epithelium loses its integrity, it does not detach from tooth surfaces.

Periodontitis

Periodontitis is the inflammatory disease that involves not only the soft tissues of the periodontium but the attachment apparatus as well. Periodontitis is usually considered to be a progression of gingivitis. However, not all untreated cases of gingivitis progress to periodontitis. The host and local factors that allow for the progression are poorly understood.

The loss of alveolar and supporting bone is accompanied by an apical migration of the gingival fiber apparatus and the junctional epithelium. The loss of osseous support can occur either as a generalized horizontal loss involving all surfaces of all teeth or as isolated areas involving single teeth or even single surfaces of single teeth. Once initiated, the bone loss tends to be progressive with time. Typically, the soft tissues will manifest the changes associated with gingivitis with one notable exception: The free gingival margin may recede in an apical direction as a result of the loss of osseous tissues. When this occurs, the cementoenamel junction and the root surface will be visible. In more advanced cases with excessive bone loss, the furcation area of multirooted teeth may be exposed to the oral environment. At times gingival recession does not accompany the bone loss, and, in fact, one may even see hyperplasia of the gingiva in the presence of bone loss. The clinical diagnosis of periodontitis therefore cannot be made only on the position of the free gingival margin relative to the cementoenamel junction; it is necessary to use radiographs or the periodontal probe or both. When one sees loss of crestal height on the radiograph and determines that a tip of a periodontal probe is 2 mm or more apical to the cementoenamel junction, the diagnosis of periodontitis can be made. The probe is used by inserting it into the sulcus parallel to the long axis of the tooth with its tip in contact with the tooth. Bleeding will invariably accompany the probing in patients with active periodontitis. The presence of purulent exudate in the pocket is a variable finding. In cases in which the bone loss has been extreme, the horizontal mobility of the teeth may increase substantially.

The earliest radiographic sign of periodontitis is a loss of definition of the crestal bone. In health, the crestal bone appears as a radiopaque line that parallels an imaginary line drawn from the cementoenamel junction of two adjacent teeth. The crestal bone is normally 1 to 2 mm apical to the cementoenamel junction. As the periodontitis advances, apical migration of the crestal bone occurs. Radiolucent areas within the furcations of the multirooted tooth also become apparent.

It is now generally believed that periodontitis develops as a sequel to a persistent gingivitis, but the factors that determine whether gingivitis will progress to periodontitis have not been thoroughly elucidated. There is some evidence that the bacterial flora present in the plaque is a determining factor. The gingival changes in periodontitis are the same as those in gingivitis. There is chronic inflammatory reaction marked by a dense infiltrate of round cells. Much of the gingival fiber apparatus is destroyed. It is interesting to note that although the crestal bone may be actively resorbing, as evidenced by extreme osteoclastic activity, there is a mass of healthy connective tissue, the transseptal fibers, immediately coronal to the bone. The inflammatory infiltrate is just coronal to this connective tissue. As the crestal bone resorbs, the transseptal fibers reattach at a more apical level on the root surfaces. It is quite likely that the transseptal fibers, which form coronal to the crestal bone, represent the union of periodontal ligament fibers from the adjacent teeth. The apical movement of the fibers allows for the junctional epithelium to move in an apical direction. The more coronal cells of the junctional epithelium detach from the tooth and become part of the sulcular epithelium, thus increasing the depth of the pocket. Bacterial plaque is seen in the pocket, almost, but not quite, in contact with the most coronal cell of the junctional epithelium. Bacteria are rarely found within the periodontal tissues. Calculus may or may not be present on the tooth surface within the pocket. With the possible exception of the periodontal abscess, the soft and hard tissues of the periodontium are not necrotic.

The mechanism for the destruction of the periodontium is poorly understood. It seems that the destructive mechanism, although triggered by the bacteria, is actually accomplished by the host. Seemingly, the host is retreating from the irritant rather than destroying it. The end point of the process, if the disease does not spontaneously arrest itself or if it is left untreated, is the loss of the tooth.

Juvenile Periodontitis

Juvenile periodontitis is a form of plaque-related disease that is seen in a young population and is characterized by a rather advanced destruction of the periodontium affecting one or more permanent teeth, usually the molars and the incisors. This entity has been known by many names since originally described by Gottlieb, and most recently it was called periodontosis. The lesion is observed after puberty and seems to be observed more often in female patients. There is a notable familial tendency. Calculus formation is not usually found on the roots of the affected teeth despite the deep pockets (10 mm and more) that are present. Plaque formation, however, is found on affected roots, and research has demonstrated certain microbial forms that seem to be pathogenic in this condition. The presence of gram-negative anaerobic rods was noted by Socransky and the genus *Capnocytophaga* has been implicated in the plaque of juvenile periodontitis.

Recently the role of *Actinobacillus actinomycetemcomitans,* or Y4, has been shown to be a very virulent component of the plaque in this infrequent form of periodontal disease. The incompetency of leukocytes to respond to chemotaxis is a phenomenon that has been noted in most cases of juvenile periodontitis.

The radiographs in this lesion usually demonstrate a vertical resorptive pattern on the first permanent molars and the incisors with the tendency to form infrabony pockets. Premolar and canine involvement may occur later.

The rationale of therapy in juvenile periodontitis is to overcome the pathogenic flora implicated in the disease process. The use of tetracycline has become part of the initial antimicrobial treatment, which is also part of the initial preparation. Culturing of the pathogenic forms to determine if they are still present has become more routine, as several laboratories have become equipped to perform this service. Pocket elimination will usually follow the inhibition of plaque flora.

Periodontal Abscess

Gingivitis and marginal periodontitis are characteristically low-grade, slowly progressive, cyclically well-contained inflammatory lesions. The remarkable containment of the lesion is largely due to the "barrier" against its spread provided by the dense collagenous nature of the gingiva and the reparative reactive fibroplasia of the connective tissues in advance of the inflammatory process (see Gingivitis and Periodontitis). Occasionally a failure or a deficiency in the resistance and reparative capacities of one or more periodontal sites may occur. In these situations an acute exacerbation of the existent chronic inflammation may result in periodontal abscess formation.

Periodontal abscesses have been initiated or excited by lodgment of foreign bodies within the tissues and by the blockage of narrow, tortuous, and constricted pockets. Common offenders may be calculus, food debris, bacterial plaque, and toothbrush bristles. Patients with diabetes mellitus (juvenile or maturity onset types) quite commonly suffer from periodic exacerbations of periodontal disease, including periodontal abscesses, because of multiple immunologic, phagocytic, microcirculatory, and cell-formative defects.

The bacterial flora of suppurative lesions of periodontal origin consists of a wide variety of gram-positive and gram-negative aerobic and anaerobic genera. In general, the histopathologic features of acute gram-negative infections resemble those associated with periodontal abscess. Endotoxin determinations of abscess exudates confirm the participation of gram-negative organisms.

The histopathologic features of periodontal abscess include (1) Pseudoepitheliomatous hyperplasia, (2) Soft tissue necrosis involving all tissue elements—structural and vascular, (3) Bone resorptive manifestations, (4) Intense tissue infiltration by neutrophilic leukocytes, (5) Pus formation, and (6) Deficiencies of reparative processes.

The periodontal abscess often drains directly into the "pocket" area through a necrotic breach in the epithelium. Lack of drainage may lead to spread of the inflammatory process, resulting in cellulitis, a localized variant of osteomyelitis, or to the formation of a fistula extending to the outer surface of the gingiva or alveolar mucosa.

The local symptoms of the periodontal abscess must be carefully studied, since diagnosis may at times be difficult. When the root apex is approached by the infection of a deep periodontal pocket, it is vital to differentiate it from the lesion of pulpal-periapical derivation. This is accomplished by pulp testing. Pulps of teeth involved with periodontal abscess are generally normal. Conversely, the periapical abscess may produce periodontal involvement, simulating a periodontal pocket, its exudate resorbing thin interdental, radicular, or interradicular bone septa along with associated periodontal ligament tissue. The exudate may continue to extend marginally, resorbing the gingival attachment to cervical cementum, and may finally "erupt" at the gingival margin. In other instances the fulminant periapical process may merge with an existing periodontal lesion, with comparable clinical manifestations. In this case the pulps will test nonvital.

The patient may experience pain ranging from slight to severe. The discomfort may be dull and continuous, sharp and piercing, or aggravated by percussion to the tooth, mastication, or occlusal contact. In many instances, especially relative to the chronic abscess of low intensity, percussion will not elicit pain, whereas gingival or mucosal palpation will do so. The periodontal soft tissues are usually edematous, shiny on the surfaces, and free of stippling. Color may be deep red, often with a purplish or bluish hue. The soft tissue distortion may be circumscribed or diffuse.

Constitutional symptoms vary with the severity of the inflammatory process, with submandibular or cervical lymph node enlargement and tenderness, and with mild fever, malaise, and anorexia. A mild granulocytic leukocytosis may be noted in the hematogram, and the erythrocyte sedimentation rate may be increased, especially with such complications as cellulitis and Ludwig's angina. Periodontal abscesses form in the soft tissue phase of the inflammatory lesion relative to suprabony, infrabony, or interradicular pockets.

Therapy is aimed at elimination of causative factors (for example, bacterial plaque), establishment of drainage of exudate from the pocket, débridement of the inner aspect of the pocket wall via curettage, cleansing by instrumentation of the root surface (which has been shown to harbor endotoxin and hydrolytic enzymes), control of infection via systemically adminstered antibiotics when required, and obviation of discomfort by analgesics and hot saline rinses. When the acute manifestations of the condition have subsided, pocket elimination is usually required.

Acute Necrotizing Ulcerative Gingivitis

Acute necrotizing ulcerative gingivitis (ANUG) is an acute infection that primarily involves the marginal gingiva. It affects a relatively young age group with an age

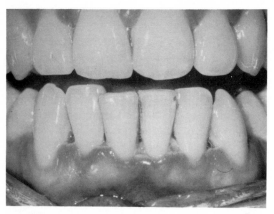

FIGURE 5–10 Appearance of Acute Necrotizing Ulcerative Gingivitis. The typical appearance of the gingival tissues affected by acute necrotizing ulcerative gingivitis. Note the "punched-out" papilla and necrotic tissue and other debris that has accumulated in the interdental area.

range of approximately 15 to 35 years. The interdental papilla is the predilected site for the destruction that takes place. The disease is characterized by necrosis of the interdental papilla, although any aspect of the marginal gingiva may be involved. Typically, the interdental papilla has a punched-out appearance. The affected tissues are covered with a gray pseudomembrane that consists of necrotic tissue, bacteria, and other oral debris (Fig. 5–10). The tissue will bleed on the slightest provocation, and it is not at all unusual for the patient to wake up with blood on the pillow or to experience bleeding during mastication. The soft tissues are acutely painful. The patient's breath is quite foul, and frequently a metallic taste is present. Oral hygiene is usually quite poor. It is not known if this is a result of the patient's inability to brush as a result of the discomfort or if the lack of oral hygiene was important in precipitating the disease. The onset of the disease is quite sudden. It is often accompanied by a low-grade fever. Lymphadenopathy in the cervical region is nearly always present. The patient may experience general malaise.

Microscopically, the lesion of acute necrotizing ulcerative gingivitis is that of an acute inflammatory process whose most striking feature is necrosis of the gingival tissues. As a result of the necrosis there are major ulcerations of both the sulcular and the oral epithelial surfaces. Unlike gingivitis and periodontitis, in which microbes are rarely found within the soft tissue, spirochetes do invade viable connective tissues subjacent to the area of acute inflammation in ANUG. No doubt the pain and spontaneous bleeding associated with ANUG are a result of the necrosis and subsequent ulcerations.

Up until approximately 1945, the disease was considered to be contagious, owing to frequent endemic outbreaks. The belief that the disease is not contagious came about largely as the result of a series of observations by Schluger in the 1940s, which have since been proved to be correct.

Although the etiology for this disease is not fully understood, two organisms, *Fusobacterium fusiforme* and *Borrelia vincentii* have been persistently cultured from the lesion. Histologic sections show the presence of spirochetes within the connective tissue beneath the active lesion. It is generally believed that in addition to the bacterial etiology, some other host modifying factors are necessary. The disease onset has frequently been associated with emotional stress. Elevated levels of 17-hydroxysteroids have been reported and may be stress related. Cigarette smokers are much more prone to ANUG than nonsmokers by a ratio of approximately 7:1.

Although the disease will spontaneously go into remission, active treatment is desirable, since the lesions of the disease do not tend to heal in an optimal fashion. In addition, treatment can rapidly and predictably manage the acute symptoms. Local treatment, consisting of débridement of the necrotic tissue via gentle curettage and débridement of calculus and plaque from the tooth surface, is extremely effective. Ultrasonic instruments are useful, since they are effective and seem to be well tolerated by the patient. The patient should be instructed in oral hygiene and placed on dilute (½ per cent) peroxide rinses. A follow-up visit should be scheduled within 2 to 4 days. By that time the acute symptoms will usually have subsided and a more complete scaling can be accomplished. Several weeks after the acute symptoms have subsided, the patient should be seen again for an evaluation of the soft tissue deformities that are frequently the aftermath of the disease. Minimal soft tissue cratering will often heal through a combination of good oral hygiene and scaling. More severe defects may require surgical management, usually a gingivoplasty or gingivectomy (Fig. 5–11).

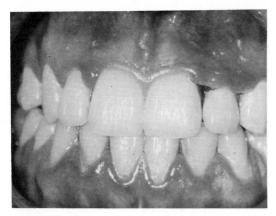

FIGURE 5–11 Acute Necrotizing Ulcerative Gingivitis Defects. Note the soft tissue craters between the maxillary left central, lateral, and canine teeth. These defects are the result of acute necrotizing ulcerative gingivitis.

The use of antibiotics should be reserved for patients who manifest systemic symptoms such as fever and malaise. On occasion, analgesics should be prescribed to alleviate discomfort, but they are rarely needed for more than a day or two after the initial débridement.

Trauma From Occlusion

Occlusal traumatism is a lesion of the attachment apparatus characterized by resorption of the alveolar and supporting bone, necrosis of the periodontal ligament, a histologic change described as hyalinization, and thrombosis of vessels within the periodontal ligament. These changes are caused by excessive forces delivered to the tooth.

Clinically, the manifestation of these changes is accompanied by an increase in the horizontal mobility of the tooth and occasional sensitivity to pressure or percussion. Radiographically, the periodontal ligament space appears widened and the lamina dura loses its definition. Currently, there is much controversy regarding this lesion. In animal studies performed in both the dog and the monkey, the aforementioned lesion does occur; however, within a period of approximately 2 weeks, the active osseous resorption ceases, the periodontal ligament is no longer necrotic, and the vasculitis disappears. The ligament space is widened, and the tooth continues to manifest increased mobility. These changes are interpreted to be a physiologic adaptation to the increased force; in other words, the combination of changes characterized by a loose tooth, a widened periodontal ligament, and a physiologic adaptation requires nothing more than longitudinal observation. It is not practical to biopsy the attachment apparatus to find out if a similar adaptation always occurs in man. It is known that if such a tooth is relieved of the excessive force, it will become more stable and radiographic changes will revert to their previous state. It is not known, however, if this treatment substantially alters the prognosis.

Before the occlusal problem is addressed, the inflammatory state of the periodontium should be brought under control. Gingivitis or periodontitis, if it exists concurrently with the occlusal lesion, should be treated. There is a twofold reason for treating the inflammatory lesion initially. First, one of the causes of increased tooth mobility is the inflamed periodontium; thus, if inflammation is minimized, mobility may return to nearly normal levels. Second, the progression of attachment loss that occurs during periodontitis may be accelerated by the occlusal lesion, and by controlling inflammation this loss can be obviated. Once the inflammation has been controlled, one can more accurately analyze the forces the teeth are receiving in relationship to the anatomy of the root, the quantity of the remaining periodontium, and the degree of mobility. When the mobility seems excessive relative to the conditions, the assumption can be made that adaptation has not occurred and treatment should be initiated to further minimize mobility. These decisions and determinations are by no means easy and require clinical judgment. In addition, the one parameter, mobility, that is crucial to the decision-making process is difficult to measure with any degree of accuracy on a longitudinal basis without the use of relatively sophisticated devices.

Additional considerations that should enter into the decision-making process include the type of treatment necessary to effect a change in mobility, the age of the patient, the level of the inflammatory control, the relative thickness or thinness of the periodontium, and if the mobility is an impediment to function or comfort. If the treatment required to manage the mobility is relatively simple and without deleterious side effects, one would be inclined toward treating the condition. If, on the other hand, the minimization of the mobility requires a major amount of treatment with potential side effects not deemed beneficial to the patient, longitudinal observation ought to be considered. One would be more prone to treat mobility in a younger patient, since the time available for the development of disease is potentially greater. Of particular concern is the possibility that at some time during the individual's lifetime, the lesion will become superimposed on periodontitis, with a potential deleterious synergistic effect.

When mobility occurs in a rather thin periodontium, its control becomes more important because there is a distinct possibility of creating an osseous dehiscence on the facial or lingual aspect of the tooth. Such a dehiscence in the uninflamed state will be masked by a soft tissue attachment to the root, but it can be diagnosed by palpating root movement under the soft tissue when force is applied to the tooth. It is suspected, but has not been proved, that such an area is more prone to rapid pocket formation if it becomes inflamed and may also be more prone to recession if inflamed or traumatized by the toothbrush. If the mobility is an impediment to function, if it is increasing with time, or if the tooth or teeth involved are moving out of function as a result of traumatic forces, occlusal intervention is mandatory. When the lesions of occlusal traumatism and periodontitis exist, the combined problem is referred to as occlusal periodontitis.

If occlusal intervention is necessary, one must select the appropriate treatment regimen. The objective of therapy is to minimize the forces that the teeth are receiving. This can be accomplished by control of parafunctional habits, by redirecting forces so that they are received along the long axis of the teeth, or by splinting teeth to one another to gain mutual stability. The treatment modalities that are useful in accomplishing these goals include occlusal adjustment by selective grinding, occlusal adjustment via the use of restorations, orthodontic tooth movement, night guards, Hawley bite plane, myofunctional therapy, the replacement of missing teeth, and splinting.

PERIODONTAL THERAPY

Oral Hygiene

Oral hygiene is directed at the removal of all supragingival plaque and subgingival plaque just apical to the free gingival margin. Effective plaque removal is an essential part of preventive dentistry, since bacterial plaque is the primary factor responsible for gingivitis, periodontitis, and caries. In the absence of plaque-retentive features, oral hygiene alone can reverse a gingivitis and very possibly control an incipient periodontitis. Oral hygiene in conjunction with periodic scaling, root planing, and curettage can effectively control most cases of periodontitis.

Technique

It is the responsibility of dentists to attempt to motivate their patients to perform thorough oral hygiene. The level of success will depend on the dentist's ability to communicate the need for this commitment to the patient and on the patient's personality and level of manual dexterity.

In the sequence of therapy, oral hygiene instruction should begin after the initial examination and should be continued in conjunction with the rest of initial therapy until satisfactory results are obtained. It is generally accepted that complete plaque removal once a day is acceptable for most periodontal patients. In fact, it may very well be that complete plaque removal every 48 to 72 hours is acceptable to keep the periodontium in a relatively uninflamed state. In the absence of appropriate studies, every 24 hours is considered to be the norm, however.

It is useful to begin oral hygiene instruction with an explanation regarding the importance of plaque control. It is often difficult for the patient to believe that plaque is not food debris but rather an accumulation

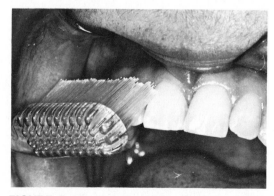

FIGURE 5–12 Toothbrushing Technique. The bristles of a soft, multitufted brush are directed into the gingival crevice at a 45 degree angle. The head of the brush is then gently moved in a mesiodistal direction.

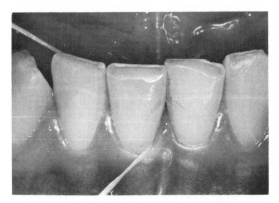

FIGURE 5–13 Dental Floss Technique. The floss is shown wrapped around the mesial aspect of a mandibular central incisor. It has been moved gently in an apical direction beneath the marginal gingiva until resistance is met. The floss is then moved coronally to the contact area. The apicocoronal movement is repeated until the tooth surface is clean.

of living bacteria. A phase-contrast or dark-field microscope is a useful tool to help convey this information. Demonstrating to the patient the relationship of plaque to disease is quite helpful. This can be accomplished by showing the patient what inflamed soft tissue looks like compared with healthy tissues and by giving the patient a disclosing solution to show the relationship of plaque to disease. While the patient uses the disclosing solution, the dentist should note on the patient's record those areas where plaque is found. It is useful to do this while the patient looks at the effect of the solution on the teeth, showing which areas were missed on this particular day. At this point it is not uncommon to hear the patient say, "I brushed this morning but didn't have time to brush

after lunch." The dentist should reassure the patient that what is being seen is not food but bacterial plaque and the result of his oral hygiene regimen. Watching the patient in action is important. Thirty seconds observing a patient brushing his teeth can reveal much about his dexterity and serve as a basis for working with him. At this point, the dentist can decide which of the various implements—brush, floss, toothpicks, or others—are most likely to be effective in the patient's hands and can introduce them to the patient at a rate that is appropriate for that patient.

Toothbrush. Currently, the modified Bass technique is considered to be not only an acceptable method of brushing but one that can be taught quite easily. A soft multitufted nylon brush should be used. The bristles are directed into the sulcus at approximately a 45 degree angle, and the head of the brush is then moved in an anterior-to-posterior motion. The bristles should not be grossly displaced as the brush head is moved back and forth (Fig. 5–12).

Dental Floss. Unwaxed or waxed floss can be used. Unwaxed floss is preferred because it frays when faulty restorative dentistry is encountered. The patient should be instructed to hold the floss by wrapping it around the third finger of each hand. This leaves the thumb and index finger free to manipulate the floss. The hands should be held close together. The floss should be gently inserted between the tooth contact and then wrapped around the mesial aspect of one tooth. The floss should then be moved apically until the soft tissue is encountered. At this point the floss should be 1 to 2 mm apical to the free gingival margin

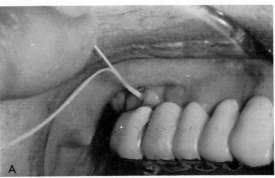
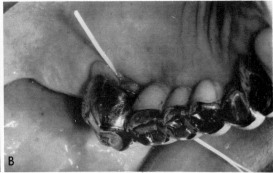

FIGURE 5–14   Floss Threaders. Floss threaders are used to facilitate dental flossing under bridges or within Class III furcations. In this illustration, a floss threader is being inserted into the facial furcation of a maxillary second molar *(A)*. In *B,* the end of the threader is exiting from the mesial furcation.

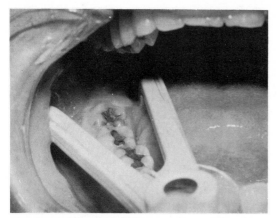

FIGURE 5–15 The Floss Holder. The Y-shaped floss holder is a useful adjunct for the patient who does not possess the manual dexterity to use floss in the more traditional fashion.

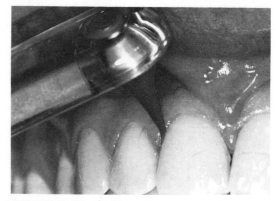

FIGURE 5–17 Rubber Tip Technique.

of the interdental papilla. It should then be moved coronally to the contact. The apical coronal movement should be repeated until the tooth surface is "squeaky" clean. This should be repeated on the distal surface (Fig. 5–13). When the gingival embrasure is abnormally large as a result of recession, it is useful to substitute dental tape for floss. When excessively wide open embrasures are encountered, 2- or 3-ply white Orlon yarn can be used in conjunction with floss.

Floss Threaders. When it is necessary to floss under splints and bridges or through Class III furcations, floss threaders can be used to manipulate the floss through the contacts. Currently one of the best floss threaders available is manufactured by Butler and consists of a monofilament loop that collapses as it passes through the contact (Fig. 5–14).

Floss Holders. The Y-shaped plastic floss threader is a helpful adjunct for patients who lack manual dexterity (Fig. 5–15).

Toothpicks and Stimulants. Toothpicks are useful for cleaning the gingival one third of the tooth surface and can be directed just apical to the free gingival margin. In conjunction with a holder, e.g., the Perio-Aid, they are particularly useful on the lingual and palatal surfaces of the posterior teeth. They can also be directed into furcation areas. Although toothpicks are probably not as efficient as floss for cleaning the interproximal areas, they are particularly useful for patients with dexterity problems (Fig. 5–16).

Rubber Tips. The rubber tip is another useful tool for cleaning the interproximal areas. The tip can also be inserted apical to the free gingival margin to clean subgingivally (Fig. 5–17).

Proxabrush. The Proxabrush is a conically shaped brush available in a variety of

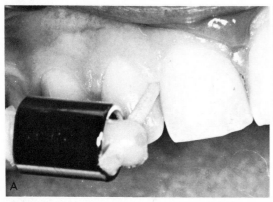

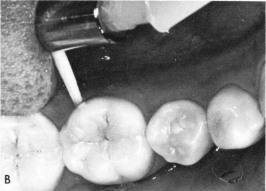

FIGURE 5–16 The Toothpick. The wooden toothpick, particularly when used in conjunction with a commercially available plastic handle, is useful for cleaning teeth interproximally (**A**) as well as for cleaning the lingual and palatal aspects of the molars (**B**).

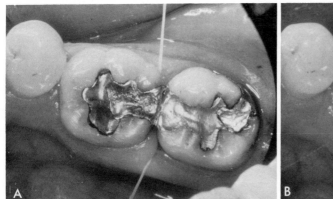 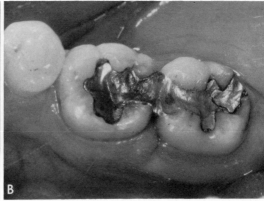

FIGURE 5–18   Oral Hygiene Trauma. The improper use of dental floss *(A)* has caused a gingival laceration on the lingual aspect of the mandibular second molar *(B)*.

sizes. It can be inserted interproximally or into furcations in areas where recession has occurred. Since the brush tips wear out quite frequently, models with disposable tips and reusable handles are preferred.

Disclosing Solutions.   There are several dye systems that will disclose supragingival plaque. The most easily obtainable is erythrosin dye, which comes in liquid or tablet form. The liquid is easier to use. The Plak-Lite system uses the dye fluorescein, which fluoresces under a light supplied with the kit. The Plak-Lite has been shown to be superior to the erythrosin dye. The disclosing solutions are useful adjuncts for some patients. They serve as a method for patients to check themselves and improve the thoroughness of their technique. Since the dyes tend to leave the mouth discolored for some time after use, it is desirable to use them at bedtime.

Toothpaste.   Any of the ADA-approved fluoridated toothpastes is an acceptable dentifrice. The toothpaste should be fluoridated not only because of the anticarious effect but also because recent studies seem to indicate that fluoride may reduce plaque accumulation. In patients in whom sensitivity to cold is experienced, one of the desensitizing pastes may be useful. Keyes advocates the use of baking soda and peroxide as a substitute for toothpaste in patients who have periodontal disease. Recently published research does not substantiate that this combination is superior to the regularly available dentifrices, although there have been a number of anecdotal reports that it is beneficial.

Oral Hygiene Trauma.   When any oral hygiene implement is used improperly, it can cause damage. The toothbrush can cause gingival recession or abrasions. The recession is most likely to occur over the roots of prominent teeth, where the periodontium tends to be thin. Common areas for this to occur are the maxillary and mandibular canines and the mesiobuccal roots of the maxillary first molars. When dental floss is not properly wrapped around the tooth, gingival lacerations can occur (Fig. 5–18). In addition, vigorous back-and-forth use of floss can also cause abrasion to occur on the tooth surface.

It is important that the patient's efforts at oral hygiene be monitored continually. Often it takes many months to bring a patient to an optimal level of oral hygiene. Occasionally it is not possible to obtain acceptable levels. The dentist should document his or her attempts in the patient's record. Not only is this important medicolegally, but it also serves as a guide in future attempts. Any one of a number of various plaque or bleeding indices is useful to monitor progress.

Conservative Techniques

Scaling and Root Planing (Root Curettage)

Scaling entails the removal of calculus from the crown and root surfaces of the teeth. Root planing, or root curettage, is the removal of residual calculus and endotoxins that are incorporated into the cementum adjacent to the pocket. Calculus is plaque-retentive. In the supragingival area, it makes plaque removal by the patient difficult, if not impossible. In the subgingival area, it acts as an impediment to healing. Not only is it a mechanical barrier to the reattachment of connective tissue fibers into the root surface, but, because endotoxins from bacteria are found within the calculus, it also acts as an irritant to the soft tissues, even after bacteria have been removed.

It has been shown that calculus attaches to the cemental surfaces by locking into irregularities within the cementum. The nature of the attachment of calculus to the root and the fact that endotoxins have also been demonstrated in the superficial surface of the cementum necessitate the removal of the outermost layer of cementum. Because the instruments used to perform these techniques are so large relative to the space between the tooth and pocket lining, invariably, part of the pocket lining is removed during the scaling and root-planing process. This inadvertent curettage does not seem to be detrimental to the healing process and may in fact be a useful part of the débridement.

As a result of scaling and root planing, some soft tissue healing will occur. The clinical manifestations of this improvement include a decrease in bleeding upon probing, shrinkage of the soft tissues so that the free gingival margin is in a more apical location, and a decrease in the clinical pocket depth. Invariably, there is a greater reduction in pocket depth than can be accounted for by shrinkage alone. Part of this decrease in depth is the improvement in soft tissue health. The tissues do not allow the probe tip to pass as far apically, an indication of improvement in the integrity of the soft tissue. On occasion, the soft tissues may actually attach to the root. When this attachment occurs, the length of the soft tissue attachment has in effect increased in apicocoronal extent. This can be the result of an increase in the width of the junctional epithelium, the connective tissue attachment, or both.

Indications.   Scaling is indicated any time there are deposits of calculus on the crown or root surfaces. Root planing is indicated whenever pockets occur apical to the cementoenamel junction.

Technique.   There are two basic ways to accomplish the removal of calculus and the planing of the cemental surfaces. One employs hand scalers and curets, the other, ultrasonic instruments. Although it has been shown that ultrasonic instruments are an effective means of removing calculus, they are not considered to be as effective for root planing.

Curets come in a wide variety of shapes and sizes. There are two basic curet designs. Some curets are considered to be universal and can be used in all areas of the mouth. There are two useful cutting edges on each end of these curets. The second type, the specific curet, is designed, as the name implies, to work only on certain tooth surfaces, e.g., the mesial aspects of molars. On these curets only one edge is designed to be effective. Specific curets are mechanically more efficient. The advantage of the universal instrument is that one needs fewer implements. Both the universal and the specific curet come in a variety of sizes. The heavier instruments are designed for scaling; the lighter, more flexible instruments are intended for root planing. Scalers are instruments designed for the removal of supragingival calculus. Many practitioners use universal curets for most of the scaling process and then switch to specific curets for root planing, particularly when pocket depths are excessive or furcations are involved. Whatever instruments the dentist chooses, it is imperative that they be kept sharp. A sharpening stone should be sterilized with the curets so that instruments can be sharpened during a visit if necessary.

Whenever scaling or root planing is contemplated, the patient should be forewarned that gingival recession may occur as a result of the procedures. It is also prudent to advise the patient that the teeth are likely to be sensitive to cold for some time after the procedure.

Scaling and root planing visits can be done in conjunction with oral hygiene instructions. The mouth can be divided in halves, quadrants, or sextants, depending on the difficulty of the scaling and root planing. Rarely should one spend much more than 45 minutes on scaling and root planing at a given visit. Soft tissue healing should be monitored constantly until optimal results are obtained. This often necessitates retreating a given area. It may be necessary to reflect the soft tissues surgically in order to gain access to the roots, particularly when very deep pockets are to be managed. Surgical procedures are discussed later in this chapter.

Recently it has been suggested that chemical adjuncts be used with root planing to make the root surface more biologically acceptable to the soft tissues. Citric acid is one of the agents that has been given considerable attention. It is felt that the acid may have the potential to degrade endotoxins incorporated in the cemental surface, but conclusive research in humans is not yet available.

Anesthesia. On occasion it is necessary to administer a local anesthetic in the areas where scaling and root planing are to be done. The dentist should try to determine if the patient's discomfort is related to the soft tissues or to the tooth. The former requires local infiltration anesthesia, while the latter may require block anesthesia. Nitrous oxide analgesia may prove useful.

Bleeding. Bleeding that occurs during the scaling and root planing procedure can be quite profuse on occasion. In most instances it can be controlled by gauze and pressure. It may be useful to remove granulation tissue purposely in the area in which the bleeding is encountered, since it is this tissue that is usually the source of the bleeding. Occasionally it will be necessary to place an interrupted suture through the interdental papilla, or to place a periodontal dressing.

Detection. Scaling and root planing are technically very difficult. One must rely a great deal on tactile sense, since the procedures are being done blindly. Sharp curets improve tactile sense. Dental explorers should be used to check the smoothness of the root surface in the subgingival area. A jet of air directed into the pocket improves visualization of the most superficial parts of the subgingival areas. A week or two after the scaling and root planing have been done, the result should be rechecked. Not only will some shrinkage have occurred, but frequently a lack of soft tissue health can indicate an area where the scaling, the root planing, or both need to be repeated.

Gingival Curettage

The periodontal pocket denotes a diseased gingival attachment to the tooth. The inner lining of the pocket is covered with ulcerated epithelium over an inflamed connective tissue. The epithelial rete ridges (pegs) elongate and tend to anastomose. The inflamed tissue bleeds readily, may produce a purulent exudate, and is frequently quite tender. Gingival curettage is a definitive surgical procedure designed to remove the ulcerated epithelial lining and the subjacent inflammatory tissue from the gingival pocket.

Gingival curettage performed without thorough removal of all deposits from the tooth ensures failure. Actually, the mechanical act of scaling the tooth surface by means of a curet to remove deposits will usually include removal of varying amounts of the pocket lining because of the proximity of the soft tissue to the tooth. Although the partial removal of the pocket epithelium during this inadvertent curettage may enhance the initial phases of healing, complete healing does not usually occur in deep pockets because of failure of the wound surface to epithelialize completely. To achieve complete wound healing, as evidenced by epithelialization and resolution of the inflammation in the gingival corium, it is necessary to accomplish complete removal of the ulcerated pocket epithelium, which is difficult to do in deep pockets.

Inflamed gingival tissues will return to health if the causative factors can be eliminated and if the area can be kept free from further insult. When gingival pockets are deep, the patient cannot cleanse the depth of the pocket and, therefore, cannot control plaque accumulation. However, where pocket depth is not severe, healing and reattachment may be augmented by definitive excision of all the ulcerated epithelium and underlying granulomatous tissue. Healing and reattachment cannot occur until removal of the ulcerated epithelium and granulomatous tissue has taken place, either surgically or biologically. When removal is accomplished surgically, a chronic wound is converted to a surgical wound, and the necessity for removal and resorption of toxic products by phagocytic and lytic actions of the body is eliminated.

Indications and Contraindications. Gingival curettage is usually employed in those instances in which healing of the gingival unit is expected to result in resolution of gingival inflammation with resultant shrinking of engorged tissues. It is expected that the gingival tissue will become firm and adherent to the tooth. Thus, the gingival tissue most amenable to treatment by curettage is soft, edematous, and flaccid and bleeds readily upon probing. The tissue is retractable and may be rolled marginally, thus enhancing retention of the plaque and debris in the area.

It must be emphasized that only shallow pockets seem to respond to this débriding technique. Once the pocket is too deep, healing may be incomplete or absent. This phenomenon may be related to the inability of the therapist to débride the deep pocket thoroughly. In addition, a deep pocket is extremely difficult to keep plaque-free. Another consideration is that a long epithelial attachment is likely to occur in a deep pocket, and this kind of attachment is more likely to break down than is a connective tissue attachment.

Although pocket elimination by gingival curettage is generally limited to relatively shallow pockets, the character and environment of which promote shrinkage, curettage is sometimes performed in deep pockets, where the resulting sulcus is likely to remain deep and where a further surgical procedure is anticipated. This allows for resolution of inflammation and the occurrence of some shrinkage, so that the tissue will be less edematous and friable during subsequent surgical procedures.

Objectives. The objectives of gingival curettage are shrinkage and a return to normal color, tone, and texture of the gingiva. Connective tissue reattachment at a more coronal level cannot be expected after gingival curettage, although it may occur on occasion. The means by which the pocket is eliminated is through shrinkage, made possible by resolution of inflammation with concomitant decrease in tissue fluid and inflammatory cells. The decrease in gingival size causes a reduction in pocket depth. Thus, the objectives of débridement are epithelialization of the wound, resolution of inflammation, and repair of the corium.

Technique. The technique of gingival curettage is not difficult, but it must be done carefully. Definitive débridement of the gingival pocket requires the use of a local anesthetic. In addition to anesthesia, the local infiltration of anesthetic aids in hemostasis and provides rigidity to the tissues, making instrumentation easier.

The movable gingiva is stabilized with a finger of the left hand, while a very sharp curet is inserted to the depth of the pocket with the blade in contact with the wall of the pocket. A circumferential stroke is used on the buccal and lingual aspects and as far interproximally as possible in order to thoroughly débride the lining of the gingival wall. The curettage is continued around each tooth until hard, fibrous tissue is encountered and the wound surface is smooth. Following débridement, the gingival tissue should be readapted to the tooth with firm pressure exerted with a gauze sponge. The gauze is held in position until the bleeding stops.

The wound may be protected with adhesive foil, periodontal surgical dressing, or not at all. Although success has been shown with all techniques, it seems rational to protect the wound from mechanical trauma and movement, as well as from debris and plaque, for 2 to 4 days.

If no dressing is used, the patient must be cautioned against disturbing and retracting the gingival margin during cleansing procedures for 4 to 5 days. Care should consist of frequent rinsing and cleansing with cotton swabs.

Ultrasonic Curettage. Débridement with an ultrasonic instrument has been investigated and reported widely during the past few years. The technique is essentially the same as that for the hand instrument. The wound surface can be thoroughly débrided, thus leaving a smooth surface. Because a diminished water spray is used, the necrotic tissues are in part coagulated by the heat and then flushed away.

Infrabony Pocket With Three Osseous Walls

The operation for new attachment is carried out under local anesthesia, which should be profound enough to allow completion of the operation without discomfort to the patient but still not interfere with the establishment of a blood clot.

A flap is raised, allowing the operative site to be opened to view. The next step in this operation is to remove the tissue from the osseous defect by using any curet or scaler. Necessarily, the instrument will have to be small, especially in a narrow defect. Often, in addition to a vertical stroke, a horizontal circumferential sweep, short and precise, may be used. After the contents of the defect have been removed, the osseous wall is examined for any soft tissue tabs. A small sharp curet serves well for their removal;

the circumferential stroke here is easily executed. The instrument is then worked toward the base of the defect between the tooth and bone, removing all the tissue until the bone wall is felt. Small bits of tissue will be removed easily; at times, a large segment will be excised.

Because of the size of the curets, even very small ones, the operator should keep the instrument against the tooth side. In this manner the head of the instrument can be inserted down to the base of the bone-tooth defect and used to remove the tissue from below the osseous process. It must be stressed that this area must be completely denuded of tissue; otherwise, an attachment apparatus will not form. A transseptal fiber group extends to the tooth in the infrabony pocket between tooth and bone. The transseptal fiber group is composed of dense connective tissue fibers running almost parallel to the tooth surface. Hence, if only the inner portion of the soft tissue wall is removed, leaving these fibers still attached, the soft tissue wall will heal covered by epithelium, preventing a new attachment. However, if all the tissue is débrided from the area, the blood clot fills the entire space between tooth and bone. After healing, a new attachment apparatus can form. Débridement of the tissue at the base (narrow portion of the infrabony pocket) must be carefully executed; the instrument must be placed deftly and removed with minimal trauma to the osseous wall.

If the lesion is chronically inflamed, the bony walls are likely to be sclerotic. In order to enhance the proliferation of repair tissue from the marrow, small intramarrow penetrations are made with a No. ½ round bur or a tapered fissure bur. These openings will permit the granulation tissue to grow into the defect.

Once this phase of the operation is performed, attention is then focused on the tooth. The cleanliness of the tooth should be checked with any suitable instrument. The operator should be sure not only that there are no deposits present but also that the surface is smooth. Also, caution should be taken not to disturb the area coronal to the operative site; otherwise, the tooth will become sensitive.

When the curettage phase is completed, a trough results, the extent of which depends upon the original topography. This area can be inspected by sponging it or by using suction to remove the blood. The lateral walls below the bone crest should be checked to ascertain whether any fragmentary tissue has been left. This surface should appear smooth.

Once this procedure has been completed, the gingival wall is sutured, ensuring a tight adaptation. The operative site over the defect is covered with a strip of tinfoil, protecting the area. This will also prevent the pack from engaging the knots of the suture. The operative site is then covered with surgical pack. The pack can be removed in 1 week; if necessary, a new pack can be placed to protect the operative site for another week.

Ellegard has suggested that the repair of an infrabony pocket may be enhanced by placing a free mucosal graft over the orifice of the osseous defect instead of suturing the buccal and lingual flaps together. This approach permits the squamous epithelium to desquamate during the first 7 days of repair and reduces the downgrowth of epithelium to re-form a pocket.

Clinical evidence seems to indicate that the reparative tissue responsible for regeneration of new cementum, periodontal ligament, and bone originates from the connective tissue of the periodontal ligament and the marrow spaces of the alveolar process rather than from the gingiva. These defects fill in from the base and gradually heal toward the orifice.

Surgical Techniques

Initial Preparation

The portion of periodontal therapy designed to diminish the inflammatory state accompanying gingivitis and periodontitis, short of surgically eliminating the pocket, and designed to improve the health and integrity of the attachment apparatus, short of permanently splinting the teeth, is often referred to as initial preparation.

Re-evaluation

After initial preparation has been completed, it is appropriate that a re-examination be conducted. This is referred to as re-evaluation. It should be done after the results obtained from scaling, root planing, and occlusal therapy are nearly optimal. In addition, the dentist should be convinced that the patient's oral hygiene is as good as it will be and that the tissues have had an adequate amount of time to heal.

The state of the soft tissues should be examined, and pocket depths remeasured and compared with the pretreatment depths. Mobility should be reassessed. If radiographic changes were anticipated, selected radiographs should be taken. If the results are not as expected, initial diagnosis, treatment plan, and therapy should be reassessed. If the results have been acceptably good, but disease still remains, future therapy should be mapped out. This is the time to decide if surgical pocket elimination is appropriate. It is also a time to finalize the restorative plan. These decisions are not always obvious, and one has the option of placing the patient on a maintenance program. This might entail periodic scaling and root planing visits over a long period of time. The intervals between these visits should be determined by the patient's response. One can start with an interval as short as 2 weeks and then increase the interval in an attempt to find out how long the patient can go without being seen.

The darkfield microscope may prove to be a practical aid in establishing the interval. Listgarten and Schifter are experimenting with such a technique. If a patient returns for a recall with what they consider to be a disproportionately high level of spirochetes and motile rods in their subgingival flora, they decrease the recall interval. If this proves to be efficacious, it will make establishing a recall interval much less subjective.

If maintenance therapy seems to be an ineffective method for controlling the patient's periodontal disease, more aggressive treatment may be indicated. At this point it is necessary for the general practitioner to assess the needs of the patient and to evaluate his or her own capabilities. If the treatment requires a greater level of expertise, a referral should be made; otherwise, the dentist can proceed with treatment.

Gingivoplasty and Gingivectomy

The gingivoplasty is a useful technique for modifying the gingival architecture without substantially altering the pocket depth. It entails removing the oral epithelium and underlying connective tissue. This procedure can be used when bulky or rolled soft tissue margins are encountered. Tissue nippers

and/or rotating diamonds are used to sculpture the gingival tissues into optimal form. The wound is dressed with a periodontal dressing that can usually be removed in 7 days. In 10 to 14 days, the tissues have re-epithelialized, and in approximately 21 days, the tissues are mature (Fig. 5–19).

The gingivectomy is one method of surgically eliminating pocket depth. Literally, it is an excision of the free gingiva. It is done in conjunction with a gingivoplasty. In fact, the two procedures are performed simultaneously. It is a useful procedure only if there is an adequate band of attached gingiva present and if there is no need to correct osseous defects. If the distance from the mucogingival junction to the depth of the pocket, i.e., the quantity of attached gingiva, is less than 2 mm, a gingivectomy is contraindicated. If there are osseous ledges or infrabony defects that require attention, the gingivectomy will not provide access and is therefore contraindicated. When the initial diagnosis is periodontitis, the gingivectomy is usually not the preferred method of surgically eliminating pockets. The gingivectomy is most likely to be useful when there have been hyperplastic changes involving the gingiva. Patients with Dilantin (phenytoin) hyperplasia can frequently be managed with a gingivectomy.

Anesthesia can be obtained via infiltration, preferably with an anesthetic solution that contains a hemostatic agent. With the use of a kidney-shaped gingivectomy knife, a beveled incision is made somewhat apical to the depth of the pocket in such a way that the knife encounters the tooth at the level of the base of the pocket. The mesiodistal extent of the incision is determined by the number of teeth to be involved. A diamond-shaped interproximal knife can then be utilized to free the tissue in the interproximal area. The free gingiva can then be removed (Fig. 5–20). At this point the pocket depth should be less than 1 mm. Curets can be used to touch up the incision line and to remove tissue tags. Tissue nippers are then brought into play to finalize the architecture. A periodontal dressing is then applied. It is usually removed in one week. Healing is almost identical to that of the gingivoplasty.

A mild analgesic, e.g., acetaminophen with 1/2 gr codeine can be prescribed to control the discomfort that is usually experienced for the first day or two following the procedure. The patient can also be in-

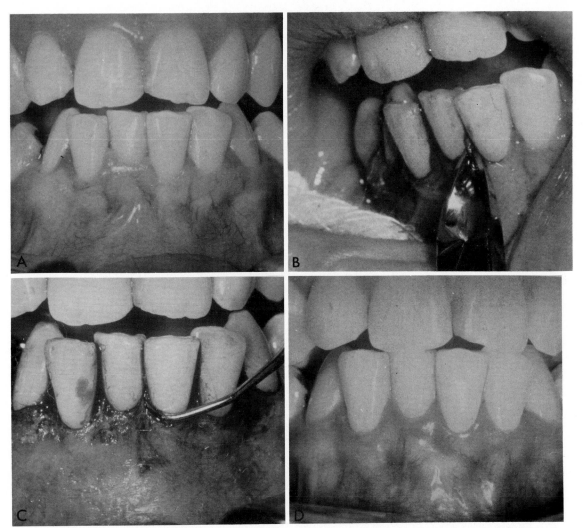

FIGURE 5–19 The Gingivoplasty. *A,* Before treatment. After injection of local anesthesia, tissue nippers *(B)* and curets *(C)* are utilized to remove the hyperplastic tissue and re-establish normal gingival architecture *(D)*.

structed to apply ice periodically (5 minutes on, 10 to 15 minutes off) for the first 12 to 24 hours. Other than gentle rinsing, no oral hygiene should be performed in the area, and the patient should take care not to dislodge the dressing.

When the dressing is removed, the teeth should be polished carefully. The patient should be instructed to begin gently brushing and flossing the teeth, unless the tissues appear to be immature, in which case the area can be redressed. It is the dentist's responsibility to remove plaque and other debris from the surgical site on a weekly basis until the tissues are mature enough for the patient to resume oral hygiene.

The Repositioned Periodontal Flap

Since the vast majority of periodontal pockets remaining after initial preparation require further management and cannot be treated with a gingivectomy, it is necessary to discuss alternative surgical procedures. These other procedures invariably require surgically created soft tissue flaps. There are a large number of flap designs and flap types that can be used; however, most do not fall within the scope of this chapter. This discussion is limited to full-thickness repositioned and apically positioned flaps.

Indications. Repositioned, full-thickness flaps are indicated when there is significant

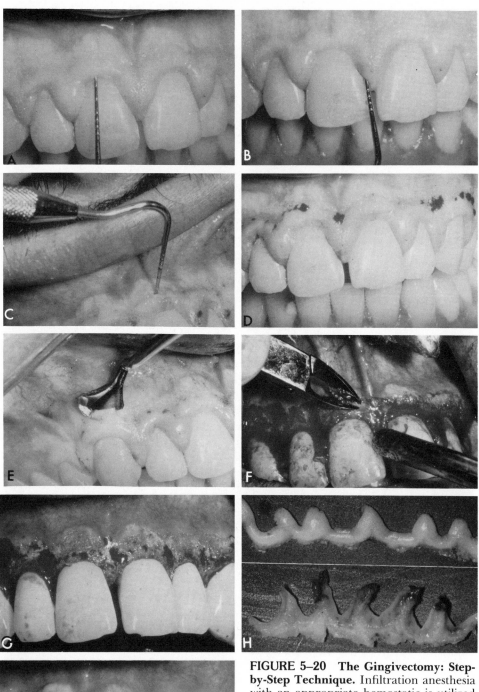

FIGURE 5–20 The Gingivectomy: Step-by-Step Technique. Infiltration anesthesia with an appropriate hemostatic is utilized for pain and bleeding control. The pockets are probed (*A* and *B*). The periodontal probe can then be used to mark the pocket depth in the oral epithelium (*C*) establishing a series of bleeding points (*D*). A beveled incision is made with a No. 11 Goldman-Fox knife (*E*). The incision is initiated 2 to 3 mm apical to the bleeding points. In this way, the knife will intersect the base of the pocket, and the resulting tissue architecture will be thin. Tissue tags are then removed with nippers or curets or both (*F*). The connective tissue wound should be nicely contoured and free of all tissue tags (*G*). The soft tissue removed from the wound can be seen in (*H*). A dressing is placed for 7 to 10 days. The wound is well healed and mature in approximately 1 month (*I*).

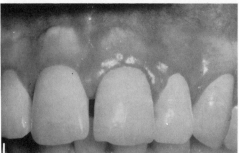

inflammation remaining after initial preparation. It is a useful way to gain access to deep pockets without creating a great deal of postsurgical recession. Although this technique may not necessarily result in complete elimination of the pockets, it will greatly reduce the level of inflammation. The remaining pockets can then be maintained through periodic scaling and root planing visits.

Technique. With a No. 15 scalpel blade, an incision is made at or just apical to the free gingival margin. The blade of the scalpel passes within the connective tissue between the oral epithelium and the sulcular

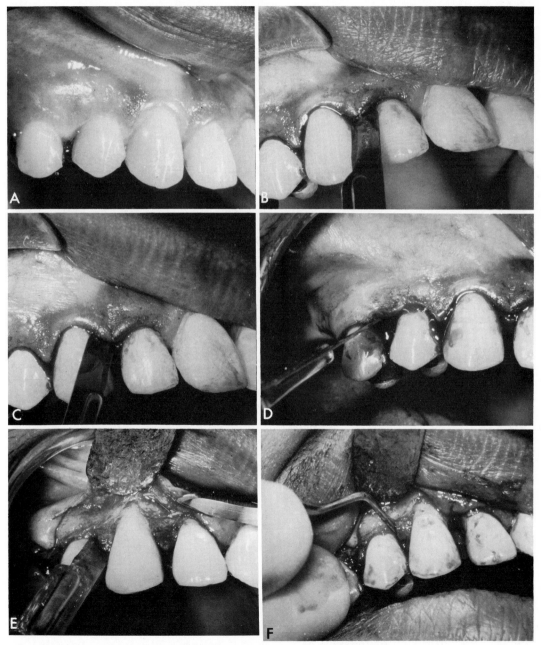

FIGURE 5–21 The Repositioned Flap: Step-by-Step Technique. Before treatment *(A)*. After appropriate anesthesia has been obtained, a No. 25 blade is used to make an inverse beveled incision. The incision is initiated at the free gingival margin and directed toward the crestal bone. Note how the knife is used to thin *(B* and *C)* and elevate *(D)* the interdental tissues. The scalpel and curet are then used to dissect free the granulation tissue *(E* to *H)*. The same technique is applied to the palatal tissues.

Illustration continued on following page

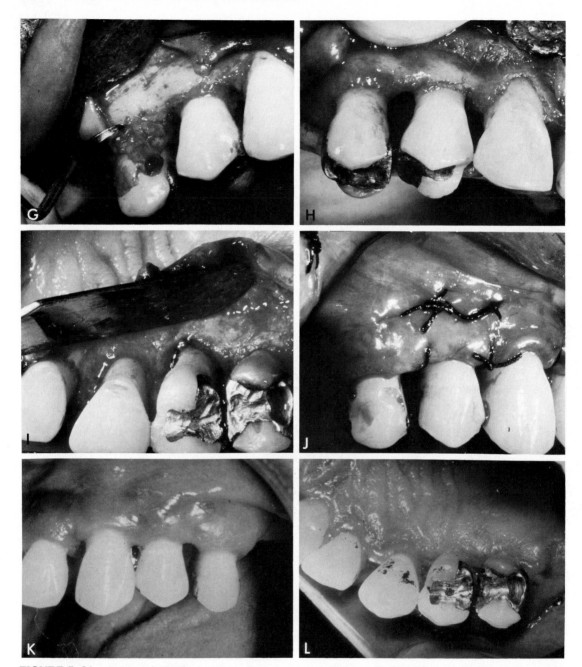

FIGURE 5–21 *Continued (I)* The tooth surfaces are carefully root planed. The tissues are then sutured back in place *(J)*. Some gingival shrinkage with resulting recession is inevitable and can be seen in the final healing *(K and L)*. (This case was provided through the courtesy of Sol Rosenberg.)

and junctional epithelium. It is directed apically to the crestal bone. The entry point of the incision should parallel the free gingival margin. This scalloped incision can include any number of teeth. When the incision has been completed, the soft tissues adjacent to the teeth are curetted away. This tissue mass includes the inflamed sulcular epithelium

and the junctional epithelium and their underlying connective tissue as well as the connective tissue attachment. This flap, which is not reflected past the crestal bone, gives the clinician access to infrabony defects, if they exist, and all root surfaces. Under direct vision, the infrabony defects can be carefully curetted and the root surfaces planed. These flaps are usually made on the facial as well as the lingual or palatal aspect (Fig. 5–21). Once the débridement is complete, the flaps can be sutured back to the original location with individual interrupted sutures in each interdental area. A periodontal dressing is then placed for 1 to 2 weeks to protect the wound during the early part of the healing process. An analgesic should be prescribed. The dressing and sutures are removed after the first week, and the teeth are carefully débrided of plaque. The dressing can be replaced for a second week. The criteria for replacement of the dressing are the maturity of the wound and the patient's ability to keep it clean. If a dressing is placed for a second week, the tooth should be débrided a second time when the dressing is removed. In fact, the teeth should be débrided at weekly intervals until the patient is able to effect good plaque control.

Healing. The flaps will predictably reattach to the tooth via junctional epithelium and connective tissue attachments. If infrabony defects were present, it is likely that some new attachment will occur. This will be the result of bony fill, cementogenesis, and the formation of a periodontal ligament. This is most likely to occur in deep narrow three-wall infrabony defects and is least likely to occur in one-wall infrabony defects. The presence of furcation involvements associated with infrabony defects greatly reduces the chance of fill. Occasionally, the apicocoronal length of the soft tissue attachment will be greater than the original length, thus further reducing the pocket depth. It is also likely that some shrinkage will occur. Because of the improved environment brought about by the débridement process as well as the reduction in pocket depth, the general level of inflammation should be very much reduced.

The Apically Positioned Periodontal Flap

Indications. Apically positioned flaps are indicated when there is significant inflammation remaining after initial preparation, owing to pockets that are inaccessible to daily oral cleansing. This procedure is of value when the pockets are apical to the mucogingival junction. Not only do the flaps created during this procedure provide a useful way of gaining access to débride root surfaces and infrabony defects, but they predictably eliminate the suprabony aspect of the pocket by surgically creating gingival recession. They have the added benefit of effectively changing free gingiva into attached gingiva. The healing process is similar to that of the repositioned flap. The apically positioned flap is also a useful method for gaining sound tooth structure for restorative purposes when caries extends below the gingival margin.

Technique. The initial incisions are made exactly as described for the repositioned flap, except where palatal tissues are to be treated. After the initial incision has been made, a periosteal elevator is utilized to lift the periosteum from the bone. The flap is elevated past the mucogingival junction. The osseous lesions are then débrided of all soft tissue. The exposed root surfaces are carefully root planed. It should be noted that the root surface in the immediate vicinity of the crestal bone does not need to be planed. This area of the tooth, which is approximately 1½ mm in apicocoronal extent, was not exposed to microbial plaque. The soft tissue attachments, i.e., the junctional epithelium and connective tissue fibers, were joined to this portion of the root; presumably, therefore, bacterial contamination of the cemental surface did not occur. The flap is then apically positioned so that the free gingival margin is placed at or just coronal to the osseous crest. The loose elastic connective tissue that makes up the alveolar mucosa allows the facial or lingual flaps to be apically positioned. Each flap is sutured separately with a continuous suture. It is the function of the suture to keep the flap from being displaced apically by the dressing. The dressing keeps the flap against the bone and, in addition, holds the flap in the apical position established by the sutures. The postoperative management is similar to that of the repositioned flaps (Fig. 5–22).

In the case of the palatal flap, the initial incision is made somewhat apical to the free gingival margin (Fig. 5–23). The exact position of this incision is based on the level of the palatal osseous tissues (assuming osseous surgery is not going to be done) and the shape of the palatal vault. Shallow palatal vaults require a more coronally placed incision, whereas deep vaulted palates require the incision to be made farther apically. As with the facial and lingual flaps, the scalpel

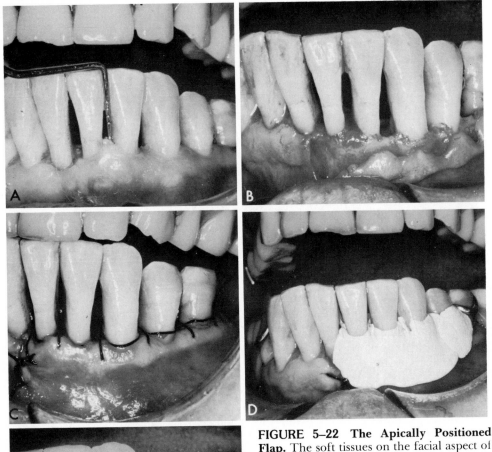

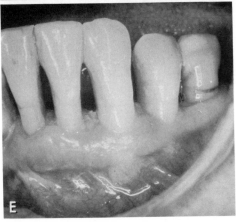

FIGURE 5–22 The Apically Positioned Flap. The soft tissues on the facial aspect of the mandibular right central, lateral, and canine teeth were apically positioned one month prior to the photograph seen in **A**. After appropriate anesthesia the pockets are measured and the initial incisions are planned. The scalpel is utilized in a fashion similar to that of the repositioned flap. Unlike the repositioned flap, the gingival tissues are reflected apical to the mucogingival junction **(B)**. After the removal of granulation tissue, the flap is sutured in an apical position so that the gingival tissues just cover the alveolar bone **(C)**. A dressing is placed **(D)**. The soft tissue result some three months later is seen in **(E)**.

is directed apically, but in the case of the palate, the blade will encounter the osseous tissue somewhat apical to the crestal bone. Essentially, the surgeon is creating a new free gingival margin in a more apical location. After the incision is made, the tissue between the scalpel and the tooth is removed. This wedge of tissue is referred to as the secondary flap. If the incision has been made in the proper location, the primary flap will fall into place at or just coronal to the crestal bone, thus eliminating all of the

suprabony aspect of the pocket. After removal of the secondary flap, the granulation tissue from all bony defects is removed. The roots are planed where necessary. The flap is then sutured, and a dressing is placed over the wound.

Osseous Recontouring

Osseous recontouring can be employed to correct abnormal bony architecture. Ledges, infrabony pockets, and reverse architecture

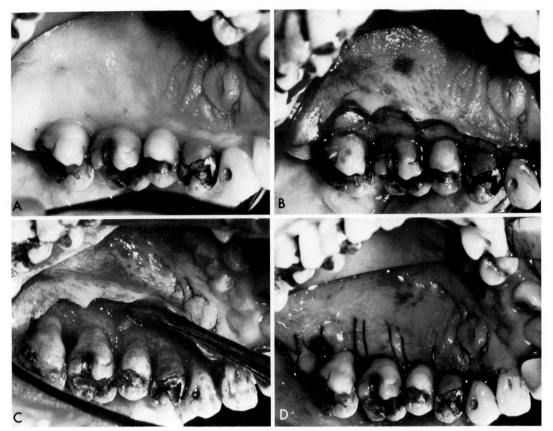

FIGURE 5–23 The Palatal Flap. Because the palatal tissues can not be apically positioned owing to the absence of alveolar mucosa, it is necessary to modify the surgical approach from the one used in the facial or lingual areas *(A)*. An inverse beveled incision is made apical to the free gingival margin *(B)*, and the wedge of soft tissue between the incision and the tooth is removed *(C)*. The new free gingival margin should just cover the crestal bone. The flap is sutured in place *(D)*.

can be effectively eliminated. These techniques do not fall within the scope of this chapter, and the interested reader can pursue this information in any one of a number of periodontology textbooks.

Free Gingival Autograft

The free gingival or mucosal autograft is composed of masticatory mucosa that has been completely dissected from its original site and consists of epithelium and connective tissue. This donor material is then transferred to a carefully prepared recipient site.

The gingival autograft is used primarily to create a wider zone of attached gingiva in areas with little or none present. It is used when there is an absence of adjacent donor tissue and in any situation in which a wider zone of attached gingiva is required. Its results are highly predictable when it is properly done. However, the gingival autograft

will not attach to denuded root surfaces predictably.

The rationale for using the gingival autograft is based on the observations that it is a highly predictable procedure for the replacement of alveolar mucosa with a dense, fibrotic gingival tissue. In addition, the procedure does not necessitate long periods of surgical exposure, is not technically difficult, and causes minimal trauma to labile tissues. In most instances bone and periosteum are completely covered, and frequently even the gingival sulcus and epithelial attachment may be left undisturbed. The postoperative course is usually benign and uneventful.

It is evident that this procedure, when indicated, causes minimal trauma, particularly when compared with alternative procedures such as periosteal retention pedicle grafts.

Disadvantages. The disadvantages of the gingival autograft must always be considered in the selection of therapy. In most instances, the donor site for graft material is the palatal masticatory mucosa. Although there are, in fact, very few instances of operative or postoperative complications with the gingival autograft procedure, the injection, incision, suturing, and dressing of the donor site may be physically and emotionally traumatic. So, the necessity for two surgical sites must be considered a disadvantage of the procedure.

In cases requiring a large graft, the stripping of a sizable area of palatal mucosa, which must heal by secondary intention, presents the potential problems of postoperative discomfort, hemorrhage, and dressing retention.

As previously mentioned, the gingival autograft cannot be relied upon to attach to denuded root surfaces predictably. In addition, the gingival autograft should not be used in any area requiring osseous surgery. Attempts to do so may compromise coverage of the osseous surgical site or may compromise preparation of the graft recipient site.

Technique. The first determination to be made is the placement of the graft. Where the marginal gingiva is inflamed and resolution cannot be fully obtained by initial therapy, where there is no attached gingiva, or where the pocket extends through the mucogingival junction, there should be complete marginal tissue replacement by the graft.

The recipient site should be planned large enough to include the affected area, while also allowing for contraction of the graft during healing. Preparation of the site must include careful and thorough removal of all muscle and connective tissue down to the firm base of periosteum. The retention of muscle fibers may lead to failure of the graft either by inhibiting revascularization, therefore resulting in necrosis, or by causing mobility of the entire graft after healing.

A graft is usually removed from the donor site after the preparation of the recipient site. This sequence is followed to minimize the amount of time that the graft is separated from a nutrient bed. This sequence also allows time for bleeding in the recipient bed to be controlled.

Although a graft may be taken from any gingival or edentulous area, the most frequently used site is the hard palate, owing to the abundance of suitable mucosa in this area. The recipient bed is measured and these measurements are transferred to the donor area. The graft material is then carefully dissected away. The objective is to obtain a graft that is thin and has a smooth undersurface. It has been suggested that optimal graft thickness is about 1.0 to 1.5 mm. It may be necessary to thin the graft to the desired thickness with a sharp scalpel after removal from the donor site.

The prime factor in the success or failure of the gingival graft is its immobilization during healing. If the graft is not immobilized, revascularization may be impaired, with resultant necrosis of the graft. One of the key factors is the proper preparation of the recipient site. Not only should the recipient site be free from muscle fibers and all other movable connective tissue but also the graft must not overlap unprepared tissue.

The usual means of immobilization is by suturing, most frequently with a 5-0 suture material. Either silk or plain gut may be used. Plain gut is preferable because it obviates the necessity for suture removal and suture protection beneath the surgical dressing. Unless the graft is unusually long, the sutures placed on either end of the graft are usually sufficient for immobilization. The inferior border of the mucosa at the recipient bed should be sutured to the underlying periosteum adjacent to the inferior border of the graft. This prevents pouching of mucosa with subsequent secondary intention healing and produces an almost entirely closed wound. Prior to dressing placement the graft should be compressed to express pooled blood and to encourage rapid formation of a fibrin clot.

Finally, the donor site should be sutured. This is recommended to help control hemorrhage, to reduce the size of the open wound, and to aid in the retention of the surgical dressing. These objectives are best accomplished by using 3-0 plain gut sutures in a continuous crisscross pattern across the denuded donor bed.

QUESTIONS

1. Pockets in excess of 6 mm (measuring from the free gingival margin to the base of the clinical pocket) are diagnostic of bone loss.
   a. true
   b. false—the free gingival margin may be in a more apical than normal position
   c. false—the free gingival margin may be in a more coronal than normal position

2. The sequence of histopathologic events in periodontitis is best described as
   a. plaque formation, gingival inflammation, crestal bone loss, and apical migration of the epithelial attachment
   b. plaque formation, crestal bone loss, gingival inflammation, and apical migration of the epithelial attachment
   c. plaque formation, apical migration of the epithelial attachment, gingival inflammation, and crestal bone loss

3. The tooth that on the average has the least gingiva (apicocoronal extent) is the
   a. maxillary first molar
   b. maxillary first premolar
   c. mandibular first molar
   d. mandibular first premolar
   e. mandibular lateral incisor

4. In a healthy dentition, the crestal bone in the interdental area should be located approximately 3½ mm apical to the cementoenamel junction. The crest should parallel an imaginary line drawn from the cementoenamel junction of the two teeth.
   a. Both statements are true
   b. Both statements are false
   c. The first statement is true and the second is false
   d. The first statement is false and the second is true

5. The surgical procedure that basically consists of an excision of the free gingiva is the
   a. free gingival graft
   b. apically positioned flap
   c. gingivoplasty
   d. gingivectomy

6. The dimension of a normal periodontal ligament space is approximately
   a. 0.02 mm
   b. 0.2 mm
   c. 1.0 mm
   d. 1.2 mm
   e. 1 to 2 mm

A 23-year-old female presents with a history that includes painful bleeding gums and spontaneous bleeding of 3 days' duration. She has a temperature of 101°F and has bilateral lymphadenopathy in the cervical area. The gingiva is extremely inflamed in the mandibular anterior region with several necrotic looking papillae. (Use this information to answer questions Nos. 7 through 9.)

7. The most likely diagnosis would be
   a. acute gingivitis
   b. menstrual gingivitis
   c. pregnancy gingivitis
   d. acute necrotizing ulcerative gingivitis
   e. acute herpetic gingivitis

8. The use of antibiotics is usually advocated for the routine treatment of this problem.
   a. true—the causative agent is penicillin-sensitive
   b. true—this disease is contagious, and appropriate antibiotic therapy is therefore indicated

    c. false—the causative agent is not sensitive to penicillin

    d. false—the disease can usually be treated solely by local therapy, i.e., scale, curettage, and so on

    e. false—antibiotics are indicated but only after culture and sensitivity testing

9. The effects of initial therapy on patients of this type are generally adequate, and if the initial symptoms subside and the patient is comfortable, no further treatment is indicated.
    a. true—the lesion heals without scars
    b. false—the bone loss that results invariably requires osseous correction
    c. false—the soft tissue architecture that remains is abnormal and often requires a surgical correction
    d. false—the lesion tends to recur, and therefore surgery should be performed

10. Pockets can occur as the result of
    a. plaque
    b. excessive forces
    c. diabetes
    d. a and b
    e. a, b, and c

11. Listgarten and Hellden demonstrated that the microbial flora associated with healthy and diseased sites within the same individual's mouth tended to be the same.
    a. true
    b. false—there was a higher proportion of cocci associated with the diseased sites
    c. false—there was a higher proportion of spirochetes associated with the diseased sites
    d. false—there was a higher proportion of spirochetes associated with the healthy sites

12. The virulent forms of microbiota that seem to be particularly harmful in rapid, destructive periodontitis are
    a. gram-positive aerobes
    b. gram-negative anaerobes
    c. streptococci
    d. veillonella

13. The rationale given for root planing is that
    a. scaled cemental surfaces may still contain calculus and therefore need to be root planed
    b. scaled cemental surfaces may contain endotoxins and therefore should be root planed
    c. scaled cemental surfaces that are rough preclude the attachment of junctional epithelium and therefore should be root planed
    d. a and b
    e. a, b, and c

14. The rationale for scaling is that
    a. calculus is plaque-retentive and therefore should be removed
    b. even plaque-free calculus has been shown to be a mechanical irritant to the soft tissues
    c. even plaque-free calculus precludes connective tissue reattachment
    d. a and c
    e. a, b, and c

15. The rationale for gingival curettage is that
    a. it débrides the inflamed soft tissue wall, thereby creating a surgical wound
    b. it débrides away the bacteria invariably found in the subsulcular connective tissue
    c. because it is an inadvertent but unavoidable part of root planing, we give it a name and say it helps healing
    d. a, b, and c
    e. a and b

16. Which of the following surgical procedures are useful for débriding an infrabony defect: (1) the gingivectomy, (2) the repositioned flap, and (3) the apically positioned flap
    a. 1, 2, and 3
    b. 1 and 2
    c. 2 and 3
    d. 1 and 3

17. The smoothness of a root-planed tooth is considered to be important because
    a. a smooth surface has been shown to be more conducive to epithelial reattachment
    b. a smooth surface has been shown to be more conducive to connective tissue reattachment
    c. a smooth surface is one of the clinical means of determining that the débridement of the root is complete
    d. a and c
    e. a, b, and c

18. It has been demonstrated in animal model systems that occlusal traumatism in combination with periodontitis may result in more attachment loss than if the periodontitis were present alone. If the periodontitis is controlled but the occlusal lesion is left untreated, the attachment loss will progress.
    a. both statements are true
    b. both statements are false
    c. the first statement is true and the second is false
    d. the first statement is false and the second is true

19. The lesion of occlusal traumatism can be differentiated from the so-called adaptive lesion by which of the following?
    a. presence of mobility in occlusal traumatism but not in the adaptive lesion
    b. presence of mobility in the adaptive lesion but not in occlusal traumatism
    c. presence of progressive mobility in occlusal traumatism but not in the adaptive lesion
    d. presence of progressive mobility in the adaptive lesion but not in occlusal traumatism

20. Increased horizontal tooth mobility can be the result of which of the following?
    a. soft tissue inflammation
    b. bruxism
    c. bone loss
    d. a, b, and c
    e. b and c only

See answers in Appendix.

REFERENCES

Epidemiology

1. Skougaard, M. R.: Oral disease prevention—its implications and applications. Keynote address from the Proceedings of the Eighth International Conference in Oral Biology. J. Dent. Res., 59 (Spec. Issue D): 2129–2130, 1980.
2. Kakehashi, S., and Parakkal, P. F.: Proceedings from the State of the Art Workshop on Surgical Therapy for Periodontitis. J. Periodontol., 53:475–501, 1982.
3. Pelton, W. J., Pennell, E. H., and Druzina, A.: Tooth morbidity experience of adults. J. Am. Dent. Assoc., 49:439–445, 1954.
4. Kegeles, S. S.: Current status of preventive dental health behavior in the population. Health Educ. Monogr., 1974, pp. 197–200.

5. Axelsson, P., and Lindhe, J.: Effect of controlled oral hygiene procedures on caries and periodontal disease in adults. Results after 6 years. J. Clin. Periodontol., 8:239–248, 1981.
6. Knowles, J. W., Burgett, F. G., Nissle, R. R., et al.: Results of periodontal treatment related to pocket depth and attachment level. Eight years. J. Periodontol., 50:225–233, 1979.
7. Lindhe, J., and Nyman, S.: The effect of plaque control and surgical pocket elimination on the establishment and maintenance of periodontal health. A longitudinal study of periodontal therapy in cases of advanced disease. J. Clin. Periodontol., 2:67–79, 1975.
8. Marshall-Day, C. D.: The epidemiology of periodontal disease. J. Periodontol., 22:13–22, 1951.
9. Schei, O., Waerhaug, J., Lovdal, A., and Arno, A.: Alveolar bone loss related to oral hygiene and age. J. Periodontol., 30:7–16, 1959.
10. Kelstrup, J., and Theilade, E.: Microbes and per-

iodontal disease. J. Clin. Periodontol., *1*:15–35, 1974.

11. Löe, H., Theilade, E., and Jensen, S. B.: Experimental gingivitis in man. J. Periodontol., *36*:177–187, 1965.

12. Socransky, S. S.: Microbiology of periodontal disease—present status and future considerations. J. Periodontol., *48*:497–504, 1977.

13. Löe, H., Anerud, A., Boysen, H., and Smith, M.: The natural history of periodontal disease in man. Study design and baseline data. J. Periodontol. Res., *13*:550–562, 1978.

14. Löe, H., Anerud, A., Boysen, H., and Smith, M.: The natural history of periodontal disease in man. The rate of periodontal destruction before 40 years of age. J. Periodontol., *49*:607–620, 1978.

15. Ramfjord, S. P., Knowles, J. W., Nissle, R. R., et al.: Longitudinal study of periodontal therapy. J. Periodontol., *44*:66–77, 1973.

16. Nyman, S., and Lindhe, J.: A longitudinal study of combined periodontal and prosthetic treatment of patients with advanced periodontal disease. J. Periodontol., *50*:163–169, 1979.

17. Hirschfeld, L., and Wasserman, B.: A long-term survey of tooth loss in 600 treated periodontal patients. J. Periodontol., *49*:225–237, 1978.

18. Becker, W., Berg, L., and Becker, B. E.: Untreated periodontal disease: A longitudinal study J. Periodontol., *50*:234–244, 1979.

19. Douglass, C. W., and Day, J. M.: Cost and payment of dental services in the United States. J. Dent. Ed., *43*:330–346, 1979.

The Soft Tissues of the Periodontium and Examination of the Periodontium

1. Ainamo, J., and Löe, H.: Anatomical characteristics of gingiva. A clinical and microscopic study of the free and attached gingiva. J. Periodontol., *37*:5–13, 1966.

2. Voigt, J. P., Goran, M. L., and Fleisher, R. M.: The width of lingual mandibular attached gingiva. J. Periodontol., *49*:77–80, 1978.

3. Bowers, G. M.: A study of the width of attached gingiva. J. Periodontol., *34*:201–209, 1963.

4. Schroeder, H. E., and Listgarten, M. A.: Fine structure of the developing epithelial attachment of human teeth. Monogr. Dev. Biol., *2*:69–78, 1977.

5. Löe, H.: The gingival index, the plaque index, and the retention index systems. J. Periodontol., *38*:610–616, 1967.

6. Listgarten, M. A., Mao, R., and Robinson, P. J.: Periodontal probing and the relationship of the probe tip to the periodontal tissues. J. Periodontol., *47*:511–513, 1976.

7. Laster, L., Laudenbach, K. W., and Stoller, N. H.: An evaluation of clinical tooth mobility measurements. J. Periodontol., *46*:603–607, 1975.

8. Listgarten, M. A., and Shiffer, C.: Differential dark field microscopy of subgingival bacteria as an aid in selecting recall interval: results after 18 months. J. Clin. Periodontol., *9*:305–316, 1982.

Etiology

1. Kelstrup, J., and Theilade, E.: Microbes and periodontal disease. J. Clin. Periodontol., *1*:15–35, 1974.

2. Socransky, S. S.: Microbiology of periodontal disease—present status and future considerations. J. Periodontol., *48*:497–504, 1977.

3. Löe, H., Theilade, E., and Jensen, S. B.: Experimental gingivitis in man. J. Periodontol., *36*:177–187, 1965.

4. Socransky, S. S.: Criteria for the infectious agents in dental caries and periodontal disease. J. Clin. Periodontol., *6* (Suppl.):16–21, 1979.

5. Listgarten, M. A., and Hellden, L.: Relative distribution of bacteria at clinically healthy and periodontally diseased sites in humans. J. Clin. Periodontol., *5*:115–132, 1978.

6. Slots, J.: Subgingival microflora and periodontal disease. J. Clin. Periodontol., *6*:351–382, 1979.

7. Lang, N. P., and Löe, H.: The relationship between the width of keratinized gingiva and gingival health. J. Periodontol., *43*:623–627, 1972.

8. Miyasato, M., Crigger, M., and Egelberg, J.: Gingival conditions in areas of minimal and appreciable width of keratinized gingiva. J. Clin. Periodontol., *4*:200–209, 1977.

9. Svanberg, G.: Influence of trauma from occlusion on the periodontium of dogs with normal or inflamed gingivae. Odontol. Revy, *25*:165–178, 1974.

10. Wentz, F., Jarabak, J., and Orban, B.: Experimental occlusal trauma imitating cuspal interferences. J. Periodontol., *29*:117–127, 1958.

11. Pennel, B. M., and Keagle, J. G.: Predisposing factors in the etiology of chronic inflammatory periodontal disease. J. Periodontol., *48*:517–532, 1977.

12. Nisengard, R. J.: The role of immunology in periodontal disease. J. Periodontol., *48*:505–516, 1977.

13. Baehni, P., Tsai, C. C., Stoller, N. H., et al.: Studies of host responses during experimental gingivitis in humans. I. Polymorphonuclear leukocyte responses to autologous plaque collected during the development of gingival inflammation. J. Periodontol. Res., *14*:279–288, 1979.

14. Kornman, K. S., and Loesche, W. J.: The subgingival microflora during pregnancy. J. Periodontol. Res., *15*:111–122, 1980.

15. Sutcliffe, P.: A longitudinal study of gingivitis and puberty. J. Periodontol. Res., *7*:52–58, 1972.

16. Cohen, D. W., Friedman, L. A., Shapiro, J., et al.: Diabetes mellitus and periodontal disease: Two-year longitudinal observations. Part I. J. Periodontol., *41*:709–718, 1970.

17. Van Dyke, T. E., Horoszewicz, H. U., Cianciola, C. J., and Genco, R.: Neutrophil chemotaxis dysjunction in human periodontitis. Infect. Immun., *27*:124–132, 1980.

Gingivitis and Periodontitis

1. Magnusson, I., and Listgarten, M. A.: Histological evaluation of probing depth following periodontal treatment. J. Clin. Periodontol., *7*:26–31, 1980.

2. Page, R. C., and Schroeder, H. E.: Pathogenesis of inflammatory periodontal disease. A summary of current work. Lab. Invest., *33*:235–249, 1976.

3. Löe, H., Theilade, E., Jensen, S. B., and Schiött, C. R.: Experimental gingivitis in man. III. The influence of antibiotics on gingival plaque development. J. Periodontol. Res., *2*:282–289, 1967.

4. Löe, H., Theilade, E., and Jensen, B. S.: Experimental gingivitis in man: J. Periodontol., *36*:177–187, 1965.

5. Egelberg, J.: Local effect of diet on plaque forma-

tion and development of gingivitis in dogs. I. Effect of hard and soft diets. Odontol. Revy, *16*:31–41, 1965.

6. Carlsson, J., and Egelberg, J.: The effect of diet on plaque formation and development of gingivitis in dogs. II. Effect of high carbohydrate versus high protein-fat diets. Odontol. Revy, *16*:42–49, 1965.

7. Egelberg, J.: Local effect of diet on plaque formation and development of gingivitis in dogs. III. Effect of frequency of meals and tube feeding. Odontol. Revy, *16*:50–60, 1965.

8. Slots, J., Möenbo, D., Langebaek, J., and Frandsen, A.: Microbiota of gingivitis in man. Scand. J. Dent. Res., *86*:174–181, 1978.

9. Löe, H., Schiott, R. C., Glavind, L., and Karring, T.: Two years of oral use of chlorhexidine in humans. I. General design and clinical effects. J. Periodontol. Res., *11*:135–144, 1976.

10. Socransky, S. S., Hubersak, C., and Propas, D.: Introduction of periodontal destruction in gnotobiotic rats by a human oral strain of *Actinomyces naeslundii*. Arch. Oral Biol., *15*:993–996, 1970.

11. Lindhe, J., Hamp, S. E., and Löe, H.: Plaque-induced periodontal disease in beagle dogs. A 4-year clinical, roentgenographical and histometrical study. J. Periodontol. Res., *10*:243–255, 1975.

12. Listgarten, M. A., and Hellden, L.: Relative distribution of bacteria at clinically healthy and periodontally diseased sites in humans. J. Clin. Periodontol., *5*:115–132, 1978.

13. Krook, L.: Periodontal disease in dogs and man. Adv. Vet. Sci. Comp. Med., *20*:171–190, 1976.

Acute Necrotizing Ulcerative Gingivitis

1. Schluger, S.: Necrotizing ulcerative gingivitis in the army: Incidence, communicability and treatment. J. Am. Dent. Assoc., *38*:174–183, 1949.

2. Giddon, D. B., Zackin, S. J., and Goldhaber, P.: Acute necrotizing ulcerative gingivitis in college students. J. Am. Dent. Assoc., *68*:380–386, 1964.

3. Listgarten, M. A.: Electron microscopic observations on the bacterial flora of acute necrotizing ulcerative gingivitis. J. Periodontol., *36*:328–339, 1965.

4. Moulton, R., Ewen, S., and Thieman, W.: Emotional factors in periodontal disease. Oral Surg., *5*:833–860, 1952.

5. Pindborg, J. J.: Tobacco and gingivitis. II. Correlation between consumption of tobacco, ulceromembranous gingivitis and calculus. J. Dent. Res., *28*:460–463, 1949.

Trauma From Occlusion

1. Polson, A. M., Meitner, S. W., and Zander, H. A.: Trauma and progression of marginal periodontitis

in squirrel monkeys. III. Adaptation of interproximal alveolar bone to repetitive injury. J. Periodontol. Res., *11*:279–289, 1976.

2. Svanberg, G.: Influence of trauma from occlusion on the periodontium of dogs with normal or inflamed gingivae. Odontol. Revy, *25*:165–178, 1974.

3. Lindhe, J., and Svanberg, G.: Influence of trauma from occlusion on progression of experimental periodontitis in the beagle dog. J. Clin. Periodontol., *1*:3–14, 1974.

4. Laster, L., Laudenbach, K. W., and Stoller, N. H.: An evaluation of clinical tooth mobility measurements. J. Periodontol., *46*:603–607, 1975.

Oral Hygiene and Scaling and Root Planing

1. Cohen, D. W., Stoller, N. H., Chace, R., and Laster, L.: A comparison of bacterial plaque disclosants in periodontal disease. J. Periodontol., *43*:333–346, 1972.

2. Keyes, P. H., Wright, W. E., and Howard, S. A.: The use of phase-contrast microscopy and chemotherapy in the diagnosis and treatment of periodontal lesions—an initial report. I. Quintessence Int. *1*:1–6, 1978.

3. Keyes, P. H., Wright, W. E., and Howard, S. A.: The use of phase-contrast microscopy and chemotherapy in the diagnosis and treatment of periodontal lesions—an initial report. II. Quintessence Int. *2*:7–14, 1978.

4. Löe, H., and Silness, J.: Periodontal disease in pregnancy. I. Prevalence and severity. Acta Odontol. Scand. *21*:533–551, 1963.

5. Muhlemann, H. R., and Son, S.: Gingival sulcus bleeding—a leading symptom in initial gingivitis. Helv. Odontol. Acta, *15*:107–113, 1971.

6. Zander, H. A.: The attachment of calculus to root surfaces. J. Periodontol., *24*:16–19, 1953.

7. Aleo, J. J., and Vandersall, D. C.: Cementum: Recent concepts related to periodontal therapy. Dent. Clin. North Am., *24*:627, 1980.

8. Nishimine, D., and O'Leary, T. J.: Hand instruments versus ultrasonics in the removal of endotoxins from root surfaces. J. Periodontol., *50*:345–349, 1979.

9. Cerra, M. B., and Killoy, W. J.: The effect of sodium bicarbonate and hydrogen peroxide on the microbial flora of periodontal pockets—A preliminary report. J. Periodontol., *53*:599–603, 1982.

10. Stoller, N. H., et al.: A comparison of scaling, root planing and traditional oral hygiene with scaling, root planing and oral hygiene utilizing baking soda and hydrogen peroxide on human periodontal disease. Clinical and microscopic observations. Presented at the Meeting of the American Academy of Periodontology, Anaheim, Calif., October, 1982.

6

ENDODONTICS IN GENERAL PRACTICE

According to the definition of the American Association of Endodontists, endodontics is "that branch of dentistry concerned with the morphology, physiology, and pathology of the human dental pulp and periapical tissues. Its study and practice encompass related basic and clinical sciences including biology of the normal pulp, the etiology, diagnosis, prevention and treatment of diseases and injuries of the pulp, and resultant pathological periradicular conditions." This definition identifies endodontics as a central and integral part of total patient care. The general practitioner, therefore, should be well trained in endo-

dontics and should be prepared to perform all types of endodontic treatment. This also means that a general practitioner should recognize the more complex conditions that should be treated in cooperation with an endodontist.

OBJECTIVES

It is often heard that endodontic treatment is technically difficult and stressful, since it is associated with pain, emergencies, and, at times, unpleasant situations for both

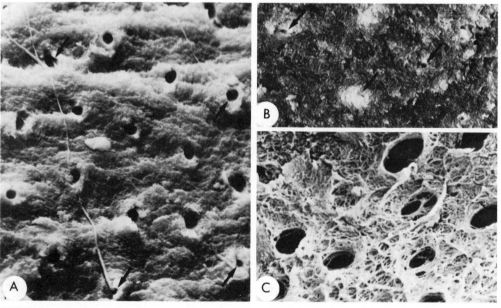

FIGURE 6–1 Scanning electron micrographs of fractured coronal dentin from a 53-year-old patient. *A,* Dentin halfway between enamel and pulp. Crosscut dentinal tubules (arrows) are seen. *B,* Mantle dentin. Note small diameter of dentinal tubules (arrows). *C,* Predentin. The unmineralized dentin matrix can be recognized. (From Tronstad, L.: Ultrastructural observations on human coronal dentin. Scand. J. Dent. Res., *81*:101–111, 1973.)

patient and dentist. Such an attitude does not necessarily reflect the anatomic intricacies of the root canal system but rather a lack of understanding of the tissue reactions and the therapeutic problems involved in endodontic treatment. The main objectives of this chapter, therefore, are to summarize some important biologic considerations in endodontics, to present a simple and practical clinical diagnostic system, and to describe the principles for modern endodontic treatment so they can become the basis for necessary therapeutic measures. At the same time, the technical difficulties involved with endodontic treatment are not ignored. The standardized technique for endodontic treatment, which is presented as the technique of choice in general practice, was, in fact, developed in an effort to simplify the instrumentation and obturation phases of root canal treatment as much as possible without making biologic compromises.

Endodontics has, as do all clinical disciplines, important preventive aspects. The pulp is surrounded by dentin, and there is a close relationship between the two tissues through the dentinal tubules (Fig. 6–1). Any lesion in the dentin may influence the health of the underlying pulp, and, just as important, all restorative treatment of lesions in the dentin may influence the pulp. Knowledge and understanding of the reaction pattern of the pulp and periapical tissues to irritants and therapeutic measures are therefore of great importance in reparative dentistry. This area is now often referred to as preventive endodontics and is an integral part of endodontics in general practice. Preventive endodontics is not treated according to its importance in this chapter. However, the point is made that biologically acceptable reparative procedures may be performed if simple pulp protective measures are applied.

BIOLOGIC CONSIDERATIONS

The Dental Pulp

The dental pulp consists of a richly vascularized and highly innervated connective tissue (Figs. 6–2 and 6–3). Typical and specific cells for the pulp are the dentin-producing cells, the odontoblasts, and cells that under certain conditions can develop into odontoblasts (Fig. 6–4).

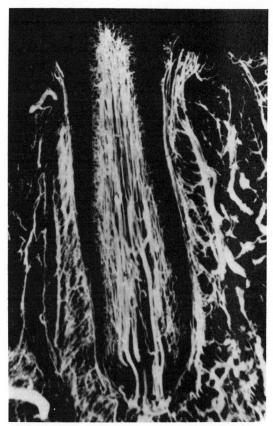

FIGURE 6–2 Microangiograph of dog premolar. The pulp is richly vascularized; note the subdentinal capillary plexus. (From Skoglund, A., Tronstad, L., and Wallenius, K.: A microangiographic study of vascular changes in replanted and autotransplanted teeth of young dogs.

The Reaction Pattern of the Pulp

As does other connective tissue in the body, the pulp reacts to irritants with inflammation (Fig. 6–5). Because of the anatomic environment of the pulp (surrounded by hard dentin walls and communicating with the rest of the organism only via small foramina near the apex of the root), the inflammatory process may take an especially serious course. Tumor (swelling) is one of the cardinal signs of inflammation. When the pulp becomes inflamed, anatomic limitations would seem to preclude an increase in tissue volume. For many years, therefore, it was assumed that even in teeth with local inflammation in the pulp, the tissue pressure would increase in the entire pulp cavity. The pressure increase was thought to result in an elevated arterial pressure followed by an increase in venous pressure. The venous pres-

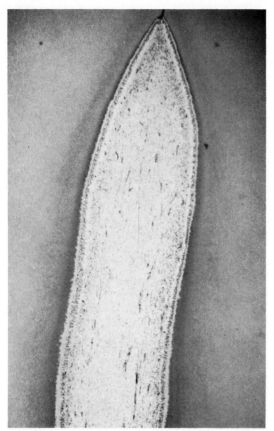

FIGURE 6–3 Paraffin section of human tooth. The connective tissue of the coronal pulp with cells and vessels is seen. Note odontoblasts lining the dentinal walls.

sure increase would again result in a new increase in the arterial pressure, continuing the cycle. The final result of the pressure increases was assumed to be a relatively rapid choking or strangulation of the pulp at the apical foramen. This theory of the development of pulp inflammation was called the strangulation theory.

Based on the results of a series of experiments using different techniques, it is currently believed that the strangulation theory is incorrect. For example, in experiments in which the tissue pressure of the pulp was measured, it was found that a pressure increase in one area of the pulp does not cause a pressure increase in the rest of the pulp. It has also been found that when a local inflammation is induced in the pulp, the tissue pressure increases only in the inflamed area and not in the entire pulp, as was previously believed.

Experiments with in vivo microscopy have confirmed that local damage in the coronal pulp may result in circulatory disturbances and, in certain cases, complete stasis in the vessels in and near the damaged area. By contrast, the circulation in the root pulp is unaffected in these experiments. These results indicate that local inflammatory changes in the pulp do not result in a complete circulatory stoppage in the entire pulp.

Thus, the modern view of the reaction pattern of the pulp is as follows. The pulp reacts to irritants with local inflammation in a larger or smaller area of the tissue that comes in contact with the irritants. The inflammation may remain as a local inflammation for years, and if the irritants are removed (for example, if carious dentin is excavated and a restoration placed in the tooth), experiments have shown that even severe local inflammation may heal. The resistance of the pulp to irritants and its ability for repair is therefore considerable.

Still, if the irritants are long lasting and

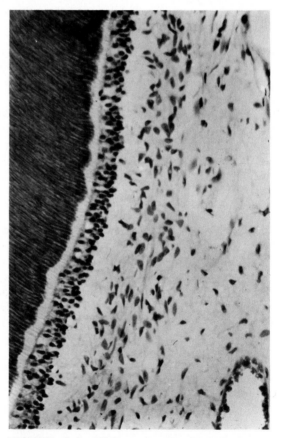

FIGURE 6–4 Higher magnification of dentin-pulp interface in Figure 6–3. Dentin, predentin (unstained), the odontoblast layer, the cell-free zone, and the cell-rich zone are recognized.

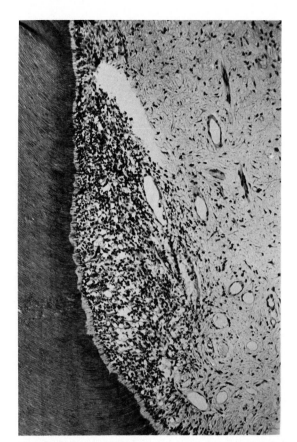

FIGURE 6–5   Paraffin section of monkey tooth. An accumulation of inflammatory cells is seen in a localized area of the pulp subjacent to the dentin wall.

strong enough, the inflammation will spread in the pulp. However, the spreading does not result in a sudden strangulation of the organ near the apex. On the contrary, the process progresses rather slowly toward the central parts of the pulp, the root pulp, and the periapical tissues (ulcerative pulpitis) (Fig. 6–6). When the damage in the pulp reaches a certain proportion, the inflammation becomes irreversible. This means that even if the original irritants that initiated the process are removed, the amount of toxic products from damaged and diseased tissue and from possible microorganisms in the tissue is so large that the inflammation is self-sustaining. Successive necrosis of the tissue in the direction of the apical foramen then takes place.

The Pathogenesis of Pulp Inflammation

The inflammation in the pulp develops in the same manner as in other tissues. It has been claimed that there is a certain difference in the cellular phase of the process, with pulpal inflammation dominated by lymphocytes (and plasma cells) from the inception and by granulocytes only during extensive tissue damage. This theory is probably not correct. It is based on studies of carious teeth and could have arisen easily from misinterpretation of chronic inflammation as the initial cellular phase of the process. In experiments in which pulp inflammation is induced experimentally, it has been shown clearly that the cellular phase is dominated first by granulocytes and that lymphocytes and plasma cells appear later. The last two cell types, however, dominate the histologic picture during pulp inflammation, which generally has the character of a chronic inflammation.

When complications that lead to a more

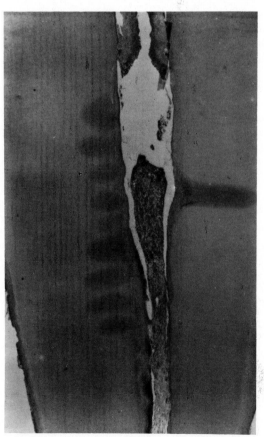

FIGURE 6–6   Paraffin section of human tooth. Because of caries, the pulp has become exposed to the oral cavity. The tissue of the coronal pulp is necrotic. Subjacent to the necrotic area, the tissue is inflamed. In the apical area, the tissue is not inflamed.

severe inflammatory response occur, infiltration of granulocytes in one or more areas of the pulp can also occur. This infiltration may cause an exacerbation of chronic pulpitis and often results in a purulent transformation of the tissue. The purulent transformation may occur as a gradual fusion of different foci but is also seen as a broad penetration through the pulp tissue. If the leukocytic breakdown takes place fairly slowly, capsuled abscesses can form. This encapsulation may, for a time, delay the further development of the inflammatory process. Sometimes even a calcification of the abscess membrane is seen, but it should never be assumed that healing will occur without treatment of the tooth.

Pulp inflammation is therefore a dynamic process. Various stages of the inflammatory process can usually be observed in different areas of the same pulp. A typical observation would be necrosis of the tissue in the area in which the inflammation started. The tissue adjacent to this area might be inflamed, dominated by cells typical of chronic inflammation. Also, in this area, one or more abscesses might be seen. Apical to the inflamed area, noninflamed pulp tissue would be present. Without treatment, the inflammation (and later the necrosis) will gradually spread in an apical direction until the entire pulp becomes necrotic. A total pulpitis, in the sense that the entire pulp is infiltrated by inflammatory cells, does not seem to occur.

Dentin Resorption. During a chronic inflammation of the pulp, dentin-resorbing cells sometimes form (osteoclasts, or, as they are also called, dentinoclasts). These cells cause resorption of the walls of the root canal, and the process is termed internal resorption (Fig. 6–7A). Internal resorption is usually a slow process, and it can even enter into a reparative phase with new formation (apposition) of hard tissue in the resorption lacunae and on the canal walls. The newly formed hard tissue is not dentin but most often resembles cementum or bone (Fig. 6–7B). However, permanent repair should not be expected, as the resorption process is progressive in character. The result can be a perforation of the root if the pulp has not become necrotic before that time or if the process is not stopped by endodontic treatment.

Internal resorption is normally seen in the root, but rapid internal resorption of the

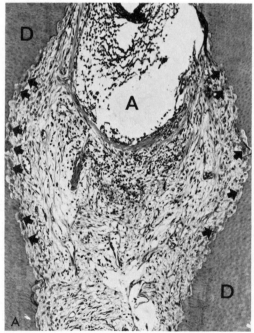
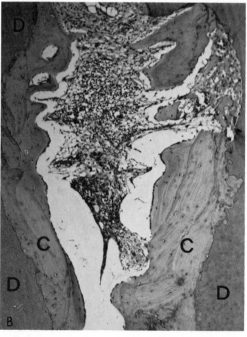

FIGURE 6–7 Paraffin sections of human primary teeth 4 years after clinically successful formocresol pulpotomy. **A,** Internal resorption with multinucleated, dentin-resorbing cells (arrows) along the dentin walls (D). A, abscess. **B,** Deposition of cementumlike tissue (C) has occurred in this area, with internal dentin (D) resorption in severely inflamed pulp. (From Rolling, I., Hasselgren, G., and Tronstad, L.: Morphologic and enzyme histochemical observations in the pulp of human primary molars 3 to 5 years after formocresol treatment. Oral Surg., 42:518–528, 1976.)

crown of the tooth can occur, especially as a result of trauma. This resorption is normally discovered because the pulp becomes visible through the enamel, and the condition is often called "pink spot" or "pink tooth."

Pulp Polyp. A seldom occurring variation in the development of pulp inflammation is the formation of a pulp polyp. Under particularly favorable circumstances, the successive breakdown of the pulp can stop temporarily when a carious attack has resulted in an opening of the pulp cavity. Instead of becoming necrotic, the pulp tissue may start to proliferate. A proliferative pulpitis or a pulp polyp then develops. On the surface the pulp polyp normally has a necrotic layer, but in about 20 per cent of the instances it becomes epithelialized. A pulp polyp may last for a relatively long time, but if treatment is not initiated, the end result will be total tissue breakdown as described above.

The Etiology of Pulp Inflammation

Inflammation of the pulp can be caused by many factors. For practical reasons, the following division can be made:
  I. Toxic-infectious pulpitis
      a. Caries
      b. Attrition, abrasion, erosion
      c. Gingival recession
      d. Periodontal disease
  II. Traumatic pulpitis
 III. Iatrogenic pulpitis
      a. Cavity and crown preparation
      b. Unsuitable restorative techniques
      c. Cements and restorative materials
      d. Cavity cleansing and disinfection
      e. Orthodontic treatment
      f. Surgical treatment

Toxic-Infectious Pulpitis

Caries. Caries is the most important cause of toxic-infectious pulpitis (Fig. 6–8). The dentinal tubules are gateways to the pulp for breakdown products, toxins, and microorganisms from the lesion, and even during early enamel caries without macroscopic loss of tissue, scattered inflammatory cells may be seen in the pulp under the involved dentinal tubules. Actual inflammatory foci with abscesses can be found under relatively superficial dentin caries. It is important to note that although there are microorganisms in the dentinal tubules of a carious lesion, the

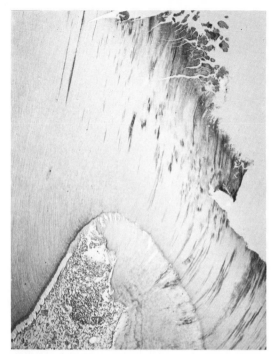

FIGURE 6–8 Paraffin section of human tooth with deep carious lesion. A severe inflammatory reaction with abscess formation is seen in the pulp. Secondary dentin, which has formed in response to the carious process, does not prevent the irritants from reaching the pulp. (From Skogedal, O., and Tronstad, L.: An attempt to correlate dentin and pulp changes in human carious teeth. Oral Surg., *43*:135–140, 1977.)

pulp is not infected as long as it is vital. If any microorganisms should reach the vital pulp, they will be destroyed quickly. Thus, it is breakdown products and the toxins from bacteria and necrotic tissue that first cause the inflammation. Not until the pulp damage is so severe that an area of necrosis has developed will it be possible to demonstrate bacteria in the pulp cavity. Bacterial colonies are then formed in the necrotic tissue, and the pulp is infected. Also, during the further spread of the inflammation in the pulp, bacteria are present only in the necrotic tissue. The "front of infection," in other words, will be at the transition zone between necrotic and vital (inflamed) tissue. The vital pulp tissue is sterile. Although marked inflammatory reactions can be observed in the pulp of teeth with relatively superficial carious lesions, it is possible to find teeth with apparently much more severe carious attacks without pulpal inflammation (Fig. 6–9). The reason for this seemingly illogical occurrence is that products from the carious process can

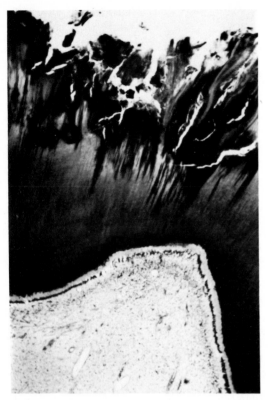

FIGURE 6–9 Paraffin section of human tooth with deep carious lesion. Only a few scattered inflammatory cells are present in the pulp. No secondary dentin has formed.

of the dentinal tubules during a carious attack.

The intratubular mineralized deposits that are formed under the influence of caries vary considerably in "quality." They may consist of small hydroxyapatite crystals that almost completely obliterate the tubules (as in age-changed dentin), of larger, irregularly arranged, needle-shaped hydroxyapatite crystals, of large rhomboidal formed whitlockite crystals, or of a combination of several or all of these. It cannot be assumed that the reaction that takes place in the dentin leads to a complete obliteration of the involved tubules. But under certain circumstances, especially if the carious process develops slowly, a barrier can be formed that prevents the passage of irritation products to the pulp so effectively that temporary repair of the pulpal inflammation may take place. A permanent repair without treatment is still unthinkable, as a carious process will proceed and gradually break through the dentin barrier so that toxic products once again can reach the pulp.

Even if the dentin barrier can be relatively effective in a carious lesion, it probably is of minor importance from a clinical point of view. The carious process spreads not only in a pulpal direction in the dentin but also in a lateral direction, especially in the area near the enamel-dentin junction. This results in toxic products reaching the pulp through newly exposed dentinal tubules, where intratubular dentin has not yet been formed. *Therefore, in practice, it must be assumed that the pulp is inflamed to some extent in all carious teeth.*

Note that the dentin barrier is formed in

stimulate the pulp to produce intratubular dentin (Fig. 6–10). In addition to this phenomenon, there is probably also a passive reprecipitation of minerals from the peripheral carious dentin in the more pulpal parts

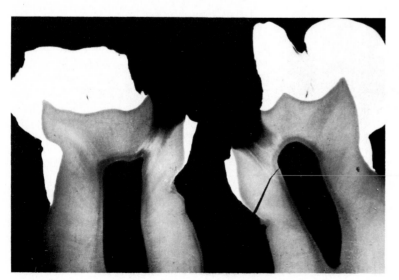

FIGURE 6–10 Microradiograph of two ground sections from human molar with deep carious lesion. A hypermineralized zone is seen in the dentin subjacent to the carious lesion. No secondary dentin has formed. (From Skogedal, O., and Tronstad, L.: An attempt to correlate dentin and pulp changes in human carious teeth. Oral Surg., *43*:135–140, 1977.)

the primary dentin. The secondary dentin, which as a rule also is formed in the pulp under a carious lesion, does not, however, constitute a barrier against the toxic products (Fig. 6–8). On the contrary, when the carious process has broken through to the secondary dentin, the pulp always appears to be inflamed. With time, the carious process will also break through to the pulp and cause a pulp exposure. At that time, the inflammation will have usually reached such a degree of severity that it is irreversible with today's treatment methods.

Exposed Dentin. Other etiologic factors leading to toxic-infectious pulpitis are conditions that contribute to the exposure of the dentin and the dentinal tubules to the oral environment. With the refinement of foodstuffs during the last generation, attrition is not as common as before. On the other hand, abrasion (particularly toothbrushing damage) is becoming a more serious problem.

In instances of gingival recession and periodontal disease and the treatment of this disease, the root cementum is often removed so that the root dentin is exposed. This means that toxic products and microorganisms from saliva and plaque may gain access to the pulp through the exposed dentinal tubules. Still, it appears that the pulp tolerates this situation quite well. Often, the pulp of such teeth is free of inflammation or only a few inflammatory cells are observed under the exposed dentin surface. Even in teeth with severe periodontitis, the pulp, as a rule, is practically free of inflammation. When a periodontal pocket reaches the foraminal area of the root, a retrograde pulpitis may develop, since irritants can enter the pulp through the apical foramen or possible lateral canals. In teeth with one root, this condition will lead to a severe disturbance of the blood supply to the pulp relatively quickly, resulting in total pulp necrosis. In teeth with multiple roots, a retrograde pulpitis in one root will spread slowly in a coronal direction, because the pulp is supplied by vessels from the other roots. It may take a relatively long time before the entire pulp becomes necrotic in such teeth.

Traumatic Pulpitis

Trauma to the teeth and jaws will often result in pulp damage and pulp death. In teeth with crown fracture and pulp exposure, a pulpitis will be established after a day

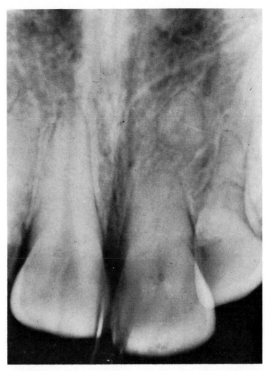

FIGURE 6–11 Radiograph of maxillary incisor with root fracture 25 years after injury. The apical fragment is separated by bone from the rest of the tooth. No periradicular inflammation is present.

or two. Without treatment this inflammation will lead to total pulp necrosis.

The majority of root fractures (75 per cent) do not result in permanent pulp damage (Fig. 6–11). The most common complication is necrosis of the pulp of the coronal fragment of the tooth. If this fragment of the tooth is treated endodontically, the pulp apical to the root fracture may remain vital, and the prognosis of the tooth is reasonably good.

Trauma often results in vascular damage with disturbances of the blood supply to the pulp. A negative sensitivity response immediately after trauma should not be interpreted as a definite sign of pulp death. The sensitivity may return within weeks or months. In teeth with open apices, a revascularization of the pulp may also occur. This process takes approximately 1 month.

Iatrogenic Pulpitis

Cavity and Crown Preparation. During preparatory work, certain iatrogenic factors are introduced that may cause pulp damage. During cavity preparation, friction may lead to considerable heat increase in the cavity. The heat increase results in a dehydration of the dentin and a flow of tissue fluid from the pulp to the dentin surface. This flow of fluid causes mechanical disturbances in the pulp, including a displacement of odontoblasts and other cells into the dentinal tubules. The results of the disturbances are tissue breakdown and inflammation (Fig. 6–12).

It is important to understand that it is not the heat of the drill by itself that causes the pulp damage. True, it has been shown that a temperature increase of 10°C in the pulp may cause inflammation. The dentin, however, is a good insulator, and cavity preparation without cooling seems to give a temperature increase of only 2 to 5°C. It is the dehydration of the dentin as a result of the drilling that causes the damage. It is of clinical importance to understand this difference because *cooling of the bur with air, cold or tempered, cannot prevent preparation damage but, rather, will make it worse.* Use of water,

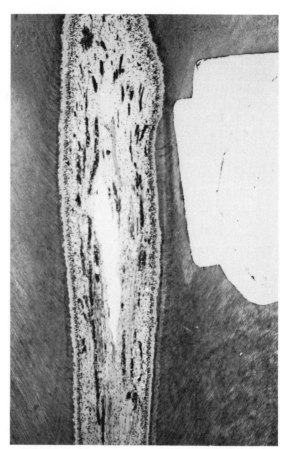

FIGURE 6–13 Paraffin section of monkey tooth with a very deep cavity prepared with ultra-high speed and a spray of water and air. The cavity was lined with a calcium hydroxide cement and filled with amalgam for 90 days. A slight amount of secondary dentin has formed; otherwise, no changes are evident in the pulp.

however, will prevent dehydration of the dentin and thereby prevent pulp damage in an effective and reliable manner (Fig. 6–13).

Unsuitable Filling Techniques. A good example of the harm that may be caused to the pulp by the placing of a restoration is the use of cohesive gold fillings. The necessary "hammering" with this technique as well as the heating of the gold foil usually causes severe pulp damage characterized by intrapulpal bleeding and inflammation. This damage is frequently irreversible. Less serious reactions in the pulp may follow other filling techniques, for instance, insertion of thermoplastic filling materials (stopping) and even machine condensation of deep amalgam restorations.

Filling Materials. Cements and filling materials used in dentistry may contain com-

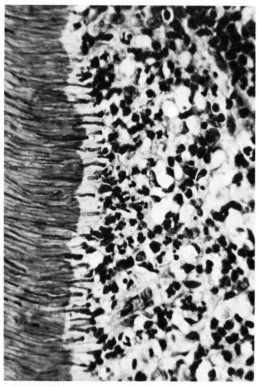

FIGURE 6–12 Paraffin section of monkey tooth showing dentin-pulp interface subjacent to a cavity prepared with ultra-high speed without water. The odontoblasts are displaced into the dentinal tubules. An accumulation of inflammatory cells, mainly granulocytes, is seen in the pulp.

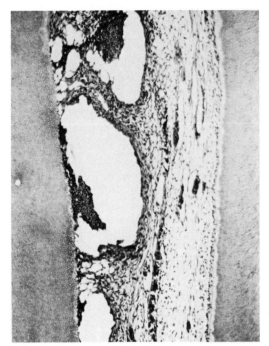

FIGURE 6–14 Paraffin section of monkey tooth showing area of pulp subjacent to a cavity filled with a methyl methacrylate resin for 8 days. Severe local inflammation with abscess formation is seen in the pulp.

ponents that are irritating the pulp. Silver amalgam, which is still the most used filling material, is, fortunately, from a biologic point of view, a fairly good material that does not cause any significant pulp reactions. It is the tooth-colored materials, the various resins and cements, that are of interest in this connection (Fig. 6–14).

Disinfection and Cleansing of Cavities. A large number of drugs have been used for cavity disinfection (phenol, silver nitrate, chloroform, alcohol, chlorhexidine). However, so far no one has been able to show that disinfection of the dentin in a cavity is necessary or even beneficial. On the contrary, several of the aforementioned preparations have been shown to be irritating to the pulp. Therefore, *cavity cleansing should involve only a thorough washing, not disinfection of the dentin.* For this purpose a spray of water and air is sufficient and probably represents the best method.

Orthodontic Treatment. During orthodontic treatment, the teeth can be exposed to forces that are strong enough to cause pulp damage. Initially, vessels may be damaged, resulting in internal bleeding. Clinically, the damage usually is discovered because the tooth becomes discolored. Internal

and, especially, external root resorption is also a common complication during orthodontic treatment.

Surgical Treatment. Oral and maxillofacial surgery may cause pulp damage and pulp death by severing blood vessels and interrupting the blood supply to the pulp. However, in such instances it must be remembered that absence of sensitivity does not necessarily mean that the tooth is nonvital. It could be the nerve supply (which lacks reserve lines) that is damaged. The blood vessels of the face and jaws have anastomoses, and the necessary blood supply could be secured in spite of the operation.

Apical Periodontitis

Etiology

In time, untreated pulp inflammation will pass through the apical foramen and attack the periodontal tissues (root cementum, periodontal ligament, bone) (Figs. 6–15 and 6–16). This inflammatory condition is called

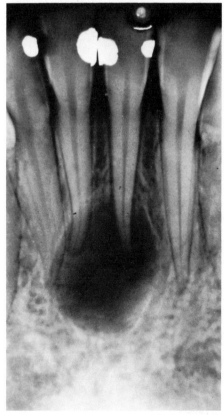

FIGURE 6–15 Radiograph of nonvital mandibular lower incisor with periapical radiolucent area, indicating apical periodontitis (apical granuloma or radicular cyst).

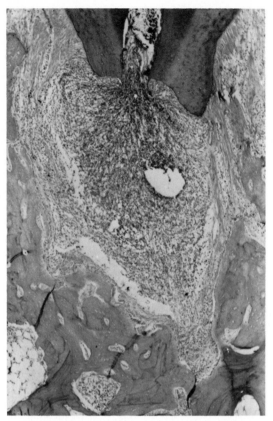

FIGURE 6–16 Paraffin section of monkey tooth with periapical granuloma. The area of inflammation is surrounded by a fibrous capsule.

apical periodontitis. The most important etiologic factors in the development of apical periodontitis are: (1) tissue breakdown products in the root canal, (2) infection, and (3) iatrogenic factors (overinstrumentation, medicaments, materials). The inflamed or necrotic pulp tissue can be considered a reservoir of toxic agents leaking out through the apical foramen and thereby provoking inflammation in the periapical area. The necrotic tissue in the root canal is usually infected, and the bacterial toxins are especially important in the development of periapical inflammation. Remember that the actual infection front (as in the pulp) occurs at the border between necrotic and vital tissues.

Apical periodontitis can also develop as a result of iatrogenic damages, such as overinstrumentation, use (and abuse) of toxic and tissue-irritating medicaments and root-filling materials as well as from overfilling of the root canal.

Pathogenesis

Apical periodontitis may be acute and symptomatic or chronic and asymptomatic. A chronic course of development is, by far, the most common, and the noniatrogenically caused inflammation is normally of an insidious asymptomatic character. Thus, there is an almost balanced condition between the defense mechanisms of the body and the factors causing the periapical inflammation.

Asymptomatic Apical Periodontitis. Typical for the asymptomatic apical periodontitis is the formation of granulation tissue at the apex of the tooth. A normally well-developed fibrous capsule forms around the granulation tissue and attaches to the root surface. When the tooth is extracted, the entire "granuloma," as it is often called, may accompany the tooth as a hat-shaped formation over the apex (Fig. 6–17). Such connective tissue encapsulation of an inflamed area should be looked upon as a protective reaction from the organism. However, repair can never take place as long as the root canal functions as a depot for inflammation-provoking agents.

The Malassez epithelial rests in the periodontal ligament can be stimulated to proliferate by the inflammatory process, and so-called epithelial islands may form in the granulation tissue. These islands may increase in size, and irregular epithelial formations, epithelial strings, may be seen in

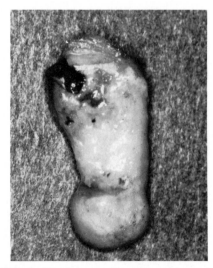

FIGURE 6–17 Extracted tooth with periapical granuloma. A continuous and uniform fibrous capsule surrounding granuloma is seen.

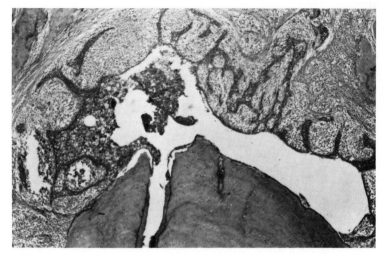

FIGURE 6–18 Paraffin section of monkey tooth with radicular cyst. Epithelium lines the cyst cavity. An area of inflammation surrounded by a fibrous capsule is seen peripheral to the epithelium.

the inflamed area. If the epithelium continues to proliferate, a cyst, i.e., a liquid-containing, epithelium-lined cavity, may develop. This type of cyst is called a radicular cyst (Fig. 6–18).

Cyst size naturally varies. Normally it is modest, but occasionally cysts reach a size such that they fill the greater part of the jaw. Traditionally, a radicular cyst has been said to be round and well delineated in a radiograph. However, cysts may be of almost any shape and cannot be distinguished radiographically from granulomas. Peripheral to the epithelium, the cyst is surrounded by granulation tissue, which may vary considerably in thickness. This tissue may contribute to the "fuzzy" appearance cysts sometimes have in radiographs.

Many histologic examinations have been performed to determine the frequency of cysts in connection with apical periodontitis, and frequencies of between 6 per cent and 43 per cent have been reported. However, none of these studies is conclusive, and at the present time no definite information about the frequency of cysts in periapical lesions is available.

Areas with increased radiographic density (osteosclerosis) sometimes are seen at the apex of the tooth. Occasionally, the formation of sclerotic bone is caused by a chronic pulpitis or by pulp necrosis. The condition is then referred to as condensing apical periodontitis (Fig. 6–19).

Symptomatic Apical Periodontitis. Apical periodontitis may begin with an acute phase.

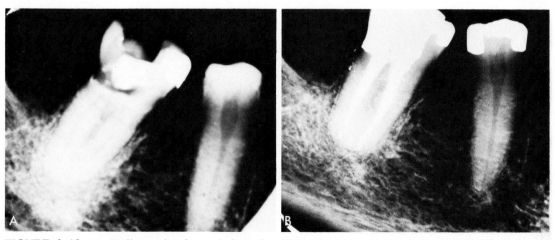

FIGURE 6–19 *A,* Radiograph of nonvital tooth with periapical radiopaque area. *B,* Radiopacity has disappeared 1 year after endodontic treatment, indicating healing of condensing apical periodontitis.

In these instances there is no radiographic evidence of inflammation, and the diagnosis is based on clinical findings and symptoms such as spontaneous pain, negative sensitivity, necrotic pulp, and tenderness to percussion. However, in the great majority of instances, a symptomatic apical periodontitis is an exacerbation of an already existing chronic inflammation. The symptoms are the same: spontaneous pain, tenderness to percussion, apical tenderness, and possible swelling. However, in these instances the diagnosis can be verified radiographically.

The most important etiologic factors for a symptomatic apical periodontitis are:

I. Increase in the amount of inflammation-provoking agents
   a. increase in the number of microorganisms
   b. increase in the virulence of the microorganisms
   c. increased tissue breakdown in the root canal
II. Lowered resistance of the individual
III. Iatrogenic factors
   a. poor root canal work (infected and necrotic material brought into the periapical tissue)
   b. overinstrumentation
   c. unsuitable medicaments
   d. excess of root-filling material

During the acute symptomatic phase of periapical inflammation, the cell picture is dominated by granulocytes. Proteolytic enzymes from these and other cells cause a breakdown of collagen, cells, and ground substance in the area. The result is pus accumulation and abscess formation. Sooner or later the abscess will drain, normally by resorbing the bone over the abscess. With time, the periosteum will also be broken through so that the abscess assumes a subcutaneous or submucous position. Gradually a fistula is formed, and the pus breaks through to a surface. The direction of the breakthrough of the abscess is generally determined by the shortest route but is influenced by the anatomy of the area. Most commonly the drainage occurs buccally in the vestibule. In the maxilla, palatal drainage may occur from the lateral incisors and from the palatal roots of the molars. Abscesses from maxillary teeth may also empty into the sinus and the nose. A spread to the brain is also possible, and it is estimated that about 10 per cent of the brain abscesses that are diagnosed are of dental origin.

Buccal drainage of an abscess is also most common in the mandible. However, lingual drainage from the molars occurs, usually under the mylohyoid muscle. Lingual drainage is a serious condition, and cooperation with a specialist should be considered, as these abscesses may continue to spread into the throat, resulting in life-threatening complications. Abscesses from incisors or molars may also break through extraorally on the chin and beneath the mandible.

MANAGEMENT OF THE ENDODONTIC PATIENT

Endodontic Diagnostic Methods

Chapters on diagnosis in endodontic textbooks generally have placed great emphasis

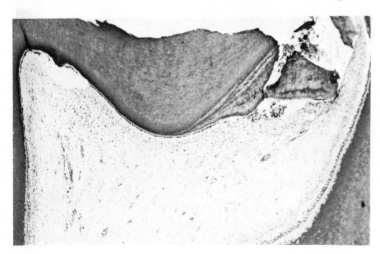

FIGURE 6–20 Paraffin section of human tooth. Pulp was exposed during excavation of caries and is virtually free of inflammation. Patient had no symptoms.

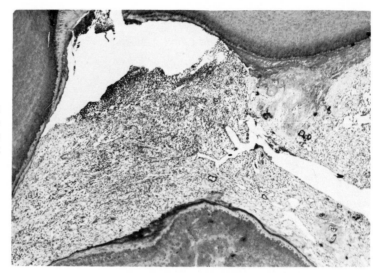

FIGURE 6–21 Paraffin section of human tooth. Pulp was exposed during excavation of caries and is severely inflamed. Patient had no symptoms.

on symptoms and their relationship to pulpal or periapical tissue damage. Histopathologic and clinical nomenclatures have therefore been combined, resulting in a number of confusing and erroneous descriptions and diagnoses. The diagnosis of *acute serous pulpitis*, for example, traditionally has meant that the patient has pain (acute), that the pulp is inflamed (pulpitis), but that as yet no abscesses have formed in the pulp (serous). Clinically it has been assumed that this condition is present when a tooth is especially sensitive to cold and reacts sooner to electrical stimulation than does a control tooth.

A great number of studies, from the classic ones by Thoma in 1928 and Greth in 1933 until today, have shown that these assumptions are incorrect in about 80 per cent of the cases. The only way to determine if the clinical diagnosis really mirrored the actual state of the pulp would have been to extract the tooth and make a histologic examination. Thus, it is impossible to determine the type and severity of possible pulp damage on the basis of clinical symptoms (Figs. 6–20 and 6–21). On the contrary, it is well known that pulpal inflammation, in most instances, develops without symptoms. Furthermore, the pulp necrotizes and apical periodontitis develops without the patient's even knowing about it. *The first condition for becoming a good diagnostician, therefore, is to accept that symptomatology usually plays only a minor role in making a clinical diagnosis.*

In order to reach as correct a clinical diagnosis as possible it is necessary to have extensive knowledge about (1) the etiology of pulpal and periapical inflammation; (2) the pathogenesis of pulpal and periapical inflammation; (3) the symptomatology of pulpal and periapical inflammation; and (4) other diseases in teeth, jaws, and adjacent tissues. Extensive knowledge of the etiology of a disease is necessary to be able to evaluate the clinical findings that are made. For example, based on our knowledge about the causes of pulpal inflammation, it is possible to reach the conclusion that if a patient arrives with a coronal fracture and an exposed pulp within a half-hour after an accident, the pulp will not be inflamed, regardless of the presence or absence of pain. It is equally definite that if the patient arrives 1 week after the pulp was exposed, the pulp is inflamed (or even necrotic), regardless of whether symptoms are present. In these instances we arrive at different clinical diagnoses and choose radically different therapy (pulp capping in the first instance, pulpectomy or root canal treatment in the second) without letting the presence or absence of symptoms influence us at all.

However, symptoms are sometimes the only reason that pulpal or periapical pathoses are discovered, and it is important to understand what different symptoms and reactions may mean. This understanding is especially important when it is difficult to localize an aching tooth; it may be possible, with certain examination methods, to get the involved tooth to react differently from its neighboring teeth and thereby arrive at the correct clinical diagnosis.

The Symptomatology of Pulpitis

As has already been stated, an inflamed pulp usually does not present symptoms, but pain is the most common symptom when symptoms do occur. Pain (toothache) may be a sign of tissue damage in the pulp, and in patients who have strong persistent pain, severe, irreversible inflammatory changes can be suspected. However, in this connection, it must not be forgotten that a pulp completely free of inflammation also may give cause for severe pain. For example, application of something sour or sweet to an exposed dentin surface may provoke severe pain: if a piece of chocolate remains in a carious lesion, the pain may persist for a considerable time. There are many examples of teeth without inflammation that have been extracted for this reason.

Patients may characterize pulpal pain as sharp, heavy, intermittent, continuous, pulsating, diffuse, or grinding; in other words, pulpal pain may be felt in many different ways. As mentioned above, many attempts have been made to relate the type of pain to the degree of tissue damage in the pulp, but without much success. Perhaps it may be said that severe, irreversible pulp damage should be suspected when a patient has heavy, continuous pain. The intensity and the duration of the pain are therefore factors that should be clarified during the examination of the patient.

It may also be important to determine the duration of the pain after tests with thermal stimuli or other stimuli (sour, sweet) that change the osmotic balance. If the pain disappears quickly after the cessation of the stimulation, the pulp may be inflamed, but it may also have been a hypersensitive reaction because of an exposed dentin surface or a similar condition. On the other hand, if the pain persists for some time after the stimulation, there would be more reason to suspect pulp damage. But it should be remembered that there is no way to determine the severity of the inflammation.

It may also be of diagnostic value to know if the pain appears spontaneously, i.e., without external stimuli. In order to reach an opinion about this it is advisable to ask the patient if he or she has been awakened by pain during the night. Spontaneous pain normally indicates serious pulp damage. Anamnestic information about repeated attacks of pain over a long period of time will also give reason to suspect serious pulp damage. Thus, when pulpal pain is used as a clinical-diagnostic aid, there are four factors that are especially important: (1) the intensity of the pain; (2) its duration; (3) its spontaneity, and (4) its occurrence. Strong, long-lasting pulpal pain that has appeared repeatedly at night over a period of time is therefore a rather definite indication of pulp inflammation. The symptoms should then be evaluated, together with other clinical findings, before the diagnosis is arrived at and the therapy determined.

The Symptomatology of Apical Periodontitis

Apical periodontitis is normally asymptomatic. The inflammation will start in the periodontal ligament and gradually lead to resorption of the hard tissues of the periodontium (especially alveolar bone, but also root cementum and dentin). The apical periodontitis can then be diagnosed radiographically.

The apical periodontitis may be acute, but more often it is an exacerbation of a chronic apical periodontitis, giving extensive and tangible symptoms. The most dramatic symptom is pain, which starts spontaneously, initially mildly, and gradually increases. The pain is continuous and, as a rule, is characterized as heavy and grinding. Especially during the first part of the process, it may be difficult or even impossible to differentiate between pulpal and periapical pain. The diagnosis must then be made based on other clinical findings, the first of these being whether the pulp is sensitive (vital or necrotic).

Tenderness of the tooth is often the patient's first complaint. The tooth feels high and tender to biting pressure or percussion because edema in the periapical tissue presses the tooth upward out of the socket. The edema may also cause abnormal mobility of the tooth.

Tenderness of the alveolar process over the apical area of the tooth is another characteristic finding during symptomatic apical periodontitis, but usually this symptom appears somewhat later. Apical tenderness is diagnosed by means of palpation. Here it is important to differentiate between apical and marginal tenderness. However, this may be difficult or sometimes even impossible, and this finding may represent what is often referred to as a combined endo-perio lesion.

The lymph glands of the region may be swollen and tender. Edema and swelling may occur relatively early in the development of symptomatic apical periodontitis. Sometimes the inflammation may cause extensive purulent breakdown, and the swelling may take on "dramatic dimensions." It is important to know that the pain during acute and exacerbating chronic apical periodontitis is strong and intense as long as exudate and pus are enclosed in the periodontium or bone; the pain is perhaps at its very strongest when the abscess is located subperiosteally (owing to the rich innervation of the periosteum). After a while, the purulent exudate will break through the periosteum and become located submucosally. This breakthrough in most regions is recognized by a dramatic relief of pain. The patient now will visit the dentist because of the swelling and not so much because of the pain. Finally, the exudate will break through to a surface and a fistula will form.

This description of apical periodontitis presents an overview of the process and its symptomatology. In the clinic, wide varieties of symptoms and combinations of symptoms will be seen. Frequently, the local symptoms are combined with general symptoms of illness, and a fever up to 102° to 104°F (39° to 40°C) is not uncommon.

Clinical Diagnosis

A simple and practical system of clinical diagnosis in endodontics follows.

Healthy Pulp. The pulp is vital and free of inflammation. This diagnosis is used, for example, during the first hours after a traumatic exposure of the pulp or when endodontic treatment of an intact tooth is indicated, perhaps for prosthetic reasons.

Pulpitis. The pulp is vital and inflamed. It is not possible to determine the degree of damage in an inflamed pulp based on symptoms or clinical examination methods. This can be done only by histologic techniques. Although it normally has no bearing on the choice of therapy, it can be of value to know if the patient had or did not have symptoms when the treatment was started. It is therefore practical to have two clinical diagnoses for the inflamed pulp.

Symptomatic Pulpitis. The pulp is vital and inflamed, and the patient has symptoms of pulpitis (pain, tenderness to percussion).

While symptomatic pulpitis can be acute, it is normally an exacerbation of a chronic inflammation. The diagnosis is made on the basis of clinical findings and knowledge of the causes and symptoms of pulpal inflammation and the reaction pattern of the pulp.

Asymptomatic Pulpitis. The pulp is vital and inflamed, but the patient has no symptoms. The diagnosis is made on the basis of clinical findings and knowledge of the causes of pulpal inflammation and the reaction pattern of the pulp.

Necrotic Pulp. This condition may be suspected when there is a negative reaction to sensitivity tests, but the diagnosis can be made with certainty only after inspection of the pulp tissue in the root canal. The pulp necrosis can be partial or total, which can be of significance for the selection of therapy, since in teeth with partial necrosis, performance of a pulpectomy should be considered.

Apical Periodontitis. Apical periodontitis is a pulp-related inflammation in the periapical area. The inflammation can be limited to the periodontal ligament, but normally the alveolar bone and often root cementum and dentin are also involved (resorption).

Symptomatic Apical Periodontitis. The apical periodontitis has started with an acute phase, or there is an exacerbation of a chronic inflammation. The diagnosis is based on clinical findings and symptoms (pain, tenderness to percussion, apical tenderness). Radiographic changes are usually present.

Asymptomatic Apical Periodontitis. The apical periodontitis has developed chronically without symptoms. The condition can be suspected when the pulp is necrotic, but the diagnosis can be made only after radiographic examination. The radiograph shows a radiolucent (in rare instances, radiopaque) area at the apex of the tooth. This is by far the most frequently occurring form of apical periodontitis.

Apical Periodontitis With Abscess. The inflammation has caused a "breakthrough" of the bone with abscess formation subperiosteally or submucosally (subcutaneously).

Apical Periodontitis With Fistula. The inflammation has caused the formation of a fistula.

Radicular Cyst. A cyst (a liquid-filled, epithelium-lined cavity) may be formed in connection with an apical periodontitis. A cyst grows expansively and therefore can be suspected when there is root deviation or thickening of the alveolar process. However, a definite diagnosis can be made only with histologic techniques.

Clinical Examination

A thorough clinical examination is necessary in order to arrive at a correct clinical diagnosis. The following aspects should be considered:
1. History
    a. Medical history
    b. Dental history
2. Visual examination
    a. Inspection
    b. Mirror and explorer examination
3. Palpation and percussion
4. Special diagnostic methods
    a. Radiographic examination
    b. Sensitivity tests

History

The history is an important part of the clinical examination. In the history, one may obtain information that gives the clinical diagnosis almost immediately. The medical history can normally be short and summary, but it is necessary to form a picture of the general health condition of the patient before treatment is started. (For a detailed discussion of this topic, see the chapter on oral medicine.) The following questions must be included in even a minimal medical history: Do you have heart problems? Are you allergic or hypersensitive to any substance? Are you diabetic? Do you have or have you had hepatitis? Are you taking any medication now? The dental history should clearly identify the reasons the patient is seeking dental care (chief complaint). The patient should be allowed to describe these reasons in his or her own words. Afterwards, the necessary leading questions may be asked.

Visual Examination

The visual examination starts with inspection of the area the patient has referred to in the history. This examination is then extended to adjacent and contralateral areas. One quick glance may be enough to make the diagnosis and to decide on the appropriate therapy. For example, it may be obvious that a tooth is so damaged by caries that the only possible therapy will be extraction. At other times, visual findings (caries, discolor-ations, swellings, or fistulae) are made that may lead to other considerations. The visual examination then continues with the aid of instruments (mirror, explorer, periodontal probe, or fiberoptics).

Palpation

Palpation is performed to ascertain tenderness, swelling, fluctuation, and crepitation in the underlying tissues. Here again it is important to make comparative contralateral examinations.

The percussion test is important in determining if the apical periodontium is inflamed. Also, with this test the response from the suspected tooth can be compared with the response of other teeth. Clinically healthy teeth may be a little sensitive to percussion, and if apical periodontitis is suspected, it is important to try to "fool" the patient by testing different teeth repeatedly without any special order. An exacerbating marginal periodontitis may also render teeth sensitive to percussion in a horizontal direction (perpendicular to the long axis of the tooth), whereas a tooth with apical periodontitis normally reacts to percussion only in a vertical direction (parallel to the long axis of the tooth).

Special Diagnostic Methods

Radiographic Examination. Modern clinical diagnosis is almost inconceivable without radiographic examination, and the final diagnosis is often based on the radiologic find-

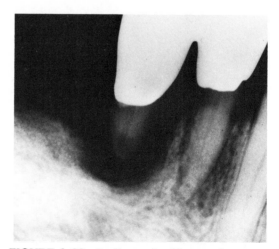

FIGURE 6–22   Radiograph of human lower premolar with periradicular radiolucency. After surgery, microscopic examination gave the diagnosis of fibroma.

ings. Note, therefore, that radiologic findings are not pathognomonic of a special disease or condition. A radiolucent area at the apex of a tooth is normally a sign of apical periodontitis but may also be indicative of a radicular cyst or another form of cyst, a cementoma, a giant cell granuloma, cancer metastasis, and several other pathologic and even normal conditions (Fig. 6–22). The radiologic findings must therefore be evaluated together with the findings from the clinical examination.

Sensitivity Tests. During the clinical examination it is not always easy to determine the vitality of the tooth. Several different sensitivity tests may be beneficial in arriving at the appropriate diagnosis. Normally, thermal (heat, cold) or electrical stimulation of the tooth is used. The response received should be compared with the response from neighboring teeth, the contralateral tooth, or both. These test methods, however, are not always reliable, and, as with the radiographic examination, the results of sensitivity tests must be evaluated together with other findings and symptoms.

Oral and Perioral Pain

The advanced toothache is often described as the most intolerable of all pain. Therefore, it becomes important for the dentist to be able to help patients with toothaches. It is also quite clear that patients who receive adequate treatment in an acute situation trust their dentist.

Pain is a subjective experience; although the transfer of pain impulses occurs in the same way in all individuals, the reaction to pain is individual and depends on psychologic phenomena. This fact makes it difficult to perform an objective examination of the physiology of pain.

A variety of pain conditions can be diagnosed in the oral and perioral regions. The pain may be caused by different factors. A practical division of these factors is: (1) regional pain, (2) neurologic pain, (3) atypical facial pain, and (4) referred pain.

Regional Pain

Regional pain encompasses pain from teeth and jaws, i.e., pain that is related to the anatomic structures of the area. Most important is pain from the pulp, the periodontium, the alveolar bone, the sinuses, and the temporomandibular joint.

Pulpalgia, or pulpal pain, is normally the most common form of pain for which a patient sees a dentist. The pain may vary in intensity, and the patient's reaction to the pain may also vary.

The first painful reaction of the pulp is referred to as hyperreactivity or hypersensitivity of the tooth. This condition is characterized by sharp but quickly disappearing pain. It is important that hyperreactive pain not be ignored. A thorough examination is indicated, as this pain (for example, in a carious tooth) may often be the first sign that serious pulp damage is developing.

Hyperreactivity of a tooth is often caused by exposure of dentin by abrasion, erosion, or root planing. The pain attack is normally set off by cold (cold drinks or ice cream) but also by heat, sweets, or probing of the exposed dentin with an instrument.

Pulpal pain of this type may also occur in teeth with incomplete crown fractures and with cracks in the dentin. When the fragments are not separated, such cracks can be very difficult to diagnose. The incomplete cusp fracture should be mentioned in this connection; it causes pain during chewing but otherwise gives no symptoms. Normally the patient can tell which tooth hurts, and by exerting selective pressure on the various cusps, the dentist usually arrives at a correct diagnosis. Transillumination of the tooth (fiberoptics) may also give valuable information about fracture lines.

Traumatic occlusion may also be the cause of pulpal hyperreactivity. The patient knows which tooth hurts, and often the presence of occlusal facets as well as other observations aids in reaching the correct diagnosis.

Typically, in the well-developed pulpalgia the patient cannot identify the painful tooth. The side of the face can always be indicated by the patient, whereas he often will not know if the pain is coming from the upper or the lower jaw. The pain is intense and the patient is often upset and difficult to deal with. It is important in these instances, therefore, to be careful to examine the patient thoroughly so that an erroneous diagnosis is not made by accepting the patient's description of the symptoms.

Pain from the apical periodontium as a result of apical periodontitis is of a somewhat different character from pulpalgia. In these instances the patient can localize the pain, and because the offending tooth always reacts to percussion, it is easy for the dentist to identify the tooth that is causing the pain. If purulent drainage occurs, the pain will normally cease instantly.

The nonpurulent exacerbation is not so common but is in many ways more troublesome. Here the development is not as dramatic, since no swelling or abscess formation can be seen, but the pain is continuous and can become intolerable. The cause (usually neuritis due to overinstrumentation or toxic medicaments or both) may be difficult to attack, and usually it will be necessary to resort to a moderate analgesic therapy.

Periodontal disease can give symptoms of pain that, from a differential diagnostic point of view, can present problems. The cause of the pain in these instances is most often a periodontal abscess. Note, therefore, that the swelling due to a periodontal abscess normally is well localized and not as widespread in the tissue as an abscess that arises from the apical periodontium.

Pericoronitis is an inflammatory condition that occurs most often in the third molar region in the lower jaw. The pain may be intense and is often accompanied by trismus.

Sinusitis, especially maxillary sinusitis, is probably the most common extraoral cause for pain in patients seeing a dentist. The patient normally complains about toothache in several or all teeth that have roots in contact with the sinus floor. The pain is constant, often relatively mild, but irritating. The patient may indicate that the teeth are too long, and pain occurs when biting together. The teeth may be sensitive to percussion and hypersensitive to cold. Sometimes it may be difficult to differentiate between pain from a sinusitis and pulpal pain. It is then important to remember that, almost without exception, in patients with sinusitis several adjacent teeth are involved. In addition, there are often extraoral symptoms such as tenderness in the bone above the sinus, increased pain when leaning forward quickly, and frontal headache.

Temporomandibular joint dysfunction syndrome also produces pain of a regional nature. The specific symptoms of this condition will not be discussed here. However, patients with temporomandibular joint (TMJ) problems will sometimes claim that the pain they are experiencing is coming from the teeth. TMJ-caused pain is always localized in the upper jaw. It is not as intense as advanced pulpalgia or pain from periapical inflammation but has a chronic, long-standing character and is therefore rather irritating.

Neurologic Pain

Patients with pain of neurologic origin do not normally see a dentist, and therefore the various conditions may be difficult to recognize. The most important conditions included in this group are trigeminal neuralgia, trigeminal neuritis, and herpes zoster neuritis.

Trigeminal neuralgia is quite different from the pain conditions referred to earlier, as it derives from intracranial changes. The changes are found primarily in the root and nucleus of the trigeminal nerve but possibly also in the semilunar ganglion. The pain is often felt in the jaws, generally in the maxillary jaw. Patients with trigeminal neuralgia may see a dentist because the pain sometimes appears to be localized in one tooth or several teeth, or because the pain can be released by touching the mucous membrane in the vicinity of the teeth ("trigger zone"). The pain attacks have a duration ranging from 10 seconds to a maximum of 2 to 3 minutes. The pain reaches maximal intensity instantly and decreases after 20 to 30 seconds. After an attack, there is a period that is free from pain. During this period, a new pain attack cannot be released (refractory period). This phenomenon is an important differential diagnostic criterion and quite characteristic for the condition. Patients who are suspected to suffer from trigeminal neuralgia should be referred to a neurologist.

Trigeminal neuritis is characterized by constant pain of relatively low intensity. It seldom encompasses all three trigeminal lines. If trigeminal neuritis is suspected, a thorough examination of the teeth and jaws must be carried out in order to exclude dental causes for the pain. If no dental cause is found, endodontic treatment or extractions will not help the patient. The patient should be referred to a neurologist.

Herpes zoster neuritis can be considered as a variant of trigeminal neuritis. It is considered to arise from an infection of herpes zoster virus in the semilunar ganglion and may cause severe pain in the trigeminal area in one half of the face. Sometimes the patient seems to localize the pain to certain teeth. Occasionally it is possible to find herpes blisters in the mouth and therefore make the correct diagnosis relatively easily. However, most often the blisters are localized in such a manner that they are not seen. Herpes zoster neuritis is difficult to treat, and the infection usually must be allowed to run its course until resolution takes place.

Intracranial tumors may cause long periods of pain without clinically visible etiologic factors.

In summary, in those instances in which it is not possible to find a dental reason for long-term pain, the patients should be referred to a neurologist.

Atypical Facial Pain

Atypical facial pain encompasses a large number of conditions of which the dentist cannot be expected to have detailed knowledge.

Psychogenic pain projected to the teeth and jaws is seen in patients suffering from atypical facial pain. This condition is observed in patients of all ages, but predominantly in adult women.

Hidden psychologic problems often will manifest themselves after a dental operation or a conversation with the dentist because of suspicion that something had been done wrong or had been planned incorrectly. Although there is no organic reason for the pain, it is real enough for the disturbed patient. The pain can be of any kind, but usually it has a constant character. Stimulation of teeth with cold or heat should not result in mentionable variation in the intensity of the pain. The distribution of the pain is important to notice. An organically related pain never crosses the midline of the face, whereas psychogenic pain is independent of all anatomic considerations.

Unfortunately, it may be difficult to get a reliable history from patients with psychogenic pain because they are often well experienced in presenting their "story of suffering." In addition, if they have seen other dentists with their problems, they may be quite familiar with the language of the dental profession and with examination methods. In these instances it is important to recognize the patient's "story" and not initiate irreversible therapy. Ideally, these patients should be referred to a psychiatrist, but this referral may not be easy, as patients of this type usually do not want psychiatric treatment. At times, the solution is referral to a neurologist. The dentist should realize that

these patients have problems and should be helped to whatever degree is possible.

Certain forms of migraine can give pain projections that cover part of the face and therefore can be suspected to be of dental origin. However, the history usually gives information that points to the correct etiology. The pain begins suddenly and lasts for a few hours. As a rule, the patients will not be able to see a dentist until the pain attack is over.

Referred Pain

In some instances pain may be localized in an area from which it does not originate. This is called referred pain. There are many such projection areas in the mouth and the face. The best-known example is pain originating in the mandibular molars and referred to an ear. It is assumed that the mechanism for referred pain is an overflow of stimuli to adjacent nerve fibers, giving the illusion of pain at the referred site.

Summary

As can be seen from this discussion, the reasons for oral and perioral pain are many. Still, dental conditions are the most frequently occurring etiologic factors, and this makes it easier for the dentist to arrive at the correct diagnosis. Obviously, it is important to know about the more atypical causes for pain so that erroneous diagnoses and inappropriate treatment can be avoided. Irreversible treatment, such as extraction or pulpectomy, should never be initiated until the diagnosis is definite. In today's well-developed health care delivery system there are rich possibilities for consultation with specialists when one's own knowledge is insufficient, and these possibilities should be used.

PRINCIPLES OF ENDODONTIC THERAPY

Treatment of Teeth With Vital Pulp

Preventive Endodontics

A close relationship exists between the dentin and the dental pulp. In teeth with hard tissue damage involving the dentin, it must be assumed that the pulp has been influenced through the dentinal tubules and is inflamed. However, it has been shown experimentally that local inflammation in a nonexposed pulp is to a great extent reversible if the tooth is treated correctly. This means that restorative measures should be carried out as carefully as possible to avoid iatrogenic irritation during treatment. In addition, methods and materials should be used that assist and accelerate the repair process in the inflamed pulp. Thus, a preventive endodontic philosophy should pervade all restorative therapy.

Cavity and Crown Preparation. Modern, ultra-speed equipment has facilitated the daily work of the dentist, but incorrect use of the equipment can easily lead to irreversible pulp damage. Ample evidence of pulp damage resulting from crown and bridge procedures is readily available. During the 1950s, when the high-speed handpiece became available, it was not fully known how important it was to flush the cavity with water during preparation. The new equipment was often used without a water spray, and the results were catastrophic in many instances. Severe internal dentin resorption in both crowns and roots occurred, with the teeth completely destroyed within 2 to 5 years when the resorptive processes were not diagnosed and stopped by endodontic treatment. However, with the use of an adequate water spray, ultra-speed equipment can be safely used (as in Fig. 6–13). It should be remembered that cold air cannot be substituted for water. The primary problem is not a heat increase in the pulp that must be prevented but dehydration of the dentin resulting in fluid flow from the pulp to the cavity through the dentinal tubules. The use of a water spray is the only effective method to prevent this dehydration, and a water spray should also be used with conventional cutting equipment. Only at 3000 rpm or lower should a bur be used in a dry cavity. This may be useful during excavation of soft caries in deep cavities.

Cavity Cleansing. Before a cavity is filled or a crown cemented, the dentin surface should be thoroughly cleansed. An effective and biologically acceptable way to do this is with water or, as is normally done in practice, with a spray of water and air. In other words, the goal is not to disinfect the dentin but to clean it well. The surface of the den-

tin can then be dried (not dehydrated) with short blasts of air and the use of cotton pellets.

Cavity Protection. There are two purposes for applying a base material to a cavity floor. The first purpose is to protect the pulp from any harmful components in a filling material and from marginal leakage. The second purpose is to influence the repair processes in the pulp in a beneficial way.

There are essentially two types of materials available for cavity protection today; zinc oxide–eugenol cement and calcium hydroxide. Most commercially available preparations rely on one of these two types of materials.

Zinc oxide–eugenol paste provides a bacteria-tight seal of the cavity. It has a good local-sedative effect, a definite antibacterial effect, and probably an anti-inflammatory effect. It is well suited for protection of the pulp in teeth with deep cavities and for cementation of temporary crowns. When used for the latter purpose, it should be remembered that the setting reaction of zinc oxide and eugenol is hydrophobic, and that the material therefore should be applied on a wet tooth in order to avoid fluid movement from the pulp resulting in hypersensitivity of the tooth. The use of zinc oxide and eugenol is contraindicated under all resin materials because eugenol interferes with the polymerization of the resin. Because of this interference, only calcium hydroxide or an acceptable commercially available calcium hydroxide cement should be used under resin fillings.

Calcium hydroxide is well tolerated by the pulp (Fig. 6–13). It does not have the sedative effect of zinc oxide and eugenol but has a good antibacterial effect, probably an anti-inflammatory effect, and has been shown to block the dentinal tubules quite effectively. Calcium hydroxide can be used under all types of filling materials.

The base material should protect the pulp against irritation from the filling material and prevent leakage between the restoration and the cavity walls. Occasionally the question arises as to the relative importance of the toxicity of the filling material and the effect of marginal leakage on the development of pulp damage beneath a restoration. It should be emphasized that silicate cement and many resin-based materials are tissue irritants and should not be used without a base material.

The importance of marginal leakage and the effect on the pulp of plaque and microorganisms in the gap between a restoration and the cavity walls are less well understood at present. For example, an amalgam restoration does not seal a cavity any better after 1 week than does a methyl methacrylate resin filling. Still, under the amalgam restoration no reaction (or a negligible one) will be observed in the pulp, whereas under the resin restoration a severe inflammatory reaction can usually be seen, often with abscess formation. Nonetheless, marginal leakage undoubtedly presents a problem in operative dentistry and should not be ignored. There is always the risk that plaque and saliva components and microorganisms and their toxins may reach the pulp through a gap between filling and tooth. But of even greater importance, the gap constitutes a definite risk for the development of secondary caries.

Marginal leakage cannot be prevented in connection with silicate cement fillings. However, the fluoride content of this material has an anticaries effect so that secondary caries generally is not a problem when silicate cement is used. With resin restorations, secondary caries was a major problem until the acid-etch technique became available. By using this technique, however, the problems with marginal leakage with resin fillings largely have been overcome. With amalgam restorations, marginal leakage can be prevented to a great extent by applying a layer of varnish in the cavity before the amalgam is inserted (Fig. 6–23). Since amalgam is rather well tolerated by the pulp, the varnish also will provide adequate pulp protection in most instances.

Thus, biologically appropriate restorative treatment can be performed with simple, routine clinical methods. One has only to think in terms of pulp protection, and the number of patients with postoperative pain, iatrogenic pulpitis, and pulp necrosis will be reduced dramatically.

Pulp Capping

Treatment of the exposed pulp by means of pulp capping has a long history. It soon became apparent that pulp wounds have a tendency to heal poorly and that pulp necrosis generally developed as a result of the exposure. Thus, in the 1920s, the thesis developed that "the exposed pulp is a lost organ." Today, more than 50 years later, pulp capping can still be a doubtful treatment form. However, a large number of experimental studies have shown that pulp capping can have a success rate of 80 to 90 per cent if specific clinical criteria are fulfilled and the treatment is performed correctly. Therefore, an exposed pulp is not necessarily a lost organ.

For a pulp-capping procedure to be successful, the following factors are of decisive importance: (1) pulp diagnosis, (2) pulp-capping material, and (3) sealing of the pulp cavity during the repair phase.

Pulp Diagnosis
Inflammation-free Pulp. In order to obtain a successful pulp capping, it is essential that the pulp be free of inflammation. An exposed pulp free of inflammation can be found with certainty only when the exposure has occurred accidentally, usually as a result of trauma. The treatment must then be performed before the inflammatory process has been established in the exposed pulp, (i.e., within 24 hours after the exposure occurred). If the treatment is then properly done, the prognosis is good (80 to 90 per cent). Thus, it is of great importance that the patient be treated as quickly as possible after the pulp is exposed.

Inflamed Pulp. Accidental pulp exposures constitute only a small portion of the teeth with exposed pulp. More frequently

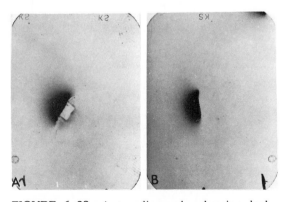

FIGURE 6–23 Autoradiographs showing leakage (Ca^{45}) around newly inserted Class V silver amalgam restoration *(A)* and prevention of leakage by application of varnish to the cavity before insertion of the amalgam filling *(B)*.

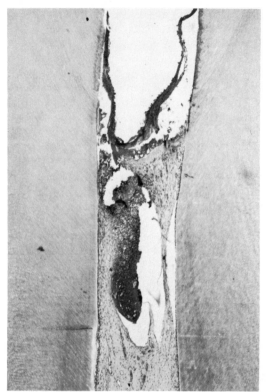

FIGURE 6–24 Paraffin section of monkey tooth with exposed, inflamed pulp. Pulp capping with calcium hydroxide; observation period, 30 days. Severe inflammation with abscess formation in the pulp.

the pulp is exposed during excavation of carious dentin. In these instances it must be assumed that the pulp is inflamed. If pulp capping is performed in such teeth, only a low success rate can be expected (20 to 40 per cent) (Figs. 6–24 and 6–25).

Capping Materials

The literature indicates that almost all possible materials and medications have been tried as pulp-capping agents. Gold and silver, different types of cements, antiseptic pastes, chemotherapeutics, ivory powder, dentin chips, plaster, magnesium oxide, calcium hydroxide, and many others have all been used. It is interesting to note that both biologically indifferent materials (gold and silver) and irritating antiseptic preparations are equally unsuitable as pulp capping agents.

The first important progress with this type of therapy was gained in the 1920s with a paste of zinc oxide and eugenol. At the beginning of the 1930s, good results were obtained by covering the pulp wound with dentin chips. But not until the later 1930s

when calcium hydroxide was introduced, was pulp capping really taken seriously. With calcium hydroxide, it became possible for the first time to obtain a hard tissue barrier (dentin bridge) covering the exposed area of the pulp and to find a healthy pulp, free of inflammation, under the dentin bridge on a routine basis.

Calcium hydroxide, $Ca(OH)_2$, is a white powder that can be mixed with physiologic saline to create a paste. The paste has a very high pH (approximately 12.5), and its application to the pulp wound results in necrosis of the pulp tissue in contact with the paste (Fig. 6–26). The necrotic area is sharply limited, and the adjacent vital pulp tissue normally shows little or no inflammation. In the transition zone between the necrotic and the vital tissue, a relatively structureless "demarcation zone" is observed after a few days. This zone is rich in collagen fibers and gradually becomes mineralized. Thus, the formation of a mineralized barrier between the necrotic and vital parts of the pulp begins. The first hard tissue formed contains no dentinal tubules, but after approximately 10

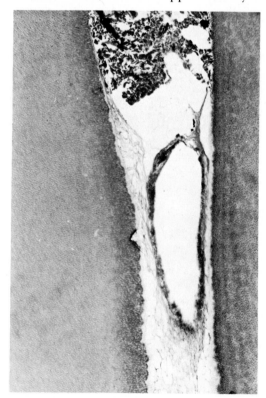

FIGURE 6–25 Paraffin section of monkey tooth with exposed, inflamed pulp. Pulp capping with calcium hydroxide. After 90 days the pulp is necrotic.

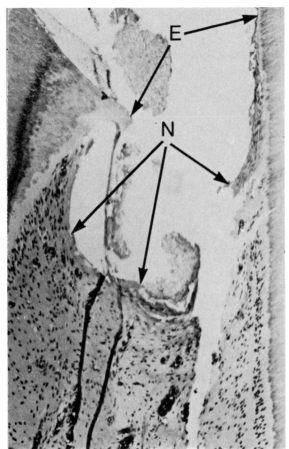

FIGURE 6–26 Paraffin section of monkey tooth with exposed, healthy pulp. Pulp capping with calcium hydroxide; observation period, 8 days. A well-delimited area of the pulp subjacent to the exposure site (E) has become necrotic (N). Only a few scattered inflammatory cells are present in the vital tissue next to the necrotic area.

days odontoblasts start differentiating from cells in the pulp and tubular dentin is formed onto the atubular mineralized tissue. The pulp is now protected by a dentin bridge and, in successful cases, will be vital and completely free of inflammation (Fig. 6–27).

In summary, the sequence of the healing process after capping of an inflammation-free pulp with calcium hydroxide is as follows. Local necrosis due to the application of calcium hydroxide develops in a limited area of the pulp, causing a mild inflammation in the adjacent vital pulp tissue. Thereafter, a mineralized barrier (dentin bridge) is formed at the transition zone between the vital and the necrotic areas of the pulp, and healing of the inflammation occurs.

This sequence represents a typical reaction to calcium hydroxide, but the reaction is not well understood. It is, for example, somewhat remarkable that the local necrosis does not spread to the rest of the pulp. Of course, in some instances (10 to 20 per cent) the treatment is not successful, and it must be pointed out that the dentin bridge formation in itself is not a criterion of pulpal repair. The pulp may become necrotic after the dentin bridge formation has started. When other materials, such as magnesium oxide, are used as pulp-capping agents, dentin bridge formation and subsequent pulp necrosis are seen routinely.

Sealing of the Pulp Cavity During the Repair Phase

In addition to the capping material and the condition of the pulp, it is of crucial im-

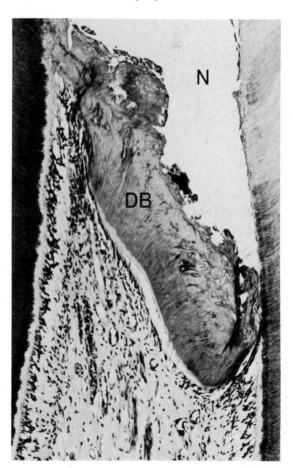

FIGURE 6–27 Paraffin section of monkey tooth with exposed, healthy pulp. Pulp capping with calcium hydroxide; observation period, 82 days. A dentin bridge (DB) has formed at the border zone between necrotic (N) and vital pulp tissue. The pulp is free of inflammation.

portance for successful treatment that the pulp cavity be sealed bacteria-tight until the dentin bridge is formed and the pulpal repair completed. If the pulp exposure occurs within a cavity, this is no great problem. The calcium hydroxide is applied to the pulp wound, and the cavity is filled with zinc oxide and eugenol, which gives a tight seal. However, if the pulp wound is located on a fractured dentin surface, it is more difficult to obtain a reliable seal. Calcium hydroxide can be applied to the wound and a temporary crown cemented with zinc oxide and eugenol. However, owing to unavoidable biting on the crown there is a great risk that leakage will occur.

The most reliable method for achieving the necessary seal is to prepare a small cavity in the area of the exposure. The cavity must be large enough to accommodate the application of calcium hydroxide on the wound surface as well as zinc oxide–eugenol paste on top of the calcium hydroxide to seal the cavity. Thereafter, a temporary crown can be applied, or, even better, the fractured surface can be covered with a hard-setting calcium hydroxide cement and a semipermanent composite-resin restoration using the acid-etch technique.

Other Factors

The size of the pulp exposure has been considered to be of importance for the prognosis of a pulp-capping procedure. In the literature it is stated that the exposure should be less than 1 mm^2 in order for the treatment to be successful. However, there is no experimental evidence to support this position. On the contrary, new findings have suggested that the size of the pulp wound is without importance for the prognosis if the pulp is free of inflammation and the treatment is carried out as described above.

The location of the pulp wound has also been considered to be important to the prognosis. Treatment of pulp wounds in the gingival third of the crown is considered by many to be contraindicated, since the tissue necrosis caused by the calcium hydroxide will be located in an area where, theoretically, the blood supply to the most coronal part of the pulp may be interrupted. However, newer findings have shown that this fear is unwarranted and that the prognosis for pulp capping in the cervical area of the tooth is just as good as that in the pulp horn, provided

that the pulp is free of inflammation and that the treatment is carried out correctly.

The age of the patient is another factor that has been considered to influence the potential success of pulp capping. In the literature it has often been stated that pulp capping is contraindicated in teeth of older patients because of poor vascularity of the pulp accompanying physiologic age changes. Since there is no scientific evidence to support this belief, it can only be assumed that the better vascularity in young teeth increases the possibilities for pulpal repair. Still, advanced age is not necessarily a contraindication to pulp capping.

Follow-up Examinations

Even with adherence to the narrow clinical indications described here (noninflamed pulp), a failure rate of 10 to 20 per cent will be observed after pulp capping; that is, the treatment will be unsuccessful in close to two out of ten teeth. Follow-up examinations should be performed 3, 6, and 12 months after the treatment and later once a year for 4 to 5 years. The control should consist of a clinical examination with a sensitivity test and radiographic examination with careful inspection for a pathologic narrowing (obliteration) of the root canal.

In summary, pulp capping is an elegant and successful treatment form, although one with rather narrow indications. An absolute prerequisite for the success of the treatment is that the pulp be free of inflammation. For this reason pulp capping is contraindicated when the pulp is exposed by caries. The main indication for pulp capping is in teeth with the pulp exposed by trauma. If capping of these teeth is performed before the inflammatory process has had a chance to establish itself in the exposed pulp, if calcium hydroxide is used as the capping material and if a bacteria-tight seal of the pulp cavity is maintained throughout the repair period, pulp capping can be expected to be successful in 80 to 90 per cent of the patients so treated.

Pulpotomy

Pulpotomy (or pulp amputation) involves partial removal of the pulp tissue. Normally, the coronal pulp is removed to the level of the orifice of the root canal, but in certain instances it can be advantageous to amputate

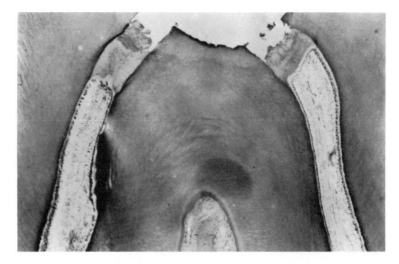

FIGURE 6–28 Paraffin section of monkey tooth. Pulpotomy with calcium hydroxide; observation period, 90 days. Dentin bridges have formed. Root pulps are free of inflammation.

the pulp even farther apically. Such a procedure is usually referred to as a high amputation. Pulpotomy developed as a logical consequence of the clinical experience that capping of teeth with inflamed pulp (carious exposures) is usually unsuccessful. The objective of the pulpotomy is the removal of the inflamed part of the pulp followed by the application of the wound dressing (calcium hydroxide) to pulp tissue free of inflammation. If this is achieved, the prognosis for pulpotomy is as good as for capping an exposed pulp free of inflammation (Fig. 6–28).

When pulpotomy is planned, the following factors should be considered: (1) the condition of the pulp, (2) asepsis, (3) wound dressing, and (4) sealing of the pulp chamber during the repair phase.

The Condition of the Pulp. The objectives of the pulpotomy are to remove all inflamed pulp tissue and to obtain repair with dentin bridge formation of the remaining uninflamed part of the pulp. The major problem with this procedure is the correct evaluation of the condition of the pulp. As we know, the degree of pulp damage cannot be determined, even after the most careful clinical examination. For that reason, inflamed tissue is frequently left in the root canal. If the wound dressing (calcium hydroxide) is then applied to the inflamed tissue, the pulpotomy will fail in the same manner as capping of an inflamed pulp fails. These diagnostic problems are well known among clinicians, and for this reason pulpotomy has never been fully accepted as a permanent form of therapy.

Asepsis. In teeth in which a pulpotomy is performed, the pulp usually has severe local damage, including inflamed areas and infected areas with necrotic tissue. After removal of carious dentin and possible fillings, a rubber dam should be applied and a thorough disinfection of the cavity and the wound surface performed. The coronal pulp is removed by means of a round bar or a sharp excavator, and the bleeding is controlled. The pulp chamber is then disinfected again, and the wound surface is lowered another ½ to 1 mm with the use of sterile instruments. Bleeding is controlled, and the wound dressing is applied.

The Wound Dressing. Historically, as in pulp capping, phenol preparations and other strong antiseptics were used routinely as wound dressings in pulpotomy treatment. However, since the late 1930s calcium hydroxide has been the dressing material of choice. The tissue reaction to calcium hydroxide in successful pulpotomies is the same as in pulp capping—development of a local necrosis subjacent to the paste, formation of a mineralized barrier (dentin bridge) between the necrotic and vital tissues, and healing of possible inflammation in the residual pulp (Fig. 6–28).

Sealing of the Root Canal. It is of crucial importance for the success of the treatment that the residual pulp, the pulp wound, and the wound dressing be protected against the oral environment during the repair phase. Contrary to what is often the case with pulp capping, maintenance of a seal does not present a problem during pulpotomy, since a temporary filling in these teeth can be retained easily in the cavity and the pulp chamber. A paste of zinc oxide and eugenol gives a bacteria-tight seal and is an excellent material for this purpose.

Indications. A number of studies have shown limited success (50 to 60 per cent) in determining when the tissue damage in the exposed pulp of a tooth is confined to the coronal pulp. Accordingly, the failure rate after pulpotomy is relatively high, and the treatment is not considered acceptable as permanent therapy. Nonetheless, pulpotomy has its place as a temporary or semipermanent treatment method in teeth in which the root development is incomplete and pulp capping is contraindicated because of diagnostic reasons. The purpose of performing a pulpotomy in these teeth is to retain as much of the pulp as possible until the root development is completed, since experience has shown that the development of the root can continue even if the pulp is chronically inflamed. However, because of diagnostic difficulties and the subsequent risk of late failures, pulpotomy should be followed routinely by pulpectomy and root filling as permanent treatment when the root development is completed.

Follow-up Examinations. Pulpotomized teeth should be followed clinically and radiologically after 3, 6, and 12 months and later once a year until a pulpectomy is performed. As the pulp is usually amputated apical to the gingival margin, a sensitivity test is of no value in these teeth. The clinical examination must therefore be limited to confirming that no signs of inflammation are present. From a radiologic point of view, the periodontal contour should be intact. Internal root resorption occurs relatively often in pulpotomized teeth and is a definite sign of inflammation in the residual pulp.

Formocresol Pulpotomy. Because experience has shown that inflammation has already reached the root pulp in many teeth considered for pulpotomy, efforts have been made to find methods to prevent the inflamed residual pulp from becoming necrotic. One approach has been to try to achieve an in vivo fixation of the tissue in the root. Formocresol, which contains formalin (the means of fixation) and various cresols (antiseptics), is the medication that has been used most often in this connection, especially in pedodontics. Clinically a success rate of 70 per cent has been reported at the

end of 3 years. Histologically, however, no repair of the pulp is seen. Chronic inflammation, internal root resorption, and, to a certain extent, apposition of hard tissue, are typical findings in these teeth, and with time their pulp becomes necrotic (Fig. 6–7). Nonetheless, necrosis, the unavoidable final result, can often be postponed by the application of formocresol to the tissue. Naturally, the formocresol pulpotomy is not a method to be used in permanent teeth, as repair of the pulp cannot be expected. *The formocresol method should be considered only as a possible last resort for maintaining primary teeth in the mouth for a limited period of time.*

Pulpectomy

Pulpectomy implies the removal of the vital pulp. This form of therapy has developed as a logical consequence of the high failure rate of pulp capping and pulpotomy in teeth with exposed, inflamed pulps.

During a pulpectomy, the pulp is severed near the apical foramen so that practically all inflamed tissue can be removed. Consequently, with pulpectomy the diagnostic problems that were unsolvable during a pulpotomy procedure do not exist. If the pulp stump that remains after pulpectomy should happen to be inflamed, it normally heals without complications because of its proximity to the periodontal ligament. In the treatment of the exposed inflamed pulp, therefore, pulpectomy is, by far, the treatment form that has the widest indications.

Amputation Level. Traditionally, *total pulpectomy,* in which the pulp tissue is removed to the periodontal ligament, has been contrasted to *partial pulpectomy,* in which the pulp is amputated within the root canal approximately 1 to 2 mm coronal to the radiographic apex. Today, it is generally accepted that partial pulpectomy has a better prognosis than total pulpectomy and is therefore the preferable treatment. For that reason, the controversy over total and partial pulpectomy has for the most part disappeared, and the term *pulpectomy,* which is identical in principle to partial pulpectomy, has been adopted.

In other words, it is important in a pulpectomy that the pulp wound be located within the root canal. Since, as a rule, the apical foramen is not located at the radiographic apex, and since it is usually not possible to decide exactly where the foramen is located, we have to be satisfied with the somewhat inexact rule that the pulp wound should be placed 1 to 2 mm coronal to the radiographic apex. With this rule in mind, and after careful study of the preoperative radiograph, it should be possible to determine the optimal level of instrumentation in each individual tooth.

By severing the pulp inside the root canal, the following advantages are achieved: (1) It is technically easier to achieve a clean wound by cutting off the pulp against the hard root canal walls. (2) A possible apical delta is left intact, and the tissue in the accessory canals will remain vital. (3) The periodontal ligament is not damaged.

Treatment Principles. The vital pulp tissue, although possibly inflamed, is sterile. Even if the pulp is exposed to the oral environment, only the superficial area of the tissue will be infected. Therefore, during pulpectomy, it is normally not a question of combating infection but of preventing contamination of the root canal during treatment. Special conditions will exist when the pulpitis has resulted in necrosis of the coronal part of the pulp. The necrotic tissue will be infected and must be removed first. The tooth and especially the pulp chamber must then be thoroughly disinfected before the vital pulp tissue is extirpated. It should be remembered that the front of infection is found at the transition between the necrotic and vital tissues.

The practical procedure advocated for pulpectomy treatment is as follows: First, a diagnosis of vital pulp must be ascertained. Anesthesia is given, and carious dentin is excavated; possible leaky fillings are removed, and cusp height is reduced. The coronal

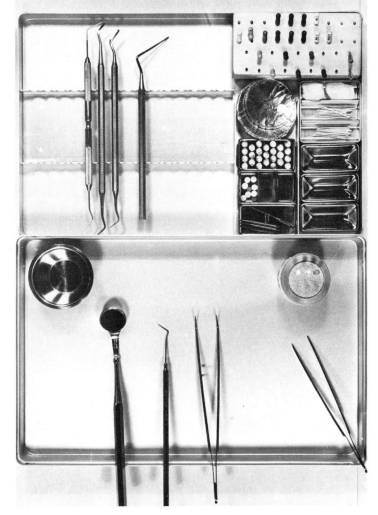

FIGURE 6–29 Endodontic tray with root canal instruments, hand instruments, paper points, cotton pellets, rubber stops, burs, and so on. Instruments in use are being placed in cover of the tray (sterile surfaced).

pulp is then removed, the canal orifices are located, and the access cavity is completed. This part of the treatment is not performed aseptically because it is difficult or even impossible to achieve asepsis as long as carious dentin and possible infected tissue in the coronal pulp are present.

When the coronal pulp has been removed, further treatment should be performed, without compromise, under aseptic conditions. Therefore, a rubber dam should be applied, and the field of operation (rubber dam, tooth, and especially the pulp chamber with the exposed pulp) should be thoroughly and conscientiously disinfected.

At this point the instruments are changed. The used, nonsterile instruments are removed, and a tray with sterile hand and root canal instruments is made available (Fig. 6–29). A tooth-length radiograph is taken with a thin, sterile instrument in the canal, and after careful measuring, the pulp tissue is removed to the optimal apical level by means of sterile instruments. The root canal is cleaned and instrumented with reamers and files under irrigation with sterile isotonic saline or a mild antiseptic solution, for example, 0.5 per cent sodium hypochlorite. The root canal is then filled permanently or temporarily (with calcium hydroxide) and a bacteria-tight temporary filling (zinc oxide and eugenol, Cavit) is applied before the rubber dam is removed from the tooth. After removal of the rubber dam, the temporary filling should be checked carefully before the patient is allowed to close the mouth.

Wound Treatment. In pulpectomy treatment, as well as in pulpotomy and pulp capping, there is a pulp wound that must be treated. Calcium hydroxide may also be used as the wound dressing in pulpectomies, resulting in the subsequent induction of a hard tissue barrier in the apical area of the pulp. However, it will take a considerably longer time for the barrier to form near the apex than in the coronal pulp, with a period of 3 to 6 months not unusual. In certain instances, especially in the treatment of teeth with incompletely formed roots, it is advantageous to delay the obturation of the canal until the apical hard tissue barrier has formed (Fig. 6–30). In the fully developed tooth, however, this waiting period is not necessary, and the canal can be filled as soon as the instrumentation is completed, preferably in the first sitting. In principle, the canal can be filled with any biocompatible material that gives a bacteria-tight seal and is not resorbed.

After the pulpectomy, healing takes place in the same manner as after implantation of an inert material in connective tissue elsewhere in the organism. A fiber-rich connective tissue capsule forms adjacent to the material, and the inflammation that always occurs in the apical area when the pulp is removed heals, usually within weeks.

Some claim that a pulpectomized tooth should not be obturated permanently in the first sitting, since the patient is anesthetized and cannot tell the dentist if the root-filling material is pushed into the vital tissue in the apical area. Overfilling of the canal and postoperative pain could easily result. These problems, however, can be avoided by using an exact and well-controlled endodontic technique (Figs. 6–47 and 6–48). First, a

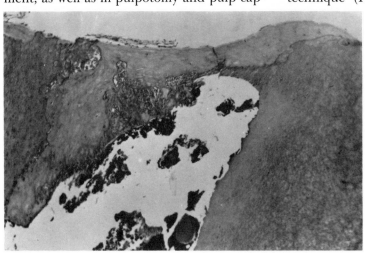

FIGURE 6–30 Paraffin section of nonvital human tooth with incomplete root formation. The root canal has been treated with calcium hydroxide for 6 months, and an apical hard-tissue barrier has formed.

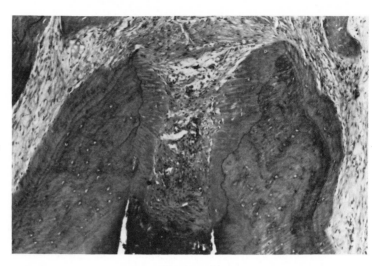

FIGURE 6–31 Paraffin section of monkey tooth. Pulpectomy; observation period, 95 days. An apical plug of dentin chips is seen in contact with the pulp stump, which is free of inflammation. (From Tronstad, L.: Tissue reactions following apical plugging of the root canal with dentin chips in monkey teeth subjected to pulpectomy. Oral Surg., *45*:297–304, 1978.)

shelf should be prepared in the root canal wall at the apical level of instrumentation. Second, the master point should be fitted in the canal as is a cork in a bottle and should reach the apical shelf of the canal. If the fit of the master point is developed properly, the canal can be obturated during anesthesia with very little risk of overfilling or other complications.

A safe and good solution to the problem of wound treatment in pulpectomized teeth is to make an apical plug of dentin chips after the instrumentation of the root canal has been completed. The plug of dentin chips is made by bringing the chips from the root canal wall in an apical direction and condensing them carefully against the apical shelf and the pulp stump. The dentin chips derive from the patient's own dentin and consequently are extremely well tolerated by soft tissue. Also, dentin chips have an ability to induce hard tissue formation. As a result of this formation, the dentin chips in the plug gradually become "cemented" together, and often a cementumlike tissue will be formed on the plug against the vital tissue in the pulp stump or in the periodontal ligament (Fig. 6–31). In this manner, a hard tissue closure of the root canal is obtained by means of a dentin chips plug similar to the closure after prolonged treatment with calcium hydroxide. The great advantage of the dentin chips plug, however, is that it permits the obturation of the root canal in the first sitting without risk of overfilling, even if techniques with soft or softened materials are used.

It should be mentioned that dentin chips may play an important part in periradicular healing after endodontic therapy, even if they are not used intentionally. Experimental findings have shown that during instrumentation of the root canal, dentin chips automatically are pushed into the pulpal ends of lateral and accessory canals. Hard tissue formation is induced, the pulpal openings of the canals are sealed off, and the peripheral connective tissue in the canals remains vital and healthy (Fig. 6–32).

Complications. During the course of treatment, observations may be made that are indicative of complications and therefore may lead to an alternative therapy. For example, in multirooted teeth with symptoms of pulpitis, the pulp tissue in one of the roots may be totally necrotic. The tooth should then be treated as a nonvital tooth. Similarly, in a single-rooted tooth, the tissue necrosis may have spread to the root pulp so that only the most apical part of the pulp is vital. In these teeth with partial pulp necrosis, it is often a question of weighing the possibilities of whether a pulpectomy and root canal obturation should be attempted in one sitting or whether the root canal infection should be dealt with in multiple visits. The rule to follow is, *If in doubt, consider the tooth as nonvital and treat accordingly.*

A common complication during pulpectomy treatment is that the pulp is not amputated within the root canal but is torn out apical to the intended level, usually in the periodontal ligament. Previously, this situation always led to a change in therapy. In these instances, the root canals were instrumented to the periodontal ligament and also

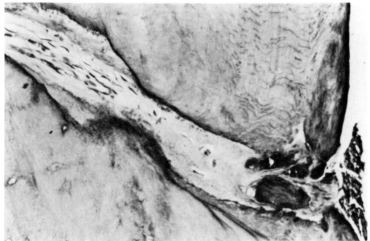

FIGURE 6–32 Paraffin section of monkey tooth. Pulpectomy; observation period, 95 days. The pulpal aspect of a lateral canal is filled with dentin chips, and hard tissue has formed on the chips. The tissue in the canal is free of inflammation. (From Tronstad, L.: Tissue reactions following apical plugging of the root canal with dentin chips in monkey teeth subjected to pulpectomy. Oral Surg., *45*:297–304, 1978.)

filled to this level (total pulpectomy). However, experimental and clinical-radiologic studies have shown that the prognosis is best if this mistake is just ignored. A shelf is prepared in the root canal wall at the optimal level decided before the extirpation was carried out, and the canal is filled to that level. The canal apical to the optimal level of obturation is not instrumented. Even if the pulp in this area has been torn out, there is normally some tissue left on the canal walls. It is important that this tissue not be disturbed further during the canal instrumentation, as it is of importance for the formation of new connective tissue in the blood clot that forms in the empty root canal space apical to the root filling. That the apical blood clot is organized to connective tissue has been shown in several studies, both in animals and in humans, and one author even claims that the new tissue is better vascularized and more resistant to irritation than the original pulp tissue.

Experiments have also been performed in which attempts were made to fill the empty apical part of the root canal with dentin chips when the pulp was totally extirpated accidentally. Here again, the instrumentation of the canal is carried out only to the optimal level of obturation. In the apical 1 to 2 mm, dentin chips are packed into the empty root canal space. Animal experiments have shown that a cementumlike tissue is formed onto the dentin chips against the vital tissue of the periodontal ligament, resulting in a "biologic" seal of the root canal (Fig. 6–33). In clinical-radiographic follow-up studies, good results have been achieved with this method.

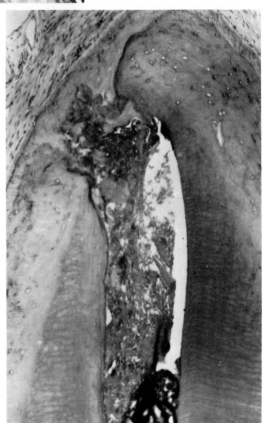

FIGURE 6–33 Paraffin section of monkey tooth. Pulpectomy; observation period, 95 days. The pulp tissue has inadvertently been removed to the apical foramen. A dentin chips plug has been made, and a cementumlike tissue has formed a deposit on the plug and has completely walled off the root canal. No periapical inflammation is seen. (From Tronstad, L.: Tissue reactions following apical plugging of the root canal with dentin chips in monkey teeth subjected to pulpectomy. Oral Surg., *45*:297–304, 1978.)

It is not yet clear if one or the other of these methods is preferable when the pulp has been totally extirpated accidentally. However, it is absolutely clear that if a total pulp extirpation does occur, the tooth should preferably be filled partially to a level 1 to 2 mm coronal to the radiographic apex.

When the anesthesia wears off, it is possible that a patient will experience discomfort after a pulpectomy, especially if the tooth was sensitive to percussion when the treatment started. Normally the discomfort is mild and will disappear within the first few hours after the treatment. Only occasionally does the pain last as much as a day or two. If necessary, analgesics should be used. It is important to know that pulpectomy with completion of the treatment in one visit does not cause additional postoperative pain in either frequency or intensity.

An unfortunate complication that occurs now and then is the loss of the temporary filling between visits. Naturally, the root canal then becomes infected and the tooth must be treated as a nonvital tooth.

Prognosis and Follow-up Examination. A number of studies from many countries, in which different techniques and root-filling materials were used, have shown that pulpectomy treatment has a very good prognosis. Furthermore, experimental and clinical-radiologic investigations have shown that the best results are achieved with this treatment when the root filling ends 1 to 2 mm coronal to the radiographic apex. A success rate of 90 to 95 per cent can be anticipated under these conditions.

However, unsuccessful cases do occur, and clinical-radiologic follow-up should take place once a year for 4 to 5 years. It is important to recognize that so-called temporary failures may occur after pulpectomy treatment. At the third-year control or earlier, however, a normal periodontal contour should be re-established.

Treatment of Nonvital Teeth

Necrotic Pulp

Pulp necrosis is suspected when a tooth does not react to thermal, electric, or mechanical stimulation, but a definite diagnosis cannot be established until inspection and probing of the pulp tissue have taken place. From a therapeutic point of view it is important to know that the necrotic pulp tissue is infected. In a tooth with a deep carious lesion or with an exposed pulp chamber, it is easily understandable that infection may be present. However, pulp necrosis also occurs in apparently intact teeth, and in such teeth the necrotic tissue is infected in close to 90 per cent of the cases. Thus, it must be assumed that any tooth with a necrotic pulp is infected and that treatment will involve the resolution of the infection.

The most important port of entry for the microorganisms to the necrotic pulp tissue appears to be exposed dentinal tubules (Figs. 6–34 and 6–35). The dentin may become exposed by caries, abrasion (tooth brushing), erosion, and the treatment of periodontal disease, in which the removal of root cementum exposes the dentinal tubules. In so-called intact teeth, (i.e., teeth without

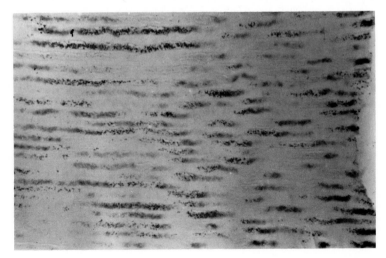

FIGURE 6–34 Paraffin section of nonvital human tooth with exposed dentin in cervical area. Microorganisms are seen in the dentinal tubules. (Brown and Brenn stain.)

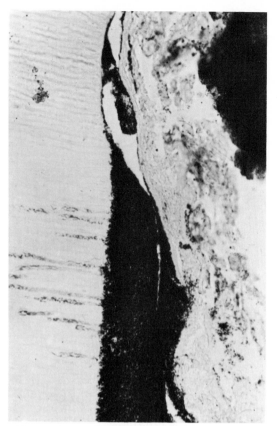

FIGURE 6–35 Paraffin section of nonvital tooth with exposed dentin in cervical area. Microorganisms are seen on the pulpal aspects of the dentinal tubules; a large colony is seen on the root canal wall. (Brown and Brenn stain.)

caries or fillings), it is normal to find exposed dentin surfaces, which may explain an infection of the necrotic pulp tissue. In addition, enamel-dentin cracks and, to a certain extent, enamel invaginations may be ports of entry to the pulp for microorganisms.

In this connection, it is important to realize that the necrosis of the pulp tissue occurs first and that the actual infection of the pulp is secondary. As long as the pulp is vital, microorganisms can be seen only superficially in the exposed dentin and in relatively few dentinal tubules. On the other hand, when the pulp has become necrotic (and notice that it may be a question of only a local necrosis in a small area of the pulp), nothing seems to prevent the microorganisms from passing through the tubules from an exposed dentin surface to the necrotic area of the pulp.

Another possible port of entry for microorganisms to the pulp is via the blood stream, the so-called hematogenous route. A bacteremia occurs easily and often (for example, after tooth brushing), but it has been shown that microorganisms that normally circulate in the blood stream are eliminated very quickly. However, they may become attached to damaged (necrotic) tissue. It is possible, therefore, that microorganisms circulating under favorable conditions may find possibilities for growth in necrotic pulp tissue.

Treatment Principles

The objectives of the treatment of teeth with pulpal necrosis are to remove necrotic tissue and tissue breakdown products from the root canal, eliminate infection, seal the root canal, and thereby establish a functioning tooth in periodontal tissue free of inflammation. The treatment may be divided into three main phases: (1) Chemomechanical instrumentation of the root canal, (2) Final disinfection of the root canal and creation of favorable conditions for periapical healing, and (3) Root canal obturation.

Chemomechanical Instrumentation. The mechanical instrumentation of the root canal supported by a chemically active irrigation solution has gained steadily in importance in the treatment of nonvital teeth. The root canal contains breakdown products from necrotic tissue and bacteria that are toxic and that may cause and maintain an inflammatory process. For this reason, it is of utmost importance that the canal be cleaned. During canal instrumentation, the necrotic tissue, with its colonies of microorganisms, is removed. Enlargement and shaping of the canal also remove possible colonies in the dentinal tubules, which, if present, are usually found close to the root canal wall. The instrumentation of the root canal is performed with reamers and files in the presence of an irrigation solution, thereby explaining the term *chemomechanical instrumentation*. Traditionally, it has been considered important that the irrigation solution be an effective antiseptic, to combat the infection in the root canal. Although the antibacterial effect is still considered advantageous today, it is probably much more important that the product have a good cleansing effect and be nonirritating to vital tissue.

One irrigation solution that fills these criteria quite well is 0.5 per cent sodium hypochlorite (Dakin's solution). Sodium hypochlorite has a good cleansing effect and, in an 0.5 per cent solution, is nonirritating yet still has a certain antibacterial effect. In addition, this product has a favorable action on the toxic proteins of the necrotic tissue, dissolving them into smaller nontoxic units. Necrotic tissue, breakdown products, blood clots, and pus are dissolved. This allows for good cleansing, even in crevices and lateral canals in which mechanical instrumentation has no effect. Since 0.5 per cent sodium hypochlorite has only a negligible effect on vital tissue, its use does not interfere with tissue repair processes.

Before the chemomechanical instrumentation is started, it is important that the exact length of the root canal be determined. Theoretically, the root canal should be instrumented to the apical foramen to ensure the removal of all necrotic tissue. However, in the treatment of nonvital teeth, as with vital teeth, it is usually not possible to determine the exact position of the apical foramen. Experimental results and clinical experience have taught us that the instrumentation should not be extended through the foramen, since this may lead to iatrogenic exacerbations, poorer repair conditions, and a compromised prognosis. Therefore, the practical rule to follow is to stop the mechanical instrumentation of the root canal 1 mm coronal to the radiographic apex. In this way the instrumentation should remain confined within the canal, and damage to the periapical tissues should be avoided.

If time allows, the chemomechanical instrumentation of the root canal should be concluded in the first visit. As a rule, however, the tooth with a necrotic pulp should not be filled at this sitting. The possibility that an exacerbation may develop after the instrumentation of the canal is always real, even if the procedure has been done carefully and correctly. Any exacerbation is normally easier to handle if the canal has not been obturated permanently. Furthermore, it is possible that the infection of the root canal system may not be completely overcome after the chemomechanical instrumentation. An antiseptic dressing in the canal for a period of time before the tooth is filled can complement the chemomechanical instrumentation and may result in eliminating the last remnants of the root canal flora.

Disinfection of Root Canal. In traditional endodontics much emphasis was placed on canal disinfection. Sophisticated disinfection methods such as diathermy and iontophoresis were advocated, and a large number of imaginative mixtures of various antiseptics were used. Today, it is known that medicaments that are effective against microorganisms also, as a rule, kill human cells and consequently cause tissue damage. The damage that may be caused by injudicious use of medicaments in the root canal can therefore greatly exceed the advantages that may be achieved with their use. Recognition of this fact led to attempts to find antiseptics that have the desired effect on the microorganisms of the root canal without causing unacceptable damage to the periapical tissues (selective toxicity). Iodine and chlorine preparations have shown the best results in these studies, and 2 per cent iodine in potassium iodide, 0.5 per cent sodium hypochlorite, and 5 per cent Chloramine-T are considered suitable medicaments in the treatment of nonvital teeth. Cresatin (metacresyl acetate) formocresol, and paramonochlorphenol are other medicaments used widely for this purpose. Although different antibiotics and sulfa preparations have also been used as intracanal medicaments with good results, their use is not recommended because of the danger of sensitizing the patient by local use of this type of medicament.

In modern endodontics, attempts have been made to find an intracanal dressing that not only disinfects the root canal but also exerts a direct favorable influence on the healing of the inflammation in the periapical area. Such a product is a paste of calcium hydroxide and isotonic saline. The use of calcium hydroxide in endodontics, as is so often the case in medicine and dentistry, developed empirically. The paste has a pH of 12.5 and has, consequently, a certain antibacterial effect. It also has an anti-inflammatory effect, as evidenced clinically by its ability to stop exudation. Although the modes of action of calcium hydroxide are largely not understood, the following factors may be of importance:

1. *pH (OH)$^-$*. Inflamed tissue has an acidic pH. Calcium hydroxide may cause a rise in the pH of a contacting inflamed area and thereby promote the repair processes. Calcium hydroxide may also have a direct influence on the acid hydrolases, enzymes with an optimal pH of 5.5 that are active in the breakdown of tissue during inflammation.

2. *Ca^{++}*. It has been reported that cal-

cium ions have a stimulating effect on certain alkaline phosphatases, enzymes connected with hard tissue formation. It is also claimed that calcium ions may have a favorable effect on the immune response.

3. *Antibacterial effect.* Calcium hydroxide has a good and, in contrast to traditional root canal antiseptics, a long-lasting antibacterial effect. Its long-lasting effect (weeks and months) makes calcium hydroxide especially well suited for root canal disinfection. A recent study found bacteria-free root canals in all teeth treated with this material.

4. *Denaturation of proteins.* Calcium hydroxide has a denaturing effect on proteins similar to that of sodium hypochlorite. Clinically, this may make it easier to obtain a clean root canal. It has also been shown that calcium hydroxide–treated tissue will be dissolved twice as fast in sodium hypochlorite as untreated tissue.

5. *"Obturation" of the root canal.* It seems that filling the root canal with a material with the consistency of calcium hydroxide is beneficial for the repair processes. A traditional antiseptic disappears from the root canal after a few hours or, at most, a few days. An exudate consisting of tissue fluid, dead cells, and possibly pus and blood will fill the canal. The exudate will be broken down and the breakdown products may conceivably maintain a periapical inflammation. Also, the exudate will be an excellent substrate for the growth of microorganisms. The possibilities for reinfection of the root canal between visits, therefore, are quite real.

Calcium hydroxide is dissolved in the tissue fluids and with time will disappear from the root canal. However, in teeth with completed root development, months will pass until so much of the material has disappeared that one can expect the unfortunate "empty canal effect" that was referred to above. This fact as well as the long-lasting antimicrobial effect of calcium hydroxide gives the dentist great freedom in scheduling the treatment ahead.

Root Canal Obturation. The permanent obturation of the canal is performed when the patient is free of symptoms and the root canal is dry, normally in the second visit. Sometimes these criteria are not achieved so quickly and the reasons for this should be determined before treatment is continued. First, one must determine if the mechanical instrumentation of the canal has been performed in a satisfactory way. Frequently the reason for the problem is thus explained. Another possible reason is infection or reinfection of the root canal. A culture may provide the answer to this question. If infection is suspected at the second visit, and the instrumentation of the root canal appears to have been carried out well, the contamination or reinfection may be the result of a leaking temporary filling, inadequate old fillings, root cracks, caries, or other similar causes. Therefore, after renewed cleansing and filling of the canal with calcium hydroxide, the new temporary filling must be carefully checked for a bacteria-tight seal. If symptoms, exudation, or fistulae persist after repeated treatment, it is useless to keep changing the intracanal dressing. An analysis of the cause of the problem must be carried out and effective measures taken.

Asepsis. When the access cavity is completed and the canal orifices are found, a rubber dam is applied to the tooth. The field of operation, including the surface of the tooth and the pulp chamber, is disinfected with an effective, surface-active disinfectant. Then the chemomechanical instrumentation of the root canal can start and is carried out with sterile instruments. A bacteria-tight temporary filling is applied before the rubber dam is removed, and the temporary filling is checked once again after the removal of the rubber dam and before the patient is allowed to close the mouth. Especially important is the maintenance of strict asepsis during the second visit, when the canal conceivably is to be filled.

Prognosis and Follow-up Examinations. Endodontic treatment of nonvital teeth has an excellent prognosis. For nonvital teeth without radiographically visible periapical inflammation, the success rate is 90 to 95 per cent, the same as for treatment of vital teeth. Still, periodic clinical and radiologic follow-up examinations are indicated following treatment. Temporary failures, occasionally seen after pulpectomies will not occur after correct treatment of nonvital teeth. Overinstrumentation of the canal and excess filling material can, however, lead to the development of periapical radiolucencies, which may disappear later.

Apical Periodontitis

The treatment of nonvital teeth with radiographically visible periapical inflamma-

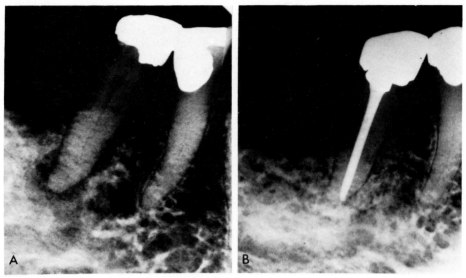

FIGURE 6–36 *A,* Radiographs of mandibular premolar with apical periodontitis. *B,* Repair 1 year after endodontic treatment (standardized technique).

tion is normally the same as that of nonvital teeth in which the apical periodontitis cannot yet be diagnosed on a radiograph. The cause for the inflammation should be removed. Normally it is not necessary to remove surgically the inflamed tissue in the periapical area for repair to occur.

Thus, the treatment of apical periodontitis is aimed at (1) Preventing the leakage of toxic products from necrotic tissue and microorganisms in the root canal to the periapical area, (2) Preventing microorganisms in the root canal from reaching the periapical area, (3) Preventing the root canal from becoming filled with exudate that serves as a substrate for microorganisms, and (4) preventing reinfection of the root canal during and after treatment. If these goals are satisfied during treatment, periapical inflammation will heal. The repair process can be followed radiographically and is characterized by the re-establishment of the bone structure of the periradicular area. When the repair is completed, a normal periodontal ligament space will be seen (Fig. 6–36). Without treatment, no repair will occur.

Asymptomatic Apical Periodontitis. Normally, apical periodontitis develops without symptoms and has an insidious, chronic character. In the treatment of chronic apical periodontitis, various methods may be used: (1) Endodontic treatment, (2) Endodontic-surgical treatment, and (3) Surgical treatment.

Endodontic treatment is without comparison the most common method used to manage asymptomatic apical periodontitis. In principle, the treatment is identical to that previously described for teeth with necrotic pulps. Only a few practical details may be different.

In teeth with large periapical radiolucent areas, prolonged treatment with calcium hydroxide may be indicated. When this method is used, the tooth is treated with calcium hydroxide for 6, 12 or even 24 months, with a change of medication normally every third month. The purpose of the treatment is to influence favorably the repair of the apical periodontitis (or a radicular cyst, which may be suspected in many of these instances). An additional benefit of the method is that the response of the periapical tissue can be determined before permanent obturation of the canal.

Prognosis and Follow-up Examinations. Endodontic treatment of teeth with chronic apical periodontitis has a good prognosis. With modern methods the success rate is 80 to 85 per cent. Despite this high rate, however, the frequency of success in teeth with this preoperative diagnosis clearly is poorer (by approximately 10 to 15 per cent) than in vital teeth or in nonvital teeth without radiographically visible apical periodontitis. Thus, good clinical (sensitivity test) and radiographic examination routines are exceedingly important. Endodontic treatment should be initiated before an apical periodontitis has had a chance to develop.

With endodontic treatment unsuccessful in 15 to 20 per cent of patients, clinical and radiologic follow-up examination of the treatment in this group is an absolute necessity. When the periapical radiolucency has disappeared and a normal periodontal ligament space has been re-established, the treatment can be considered successful, and subsequent follow-up examinations are not indicated. Periapical repair may occur relatively quickly and be completed within 6 to 12 months, but sometimes several years may pass before even small periapical radiolucencies disappear. If a radiolucency remains after 5 years in a symptom-free tooth with an adequately filled root canal, it will be necessary to make a decision as to whether the root filling should be revised, whether sur-

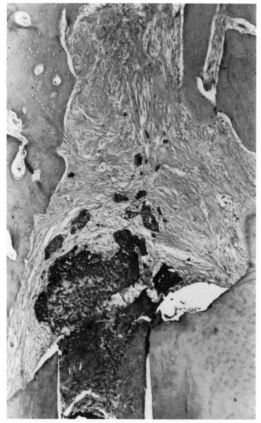

FIGURE 6–37 Paraffin section of monkey tooth with experimentally induced apical periodontitis. Periapical fibrous repair is evident 90 days after endodontic treatment. Dentin chips plug in foraminal area, with some chips beyond the apex.

gical treatment should be performed, or whether the treatment should be considered successful. Periapical repair with formation of fibrous connective tissue instead of bone does occur and makes this decision difficult in certain instances (Fig. 6–37). The general rule is, however, that in healthy, adult patients restraint should be exercised in performing surgical treatment if small periapical radiolucencies do not increase in size. Long-term follow-up examinations are indicated for these patients at 2- to 3-year intervals.

Endodontic-Surgical Treatment. In certain instances endodontic treatment must be combined with a surgical operation. Combined therapy is indicated in the treatment of osteolytic processes of the jaws when routine endodontic treatment has proved ineffective. In addition, clinical experience has shown that a surgical approach should be used in teeth with extensive and persistent exudation that does not respond to prolonged treatment with calcium hydroxide. Surgical treatment may also be of value when complications arise during the endodontic treatment, as, for example, with root perforations and instrument fractures and in the case of a large excess of root-filling material.

Surgical Treatment. In principle, surgical treatment of apical periodontitis as the primary treatment form is performed only by extraction of the tooth. Primary surgical treatment may, however, be the last resort in certain teeth in which an obliteration of the canal (usually after trauma or orthodontic treatment) makes it impossible to negotiate the root canal. Such teeth may be treated tentatively with a retrograde root filling (Fig. 6–38). However, it must be understood that even if a canal is clinically and radiographically obliterated, there is necrotic tissue in microscopic spaces in the root. This tissue is left in the tooth with this method, and leakage of breakdown products may occur in spite of the retrograde filling. On the other hand, surgical treatment of apical periodontitis is important when the endodontic treatment has failed for one reason or another. (This will be discussed in the section on retreatment.)

Symptomatic Apical Periodontitis. The first phase of the treatment of symptomatic apical periodontitis is to relieve the patient of

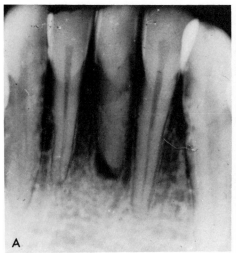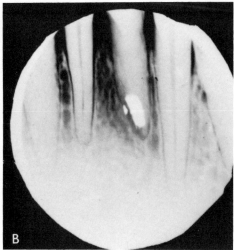

FIGURE 6–38 *A,* Radiograph of lower incisor with obliterated root canal and periapical radiolucency (apical periodontitis). *B,* Repair 1 year after apicoectomy and retrograde amalgam filling.

pain and take care of possible medical complications caused by the inflammation. (This will be discussed in the section on emergency treatment.) When the acute phase and the symptoms are under control, the treatment should be continued as described for an asymptomatic apical periodontitis.

Retreatment

Revision of endodontic treatment may be necessary when repair does not occur. If the technical quality of the root filling is not satisfactory, retreatment may become necessary even if repair has taken place.

The most common error in the technical quality of the root canal filling is that it does not seal the canal properly. Another error is the failure of the obturation to end at the optimal apical level. It is not unusual for both of these errors to occur simultaneously. In certain instances an unsuccessful technical result may result from complications such as instrument fractures or root perforations.

The prognosis of endodontic treatment becomes significantly poorer if the technical quality of the root filling is not satisfactory, and especially if the canal is inadequately sealed. In principle, therefore, all teeth in which the root canal obturation is not technically satisfactory should be retreated. An exception to this rule may be teeth treated more than 5 years previously in which repair has occurred in spite of inadequacies in the

canal obturation. However, regardless of age, a technically unsatisfactory root filling should always be revised if a post is to be prepared for the tooth.

Occasionally periapical repair will not occur even if the technical standard of the canal obturation appears satisfactory radiographically. One must remember there are limitations to the radiographic examination, and the root canal may be inadequately filled even when the radiograph indicates the opposite. Correct treatment in such instances is the removal of the root filling and further chemomechanical instrumentation of the canal. The objective of such treatment is the removal of the causal factors and the establishment of an adequate seal to promote periapical repair. Controlled follow-up studies have shown that about 60 per cent of unsuccessful cases will be successful after retreatment.

Surgical-Endodontic Retreatment. In a variety of situations involving unsuccessful endodontic treatment, surgical-endodontic retreatment represents the only alternative to conventional retreatment. The indications for surgical retreatment follow.

Unsuccessful Conventional Endodontic Retreatment. When the apical periodontitis has not healed despite a revision of the root filling, surgical intervention is indicated.

The apical 2 to 5 mm of the root end are cut off in order to remove the part of the root most likely to contain accessory canals conceivably responsible for the failure of the

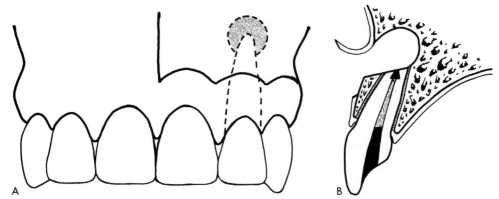

FIGURE 6–39 Diagrams indicating a suitable technique for periapical surgery. The scalloped, horizontal, full-thickness flap includes at least one tooth on each side of the one to be operated on and a mesial vertical incision. **A,** This flap design is suitable in most areas of the mouth. After removal of the granulation tissue, 2 to 5 mm of the root tip is cut off. **B,** The apical root surface is beveled in a buccal direction to facilitate the preparation of a cavity and insertion of a retrograde amalgam filling.

conventional treatment. The root canal is then sealed by an orthograde root filling during the operation. If the canal obturation appears adequate both radiographically and clinically, a retrograde filling is placed in the root (Fig. 6–39).

Post in the Canal. When the apical periodontitis has not healed, and conventional endodontic retreatment is made difficult or impossible because the root canal is blocked coronally by a post, surgical retreatment may become necessary.

The possibilities of removing the post and thus avoiding surgical treatment should be evaluated carefully, especially in teeth in which the root filling is short or in some other way technically inadequate. The technical quality of the root filling must then be evaluated against the type and size of the post and the risk of root fracture and other complications.

In teeth with a blocked root canal, in which an orthograde root filling cannot be placed, the surgical treatment should always be concluded with a retrograde root filling. In spite of its inadequacies, zinc-free silver amalgam is the material of choice for retrograde root fillings. It is good clinical practice to place a retrograde amalgam filling in all teeth if the orthograde filling has not been revised during the operation, even if the old orthograde filling appears to be satisfactory radiographically.

Follow-up examinations have indicated a success rate of 50 to 60 per cent after surgical-endodontic retreatment of unsuccessful cases, about the same success rate as is seen after conventional endodontic retreatment of unsuccessfully treated teeth.

Instrument Fragment in the Canal. Fractures of instruments occur, and the fragments are normally impossible to remove from the root canal. The canal should be filled to the level of the instrument fragment in the hope that repair will take place in spite of the inadequacy of the obturation. Often healing occurs, especially in vital teeth, but instrument fragments in the root canal have proved to have a negative effect on the prognosis of endodontic treatment, and failures must be expected. Surgical-endodontic treatment is then usually the only alternative. Ideally the instrument fragment is removed apically, and an orthograde root filling is placed in the canal during the operation. If it is impossible to remove the instrument fragment, a retrograde filling is placed.

Root Perforations. A perforation of the root can sometimes be managed by conventional endodontic methods. However, in many instances a surgical approach may be the best or the only alternative. Typical indications for surgical retreatment include perforations in the apical area of curved roots when it is impossible to gain re-entry into the original root canal. An apicoectomy with orthograde and retrograde fillings may save such teeth. Perforations are also seen in conjunction with post preparations. A surgical exposure of the perforation and placement of an amalgam filling is usually the treatment of choice.

External Root Resorption. Generally, ex-

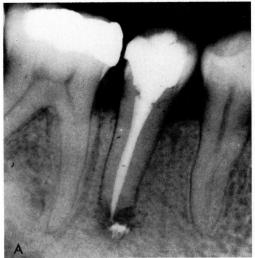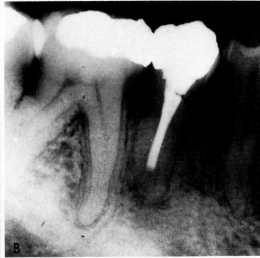

FIGURE 6–40 *A,* Radiograph of tooth with apical resorption in conjunction with endodontic treatment and overfilling of root canal. *B,* Repair as it appears six months after apicoectomy and removal of excess filling material.

ternal root resorption should be treated endodontically. In certain instances surgical treatment can be helpful, especially in teeth with resorption in the apical area. The periapical inflamed tissue is removed, the apical part of the root where the resorption lacunae are diagnosed is resected, and the root canal is sealed.

A very rapid apical resorption is occasionally seen in connection with large excesses of root-filling material. In these instances surgical removal of the excess material is an effective treatment method and should be considered (Fig. 6–40).

Root Fracture. In teeth with a horizontal fracture of the root, the pulp in the apical fragment may become necrotic and cause an apical periodontitis. Endodontic treatment can then be attempted but will usually be unsuccessful because of the fracture. Surgical removal of the apical fragment may then be a possible treatment method, especially if the fracture is in the apical third of the tooth.

In summary, surgical-endodontic treatment is a useful and valuable complement to conventional endodontic treatment, especially in "problem cases" as described above. Nonetheless, it is a grave error to burden the patient with unnecessary surgery. Surgical treatment should not be performed if conventional endodontic treatment can lead to success.

Prophylactic Use of Antibiotics

Prophylactic use of antibiotics has limited, but important, indications. It should be used for a select group of patients during treatment in which bacteremia might be expected, for example, during endodontic treatment of nonvital teeth. This group consists of patients with heart valve damage, acute glomerulonephritis, difficult-to-control diabetes, patients on steroid therapy, and a new, steadily increasing group of patients who have had open heart surgery. Patients with implants and pacemakers should also be included in this group.

Prophylactic antibiotic treatment should be performed with bactericidal products, normally penicillin. The treatment starts immediately (½ hour) before the operation; that is, the patient should receive the medicament while in the waiting room. High dosages should be used (at least two times normal dosage), and the treatment should continue for 24 hours.

Emergency Treatment

Approximately 60 to 70 per cent of patients with oral or perioral pain need some form of endodontic emergency treatment. The immediate goal of the emergency treatment should be the relief of the patient's symptoms. If possible, emergency treatment should also become the first phase in the permanent treatment of the condition. Since emergency treatment, as a rule, takes place "between patients" in a busy schedule, the therapeutic procedures should be as simple as possible in keeping with the objective of relieving the patient of pain.

Emergency Treatment of Vital Teeth

Approximately 90 per cent of the vital teeth that need endodontic emergency treatment will be carious or will be teeth previously restored because of caries. About 5 per cent of the teeth will have symptoms because of occlusal traumatism. Exposed, hyperreactive dentin and tooth fractures are other conditions causing pain in vital teeth.

Hyperreactive dentin can often be treated successfully with fluoride preparations and good oral hygiene. However, sometimes a filling may have to be placed and, on rare occasions, the pulp may have to be extirpated to give the patient necessary relief. Symptoms from exposed dentin because of a fracture can be controlled by restoring the tooth or simply covering the exposed dentin surface with a paste of zinc oxide and eugenol. If the fracture is incomplete, the fragment should usually be removed. In cases of occlusal traumatism, relief is usually obtained after simple occlusal adjustment. On rare occasions, however, the pulp may have to be extirpated.

In symptomatic teeth with carious lesions or restorations, the carious dentin should be excavated and existing restorations removed. If the pulp is not exposed, filling the cavity with a dry mix of zinc oxide and eugenol will give relief of pain in 90 to 95 per cent of patients. This is a simple and rapid procedure, and it should be the treatment of choice in these teeth. One should remember, however, when the final treatment is planned that the absence of symptoms does not guarantee a healthy pulp.

If the pulp is exposed after excavation of caries, removal of restorations, or both, three possible procedures exist for emergency treatment. Although the three procedures are not equally effective, they are all good enough to provide a reasonable choice according to the time available for the emergency treatment.

The simplest method of treatment is to apply a cotton pellet with a medicament with an anodyne effect, such as Cresatin or camphorated phenol, directly on the pulp exposure. The cavity is then sealed with a temporary filling material, preferably a dry mix of zinc oxide and eugenol. This treatment will give relief of pain in more than 80 per cent of patients until a pulpectomy can be performed.

The second method is to remove the coronal pulp of the symptomatic tooth and apply the cotton pellet with the medicament on the remaining pulp stump. The tooth is then sealed as described above. This method will give relief of pain in more than 90 per cent of patients. It is simple and rapid and should probably be regarded as the routine method in emergency treatment of vital teeth with exposed pulp.

The third method is to do a pulpectomy immediately and to fill the canal temporarily with calcium hydroxide paste. This is the most reliable method and gives relief of pain in 99 per cent of patients. However, it is considerably more time-consuming than the two other methods and, for that reason, usually cannot be carried out in the emergency situation. It should also be noted that if a pulpectomy is attempted but for some reason cannot be carried through and tissue remnants are left in the root canal, the effectiveness of the treatment to relieve pain is greatly reduced (to about 80 per cent). Thus, the effectiveness of an "incomplete" pulpectomy with the placement of a medicament in the root canal is no greater than when the medicament is placed directly on an exposure in the cavity.

Emergency Treatment of Nonvital Teeth

In nonvital teeth, pain is associated with symptomatic apical periodontitis. The following factors are of special importance in obtaining relief of pain in this condition.

Drainage. Probably the most important cause for the symptoms present during symptomatic apical periodontitis is elevated pressure in the tissues. Accordingly, the treatment must be aimed at normalization of the tissue pressure, which, as soon as it is achieved, results in rapid relief for the patient. Therefore, drainage must be provided if at all possible. First, the pulp chamber is opened through the crown of the tooth; direct drainage of pus through the root canal may then take place. However, sometimes the purulent breakdown occurs in a periapical area that does not have contact with the tooth such that drainage through the root canal will take place. It is then important to remember that the toxic content of the root canal has caused the apical periodontitis. Thus, to instrument and clean the root canal is also good therapy in the attempt to obtain relief from pain.

When exudation from the root canal has stopped or has been reduced significantly (it is often impossible to stop the exudation completely during the first visit), the root canal is filled with a suitable dressing, such as calcium hydroxide, and the tooth is sealed with a bacteria-tight temporary filling.

Some endodontists believe that a tooth should not be sealed in an acute situation but should remain open in order to achieve relief of pain more quickly. Controlled clinical experiments, however, seem to indicate that this procedure at best only postpones the problems at hand. An open root canal will be filled with saliva, plaque, and the microflora of the oral cavity, and a new, more severe exacerbation is often the result when a tooth that has been left open is instrumented and sealed. However, on rare occasions, when the exudation is so severe and persistent that it is not possible to seal the canal, it may be advisable to allow the canal to remain open. In these instances it is a good practice to seal the canal as soon as possible (after 24 hours), so that the downgrowth of plaque into the canal is limited to a minimum.

Effective drainage can be provided further through an incision of a fluctuant abscess. In many instances, incision and drainage will lead to a dramatic relief of pain for the patient. The incision should be performed in addition to, not as a substitute for, the chemomechanical instrumentation of the root canal if the patient's condition allows access to the guilty tooth.

Occlusion. During symptomatic apical periodontitis, the tooth is usually pushed somewhat out of the socket by the edema in the periapical tissues. Consequently, each time the patient closes on the tooth, the periodontal tissues, already hypersensitive because of the inflammation, are traumatized. Careful reduction of the crown of the tooth to avoid the traumatic occlusion normally has a palliative effect on the patient's symptoms. Actually, the tooth is "immobilized," and this is a correct and an effective therapy in such a situation.

Antibiotics. Symptomatic apical periodontitis can usually be treated without antibiotics. If good drainage has been provided, the symptoms will disappear relatively soon, and the situation can be corrected with routine endodontic treatment. However, there are situations in which the use of antibiotics is absolutely indicated. As a general rule, if the patient's general health is influenced by the periapical inflammation or if the patient's medical status is poor, antibiotics should be given. Furthermore, antibiotics should be used for abscesses in the floor of the mouth, for perimandibular abscesses, or for any other dramatic inflammatory situation with severe swelling, especially when it is impossible to perform a surgical incision. One should remember that the inflammatory process involved in these situations occurs in the face-throat region, with anatomically determined routes of spread to the brain as well as to the mediastinum. In the actual situation, it does not help much to think about statistics or to worry about general abuse of antibiotics. On the contrary, the clinician assumes the responsibility for the patient's health and must provide the very best treatment that can be offered.

If the decision is made to administer antibiotics, penicillin is normally the medicament that has the best effect on this type of infection. Since penicillin sensitivity is becoming increasingly common, the patient should be questioned about previous antibiotic experiences before antibiotics are prescribed. Erythromycin is a good replacement if penicillin sensitivity is suspected. Finally, antibiotics should be considered as replacement therapy for the chemomechanical instrumentation of the root canal or an incision of a possible abscess when the involved tooth is not accessible or when there is a threatening abscess in the floor of the mouth.

Analgesics. In addition to local treatment (and possible antibiotic therapy), most patients with symptomatic apical periodontitis should receive pain-soothing medication. Because of attitudes toward narcotics and medication abuse, patients are often afraid to take analgesics, even when they have severe pain. It is therefore important to explain to them that they can take the prescribed medicine safely, and that mild analgesics can help them through the period when they experience the most severe symptoms. In some instances sleeping pills may also be indicated.

It is important to realize that patients with symptomatic apical periodontitis may not only have severe pain but may also have fever and generally feel sick. Because of swellings in the facial region, that fortunately, as a rule, look more dramatic than they actually are, patients may also be quite anxious and uneasy. Consequently, an important part of the treatment is that the dentist exhibit security and authority as well as warmth and understanding for the problems of the patient. The dentist's behavior can make an uneasy patient calm and confident. If this is achieved, the patient will be better prepared to tolerate the potentially painful treatment and the often unavoidable postoperative period of discomfort.

Root-Filling Techniques

When examining the root-filling materials available today, it seems that there are no real alternatives to obturation techniques using silver or gutta-percha points in combination with a sealer.

Root Filling with Silver Points

Traditionally, silver points are used together with a zinc oxide–eugenol sealer (e.g., Grossman's sealer). The sealer is brought into the canal with a spiral filler or a similar instrument, and a silver point that fits in the canal as well as possible is inserted to the predetermined apical level. During insertion into the canal the point acts as a piston, pressing the sealer in apical and lateral directions. This relatively simple procedure achieves a good filling and seal of the root canal. The zinc oxide–eugenol sealer has good dimensional stability but may be resorbed from the canal so that the apical seal becomes inadequate. This may lead to an exposure of the silver point to the tissue fluids, corrosion of the point, formation of toxic corrosion products, and, in many instances, failure of the treatment several years after the endodontic therapy is completed (Fig. 6–41).

In view of the potential for late postoperative failures, the use of silver points is be-

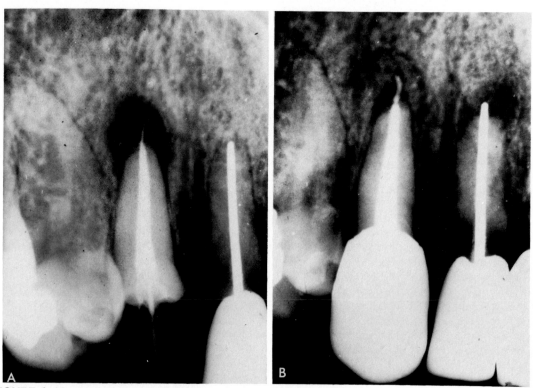

FIGURE 6–41 Radiograph of maxillary right lateral 8 years after endodontic treatment and root canal obturation with silver point (tooth to the right in **A**). **B,** After 13 years, apical periodontitis had developed on this tooth.

coming less popular, and today silver points are generally considered to have only very minor indications. The indications might be those instances in which silver points, with their special physical characteristics (they are stiff but still soft and flexible), can possibly be the best solution for special clinical problems. For instance, silver points may be indicated in teeth with narrow, severely curved canals in which an enlargement of the canals might result in a fracture of the instruments. They may also be indicated when mechanical obstructions are present in the canal (e.g., ledges, instrument fragments, or perforations), which may be difficult to bypass with gutta-percha points.

However, if silver points are to be used, special precautions have to be taken to protect them against corrosion. This protection can be achieved most effectively by means of an apical dentin-chips plug.

Root Filling With Gutta-percha Points

Today, without question, gutta-percha points are the most widely used root-filling material throughout the world. There are no contraindications for the use of gutta-percha except those associated with its physical properties. Gutta-percha points are used in different ways and with various techniques. The most important techniques are: (1) the dipping technique, (2) the warm gutta-percha technique, (3) the lateral condensation technique, (4) the standardized technique, and (5) the two-step technique.

The Dipping Technique. Gutta-percha softens when dipped in chloroform, eucalyptol, or other organic solvents, and the dipping technique is based on this property. When softened, a gutta-percha point may be given the exact, three-dimensional form of the root canal space. Unfortunately, the dipping technique has been advocated by some for use without a sealer. This is a misunderstanding due to the presence of a certain stickiness of the gutta-percha point in the softened condition. However, without a sealer, gutta-percha cannot seal the root canal permanently. When the solvent evaporates, the point loses its stickiness and spaces occur between the point and the root canal wall. Thus, the use of a sealer is necessary with the dipping technique.

All types of sealers may be used, but the most homogeneous root filling with the dipping technique is achieved with the use of Kloroperka N-Ø or similar material. The sealer is applied sparsely on the root canal wall and a master point, which has a somewhat larger apical diameter than the root canal, is dipped in chloroform and inserted into the root canal under pressure until it reaches the apical level of instrumentation. The apical part of the root canal is now tightly sealed. In the more coronal parts of the canal, accessory points dipped in chloroform are inserted next to the master point, and by lateral condensation the canal is filled completely with gutta-percha. If the condensation is successful, a biocompatible, homogeneous, and bacteria-tight obturation of the root canal is achieved (Fig. 6–42).

The disadvantages of the dipping technique are that it is relatively difficult to perform and even more difficult to control. Overfilling of the canal frequently occurs during the insertion of the softened master point. If the master point is softened too much, filling material may also be pushed through the apical foramen during the lateral condensation. Furthermore, there are the problems with the shrinkage of gutta-percha that has been softened in chloroform. A common result of the dipping technique is, therefore, an excess of root-filling material and, after some time, a leaky root filling (Fig. 6–43). The technique should not be used without special training.

The Warm Gutta-percha Technique. This technique uses heat-softened gutta-percha, and as with the dipping technique, the goal is to achieve a tight, three-dimensional filling of the root canal space with gutta-percha.

A sealer is applied sparsely to the root canal walls. A zinc oxide–eugenol sealer is commonly used, but logically a more homogeneous result would be obtained by using a material such as Kloroperka N-Ø, which will unite with the gutta-percha. Gutta-percha points 2 to 5 mm long are introduced into the root canal. Pluggers (heat carriers) especially made for this technique are heated over a gas flame until they are cherry red. They are then inserted into the gutta-percha and quickly withdrawn before the material adheres to the instrument. Cold pluggers are then used to condense the heated and softened gutta-percha in the canal by vertical condensation. The heating and the con-

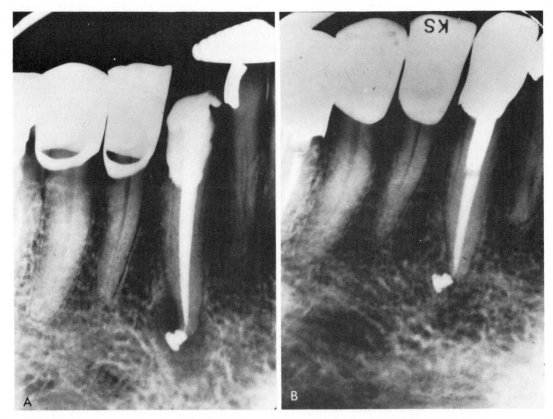

FIGURE 6–42 *A,* Radiograph of mandibular canine with apical periodontitis. The tooth was treated endodontically, and the root canal was filled with gutta-percha softened in chloroform (dipping technique). *B,* Repair after 1 year. The excess root-filling material is typical for this technique.

densing of the gutta-percha are repeated, and new gutta-percha points are applied until the entire canal is filled (Fig. 6–44).

The advantage of the warm gutta-percha technique over the dipping technique is that gutta-percha softened by heat does not shrink nearly as much after hardening as when it is softened chemically. The disadvantage of this technique is that it is rather difficult to carry out and even more difficult to control. Owing to the vertical condensation, overfilling of the canal is a regularly occurring phenomenon, and longitudinal cracks and fractures of teeth treated with this method have been reported. Also, it appears that the apical part of the canal often is not well filled with gutta-percha in spite of the vertical condensation.

The warm gutta-percha technique is an ambitious technique, but so far no controlled studies of the long-term results of teeth treated with this technique have been published. The technique should not be used without special training.

The Lateral Condensation Technique.
With the lateral condensation technique, the root canal is filled with gutta-percha without softening of the points with chemicals or heat. It was hoped that this technique would be easy to control and result in a dimensionally stable, bacteria-tight seal of the canal.

The instrumentation is carried out so that the apical part of the root canal is given a cone-shaped form with the foramen at the apex of the cone. A gutta-percha point is selected and fitted so that it reaches to and stops at the desired apical level of the canal. The point is removed, sealer is applied (any sealer may be used), and the point is reinserted without being softened. A spreader (or finger plugger) is then introduced into the canal to a level 1 mm shorter than the apical end of the first gutta-percha point. The spreader is removed and an unsoftened accessory point is inserted into the canal to the level of the spreader.

The spreader is used again, this time to a

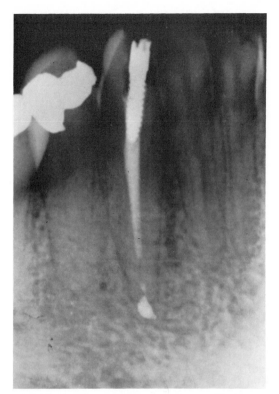

FIGURE 6–43 Radiograph of mandibular canine 6 months after endodontic treatment and root canal obturation according to the dipping technique. In spite of overfilling of the canal as evidenced by excess material, the gutta-percha in the apical part of the canal has disappeared, presumably because of oversoftening in chloroform.

level 1 mm short of the second point; the spreader is removed, and a third point is inserted. The sequence is repeated until the canal is completely filled with gutta-percha at all levels (Fig. 6–45).

This is an excellent technique when mastered. However, experience has taught that lateral condensation in the apical area of the canal is far from an easy procedure, and experimental results have indicated that each accessory gutta-percha point should reach a level only 1 mm shorter than the preceding point if the canal is to be tightly sealed. What is often seen, however, is that the apical part of the canal is filled mostly with sealer because the lateral condensation technique was not mastered. Thus, the long-term success of this technique is often dependent on the properties of the sealer. If the sealer shrinks or becomes resorbed, the root filling will become leaky, and the possibilities of an unsuccessful result increase.

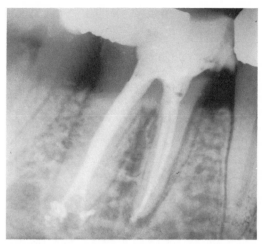

FIGURE 6–44 Radiograph of mandibular molar treated according to the warm gutta-percha technique. Note enlargement of root canals in the cervical area to facilitate vertical condensation of gutta-percha apically in the canal. Excess of root-filling material is commonly seen with this technique. (Courtesy of Dr. Peter Brothman.)

The sealer is a weak point with all root-filling methods, and the amount used should be minimal. Based on the lateral condensation technique, a new technique has been developed in which the weaknesses of the old method have been largely overcome through an exact adjustment of the first gutta-percha point (master point) to the apical root canal space. The amount of sealer in the apical area can then be reduced to a

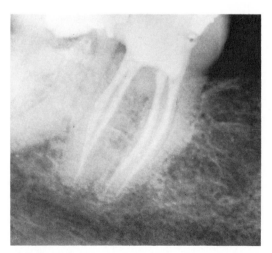

FIGURE 6–45 Radiograph of mandibular molar treated according to the lateral condensation technique. Note step-back instrumentation of root canals. (Courtesy of Dr. Frederic Barnett.)

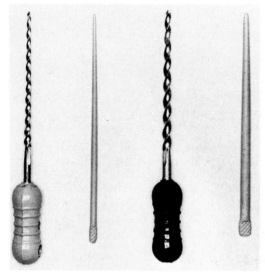

FIGURE 6–46 Photograph showing reamers (Nos. 40 and 80) with matching gutta-percha points (Nos. 40 and 80).

minimum. This technique is called the standardized endodontic technique.

The Standardized Endodontic Technique. The standardized technique has been made possible through the development of standardized root canal instruments and standardized gutta-percha points (and silver points) (Fig. 6–46). The standardized instruments and points are manufactured according to strict norms set by the International Standardization Organization (ISO); the variation in diameter between the instrument (and points) of the same size (number) can be at most ±0.02 mm. Thus, with the standardized instruments it has become possible to give the apical 1 to 5 mm of the root canal a circular shape with known diameter (Fig. 6–47A).

Morphometric studies have shown that a "standardization" of the canal may be achieved in most of the teeth in all groups. In order to obtain a circular cross section of the canal only, instruments that are used with rotating movements, reamers and K-files, should be used in the apical part of the root canal. The Hedström type of instruments, which are used with rasping, longitudinal movements, should therefore be used only in the more coronal parts of the canal, where a circular form is not required.

When the preparation of the root canal is completed, a gutta-percha point (master point) with the same size and form (same number) as the last reamer used is selected (Fig. 6–47B). The point will fit in the apical part of the root canal as does a cork in a bot-

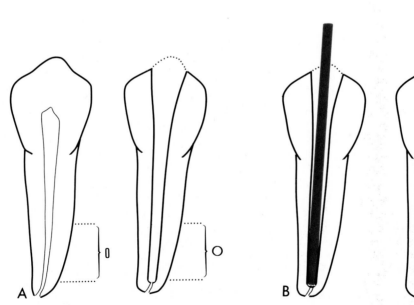

FIGURE 6–47 Diagrams showing principles for endodontic treatment with the standardized technique. The apical part of the root canal is prepared with rotating instruments (reamers) to obtain a circular form *(A)*. A gutta-percha masterpoint with the same diameter fits in the apical part of the canal as does a cork in a bottle *(B)*. Further coronally, additional points are used to fill the canal completely.

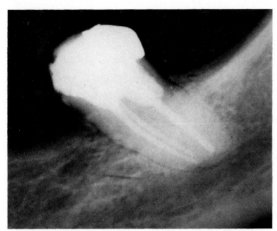

FIGURE 6–48 Radiograph of mandibular molar treated according to the standardized technique. Note enlargement of the root canals in the apical area. In the mesial canals, masterpoint No. 40 was used, and in the distal canal, masterpoint No. 80 was used.

tle. When the fit of the point has been established radiographically, the point is removed and a sealer is applied sparsely on the root canal wall (any type of sealer may be used). The master point is then reinserted into the canal without being softened. In the coronal parts of the canal that are not entirely filled by the master point, accessory points are inserted and lateral condensation is used to completely fill the canal with gutta-percha (Figs. 6–47B and 6–48).

This technique has many advantages. The greatest advantages are the systematization that a standardized system offers and the ease of carrying out and controlling the technique. The final outcome of the treatment is the result of well-planned and well-controlled therapeutic measures.

The master point is applied without being softened. Therefore, it does not shrink. Furthermore, in principle, the master point fits the root canal space exactly at the apex. The precise fit reduces the amount of sealer needed to a thin film between the point and the canal wall. A further advantage of the method is that overfilling of the canal is easily avoided because the master point is not softened, and for the same reason, overfilling during the lateral condensation phase does not occur. A 5-year follow-up study of teeth treated with the standardized technique showed that the root fillings were dimensionally stable and adequately sealed the root canal after a long time.

The disadvantage of the method is related to root canal anatomy. It has been shown that within all groups of teeth there may be root canals that cannot be prepared according to the standardized technique. Canals may have a largest diameter larger than the root's smallest diameter or they may have a diameter larger than the diameter of the largest standardized instrument (No. 140, 1.4 mm). Canals in the maxillary lateral incisors and first premolars and in the mandibular incisors and mesial roots of the mandibular molars may create problems when the standardized technique is used. But even in these groups of teeth, problem canals are exceptions, and follow-up studies have shown a success rate of more than 90 per cent in both one-, two-, and three-rooted teeth treated with this technique.

Furthermore, it may sometimes be difficult, or even impossible, to prepare the root canal according to the standardized technique in severely curved roots. Fortunately, the roots that most frequently are curved have narrow canals that can be given the desired apical circular shape with reamers Nos. 30 to 40. Flexible instruments are now available that can be used without too great a risk of fracture in such canals. In wider curved canals, as seen in maxillary lateral incisors, a modification of the technique may be necessary so that files are used more in the apical area. A master point of the same size as the last reamer used (for example, No. 35) should still be used, but accessory points and lateral condensation using flexible instruments (reamers or files) in the apical area of the canal may be necessary.

An overall evaluation of advantages and disadvantages seems to indicate that with the materials available today, the standardized endodontic technique is superior to other accepted techniques. The standardized technique is certainly simple compared with other techniques. It is easily controlled and can be performed with a minimum of complications. Technically, it gives bacteria-tight obturations that are dimensionally stable for a long time, and most important, a success rate of 90 per cent or higher can be expected in all groups of teeth.

The Two-Step Technique. Occasionally during endodontic treatment, routine methods will have to be modified for teeth with special problems. In some instances, such as in a tooth whose root canal divides into two canals in the apical part of the root or in teeth with internal resorptions, a technique in which the tooth is filled in two steps may be practical. In a tooth whose canal divides, both canals are prepared according to the standardized technique. Thereafter one of the canals is obturated. When this is completed, a heated reamer is brought to the level at which the root canal divides and the gutta-percha coronal to this level is removed. Then the second apical canal and the main canal are filled in the customary way.

Similarly, in teeth with internal resorption, the root canal apical to the resorption defect is filled first. Thereafter, it is possible by means of vertical and lateral condensation of softened gutta-percha to obturate the resorption defect without risk of overfilling the canal apically.

Sometimes, especially in teeth with incomplete root formation (in children younger than 13 years of age), the diameter of the root canal is wider than the widest standardized gutta-percha point. In such teeth it may be a good alternative to custom make a master point that fits in the apical part of the canal. This is done by heating several gutta-percha points and rolling them between two glass slabs until they become one point slightly larger than the canal to be filled. The master point is then carefully softened in warm water and inserted into the root canal to the desired apical level. After hardening, the point is removed from the canal, sealer is applied, and the point is reinserted to seal the apical part of the canal. Farther coronally, the canal is filled with necessary accessory points, and a lateral condensation technique is used.

Other Techniques

Paste Techniques.   Pastes mixed from a powder and a liquid to obturate the root canal are available on the market. The pastes are inserted into the root canal by means of spiral fillers or by injection. At first glance, this may seem to be a simple and attractive technique, but in reality it is difficult. Overfilling of the canal is the rule and not the exception. The homogeneity of the fillings is often not satisfactory, and the canal may be inadequately sealed in spite of the overfilling.

Some of the pastes will shrink after setting, and most of them are resorbable. The physical properties of the resin-based pastes Diaket and AH-26 are the most interesting.

However, the fact that these materials are almost impossible to remove from the root canal after setting is reason enough that they cannot compete with a good gutta-percha and sealer technique.

All pastes with so-called therapeutic effects are too toxic to be used in modern endodontic therapy.

"Biologic" Techniques.   During the past 50 years, there have been numerous attempts to develop so-called biologic obturation techniques, that is, techniques aimed at inducing hard tissue closure of the canal or ingrowth of new connective tissue into the canal from the periapical area. Best known in this connection are the experiments with calcium hydroxide as a root-filling material. It was thought that filling the root canal with calcium hydroxide might lead to precipitation of calcium salts, which ultimately would result in obturation of the canal. Although this did not happen, it was learned during these experiments that calcium hydroxide does have a hard tissue–inducing effect. This effect has been taken advantage of in many areas in modern endodontic therapy, first in pulp capping and later in apexification treatment of teeth with incompletely formed roots.

An apical hard tissue barrier may be induced by means of calcium hydroxide in both vital and nonvital teeth. In vital teeth the barrier usually is achieved after 3 to 6 months, whereas in nonvital teeth a treatment period of 6 to 24 months may be required (Fig. 6–30). The calcium hydroxide in the root canal should be changed every 3 months during this time. When the apical hard tissue barrier is formed, the canal may be filled according to the standardized technique. If the canal is too wide, which usually is the case in children under 13 years of age, a customized master point should be used.

An apical barrier can also be achieved by means of dentin chips from the root canal wall. Dentin chips have a hard tissue–inducing effect, and a cementumlike tissue may form on the dentin chips and close off the root canal completely (Fig. 6–33).

Lately, interesting animal experiments have been reported in which a gel of collagen and biologically active chemicals ($CaCl_2$, K_2HPO_4) has been applied in the root canal. With this method, both ingrowth of tissue and apical and intracanal calcifications have been observed. However, the most interesting experiments in this area are the attempts, by means of a blood clot in the root canal, to induce the formation of new connective tissue in the canal. The root canal was instrumented through the apical foramen but otherwise was prepared in the normal way. Periapical bleeding was then provoked. When the canal was filled with blood, it was sealed in the cervical area. From an experimental point of view, this method led to excellent results in vital teeth. New connective tissue, or "a new pulp," was formed routinely in the canal as far as 12 to 13 mm from the apical foramen. In nonvital teeth, however, the new connective tissue was achieved only in exceptional cases. Despite the questionable results in nonvital teeth, the findings of these experiments were promising and are already in clinical use. In pulpectomy treatment, canals are now consistently filled to a level 1 to 2 mm coronal to the radiographic apex, even if the entire pulp has been extirpated. The unfilled space apical to the root filling will automatically be filled with tissue fluids and blood, which will organize to form new connective tissue.

The good results achieved with calcium hydroxide, the blood clot, and other experiments of this type have resulted in a wave of enthusiasm, and almost every month new results of experiments with "biologic" methods in endodontics are published. Therefore, there is good reason to believe that root-filling techniques may change radically within the forseeable future. Until then, however, the goal must be to achieve a bacteria-tight seal of the root canal with biologically acceptable materials.

The Prognosis of Endodontic Treatment

A number of good prognostic studies have shown the success rate of endodontic treatment to be 85 to 95 per cent. One study, which particularly dealt with the results obtained with the standardized endodontic technique, found a success rate of 91 per cent. It is conceivable that the following factors might influence the prognosis of endodontic treatment.

Age. No difference has been found in the results of endodontic treatment in younger (under 35 years) or older (over 35 years) patients.

Health. It has not been shown that an impairment of the general health implies a prognostic risk for endodontic treatment.

Root Canal Morphology. It seems logical that the root canal morphology should be of

importance for the prognosis of endodontic treatment. One might assume that the results would not be as good in molars, whose root canals may have a complicated anatomy, as in incisors, whose anatomy is less complicated. However, several studies have shown the opposite results, namely, that endodontic treatment is more successful in a tooth with three roots than in a tooth with two roots and is better in a tooth with too roots than in a tooth with one root. There are no biologic explanations for these somewhat surprising results. Probably they are due to the fact that the relatively narrow canals in multirooted teeth are more thoroughly cleansed than the wider canals in single-rooted teeth. The results of a study with the standardized technique, in which the root canals were enlarged considerably more than with other accepted techniques, support this hypothesis. In this study the results were the same in all groups of teeth, and all studies support the view that endodontic treatment may be performed with a high success rate in all groups of teeth.

Preoperative Diagnosis. There is no difference between the results of endodontic treatment of vital teeth (pulpectomy) and nonvital teeth without radiographically diagnosed apical periodontitis. The success rate drops about 10 to 15 per cent in nonvital teeth with periapical radiolucencies. There also appears to be a tendency for the size of the radiolucency to be of importance to the prognosis.

There is no difference in the results of the treatment of asymptomatic apical periodontitis or symptomatic apical periodontitis nor does the presence of a fistula from an apical periodontitis influence the prognosis.

Canal Instrumentation. The technical aspects of endodontic treatment have great influence on the prognosis. A prerequisite for a successful obturation of the root canal is adequate instrumentation of the canal. It has been claimed that it is impossible to determine clinically if a canal is adequately instrumented or not. In one study, therefore, the success rate of teeth with root canals prepared with reamers Nos. 20 to 40 was compared with that of teeth with canals prepared with reamers Nos. 45 to 100. The success rate was the same in both groups, indicating that an experienced dentist is able, to a great degree, to decide when a canal is adequately instrumented.

Another factor in the canal instrumentation that may be of prognostic importance is the degree of enlargement of the apical foramen. Preparation of the foramen with reamers larger than Nos. 20 to 25 seems to influence the prognosis negatively; in other words, the canal preparation should not include the foraminal area but should terminate inside the root canal (short of the apex).

Teeth with root canals that cannot be instrumented to the desired apical level owing to canal obliteration have a good prognosis, even better, actually, than roots that are instrumented through the foramen. This teaches us that in such teeth one should not try to force one's way in an apical direction but to instrument and fill the canal as far apically as it is accessible.

Antibacterial Treatment. Several studies have shown that the prognosis of endodontic treatment will be 10 to 15 per cent poorer if the canal is infected at the time of obturation. For the time being these results are widely discussed, as other studies have indicated that periapical healing cannot be related to the state of bacterial cultures from the root canal. There is, however, full agreement about the treatment goal—namely, that root canal infection is to be eliminated, and that, if this is not possible, the number of microorganisms in the root canal should be reduced as much as possible before the canal is filled. The chemomechanical instrumentation of the canal is the most important factor in this process but is usually not enough to give a bacteria-free canal. Additional treatment of infected canals with antibacterial agents should therefore be performed.

Root-Filling Materials. In all good follow-up studies, acceptable root-filling materials have been used. From experimental studies, however, the conclusion can be drawn that it is important for the prognosis of endodontic treatment to use tissue-compatible materials that do not irritate the periapical tissues. In addition, it is important

that the materials be dimensionally stable for a long time.

The Technical Standard of the Root Filling. The technical standard of the root filling has been found in all studies to have a great influence on the result of the treatment. The most important aspect seems to be that the root filling seals the canal in an adequate manner. It has been found that an inadequate seal results in approximately 20 per cent poorer prognosis of endodontic treatment. Thus, inadequate seal of the canal is the one factor that has the greatest negative influence on the prognosis. An excess of root-filling material larger than 1 mm causes a reduction of about 10 per cent in the success rate.

Clinical Complications. The occurrence of an excerbation of an apical periodontitis during the treatment seemingly has no influence on the prognosis of endodontic treatment.

Technical Complications. The most common and, from a prognostic point of view, the most influential technical complication is the fracture of an instrument in the root canal. A negative effect on the prognosis of 19 per cent was observed in one study. Especially doubtful is the prognosis of nonvital teeth with apical periodontitis if an instrument fracture has occurred. To a certain extent, the prognosis is dependent on where in the canal the instrument fragment is located and during which stage of the canal instrumentation the fracture occurred. It may be necessary to resort to surgical-endodontic treatment in such instances.

Another technical complication is root perforation. The treatment of root perforations has a poor prognosis despite the fact that newer treatment methods using calcium hydroxide or dentin-chips plugs have made the picture somewhat brighter.

As is evident, a relatively clear picture has been established about the therapeutic factors of importance for the results of endodontic treatment.

QUESTIONS

1. A tooth is hypersensitive to cold. What is the actual state of the pulp in this tooth?

2. A patient complains that a molar tooth is sensitive when he bites on one of the cusps in a certain direction. What is the likely cause for the sensitivity?

3. A patient complains that several teeth on the maxillary right side are sore when biting and are hypersensitive to cold. What is the most likely diagnosis?

4. A patient complains that the right maxillary first premolar is hyperreaction to cold and heat. A radiograph shows that the tooth has a nickel-sized periapical radiolucency. How do you explain these findings?

5. What is the most important etiologic factor in the development of apical periodontitis?

6. How can you radiographically distinguish between a periapical granuloma and a radicular cyst?

7. What are the two main objectives for using a base material underneath the restorative material?

8. How can marginal leakage be prevented around an amalgam restoration?

9. What is the success rate for pulp capping under optimal conditions?

10. To obtain this success rate with pulp capping, which criteria must be met?

11. What will the success rate for pulp capping be if you use this treatment form routinely in teeth with carious exposures?

12. In pulpectomy treatment you are supposed to sever the pulp 1 to 2 mm coronal to the radiographic apex. Why is that important?

13. What do you do if, during pulpectomy treatment, you inadvertently extirpate the whole pulp and instrument beyond the apex?

14. What is an apical dentin-chips plug?

15. How can dentin chips be useful in endodontic treatment, even if the dentist does not actively attempt to make apical dentin-chips plugs?

16. Why should a pulpectomy (with canal obturation) preferably be completed in one visit?

17. Why should a dentist preferably treat a nonvital tooth in two (or more) visits?

18. Calcium hydroxide is being used as an intracanal medicament in endodontic treatment. What are the main differences between the effects of calcium hydroxide and the traditional intracanal medicaments like Cresatin, formocresol, and others?

19. What are the principles for the standardized endodontic technique?

20. What single factor has the greatest negative influence on the prognosis of endodontic treatment?

See answers in Appendix.

REFERENCES

1. Baume, L.: Dental pulp conditions in relation to carious lesions. Int. Dent. J., *20*:308–319, 1970.
2. Bender, I. B., Sletzer, S., and Yermish, M.: The incidence of bacteremia in endodontic manipulation. Oral Surg., *13*:353–360, 1960.
3. Cvek, M.: Treatment of non-vital permanent incisors with calcium hydroxide. Odontol. Revy, *23*:27–33, 1972.
4. Cvek, M., Hollender, L., and Nord, C. E.: Treatment of non-vital permanent incisors with calcium hydroxide. Odontol. Revy, *27*:93–99, 1976.
5. Frank, R. M., Wolff, F., and Gutmann, B.: Microscopie electronique de la carie au niveau de la dentine humaine. Arch. Oral Biol., *9*:163–179, 1964.
6. Grossman, L. I.: Endodontic Practice. Philadelphia, Lea & Febiger, 1981.
7. Heithersay, G. S.: Calcium hydroxide in the treatment of pulpless teeth with associate pathology. J. Br. Endodont. Soc., *8*:74–81, 1975.
8. Kakehashi, S., Stanley, H. R., and Fitzgerald, R. F.: The effect of surgical exposures of dental pulps in germ free and conventional laboratory rats. Oral Surg., *20*:340–349, 1965.
9. Kerekes, K., and Tronstad, L.: Long-term results of endodontic treatment performed with a standardized technique. J. Endont., *5*:83–90, 1979.
10. Langeland, K.: Tissue changes in the dental pulp. Odontol. Tidskr., *65*:239–385, 1957.
11. Langeland, K.: Histologic evaluation of pulp reactions to operative procedures. I. and II. Oral Surg., *12*:1235–1248 and 1357–1369, 1959.
12. Langeland, K.: The histopathologic basis in endodontic treatment. Dent. Clin. North Am., 1967, pp. 491–520.
13. Langeland, K., Rodriques, H., and Dowden, W. E.: Periodontal disease, bacteria, and pulpal histopathology. Oral Surg., *37*:257–270, 1974.
14. Massler, M.: Pulpal reactions to dental caries. Int. Dent. J., *17*:441–460, 1967.
15. Mjor, I. A., and Tronstad, L.: Experimentally induced pulpitis. Oral Surg., *34*:102–108, 1972.
16. Mjor, I. A., and Tronstad, L.: The healing of experimentally induced pulpitis. Oral Surg., *38*:115–121, 1974.
17. Nyborg, H.: Healing processes in the pulp on capping. Acta Odontol. Scand., *13*:Suppl. 16, 1955.
18. Nygaard-Ostby, B.: Introduction to Endodontics. Oslo, Universitetsforlaget, 1971.
19. Nygaard-Ostby, B., and Hjortdal, O.: Tissue for-

mation in the root canal following pulp removal. Scand. J. Dent. Res., *79*:333–349, 1971.

20. Rolling, I., Hasselgren, G., and Tronstad, L.: Morphologic and enzyme histochemical observations in the pulp of human primary molars 3 to 5 years after formocresol treatment. Oral Surg., *42*:518–528, 1976.

21. Seltzer, S., Soltanoff, W., Sinai, I., and Smith, J.: Biologic aspects of endodontics, IV. Periapical tissue reactions to rootfilled teeth whose canals had been instrumented short of their apices. Oral Surg., *28*:724–738, 1969.

22. Seltzer, S., Soltanoff, W., and Smith, J.: Biologic aspects of endodontics. V. Periapical tissue reactions to root canal instrumentation beyond the apex and canal fillings short and beyond the apex. Oral Surg., *36*:725–737, 1973.

23. Selvig, K. A.: Biological changes at the tooth-saliva interface in periodontal disease. J. Dent. Res., *48*:846–855, 1969.

24. Skogedal, O., and Tronstad, L.: An attempt to correlate dentin and pulp changes in human carious teeth. Oral Surg., *43*:135–140, 1977.

25. Spangberg, L.: Cellular reactions to intracanal medicaments. *In* Transactions of the Fifth International Conference on Endodontics. L. I. Grossman (ed.). Philadelphia, University of Pennsylvania, 1973, pp. 121–130.

26. Stafne, E. C. and Gibilisco, J. A.: Oral Roentgenographic Diagnosis. Philadelphia, W. B. Saunders Company, 1975.

27. Strindberg, L. Z.: The dependence of the results of pulp therapy on certain factors. Acta Odontol. Scand., *14*:Suppl. 21, 1956.

28. Sundquist, G.: Bacteriological Studies of Necrotic Dental Pulps. Umeå, University of Umeå, 1976.

29. Torneck, L. D.: Reaction of hamster tissue to drugs used in sterilization of the root canal. Oral Surg., *14*:730–747, 1961.

30. Tronstad, L.: Ultrastructural observations on human coronal dentin. Scand. J. Dent. Res., *81*:101–111, 1973.

31. Tronstad, L.: Tissue reactions following apical plugging of the root canal with dentin chips in monkey teeth subjected to pulpectomy. Oral Surg., *45*:297–304, 1978.

32. Tronstad, L., and Mjor, I. A.: Capping of the inflamed pulp. Oral Surg., *34*:477–485, 1972.

33. Tronstad, L., Andreasen, J. O., Hasselgren, G., et al.: pH changes in dental tissues after root canal filling with calcium hydroxide. J. Endodont., 7:17–21, 1981.

34. Verniehs, A. S., and Messler, L. B.: Calcium hydroxide induced healing of periapical lesions: A study of 78 non-vital teeth. J. Br. Endodont. Soc., *11*:61–69, 1978.

HENRY W. FIELDS
WILLIAM R. PROFFIT

7

ORTHODONTICS IN GENERAL PRACTICE

OBJECTIVE

This chapter has two major purposes: (1) to present diagnostic and treatment methods that can be employed by general practitioners of dentistry to produce sound treatment results for certain patients, and (2) to provide a general background of modern orthodontic treatment procedures for all types of patients, which will assist the generalist in appropriately referring patients for treatment by the orthodontic specialist. Since a sound diagnostic approach is necessary to select patients for treatment or for referral, emphasis is placed on diagnostic considerations. Efficient, successful orthodontic treatment procedures are certainly within the scope of general practice. The treatment procedures presented in this chapter are based upon sound physiologic and biomechanical principles and, if used appropriately, will enable a generalist to provide an important service for his patients.

THE ROLE OF THE GENERAL PRACTITIONER IN ORTHODONTICS

Until the past decade, there were no good data for the incidence of orthodontic problems in the United States. In the 1970s, two major studies carried out by the Division of Health Statistics of the United States Public Health Service were published. These studies provide by far the best picture of the occlusal status of American children and youths that has ever been available. From an epidemiologic point of view, both the United States Public Health Service (USPHS) studies used a very large sample, approximately 8000 children in each group. In addition to cataloguing the incidence of various kinds of problems, the USPHS studies used the Treatment Priority Index (TPI) to gain an estimate of the severity of malocclusion. Since the TPI does not take into account radiographic and other findings but is based entirely on the dental occlusion itself, it is not a perfect estimator of malocclusion severity. It does seem clear, however, that it is the best single index for this purpose, especially for large-scale studies. Data from the USPHS studies for children aged 6 to 11 years and youths aged 12 to 17 years are summarized in Tables 7–1 and 7–2.

From these data, it can be seen that approximately 40 per cent of American children and youths (and presumably, adults) have an occlusion close enough to ideal that it can be called entirely normal. These fortunate individuals possess a functional and esthetically pleasing dentition, one that is more likely to remain healthy. At the other

TABLE 7–1 Per Cent Incidence of Types of Malocclusion

	Age 6–11 (%)	Age 12–17 (%)
Overbite, 6 mm or more	6.6	10.3
Open bite, 2 mm or more	2.5	2.3
Overjet, 6 mm or more	16.7	14.9
Reverse overjet	0.8	0.9
Posterior crossbite, 4 or more teeth		
Lingual	1.1	1.5
Buccal	0.1	0.1
Malalignment	42.2	86.6

249

TABLE 7–2 Distribution of Treatment Priority Index Scores

	Age 6–11 (%)	Age 12–17 (%)
0 (normal)	24.4	11.0
1–3 (minor malocclusion)	39.0	34.8
4–6 (moderate malocclusion)	22.4	25.2
7–9 (severe malocclusion)	8.7	13.0
10 or more (very severe malocclusion)	5.5	16.0

end of the spectrum, a surprisingly large percentage of the United States population has a rather severe malocclusion. As can be seen from Table 7–2, a TPI score of 7 or greater, which indicates a severe malocclusion, occurs in 14.2 per cent of children and 29 per cent of youths. This high rate of malocclusion reflects, in part, the genetic diversity of the United States population. Malocclusion is less common in countries that have not experienced the mixing of population groups that is characteristic of this country.

Severe malocclusion may be due to malrelationships of the jaws or, less commonly, may result only from discrepancies in the dentition itself. Whether severe problems are skeletal, are dental, or are due to a combination of both, treatment is likely to require complex and prolonged procedures. Such patients are best treated by specialists in orthodontics.

There remains a rather sizeable number of individuals who have moderate irregularity or malpositioning of teeth. They cannot be said to have ideal or even reasonably normal occlusion, yet they do not have severe orthodontic problems. For some, treatment is not indicated. When orthodontic treatment is indicated, the treatment itself (though not necessarily the diagnosis) is likely to be straightforward and uncomplicated. These patients can and should receive orthodontic treatment within the framework of the general practice of dentistry. As we will point out later, this group includes both adults and children. The opportunity to provide orthodontic treatment services for adults as a part of the general practice of dentistry should not be overlooked.

If orthodontics is to be successfully incorporated into a well-run general practice, two things are necessary: (1) Diagnostic skill must be developed to the point of differentiating between relatively simple and relatively complicated orthodontic problems, a task that is not always easy; and (2) treatment skills in the use of effective appliances for movement of teeth must be developed. Of the two, diagnostic skill is more important. The general practitioner who is interested in orthodontics must be able to make difficult diagnostic decisions (with help, if needed, from referral and consultation), but he does not have to master difficult and complex treatment techniques.

Two different groups of patients requiring orthodontic treatment fit particularly well into general practice. The first group are adults who need tooth movement to facilitate and perhaps to make possible other dental treatment, as, for instance, in conjunction with fixed prosthodontics or periodontal care. Producing ideal occlusion through major orthodontic tooth movement is not the treatment objective for many adults. Typically, these patients require uprighting of molar teeth or repositioning of incisors to produce a better environment for periodontal maintenance and to allow the fabrication of more satisfactory splints and fixed bridges. Many of these patients can be treated within the framework of general practice rather than by orthodontic specialists.

The second major group who are potential candidates for orthodontic treatment within the framework of general practice are children with mixed-dentition space prob-

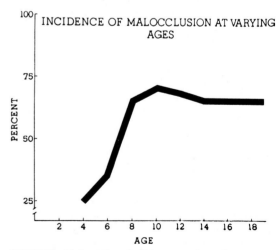

FIGURE 7–1 The incidence of malocclusion shows a dramatic increase from age 6 to 10 as crowding of permanent teeth becomes apparent. Malocclusion decreases slightly during the period of adolescence.

lems. As can be seen from Figure 7–1, the incidence of malocclusion increases sharply at the time the transition from the primary to the mixed dentition begins. The increase is due to the appearance of crowding and malalignment as the larger permanent incisors replace their primary predecessors. As with all types of orthodontic problems, space problems can be quantified as mild, moderate, or severe. A conscientious general practitioner can provide an important service by differentiating the less severe from the more severe space problems and by working with the children in his practice who have less severe problems that are amenable to relatively simple treatment. This is the type of care that in the past has been characterized as "preventive and interceptive orthodontics."

Widely differing opinions as to the value of preventive and interceptive orthodontic treatment continue to be offered. Some practitioners feel that early preventive and interceptive treatment can be helpful for a majority of children with malocclusion. Others feel equally strongly that early mixed-dentition treatment is not cost effective. Two recent studies, one carried out in conjunction with a Canadian growth study in Burlington, Ontario, the other based on the results of a special clinic at the University of Pennsylvania, shed some light on the role of preventive and interceptive treatment. The results from both studies are remarkably similar. In both, the conclusion was that about 15 per cent of all children would receive a satisfactory occlusal result from preventive and interceptive treatment alone. Since this is the type of treatment that reasonably can be provided in general practice, it appears that approximately one child in six in the typical general practice might be a candidate for some mixed-dentition orthodontic treatment.

In the final analysis, the decision as to which patients to select for treatment and the types of orthodontic treatment to be offered in a general practice is an individual one. The amount of orthodontics included in the general dental curriculum has increased at almost all schools in recent years but remains at a relatively basic level compared with subjects such as restorative dentistry. The principles of orthodontics are not readily grasped. Development of clinical judgment in orthodontics requires clinical experience. There is no way to develop "in-

stant orthodontics." It is unfair to the patient to attempt treatment without specific goals or the required expertise. Extensive, unproductive treatment of a child can reduce the child's potential for cooperation in definitive treatment at a later stage. Periodontal damage is a real possibility for adults in whom overly ambitious treatment is attempted. These considerations merely reinforce the importance of carefully selecting patients for orthodontic treatment. With mastery of the principles involved, both orthodontic care and intelligent orthodontic referral can become a rewarding part of the general practice of dentistry.

BIOLOGIC CONSIDERATIONS IN ORTHODONTIC THERAPY

Skeletal Growth and Development

For a review of the nature of craniofacial skeletal growth in the major growth sites, the reader is referred to Enlow's *Handbook of Facial Growth* and to the standard orthodontic texts. Three pertinent and frequently misunderstood points selected for special emphasis follow.

Dentofacial Proportions

1. *Dentofacial proportions are established at an early age and with few exceptions are maintained thereafter.* If a child has good facial proportions at age 3 years, it is highly likely that this also will be true at age 12 years and in adult life (Fig. 7–2). Conversely, if there is evidence of disproportionate or dysplastic growth at an early age, it is quite likely that this pattern will continue also. A number of exceptions to the general rule of this "constancy of the pattern" have appeared in the recent literature, and this in turn has led to confusion as to how often growth patterns change spontaneously or can be changed by treatment. Spontaneous change in growth pattern occurs and can be documented in individual cases, yet it is important to remember that this is a rare phenomenon. Only a small proportion of children, probably less than 5 per cent, who have good facial proportions at an early age develop skeletal jaw problems as they continue to grow. An even smaller number, probably 1 per cent or less, show spontaneous recovery from jaw dis-

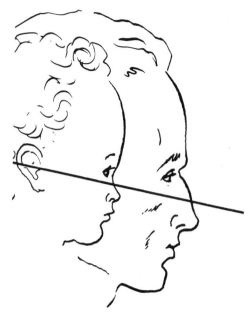

FIGURE 7–2   Illustration of the relative proportions of the face and cranium of the child and the adult. Note the great vertical change in the lower face from infancy to adulthood as the alveolar processes develop.

crepancies that were apparent at an early age. The moral of the story is that there is no reason to be greatly concerned that a child who does not have a skeletal Class II or Class III malocclusion at an early age will develop one. On the other hand, there is

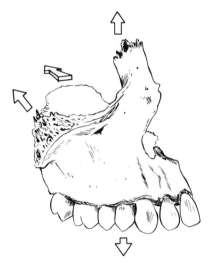

FIGURE 7–3   This three-quarter view of the maxilla indicates the direction of growth of this bone. The apparent downward and forward growth is actually due to translation of the maxilla as it "pushes off" the cranial base.

also no reason to suggest to a concerned mother that a child with a severe skeletal jaw discrepancy will "grow out of it," since the chances of this happening are extremely remote.

2. *Orthodontic treatment methods can alter jaw proportions by redirecting growth, but only when active growth is occurring.* Skeletal jaw discrepancies in children can be approached in two different ways conceptually, either by attempting to retard growth in areas that are growing too much or by stimulating the areas showing deficient growth. Until recently, although effective treatment based on restraining maxillary growth with extraoral force was well documented, there was little evidence for successful stimulation of maxillary (Fig. 7–3) or mandibular growth (Fig. 7–4). Recent results with forward traction to the maxilla appear to have demonstrated growth stimulation in this circumstance, and functional appliances that propel the mandible forward also may produce some growth changes. However, it is important that these findings be kept in perspective. Obviously, growth restriction works only when active growth is occurring. Even the most ardent advocates of growth-stimulating appliances admit that if effects are produced at all in older individuals, these effects are minimal. In short, despite encouraging results with some new types of appliances in recent years, it remains true that the only way to correct skeletal problems of any severity in adults is with surgery. An appliance that might produce significant growth changes in a 10-year-old child will have little or no result when used at 20 years of age.

3. *There is relatively more mandibular than maxillary growth at the time of the adolescent growth spurt.* Since the great majority of skeletal jaw discrepancies are Class II, the fact that the mandible tends to grow later than the maxilla can be very helpful. Any force system that impedes maxillary growth at the time that good mandibular growth is occurring can correct a skeletal Class II malocclusion. Extraoral force against the maxilla corrects a Class II problem in just this way. It is not so obvious but can be demonstrated easily that the functional appliances also have a headgearlike effect on the maxilla, effectively restraining maxillary growth. It is not necessary to stimulate mandibular growth to correct a Class II malocclusion when taking advantage of the naturally occurring differential between the maxilla and mandible.

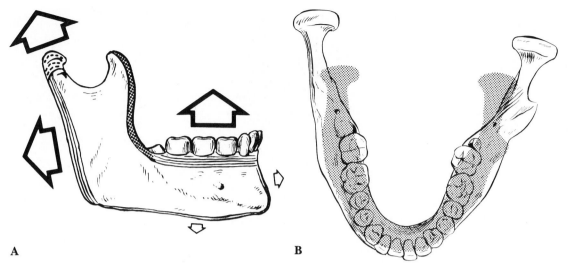

A   **B**

FIGURE 7–4 **A,** Schematic representation of mandibular growth, indicating the relative amounts of growth at various areas. The crosshatching on the anterior border of the ascending ramus indicates resorption to accommodate the erupting teeth. **B,** The sketch represents anteroposterior growth of the mandible. The general form is that of an expanding V, with minimal changes in the anterior region.

This same effect of greater mandibular than maxillary growth, however, makes it extremely difficult to control a Class III mandibular excess tendency in a child. A borderline Class III malocclusion present at age 10 or 11 can be easily converted to a true Class III malocclusion by the normal tendency for slightly greater mandibular (as opposed to maxillary) growth. Similarly, a Class III tendency that apparently has been controlled by treatment in the early teens may recur because of continued differential excess mandibular growth in the late teens.

If treatment to correct a skeletal malocclusion is to succeed, it must be carried out while active growth is continuing. Treatment of skeletal problems requires careful analysis of cephalometric films. Cephalometric diagnosis is highly desirable; cephalometric monitoring of treatment effects is mandatory for proper treatment. Treating skeletal growth problems without following the results cephalometrically is indefensible neglect of the patient. Although it is not likely that patients with skeletal growth problems will be selected for treatment within the framework of general practice, it is important for all practitioners to understand the appropriate timing for treatment, the importance of evaluating the patterns of growth at an early age, and the possibilities and limitations of growth modification treatment.

Dental Arch Growth and Development

It is important to understand the changes in arch dimension that occur during the development of the primary and permanent dentitions before one attempts to render treatment. Since it is apparent that faces increase in size, it is often mistakenly assumed that the arches increase in size in a similar and proportionate manner. In fact, the head and face do become larger, but not significantly in the areas of the dental arches between the first permanent molars that will accommodate the succedaneous teeth. The degree of accommodation of the permanent teeth and interarch adjustments also play important roles in determining the resultant spacing or crowding and occlusal relationships. Statistical descriptions of samples can describe mean development with some variation. Caries, restorative and surgical treatment, hard and soft tissue pathology, eruption disturbances, and aberrant tooth number superimposed upon these data describe the spectrum of clinical variability that lies beyond the scope of these longitudinal studies. Judgments based on these factors are the responsibility of the clinician.

Dental Arch Width Development

Dental arch width is usually measured from the cusp tip or mesiolingual cusp of

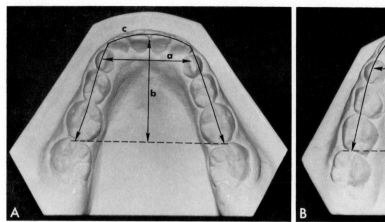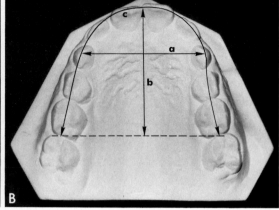

FIGURE 7–5 These casts (*A,* mandibular arch and *B,* maxillary arch) demonstrate *a,* arch width, *b,* sagittal arch length, and *c,* arch circumference in the mixed dentition.

antimeres or at the crest of the gingival tissue on the facial surface of the tooth (Fig. 7–5). During the primary dentition years there is some increase in the canine and primary molar arch widths. The maxillary intercanine width increases during permanent incisor and canine eruption by as much as 5 mm. This increase is partially due to some facial tipping of the crown of the permanent canine. Sizeable increases in mandibular intercanine width are confined to the period of eruption of the mandibular permanent incisors. At this time there may be as much as 3 mm of intercanine width increase. The intercanine width increases take place as a result of lateral and distal positioning of the primary canines into the mandibular primate space. In the primary molar and premolar region there is a consistent and steady increase in width throughout the primary-dentition and mixed-dentition years that is not necessarily associated with adjacent tooth eruption. Because of the lateral inclination of the maxillary alveolus, some changes result from skeletal growth of the arches combined with vertical tooth movement. Therefore, it appears that the maxillary and mandibular arches are somewhat wider in adolescence than they are in early childhood. These changes are not dramatic but will help accommodate the larger permanent teeth.

Dental Arch Anteroposterior Development

Dental arch length customarily has been measured from the midpoint or the most la-

bial point of the central incisor sagittally to the distal surface of the primary second molar or permanent premolar (Fig. 7–5). Initially, there is a decrease in arch length during the primary dentition years. When the permanent incisors erupt, there is a slight increase in arch length owing to their facial positioning. Finally, there is another decrease in arch length in both arches when the primary molars are replaced by the permanent premolars. Although arch length both decreases and increases, overall there is a decrease from the primary-dentition years to the permanent dentition.

Dental Arch Perimeter Development

The dental arch perimeter is the arch circumference or arc that the teeth will occupy over the alveolus. Arch circumference has been measured on the curve described by the incisal edges or facial cusp tips of the teeth between the second primary molars or permanent premolars (Fig. 7–5). This dimension consistently has been found to increase slightly in the maxillary arch and to decrease in the mandibular arch. Most of the decrease in mandibular arch circumference reflects the mesial shift of the molars and loss of the leeway space, which is the space differential between the large primary molars and the smaller premolars. These data imply that there is a change in arch form in both arches. The arches are shorter anteroposteriorly, wider and of slightly greater circumference in the maxillary arch, and of noticeably less circumference in the mandibular arch. The larger permanent teeth are accommodated by the small increase in arch width, developmental and primate spaces, and facial positioning of the incisors. One problem with these data is that it is tempting for the clinician to consider the dentition as an isolated entity. It must never be forgotten that the dentition resides within the face and is affected by facial changes.

Soft Tissue Growth and Development

It appears that the size and contour of the nose, lips, and chin also change during the adolescent and postadolescent periods. This development has not been examined carefully in the past, but currently some information is emerging. It is now apparent that the soft tissue development lags behind the growth of the face. Therefore, in the postadolescent period there is a noticeable amount of nose growth, especially in males. There are also hard and soft tissue changes at the chin, again predominatly in males. The vertical growth of the lips lags behind the vertical growth of the face, but it is ultimately of a greater magnitude than the vertical skeletal development. This results in an increased incidence of competent lips (lips that approximate at rest) in the postadolescent age group. The thickness of the lips also decreases in the postadolescent period and is more noticeable in females than males. The entire dental complex is encompassed by the soft tissue of the lips and cheeks. The influence of these soft tissues is interesting but not understood. Treatment changes that are accomplished by modification of the resting posture of these tissues have not been demonstrated in the posttreatment and postretention periods. It may be possible that this soft tissue matrix is a more important morphologic and functional factor than previously was believed.

The Integrated Final Form

Although some of the form of individual bones and the relationships of skeletal units are under genetic control, many effects of environmental forces on dental occlusal relationships may be observed. There is always an interaction between form and function, with each influencing the other.

A primary function of the oral-pharyngeal complex is respiration, and respiratory needs may ultimately influence dental occlusion. There is reason to believe that, in many individuals, tongue posture and perhaps the postural relationships of the head to the neck are influenced by reflex mechanisms that serve to maintain an adequate airway, and although it is true that the major function of oral structures is chewing and swallowing food, these movements also may be related to postural relationships dictated by respiratory needs. Similarly, speech may be affected by adjustments of the musculature required for respiration and swallowing.

Both experience and logic indicate that teeth are guided as they erupt by the normal position of the tongue and lips. Forces generated within the periodontal ligament also may be important. This concept is expressed formally in "equilibrium theory," which states that teeth assume positions in which forces acting on them are balanced, so that no tooth movement will occur (Fig. 7–6).

From the moment a tooth begins to erupt, it is subject to environmental forces that direct its eruptive path. As eruption continues, the teeth and alveolar processes grow vertically to an amount compatible with occlusal forces. Erupting teeth are also deflected buccally or lingually in response to tongue and lip activity. This mechanism allows the functional environment to influence dental arch form and occlusal relationships directly and ensures that teeth assume positions that are in harmony with the musculature. Malocclusions, however undesirable the arrangement

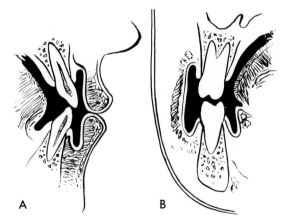

A   B

FIGURE 7–6 Diagrams indicating the opposing muscular forces on the dentition. Teeth and alveolar bone are positioned during growth by labial or buccal and lingual forces. If the muscular balance is altered at any time of life, stability of the teeth will be affected and tooth movement may occur.

of teeth may seem, are stable. The teeth are in positions of balance between the forces that operate on them.

PRINCIPLES OF ORTHODONTIC DIAGNOSIS

Profile Relationships

One important obligation of the dentist who is performing an orthodontic diagnosis is the assessment of the face in all planes of space. The anteroposterior conformation of the profile and lip protrusion is usually examined first. Unfortunately, less frequently, the total face is considered in the vertical and transverse dimensions. A complete evaluation includes all aspects of the face that will envelop the skeletal and dental components that must reside within the soft tissue.

Skeletal Relationships

Many times the face reflects the underlying skeletal components. Therefore, a thorough facial analysis should provide clues to the skeletal relationships. The Angle classi-

fication of malocclusion, which was originally based solely on the relationship between the permanent first molars, has served long and well, primarily because of the simplicity with which it can be used. It could not have survived, however, if it had not been compatible with newer findings regarding skeletal relationships. Terms such as "skeletal Class II" and "mild skeletal Class II relationships with Class I molars" are in common use. This descriptive terminology has arisen from the custom of describing skeletal maxillomandibular relationships in terms of the molar relationships that normally accompany them.

It is important in classifying malocclusion to evaluate not only the molar relationship but also the skeletal relationship that underlies it. Treatment procedures correlate with the skeletal situation, not just with the arrangement of the teeth in relation to each other. From the point of view of skeletal classification, both normal occlusion and Class I malocclusion are characterized by a correct relationship of the maxilla and mandible and are accompanied by a somewhat straight or mildly convex profile (Fig. 7–7).

A skeletal Class II malocclusion is one in

CLASS I

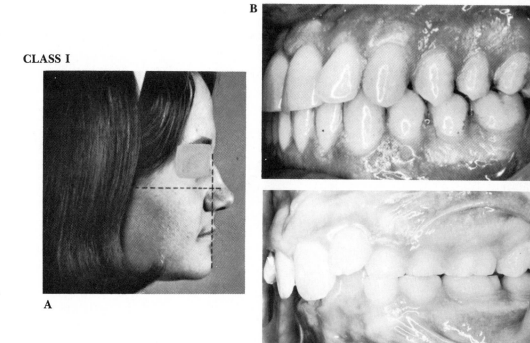

FIGURE 7–7   *A,* A Class I, or orthognathic, profile and *B,* the normal molar relationship and occlusion or *C,* the malocclusion that accompanies it.

Illustration continued on opposite page

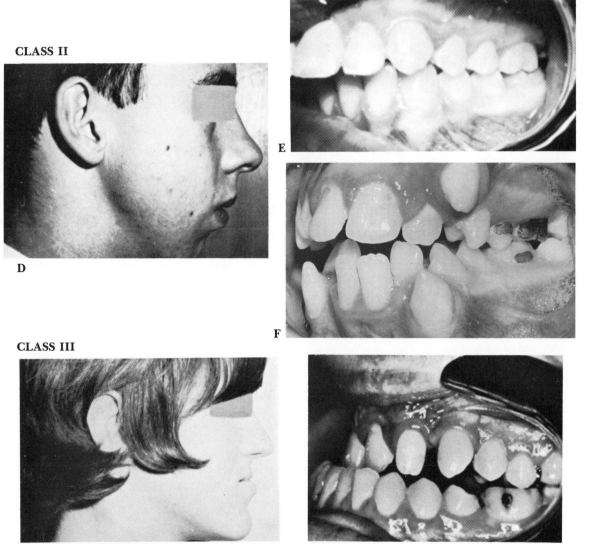

CLASS II

D

E

F

CLASS III

G

H

FIGURE 7–7 *Continued D* represents a Class II, or retrognathic, profile, accompanied by either *E* Class II, division 1 malocclusion (protrusive maxillary incisors) and Class II molar relationship or *F* Class II, division 2 malocclusion (upright central incisors and protrusive lateral incisors) and Class II molar relationship. *G* represents the Class III, or prognathic, profile and *H* the Class III molar relationship that accompanies it.

which the mandible is small or positioned posteriorly in relationship to the maxilla, one in which the maxilla is large or positioned anteriorly in relation to the mandible, or one in which some combination of the two has occurred. A retrognathic or very convex profile usually is found in conjunction with this type of skeletal relationship.

The same type of skeletal classification applies to Class III malocclusion. A skeletal Class III relationship is one in which the mandible is large or positioned anteriorly

relative to the maxilla and is, therefore, anteriorly positioned; or in which the maxilla is small or positioned posteriorly to the mandible; or in which some combination of the two has occurred. This profile is prognathic or concave with a very prominent chin.

Dentoskeletal Relationships

The appropriate Angle molar classification usually accompanies the compatible skeletal pattern. Edward Angle originally based his classification on the premise that the anteroposterior position of the maxillary first molar in the maxilla was constant. It is known now that, although the position of the maxillary first molar is indeed remarkably stable, this tooth, or any other, can be positioned forward or backward on the bone that supports it. Both normal occlusion and Class I malocclusion have Class I molar relationships. Class I malocclusion, which represents 60 to 70 per cent of all malocclusions, is due to a poor relationship of the teeth to the jaws and to each other.

Class II malocclusions appear as either Division 1 or Division 2, a notation that describes the position of the anterior teeth. Class II, Division 1 malocclusions have proclined maxillary central and lateral incisors and make up approximately 20 per cent of malocclusions. Class II, Division 2 malocclusions have upright maxillary central incisors and proclined maxillary lateral incisors and represent less than 5 per cent of all malocclusions. A Class II molar relationship, as Angle described it, is sometimes found when the maxilla and mandible are quite well related, the problem being due solely to the relationship of the teeth. In this situation there has usually been space loss that allowed the maxillary posterior teeth to move anteriorly. A good key to this type of discrepancy is obtained by observing the canine relationships. Since tooth loss in the posterior segments sometimes does not disturb the original canine relationships, the canines may provide a clue to the original malocclusion.

A Class III molar relationship generally accompanies a Class III skeletal pattern and occurs as 3 to 7 per cent of malocclusions. It is possible that normal skeletal relationships can be present when Class III molar relationships exist. Usually this patient has had tooth loss and movement of the mandibular posterior teeth in an anterior direction. Once again the clue that this type of situation is not a true Class III malocclusion sometimes can be obtained from the canine relationship.

The relationship of teeth in each dental arch to the bone that supports them must also be considered in the orthodontic diagnosis. This refers to the relationship of the maxillary teeth and their alveolar process to the basal or supporting bone of the maxilla and of the mandibular teeth to the bone of the mandible. The relationship of teeth to supporting bone is particularly important in the anterior regions of both dental arches. The incisor teeth may assume a variety of anteroposterior positions, leaning forward or backward, depending upon two factors: the amount of room available to support the teeth and the degree of protrusion or forward positioning of the teeth that the musculature will accept. This leads to an important yet confusing concept: Crowding of incisor teeth and protrusion of incisors are different aspects of the same problem.

Imagine that 60 mm of space is available around the dental arch from first molar to first molar if the teeth are positioned upright over the ridge. If the sum of the widths of the teeth that will occupy that space is 64 mm, there are three possibilities for arranging these teeth: (1) The teeth may remain upright over the ridge, in which case there will be 4 mm of crowding, probably in

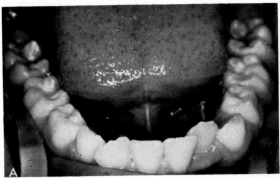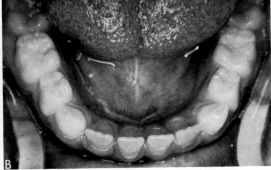

FIGURE 7–8   Both children have the same amount of mandibular space for the permanent teeth. *A* shows lower anterior crowding (4 mm discrepancy) with the teeth generally upright. *B* shows lower teeth in alignment, but protrusion of the incisors. If these teeth were brought back to an upright position, they would also be crowded. (Courtesy of Dr. M. Gellin.)

the anterior region; (2) the incisor teeth may lean forward, so that they no longer stand upright but protrude along the arc of a larger circle, in which case no crowding will be observed; or (3) there may be a combination of protrusion and crowding (Fig. 7–8). The size of the teeth and the amount of space available to accommodate them remain the same in all three situations, yet the arrangement of teeth varies from considerable crowding to no crowding at all. The difference in the three cases lies in the environmental influences on the dentition. If the musculature is such that the balance of forces on the teeth hold them upright, crowding occurs. If the musculature will tolerate protrusion rather than crowding, then the teeth can lean forward, aligning themselves. Many individuals who have crowding of incisors also have some degree of protrusion, and in the diagnosis this must be evaluated before the amount of space available over basal bone can be estimated.

To a certain extent the evaluation of protrusion is subjective. One of the reasons for concern about excessive protrusion is its detrimental effect on facial appearance. The amount of dentoalveolar protrusion that is usually found, and which is therefore esthetically acceptable, varies greatly from one racial or ethnic group to another. Nonetheless, an evaluation of the amount of protrusion is essential when one is making an orthodontic diagnosis.

It may be assumed that when crowding

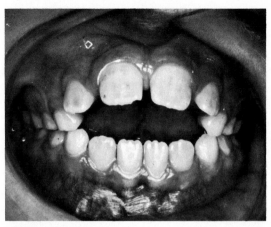

FIGURE 7–10 Open bite due to finger-sucking habit in a child.

and protrusion occur together, further expansion (enlargement) of the dental arches is not likely to be tolerated by the musculature. On the other hand, if minor crowding occurs without protrusion of the teeth, moderate expansion may very well be a possible form of orthodontic treatment.

In addition to determining the anteroposterior relationship of the dentition to the underlying facial skeleton, it is necessary to look at the vertical relationship of the dental arches. A deep anterior overbite is often accompanied by an exaggeration of the curve of Spee in the lower arch, with lower incisors being relatively supererupted while eruption of the premolars is inhibited (Fig. 7–9). Overbite problems typically accompany Class II malocclusions, but they also occur in situations in which no skeletal problem exists. When open bite malocclusions occur, the lower arch is usually flat, whereas the upper arch has an exaggerated curve of Spee (Fig. 7–10). In this situation, the eruption of upper incisors is impeded, but the eruption of posterior teeth is facilitated. Open bites may accompany any type of malocclusion.

In both instances in which problems of anterior vertical relationships occur and there is no evidence of skeletal malrelationships, habit patterns may be implicated in the cause. The relationship of anterior open bite to thumb-sucking is well known. In such cases the anterior open bite tends to develop over a period of time, as eruption of anterior teeth is impeded by the presence of the thumb in the anterior part of the mouth. Concurrently with this, the mouth is typi-

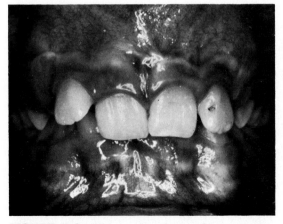

FIGURE 7–9 This patient has a deep anterior overbite with an excessive curve of Spee in the lower arch. The lower arch is completely hidden by the upper anterior teeth in this view.

cally held open while at rest, and excessive eruption of posterior teeth occurs. The relationship of deep overbite problems to habit patterns is not so clear-cut. Speech problems are frequently associated with open bite malocclusions but are less common when deep overbite occurs. There is little reason to believe that speech per se can be a factor in producing malocclusions, but normal speech may be difficult in the presence of either a severe anterior open or closed bite.

Dental Relationships

Most cases of malocclusion arise from problems of tooth to jaw (dentoskeletal) or jaw to jaw (skeletal) relationships. It is also possible to have malocclusions due solely to dental factors. These malocclusions occur most commonly when some teeth are congenitally missing or reduced in size. The presence of supernumerary teeth may lead to the same problem, as in many situations in which individual teeth exhibit unusual

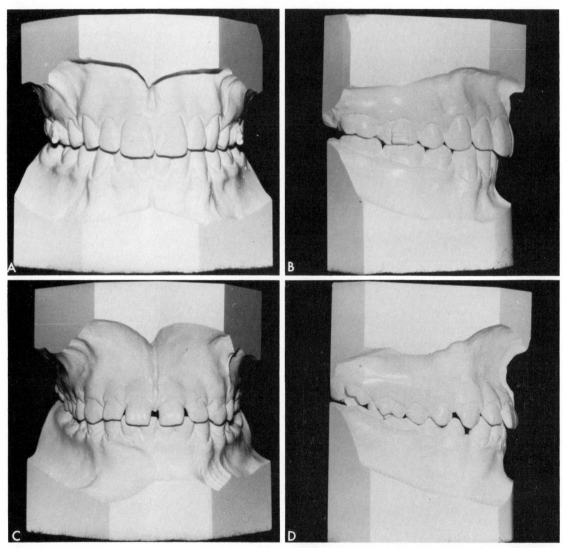

FIGURE 7–11 These casts show relative maxillary anterior excess tooth size discrepancy (**A** frontal and **B** lateral view). The molar and canine relationships are Class I, but the upper teeth are too large mesiodistally for the lower teeth, resulting in excessive overbite and overjet. **C,** frontal view and **D,** lateral view casts demonstrate a relative mandibular anterior excess tooth size problem. Again the molar and canine relationships are Class I, but the mandibular teeth are relatively too large for the maxillary teeth, and spacing of the maxillary anterior teeth results.

shape, enamel hypoplasia, or other types of pathologic change.

A more subtle type of malocclusion due solely to dental factors is malocclusion caused by "tooth size discrepancy" (Fig. 7–11). Some individuals have dentitions that simply cannot be made to occlude well because of the discrepancies in relative sizes of the teeth, either within one arch or in both arches. The effect is similar to that seen when a denture set-up is attempted with one mold for the upper teeth and a mold of a different size for the lower teeth. Minor tooth size discrepancies, seen in most natural dentitions, have no serious effects on occlusion. A small percentage (perhaps 5 per cent) of more severe malocclusions, however, are related to teeth that simply cannot be made to fit together in an ideal relationship or even an approximation of it.

There are two ways to check for tooth size discrepancies in the natural dentition. The best and most straightforward way is to do a "diagnostic set-up" with casts of the natural teeth by cutting the teeth off a cast (being careful not to reduce the dimensions of the contact point) and then setting the teeth in wax to see how they can be made to fit together (Fig. 7–12). A less time-consuming method is to check the sizes of the teeth of the individual patient again and prepare tables of proportional relationships (Table 7–3).

A diagnostic set-up simplifies treatment

TABLE 7–3 Tooth-size Ratios*

If the Sum of the Widths of the Six Mandibular Incisors Is:	The Sum of the Widths of the Six Maxillary Incisors Should Be:
31 mm	40.1 mm
32	41.4
33	42.7
34	44.0
35	45.3
36	46.6
37	47.9
38	49.2
39	50.5
40	51.8
41	53.1
42	54.4

If the Sum of the Widths of the Twelve Mandibular Incisors, Canines, and Premolars Is:	The Sum of the Widths of the Twelve Maxillary Incisors, Canines, and Premolars Should Be:
78 mm	85.6 mm
80	87.8
82	89.9
84	92.0
86	94.2
88	96.4
90	98.6
92	100.8
94	103.0
96	103.0
98	105.2
100	107.4

*Discrepancies of less than 2 mm from these ratios are not significant. (From Bolton, W. A.: Disharmony in tooth size and its relation to the analysis and treatment of malocclusion. Angle Orthodont. *28*:113–130, 1958.)

planning in cases of tooth size discrepancy. Orthodontic correction of such malocclusions is difficult. It often involves asymmetric extraction of teeth (for example, two upper premolars and one lower incisor), reduction in size of some teeth by interproximal stripping, or increase in the size of some teeth with resins or crowns (Fig. 7–13).

Supporting Structures

An evaluation of the supporting structures is critical to the diagnosis. Not only are the usual periodontal criteria important, such as the kind and amount of tissue present, but additional considerations, for example, the height and quality of frenal attachments and the thickness and shape of the alveolus, play critical roles in future treatment. The quality of oral hygiene also must be considered.

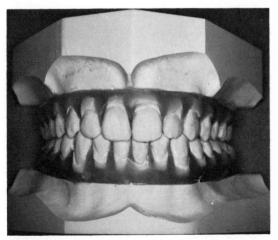

FIGURE 7–12 A diagnostic set-up is made by carefully cutting the teeth from a plaster cast and remounting them in wax to the best possible occlusion. This procedure is particularly useful in tooth size discrepancy problems.

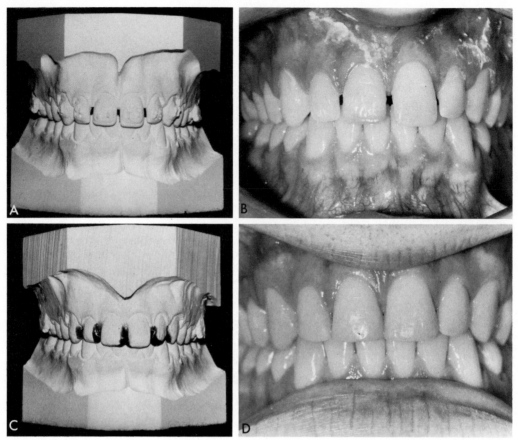

FIGURE 7–13 *A,* the finishing stages of orthodontic treatment and *B,* a relative mandibular anterior excess and maxillary spaces at debonding. *C,* This cast shows the proposed resin build-ups, represented by blue inlay wax, that will increase the size of the maxillary teeth. *D,* the intraoral view of the completed resins. This semipermanent solution to tooth size discrepancies can be quite helpful in the young permanent dentition when other treatments are impractical.

DIAGNOSTIC METHODS FOR CHILDREN

Selection of Patients and a Framework for Diagnosis

Success or failure in orthodontics in general practice depends on intelligent case selection. A dentist in general practice typically expects to treat 80 to 90 per cent of restorative and prosthetic problems and refers only a small percentage of patients to a specialist in these areas. A much higher percentage of potential orthodontic patients will be referred. If the practitioner is able to select the easier problems to treat himself, referring more difficult cases to an orthodontist, he will enjoy providing orthodontic care and will do a good job. If he unwittingly se-

lects the difficult cases to treat himself, both he and his orthodontic patients will soon be in trouble.

General dentists can improve the chances of successful orthodontic treatment by the use of a framework that helps them first to focus objectively on the patient's orthodontic problems and then to focus on the best treatment. Simple but complete records that meet the needs of limited treatment are necessary. These records help ensure that any problems presented by the patient are not overlooked. Orthodontic diagnosis requires the following minimum records: (1) medical and dental histories, (2) profile and extraoral examinations, (3) intraoral examination, (4) full-mouth radiographs, and (5) dental casts.

The patient's problems are best assessed

by using a systematic approach to diagnosis. One useful approach is the Ackerman-Proffit system, which covers each plane of space or component of malocclusion (profile, perimeter, anteroposterior, transverse, and vertical). After these problems have been identified, reasonable treatment solutions can be listed for each problem. Interestingly, many times a common solution will remedy several problems. A systematic diagnosis will direct the practitioner's thinking and aid in effective treatment planning. Although one or more problems may exist, the general practitioner should address problems whose correction will definitely benefit the patient. Limited treatment is not a substitute for necessary full treatment.

Medical and Dental Histories

As with all dental procedures, medical and dental histories are required before orthodontic treatment is begun. Since the orthodontic patient has usually been seen previously for other reasons, much of the necessary information may have already been obtained. A medical history should include a brief review of organ systems and birth defects, serious illness, allergies, immunizations, and accidents.

Although many medical problems do not contraindicate orthodontic treatment, special precautions are often necessary. The presence of any condition that would make the practitioner reluctant to perform oral surgery for the patient is also a signal for consultation or referral for orthodontic care.

Three relatively common situations illustrate the effect of medical problems on orthodontic treatment. A patient with a history of congenital heart disease or rheumatic fever will probably require antibiotic coverage during the fitting, cementation, and removal of bands. Gingival hyperplasia may develop in response to the use of orthodontic appliances in a child who is taking phenytoin (Dilantin) to control seizures. Even if hyperplasia has not previously been a problem, repeated gingivectomies may be required. Tooth movement in the presence of severe gingival hyperplasia is almost impossible. Patients with metabolic disease (of which diabetes is the most frequently seen) may show abnormal tissue response to the orthodontic forces and must be carefully observed. Such patients represent a poor treatment risk for orthodontics in general practice.

In the dental history it is important to note any episode of dental trauma, endodontic treatment, ankylosis of teeth, or temporomandibular joint problems. A nonvital tooth observed after orthodontic treatment has begun may be difficult to explain even if it is unrelated to tooth movement. An endodontically treated tooth may be moved, but the risk of tooth resorption is increased. Ankylosed teeth will not respond to orthodontic forces. If a patient has a history of ankylosis, the dental x-rays should be carefully studied for additional bony bridges. Great care must be taken in planning force application in these patients. Finally, the changing occlusion during tooth movement may exacerbate an old temporomandibular joint disorder, and the dentist who has adult orthodontic patients must be prepared to cope with this problem.

Profile Analysis

The initial steps in orthodontic diagnosis should be: (1) an estimate of the skeletal maxillary and mandibular position; (2) an estimate of the skeletal relationship between the maxilla and mandible; (3) an evaluation of the relationship between the teeth and each jaw and their supporting bone (dentoskeletal relationship); (4) an assessment of the vertical facial relationships; and (5) an appraisal of the transverse facial relationships.

Profile photographs of several children are shown in this section. It is apparent that some information is available from these extraoral views that will enable one to evaluate the skeletal composition. First, one needs to determine the position of the maxilla and mandible as retrusive, normal, or protrusive. This is best accomplished when the patient is in an upright position in the dental chair. Figure 7–7A shows a Class I patient with good maxillary and mandibular position. When a line is extended from the soft tissue bridge of the nose perpendicular to Frankfort horizontal for this patient, it passes through the anterior extent of the maxilla and the mandible. If the maxilla or mandible are behind this line, they are retrusive. If they are anterior to this line, they are protrusive. When the maxilla is anterior to the mandible, a Class II skeletal relationship is present (Fig. 7–7B). If the mandible is anterior to the maxilla, a Class III skeletal pattern is present (Fig. 7–7C). From this analysis one can describe the position of the

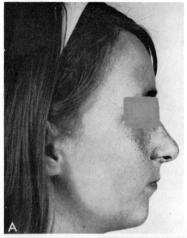

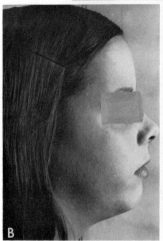

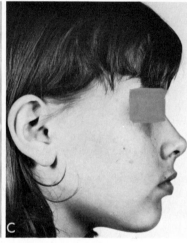

FIGURE 7–14 *A, B,* and *C,* All three girls have a normal skeletal relationship but exhibit increasing dental protrusion. The profile in *C* is typical of bimaxillary dental protrusion.

maxilla and mandible and their relationship to each other. It is also evident that skeletal relationships can be caused by either the upper or the lower jaw or both. Therefore, as mentioned, each jaw must be evaluated.

Similarly, especially if the denture bases are palpated, the relationships between the teeth and their bony bases can be established with reasonable accuracy by observing the lip profile. Here, the key is the relationship of the lower lip to the chin and the upper lip to the nose and the anterior maxilla. If the lower lip is well ahead of the chin so that it is protruding forward even at rest, the incisors are probably protruding to support the lip. The same is true for the upper lip; the incisors are positioned forward on the maxilla if the upper lip is prominent relative to the nose and the rest of the face (Fig. 7–14). It may be useful to use a prepared form to guide one's analysis until this process is automatic (Fig. 7–15).

Another factor to consider is the relative size of the nose and chin button. A small nose or chin button can make the lips appear to be more prominent. Alternatively, a large nose and chin button can cause the lips to appear to be less prominent or allow a more prominent lip posture to be acceptable. These relationships are critical not only at the time of diagnosis in childhood but also when projecting future appearance. It appears that most individuals develop larger noses and chin buttons in the postadolescent period. This is especially true of males who also have bony apposition at the brow ridge areas. At the same time, the soft tissue overlying the lips is becoming thinner. Therefore, the soft tissue profile will change with or without treatment. Potentially problematic contours should be recognized and treatment aimed at not worsening the appearance.

It is also important to evaluate the patient's vertical facial relationships. The mid-

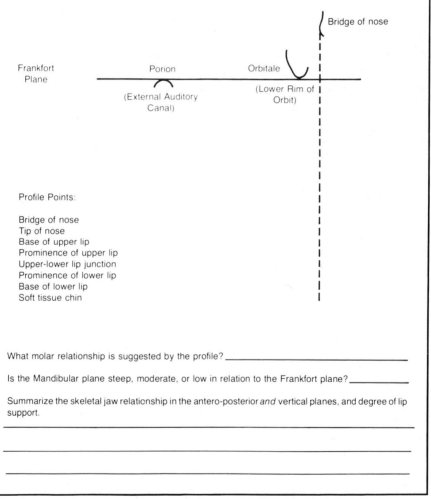

UNIVERSITY OF NORTH CAROLINA AT CHAPEL HILL
SCHOOL OF DENTISTRY

FACIAL PROFILE ANALYSIS

Draw the patient's profile. Mark the position of each profile point relative to the imaginary vertical reference line, which is perpendicular to the visual axis or Frankfort plane; then connect your points to complete the profile drawing.
For the drawing, the patient should be in, or very near, the terminal hinge position.

Bridge of nose

Frankfort Plane

Porion

Orbitale

(External Auditory Canal)

(Lower Rim of Orbit)

Profile Points:

Bridge of nose
Tip of nose
Base of upper lip
Prominence of upper lip
Upper-lower lip junction
Prominence of lower lip
Base of lower lip
Soft tissue chin

What molar relationship is suggested by the profile? _____

Is the Mandibular plane steep, moderate, or low in relation to the Frankfort plane? _____

Summarize the skeletal jaw relationship in the antero-posterior *and* vertical planes, and degree of lip support.

_____

_____

_____

FIGURE 7–15 A facial profile analysis may be completed by drawing the patient's soft tissue profile relative to the Frankfort horizontal plane and vertical perpendicular to Frankfort horizontal through the bridge of the nose; this helps to assess the relative position of the maxilla and the mandible. The vertical reference line usually contacts the soft tissue of the maxilla and mandible in Class I patients. Patients whose maxillas and mandibles lie anterior or posterior to the vertical reference line have protrusive or retrusive problems with their respective jaws.

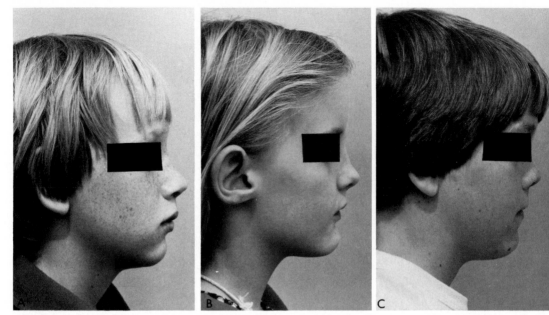

FIGURE 7–16 These three children demonstrate different vertical facial proportions. *A,* This boy has normal relationships, since the middle third of his face (the distance from the bridge of the nose to the base of the nose) is equal to the lower third of his face (the distance from the base of the nose to the bottom of the chin). The outline of his mandibular plane (lower border of the mandible) also appears to have a normal inclination. *B,* This girl demonstrates a reduced lower facial third and a flat (more horizontal) mandibular plane. *C,* This boy demonstrates an increased lower facial third and a steep (more vertical) mandibular plane.

dle third of the face and the lower third of the face should be approximately equal, or the lower third may be slightly smaller than the middle third. Another method of evaluating the vertical relationships is to consider the mandibular plane, which describes the lower border of the mandible. This plane is usually steep in cases of long lower-face height and flat in short lower-face height (Fig. 7–16).

The transverse relationship should be assessed with the patient reclining and observed from above. This enables one to evaluate the upper face to the cranium and the mandible to the upper face (Fig. 7–17). Although all people exhibit minor amounts of asymmetry, this systematic evaluation technique will demonstrate significant deviations. At this time the maxillary and mandibular dental midlines should be assessed to their respective jaws.

Dentists who have been trained to use this systematic method of facial profile analysis can do it reliably with patients of all ages, but the technique is more useful with adolescent patients than with younger patients. Patients who have maxillary retrusion and

Class III skeletal relationships are hard to evaluate by this technique. This probably reflects the lack of attention to the maxillary skeletal position. Patients with long lower face height are also difficult to evaluate. It would probably be wise to request an orthodontic consultation for those patients with vertical discrepancies in order to accurately evaluate the underlying skeletal relationships.

Intraoral Examination

It is not possible to diagnose all conditions from either an intraoral examination or diagnostic casts. Therefore, an intraoral examination is necessary to complement the diagnostic cast. It is essential to carefully count the teeth and to distinguish between primary and permanent dentitions. This procedure will help identify missing, extracted, supernumerary, fused, or geminated teeth. The size of the teeth should also be evaluated. As described previously, although generalized large or small teeth may be a problem, inconsistencies in one dentition, especially in one arch or between two arches, may preclude a good occlusion with-

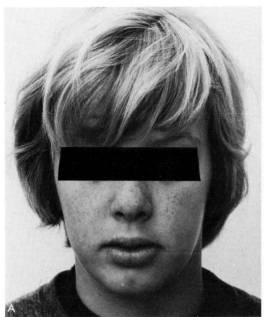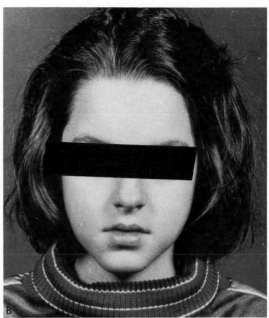

FIGURE 7–17 *A,* The boy shows normal transverse relationships, whereas *B,* the girl demonstrates facial asymmetry. Note that her upper face is symmetric but that the center of her chin is approximately 3 mm to the right of her upper facial midline.

out carefully planned tooth movement. Identification of hypoplastic teeth or teeth with aberrant shape is necessary. Most often, maxillary lateral incisors and mandibular second premolars exhibit problematic morphology.

Molar and canine relationships should be noted in the primary, mixed, or permanent dentitions. These two relationships will help solve diagnostic problems even when teeth have migrated to new positions following tooth loss. The accuracy of the diagnostic casts can also be verified by this information. Overbite and overjet should be measured or carefully estimated.

Midlines have already been evaluated in relation to the face. As part of the intraoral examination, they should be related to each other in centric relation and centric occlusion. This type of evaluation identifies these static relationships and the differences between them. Midline changes from centric relation to centric occlusion are related to mandibular shifts. Since lateral shifts and posterior crossbites are intimately related, it is necessary to evaluate the teeth in crossbite in centric relation and centric occlusion. This will diagnose definitively the type of posterior crossbites.

Owing to a shift of the mandible from centric relation to centric occlusion, a unilateral crossbite may be caused by bilateral constriction. To distinguish the difference between unilateral and bilateral problems, a careful clinical examination is necessary. By guiding a patient's mandible to the centric relation position and closing the teeth to initial contact, the dentist can observe the buccolingual relationships of the posterior teeth and canines as well as the maxillary and mandibular midline relationships. When the patient closes to the centric occlusion position, the relationships of the posterior teeth, the canines, and the midlines are again observed. If there is a bilateral crossbite in centric relation and centric occlusion, the patient usually has a bilateral maxillary constriction (Fig. 7–18). If there is a bilateral crossbite in centric relation accompanied by a lateral shift of the mandible, a change in midline relationships, and a unilateral crossbite in centric occlusion, the patient also has a bilateral maxillary constriction (Fig. 7–19). Facial asymmetry in centric occlusion and excessive muscle tension on one side of the face may also be clues to a mandibular lateral shift. If the patient has a unilateral crossbite in centric relation and centric occlusion, he usually has a true unilateral maxillary constriction (Fig. 7–20).

Anterior shifts from centric relation to centric occlusion are also important. Some

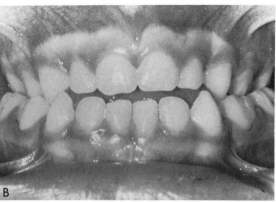

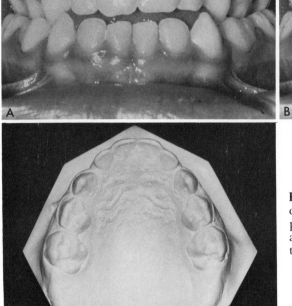

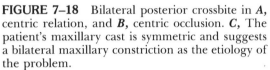

FIGURE 7–18 Bilateral posterior crossbite in *A,* centric relation, and *B,* centric occlusion. *C,* The patient's maxillary cast is symmetric and suggests a bilateral maxillary constriction as the etiology of the problem.

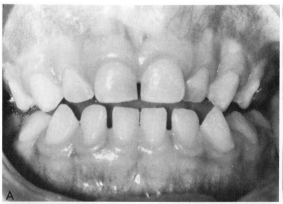

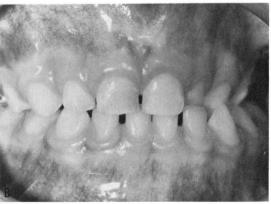

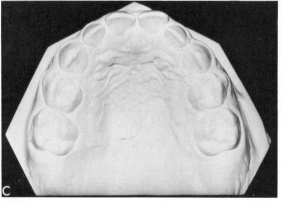

FIGURE 7–19 *A,* Bilateral edge-to-edge posterior occlusion in centric relation with a shift of the mandible to the left and *B,* a unilateral posterior crossbite in centric occlusion. *C,* The symmetric maxillary casts suggest a bilateral maxillary constriction as the etiology of the problem.

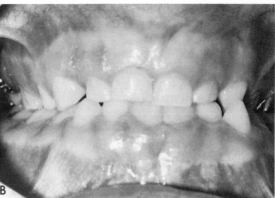

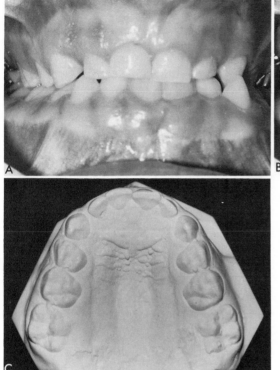

FIGURE 7–20 Unilateral left posterior crossbite in *A*, centric relation, and *B*, centric occlusion. *C*, The maxillary cast confirms a true unilateral constriction of the patient's primary left canine and primary first and second molars.

individuals exhibit Class I molar and canine relationships and an edge-to-edge incisor relationship. Because of the incisor interference, an anterior shift is necessary for these patients to reach a comfortable centric occlusion position. This centric relation to centric occlusion shift results in an anterior crossbite and Class III molar and canine relationships. This is defined as a pseudo–Class III relationship (Fig. 7–21) and is not indicative of a true Class III skeletal or dental problem.

Finally, the quality and amount of keratinized tissue must be evaluated. The dentition is no more sound than the supporting struc-

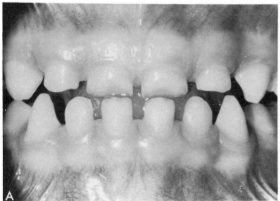

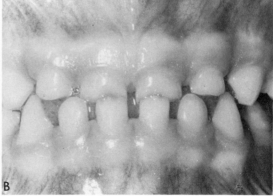

FIGURE 7–21 The complete primary dentition of this patient illustrates a pseudo–Class III relationship. In *A*, centric relation, the canines are in a Class I relationship but there is incisal interference, which results in *B*, an anterior shift of the mandible, an anterior crossbite, and a Class III canine relationship in centric occlusion.

tures. A band of attached keratinized tissue should be present that is not under the stress of an adjacent frenum. It is also important that erupting teeth emerge through a band of keratinized tissue. Absence of this tissue at eruption will be followed by periodontal pathology. Inflammation of the tissue should also be noted prior to orthodontic treatment. This condition usually worsens during therapy, especially when it is present in the pretreatment period. A score that documents oral hygiene and soft tissue inflammation or a bleeding point index helps to assess the conditions objectively. The risk of permanent loss of or decrease of attachment is not merited as a result of orthodontic treatment.

Record Analysis

Radiographs

A complete radiographic examination of the mouth is essential to document and diagnose possible complicating conditions related to the orthodontic treatment. Detection of pathology should be the first use of the radiographs, but several other factors are also important. First, the number and position of all teeth present and forming can influence the timing and direction of treatment. It is frequently important to predict from radiographs how long it will be before primary teeth exfoliate and permanent teeth erupt. The remaining root structure of the primary tooth can serve as a partial guide, since a primary tooth is usually not exfoliated until its root is almost completely resorbed. The best guide, however, is the degree of root formation of the permanent tooth.

Eruption of the permanent tooth usually takes place when its root is approximately one-half to two-thirds completed. About 1 year is required for completion of each third of the roots of the canine and premolar teeth. If only the crown of a premolar tooth is completed, it may be estimated that approximately 2 years will be required for completion of two thirds of the root and that the tooth will not erupt under normal circumstances until this period has elapsed. Similar calculations may be done for other teeth.

It is also important to be able to predict when the permanent successor will erupt after a primary tooth has been lost prematurely. In this situation, two factors may be used as a guide: the degree of completion of the root of the permanent successor (as mentioned previously) and the amount of alveolar bone overlying the permanent successor. Early removal of a primary tooth will accelerate the eruption of the permanent successor (1) if the permanent tooth is within 12 months of normal eruption, as determined by its degree of root formation, or (2) if periapical infection or other causes have resulted in the destruction of much of the alveolar bone overlying the permanent tooth. In the first instance the permanent tooth is approaching "alveolar emergence," with the crown having penetrated or almost penetrated the alveolar process. In the second instance, in which there has been destruction of overlying alveolar bone, an artificial "alveolar emergence" has been produced.

The general rule is that loss of an overlying primary tooth 6 to 12 months early (at a time when its permanent successor has nearly penetrated the alveolar bone and has one half to two thirds of its root completed) will accelerate the eruption of the permanent tooth. If, however, a primary tooth is lost prematurely at a time when its permanent successor is not well formed and is nowhere near alveolar emergence (as, for instance, in the case of an primary central incisor avulsed at 3 years of age), the eruption of the permanent successor may be delayed rather than accelerated. This delay may be related to slow resorption of the bone over the unerupted permanent tooth.

Eruption of permanent teeth in an unusual location, "ectopic eruption," sometimes occurs and is a cause of considerable concern when it appears. Ectopic eruption of a permanent first molar may be the cause of early loss of a primary second molar or impaction of the permanent first molar (Fig. 7–22). Ectopic eruption of permanent incisors is also seen. Many cases of so-called ectopic eruption of incisors are merely instances in which permanent incisors have been displaced from their normal position because of crowding in the dental arch (Fig. 7–23).

In some instances one or two primary or permanent teeth in a quadrant fail to erupt; this is due to ankylosis. The clinical manifestations of this entity are: (1) location of the occlusal position of the questionable tooth

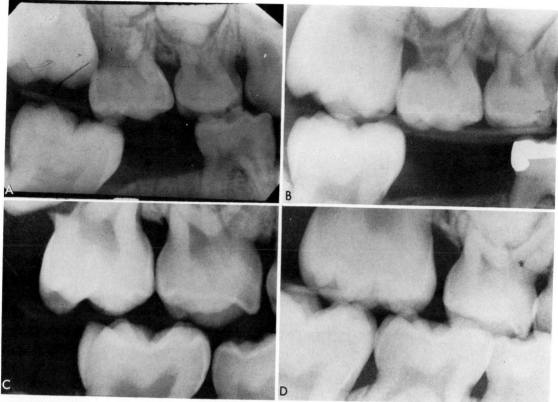

FIGURE 7–22 *A,* Ectopic eruption of the permanent maxillary first molar caused resorption of the distal root structures of the primary second molar. *B,* Since the amount of resorption was minimal, the eruption continued and the condition "self-corrected." Radiograph *C* shows the permanent maxillary first molar causing resorption of the distal root of the primary second molar and *D* shows subsequent loss of the primary molar and space. Watchful waiting may be indicated in some cases that demonstrate minimal resorption, but tooth loss and space loss may occur in some cases.

below the occlusal plane, (2) no detectable mobility of the tooth, and (3) a firm sound upon percussion. Occasionally a lack of periodontal ligament space can be discerned on a radiograph (Fig. 7–24). Many times this is impossible, however, since the area in which cementum and alveolar bone are joined is very narrow. Although ankylosed primary teeth usually exfoliate in a normal fashion, it is possible to have delayed exfoliation and defection of the erupting permanent tooth. The opposing tooth may supererupt to maintain contact with the ankylosed tooth, which can lead to occlusal irregularities.

Study Casts

Study casts for orthodontic purposes allow study of the patient's alignment and space problems. By forcing excess impression material to flow into the vestibular areas, impressions for orthodontic casts include as much as possible of the alveolar processes. Casts are most useful when a symmetric base aids the eye in detecting asymmetries in the dentition (Fig. 7–25). These records also are helpful in case presentations and during treatment to evaluate progress.

The occlusion, posterior alignment, and arch form should be evaluated from the casts. Transverse asymmetries and the location of arch constrictions measured from casts are key diagnostic criteria for posterior crossbite correction. When evaluating alignment, rotations versus faciolingual positioning is an important distinction. Careful observation of the relationships of central groove and facial surfaces of adjacent posterior teeth can aid in the evaluation of alignment. Also, the faciolingual positioning needs further classification as a tipped tooth or a bodily malpositioned tooth. This is also

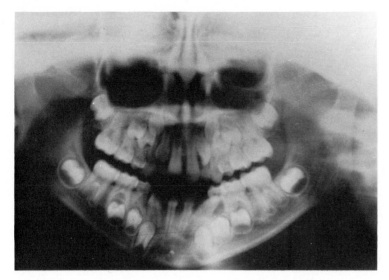

FIGURE 7–23 Ectopic eruption of the permanent mandibular lateral incisors resulted in the loss of the primary lateral incisors and canines and the imminent loss of the primary left first molar. The patient also had a severe space discrepancy.

an important distinction since the method of correction will be completely different.

Space Analysis

Probably the most common use of the casts is for a space analysis. Most interceptive orthodontic treatment provided by the general practitioner is performed for patients whose problems lie in the relationship of teeth to supporting bone but who have no skeletal abnormalities. Such problems typically involve crowding or the threat that it will occur.

In order to evaluate crowding during the mixed-dentition period, it is necessary to be able to predict how much room will be available for the remaining permanent teeth when they erupt and how much space will be required to align them in a good occlusal relationship at that time. This space analysis prediction is usually needed after the first permanent molars and the permanent incisors have erupted but before the permanent canines and premolars have erupted.

Early loss of a primary molar normally calls for placement of a space maintainer to prevent mesial drift of posterior teeth and posterior drift of anterior teeth with subsequent space closure. If any drift of teeth has occurred before the child is seen for dental treatment, placement of a space maintainer is not enough. Only by means of a space analysis procedure can one determine if

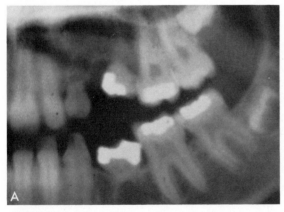
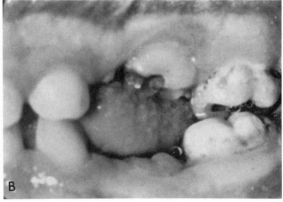

FIGURE 7–24 *A,* This radiograph demonstrates ankylosed maxillary and mandibular primary second molar teeth below the occlusal plane and obliteration of the periodontal ligament space. *B,* The corresponding clinical photograph also points out the lack of continued eruption of the primary molars.

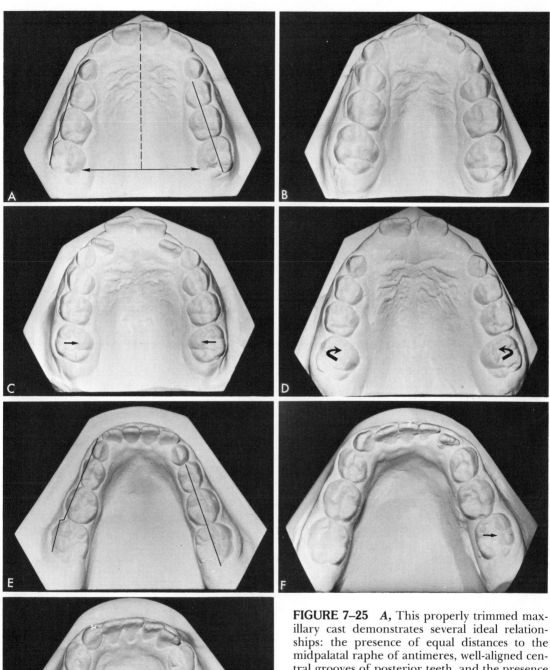

FIGURE 7–25 *A,* This properly trimmed maxillary cast demonstrates several ideal relationships: the presence of equal distances to the midpalatal raphe of antimeres, well-aligned central grooves of posterior teeth, and the presence of a facial offset of the permanent first molars. Absence of these relationships should be clues to the etiology of malocclusion. *B,* This cast demonstrates maxillary skeletal constriction and a reduced palatal transverse dimension. *C,* These maxillary first permanent molars lack the proper facial offset and are lingually positioned. *D,* This cast reveals a lack of facial molar offset due to mesiolingual rotation of the permanent maxillary first molars. *E,* This mandibular cast reveals ideal relationships of a facial offset of the permanent mandibular first molars and well-aligned central grooves. The casts in *F* and *G* demonstrate permanent mandibular first molars that are facially positioned and distofacially rotated, respectively. Discriminating between these problems will aid in the choice of effective therapy.

UNIVERSITY OF NORTH CAROLINA AT CHAPEL HILL
SCHOOL OF DENTISTRY

SPACE ANALYSIS FORM

Patient's Name: _____   Date: _____

SECTION 1
AVAILABLE MANDIBULAR SPACE

RIGHT   LEFT   *Arch Segment*
                            Lengths

a: _____ mm

b: _____ mm

c: _____ mm

d: _____ mm

TOTAL: _____ mm

SECTION 2
MANDIBULAR INCISOR WIDTH

#23: _____ mm

#24: _____ mm

#25: _____ mm

#26: _____ mm

TOTAL: _____ mm

SECTION 3
AVAILABLE MAXILLARY SPACE

Arch Segment
Lengths

e: _____ mm

f: _____ mm

g: _____ mm

h: _____ mm

RIGHT   LEFT   TOTAL: _____ mm

SECTION 4
MAXILLARY INCISOR WIDTH

#7: _____ mm

#8: _____ mm

#9: _____ mm

#10: _____ mm

TOTAL: _____ mm

SECTION 5
MANDIBULAR SPACE ANALYSIS

a. **TOTAL SPACE AVAILABLE** *(from Section 1)* _____

b. **SUM OF MAND. INCISOR WIDTHS** *(from Section 2)* _____

c. **SUM OF LEFT CANINE & PREMOLARS** *(estimated below from mand. incisors)* _____

d. **SUM OF RIGHT CANINE & PREMOLARS** *(estimated below from mand. incisors)* _____

e. **TOTAL SPACE REQUIRED** *(b + c + d)* _____

f. **DISCREPANCY** *(a − e)* _____

SECTION 6
MAXILLARY SPACE ANALYSIS

a. **TOTAL SPACE AVAILABLE** *(from Section 3)* _____

b. **SUM OF MAX. INCISOR WIDTHS** *(from Section 4)* _____

c. **SUM OF RIGHT CANINE & PREMOLARS** *(estimated below from mand. incisors)* _____

d. **SUM OF LEFT CANINE & PREMOLARS** *(estimated below from mand. incisors)* _____

e. **TOTAL SPACE REQUIRED** *(b + c + d)* _____

f. **DISCREPANCY** *(a − e)* _____

SECTION 7
SKELETAL JAW RELATIONSHIP
(from Facial Profile Analysis)

( ) CLASS I;   ( ) CLASS II;   ( ) CLASS III

SECTION 8
OCCLUSION OF PERMANENT FIRST MOLARS

RIGHT SIDE ( )   ANGLE CLASS I ( ) LEFT SIDE
           ( )   END-TO-END   ( )
           ( )   ANGLE CLASS II ( )
           ( )   ANGLE CLASS III ( )

SECTION 9
MOLAR SHIFT *(From end-to-end to Class I)*
For Skeletal Class I only

RIGHT SIDE + LEFT SIDE = TOTAL SHIFT
_____ mm + _____ mm = _____ mm TOTAL

SECTION 10
LIP POSTURE *(from Facial Profile Analysis)*
( ) ACCEPTIBLE;   ( ) PROTRUSIVE;   ( ) RETRUSIVE

MANDIBULAR INCISOR POSITION
(from Facial Profile Analysis and casts)
( ) ACCEPTIBLE;   ( ) PROTRUSIVE;   ( ) RETRUSIVE

INTERPRETATION OF NUMERICAL RESULTS *(based on observations in Sections 7 — 10)*

ESTIMATES FROM: Moyers, R. E., Handbook of Orthodontics. 3rd Ed. Chicago, Yearbook Medical Publishers, Inc., 1973.

Total Mandibular Incisor Width *(from Section 2)*		19.5	20.0	20.5	21.0	21.5	22.0	22.5	23.0	23.5	24.0	24.5	25.0	25.5	26.0	26.5	27.0	27.5	28.0	28.5	29.0
Predicted Width of Canine & Premolars	MX *(75%)*	20.6	20.9	21.2	21.3	21.8	22.0	22.3	22.6	22.9	23.1	23.4	23.7	24.0	24.2	24.5	24.8	25.0	25.3	25.6	25.9
	MN *(75%)*	20.1	20.4	20.7	21.0	21.3	21.6	21.9	22.2	22.5	22.8	23.1	23.4	23.7	24.0	24.3	24.6	24.8	25.1	25.4	25.7

FIGURE 7–26   Step-by-step space analysis form helps to calculate the space discrepancy and includes other relevant factors that the clinician needs to consider when evaluating space problems.

space maintenance will be adequate, if an active orthodontic appliance must be used to regain space lost through drift, or if no treatment is indicated.

When completing a space analysis, the dentist makes several assumptions that must be recognized. One assumption is that all permanent teeth are forming and that the unerupted teeth have a size correlated with the erupted incisors. Another assumption is that prediction tables apply to the patient under examination. Differences in ethnic backgrounds make application of these prediction tables very risky. The size of the dental arches measured on the casts is considered to be stable and unchanging. This leads to the assumption that all growth in the mandible will occur away from the alveolar ridge and that the incisors are in a fixed position. Although some canine width increase does occur, these small changes in arch circumference can be ignored. On the other hand, in Class II and Class III occlusions, incisor positions have been documented to change owing to compensation of the dentition for the skeletal growth pattern. This movement of incisors can have an effect on the arch circumference that needs to be considered. With these assumptions in mind, one can proceed to the execution and interpretation of the space analysis. The following five steps are necessary in making a mixed-dentition space analysis. A prepared form is helpful to outline these steps (Fig. 7–26).

1. *Determination of the amount of space available for the permanent teeth.* The technique for measuring available space is illustrated in Figure 7–27. The arch length is measured with dividers, or a sharpened Boley gauge, from the mesial of one first permanent molar to the mesial of the first permanent molar on the opposite side of the arch. Each arch is measured in four segments.

2. *Estimation of the size of the unerupted permanent teeth.* This may be done in several ways. One method is to obtain the size of unerupted canines and premolars from published prediction tables, which give the cor-

relation between the size of lower incisors and canines and premolars. Estimates from the table are accurate (in most cases) to ±1 mm.

In lieu of the extensive prediction table, another form of prediction is also possible. This method, developed by Tanaka and Johnston, uses the sum of the mesiodistal width of one mandibular central and lateral incisor plus 10.5 mm to predict the size of the unerupted canine and two premolars in one mandibular quadrant. For the maxillary arch, the sum of the mesiodistal width of one mandibular central and lateral incisor plus 11.0 mm will predict the size of the unerupted canine and two premolars in one maxillary quadrant. This method sacrifices some accuracy but is very easy to employ.

The size of the unerupted teeth also may be measured directly from the radiographs. This method is especially useful with racial groups for whom the tables do not apply. Because the rotation and severe tipping of unerupted teeth can cause significant errors despite correction for magnification, it is probably better as a rule to use radiographs as a guide in interpreting the prediction tables. Even if radiographs of excellent quality are available, it is wise to check the tables and films against each other.

3. *Determination of the total space required for the succedaneous permanent teeth.* This is the sum of the widths of individual permanent incisors, which can be measured directly on the casts, plus the estimated size of unerupted canines and premolars.

4. *Initial calculation of arch circumference*

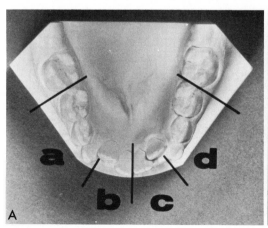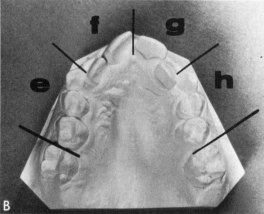

FIGURE 7–27 The space available is determined by adding the sum of the space in segments a, b, c, and d in the mandibular arch *(A)* and segments e, f, g, and h in the maxillary arch *(B)* as measured over contact points and cusp tips.

discrepancy by subtracting space required from the space available. This step is completed on the prepared form and is subsequently corrected on the basis of several important variables.

5. *Application of the necessary corrections to the amount of space available.* The interpretation of these figures is the most important factor in this diagnosis. Although the amount of space available around the dental arches can be measured directly, two corrections must be made in many cases. The first of these is the correction for space that may be required in a Class I skeletal patient to shift the lower molar forward from end-to-end to a Class I molar relationship (Fig. 7–28). An end-to-end molar relationship is normal in the primary and mixed-dentition periods, although a shift of the molars into a Class I relationship may take place any time after the eruption of the permanent first molars. The amount of space required for molar shift should be calculated on an individual basis. There is a great deal of individual variation in the space required to correct the molar relationship, and the use of averages leads to unnecessary errors.

It is also necessary to note the effect on available space of any anterior or posterior movement of incisors. If incisors are highly protrusive, it may be desirable to retract them to a less protrustive position. This will mean arranging them along the perimeter of a smaller arc and will thus decrease the amount of available space, thereby increasing the crowding. If incisors have been displaced lingually as a result of sucking habits or other causes, it may be equally desirable to allow them to come forward into a more normal position. This would increase the amount of available space. Arch circumference is said to be adequate when sufficient space exists around the arch, from the mesial of one first permanent molar to the other, to accommodate the intervening teeth without crowding and without excessive protrusion of the teeth and the alveolar process; otherwise, an arch circumference discrepancy exists.

Because the lower arch is enclosed by the upper, mandibular arch circumference is critical in the determination of arch circumference. Adequate lower arch circumference will mean adequate upper arch circumference if molar relationships are symmetric and if correct size relationships exist between the upper and lower teeth. Space analysis, therefore, should always be done for the mandibular arch if questions about space arise. Analysis of the maxillary arch may be omitted if there are no questions of asymmetry or unusual space loss in the maxilla.

When an arch circumference discrepancy is discovered, it indicates that some treatment procedure will be needed to prevent crowding of the permanent teeth. Movement of teeth to increase arch circumference (arch expansion) is one possibility; reducing the required space, by extracting teeth and closing excess space, is the other. The position of the first molars and the amount of intervening space around the arch are the diagnostic keys.

Cooperation and Hygiene

An evaluation of the patient's potential for cooperation with appliance wear and oral hygiene is also essential. An immature patient or one with poor oral hygiene can affect not only the type of appliance selected but also the decision of whether or not to initiate treatment. It is important that this appraisal be made before treatment is begun.

DIAGNOSTIC METHODS FOR ADULTS

The observations made for orthodontic diagnosis in an adult are the same as for a child, i.e., evaluation of profile, skeletal,

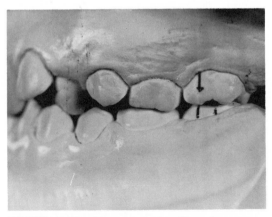

FIGURE 7–28 Space must be allowed to correct the molar relationship from end-to-end to complete cuspal interdigitation in patients with Class I skeletal patterns. The amount of space needed for this correction should be calculated for each individual and entered on the space analysis form.

dentoskeletal, and dental relationships and of supporting structures. The chief difference in an interpretation is that growth changes are no longer a factor to be considered. All changes will therefore have to be produced through tooth movement or through surgical repositioning of jaws or alveolar segments. Orthodontic diagnosis for an adult may be considerably simpler than for a growing child, but treatment (which is discussed in detail later) is likely to require a more direct attack on the relatively static adult problem than would be employed in treating children.

TREATMENT PLANNING

Treatment should be aimed at a specific goal that has been identified on the problem list. The treatment goal should be a specific end point that is easily recognizable by the practitioner. Goal identification will tend to eliminate "creeping ambition," which extends treatment for an unreasonable amount of time with little therapeutic benefit. Treatment should be aimed at an existing or imminent problem. Limited treatment offered by the general practitioner probably should not extend over 6 to 9 months. Treatment demanding more time than this could be part of an efficient full-treatment approach. When the treatment decision has been made, a simple and efficient appliance should be chosen. It is also wise to set a re-evaluation date, a point by which treatment should be completed or a significant amount of improvement in the condition should be observable. If treatment is not proceeding as planned, or if the anticipated treatment completion date is rapidly approaching without resolution of the problem, a systematic reappraisal of the problems, goals, and appliance design is needed. This will eliminate unrealistic and lengthy treatment due to misdiagnosis or poor cooperation. If careful thought and imagination are applied, treatment planning can be one of the most stimulating aspects of orthodontic therapy.

PRINCIPLES OF ORTHODONTIC THERAPY

The Nature of Orthodontic Tooth Movement

Orthodontic tooth movement is made possible by metabolic changes in the periodontal ligament in response to pressure or tension directed against it. The metabolic changes in the ligament, in turn, lead to remodeling of the adjacent alveolar bone, which ultimately allows the tooth and its attachment apparatus to move slowly through the bone.

Two major variables determine the response to orthodontic force: the duration of the force and its magnitude. Although discussions of force response usually begin with magnitude, duration is probably more important and deserves to be discussed first.

Force Duration

The periodontal ligament is well adapted to withstand forces, light or heavy, that are applied for short periods of time. Short force applications occur normally during mastication of food, when heavy biting force may be brought to bear for an instant during each cycle of chewing movements. Periodontal ligament fibers are arranged to resist occlusal force. To a large extent, the vascular network within the periodontal ligament space serves to cushion the force of chewing. This cushioning occurs as blood and tissue fluids are expressed from the periodontal ligament area when tissues are compressed, returning an instant later when the pressure is withdrawn. Even when a tooth is in traumatic occlusion and is repeatedly stressed by occlusal forces, orthodontic tooth movement does not occur in response to these intermittent pressure applications.

Just as examination of patients with traumatic occlusion demonstrates that intermittent forces of short duration are not effective in moving teeth, experience with removable appliances that are not worn all the time clearly shows that constant force is not necessary for tooth movement. If a removable appliance is worn 24 hours a day, tooth movement will occur more rapidly than if the same appliance is worn only 12 hours a day, but there will be a response to 12 hours of force application. Recent experimental work with animals indicates that after approximately 4 hours of force application to a tooth, chemical changes, including elevated levels of cyclic nucleotides, can be detected in the periodontal ligament space. The signal to begin differentiation of osteoclasts and osteoblasts probably is closely related to these chemical changes, so it seems reasonable that the absolute minimum time of force application to produce any result is in the vicinity of 4 to 6 hours. Results with human patients wearing removable appliances corroborate this experimental result. For all practical purposes, a patient must wear a removable appliance approximately half the time if it is to have any real effectiveness in producing tooth movement.

Force Magnitude

The other major variable in orthodontic tooth movement is the amount of orthodontic force. If a light force is applied to the tooth so that the periodontal ligament is compressed but blood flow is not completely eliminated, cells within the periodontal ligament space differentiate into osteoclasts rapidly (within 48 to 72 hours). These cells produce dissolution of bone mineral and destruction of bone matrix. When osteoclastic activity has removed bone adjacent to the periodontal ligament, movement of the tooth in that direction can occur. On the opposite side, where the periodontal ligament was stretched rather than compressed, a similar phenomenon takes place, except that in this instance new bone is laid down adjacent to the periodontium through the action of osteoblasts. The tooth moves, as resorption of bone occurs on one side of the root and deposition occurs on the other, until it has reached a position where there is no longer significant net force against it.

If force against the tooth is so heavy that blood flow in the affected parts of the periodontal membrane is completely cut off, death of cellular elements within the membrane in this area occurs, and differentiation of cells within the periodontal membrane into the needed osteoclasts and osteoblasts is prevented. After a delay of several days, osteoclasts differentiate within the marrow spaces of the alveolar bone adjacent to the cell-free areas of the periodontal membrane. Alveolar bone is then removed by "undermining resorption," with the osteoclastic attack coming from the underlying marrow spaces rather than from the periodontal membrane side. Eventually, large bony spicules are removed, and tooth movement can occur.

When heavy force causes undermining resorption, tooth movement may occur quite rapidly after an initial period of no response and will usually be accompanied by marked looseness of the teeth due to excessive widening of the periodontal membrane space. Tooth movement is least traumatic and most effective when orthodontic forces are light enough so that direct, rather than undermining, resorption occurs.

The absolute magnitude of force is of course important, but the most significant factor in determining the periodontal reaction is the pressure, or force per unit area, that is developed in the periodontal ligament. The area of the periodontal membrane over which force is distributed is determined by the manner in which force is delivered to the tooth. Application of force against a single point on the crown of the tooth will cause the tooth to begin to tip around a center of rotation located approximately one third of the way up the root from the apex, and relatively small areas of compression and tension in the membrane will develop. Such tipping forces must be kept light in order to prevent undesirable periodontal membrane changes. If, however, force is applied at two points on the crown of the tooth (through a "couple") so

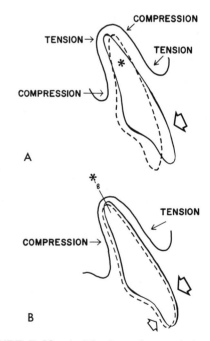

FIGURE 7–29 *A,* Tipping of a tooth is caused by application of a simple force to the crown. Note the areas of tension and compression of the periodontal membrane. The center of rotation is indicated by an asterisk. *B,* This illustration shows the application of force for bodily movement. In order to achieve bodily movement, a "couple" is necessary; that is, a force in the desired direction of movement must be coupled with a smaller force opposing the direction of movement.

that the tooth is moved bodily (Fig. 7–29), the force is distributed throughout the periodontal membrane. It follows that a greater amount of absolute force will have to be used in order to create the same amount of force per unit area within the periodontal membrane. Thus, light force should be used while tipping movements of teeth are being produced, but heavier forces are likely to be required during the production of bodily movement or other movement of roots of teeth, as in paralleling roots after extraction of teeth or backward movement (torque) of roots of anterior teeth.

Light force applied continuously (which requires that springs remain active after teeth begin to move) is quite effective in producing tooth movement because the periodontal membrane is constantly kept in a state leading to the production of bony changes. With this type of force, tooth movement continues without frequent appliance adjustments. It can be seen, then, that from the point of view of the patient's welfare and from that of efficient practice, light continuous forces are best for producing tooth movement. In rare situations, heavy intermittent force may be useful. It is important that heavy forces be relieved after very slight tooth movement so that periodontal damage does not occur.

If tooth movement is accomplished carefully, minimal pain and discomfort accompany it. In most instances, teeth that are being moved orthodontically become somewhat sore (and particularly sensitive to pressure during chewing) for a few days after activation of the appliances. As tooth movement proceeds, radiographs reveal a widened periodontal membrane space, accompanied by an increase in mobility of teeth. Neither severe pain nor marked looseness of teeth should ever be associated with orthodontic therapy. If these symptoms occur, excessive force is probably being used.

A mild pulpal reaction, usually the result of mild hyperemia, often follows (or accompanies) orthodontic tooth movement, producing an increased sensitivity of the tooth or teeth to thermal stimuli. Severe pulpal reactions are almost never associated with orthodontic tooth movement, even when excessive force is used.

Concepts of Anchorage

Anchorage may be defined as the resistance areas (teeth or other structures) against which a reactive force will be placed as teeth are moved. Whenever orthodontic tooth movement is undertaken, anchorage is an important consideration, for the laws of motion are as valid in this situation as in any other: "For every action there is an equal and opposite reaction."

When the resistance to the movement of one tooth comes solely from resistance to tipping by another tooth, it may be said that simple anchorage exists. Often simple anchorage is at the same time reciprocal anchorage, in which the movement of one tooth serves simultaneously as the anchorage for the movement of another. This occurs, for instance, when central incisors are being tipped by a rubber band pulling their crowns together. Simple anchorage, represented by the left central incisor, serves as resistance for the orthodontic movement of the right central incisor, and vice versa, in this reciprocal situation.

Ordinarily, simple anchorage is not enough unless reciprocal tooth movement is desired. Reinforced anchorage of some sort must be obtained. This may be done in several ways. One method is to incorporate several teeth into the anchor unit opposing a tooth that is to be moved. If one central incisor is pitted against another, both will move in approximately equal amounts. However, if one central incisor is pitted against an anchor unit composed of the other central incisor, lateral incisor, and canine, the unit with three teeth has been reinforced, so that it has more anchorage value than the single incisor. The single tooth will obviously move a great deal more than the three-tooth unit; however, it is important to realize that, even in this situation, both units will move.

A second way of increasing anchorage is to arrange appliances so that the tooth or teeth that are to be tipped are balanced by an anchor unit of teeth that must be moved bodily if the teeth are to be moved at all. Since it is much more difficult to move a tooth bodily than to tip it, this maneuver can greatly increase anchorage value. This type of anchorage reinforcement is produced typically by ligating anchor teeth to a tightly fitted rectangular arch. (See, for example, the section on molar uprighting, p. 326.)

A third method of reinforcing anchorage is to include teeth in the opposing dental arch or in structures outside the oral cavity. With removable appliances, the soft tissues covered by the appliances may contribute slightly to reinforcement of anchorage. In

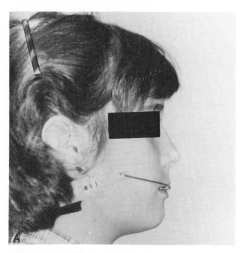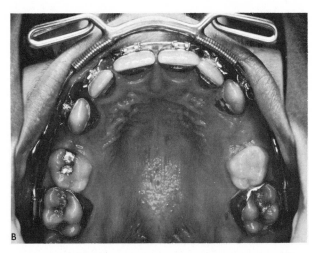

FIGURE 7–30 *A,* The cervical (Kloehn) headgear is an extraoral device with the outer bow worn outside the mouth attached to a neck strap. *B,* The outer bow attaches anteriorly to an inner bow of smaller wire diameter. The inner bow has a stop either bent or soldered to it that rests against tubes on the molar bands. The inner bow should not contact the maxillary incisors.

many situations, desired tooth movements are impossible unless some sort of extraoral anchorage can be obtained. This is possible through the use of facebow or headgear appliances, which attach to the teeth, extend out of the corners of the mouth, and are fastened behind the head or neck (Fig. 7–30).

The dentist who ignores anchorage runs the risk of finding that he has accomplished tooth movement, but into areas other than those where it was wanted. The laws of action and reaction, not the dentist's wishes, determine which teeth move and which ones do not.

Orthodontic Forces

Differential Forces

It has already been pointed out that optimal tooth movement is obtained with light continuous forces, which stimulate the periodontal membrane to react but do not cause changes of such magnitude in the membrane that it cannot function. Excessive force applied against teeth produces responses from outside the periodontal membrane and delays tooth movement while undermining resorption occurs. This explains what might otherwise seem a paradoxical situation: The degree of force applied to units of teeth may determine which units move and which units do not, in a manner that would seem to confound classic concepts of anchorage.

Differential force can best be explained by an example. Suppose that a canine tooth is to be retracted distally into a space available for it, and that the second premolar and first permanent molar are available as anchor units. The appliances are arranged so that the canine will be tipped distally, and reinforced anchorage will be provided by the molar and premolar, which must move bodily. If a spring is now placed between the canine on the one hand and the molar and premolar on the other and is activated correctly, optimal force levels will produce compression and tension in periodontal membrane areas around the canine so that its tipping is facilitated. The same force will be distributed through the periodontal membranes of the molar and premolar in a way that will cause minimal response in any single area around these teeth. The canine will move, whereas the molar and premolar will remain in relatively constant position.

With the same appliances, if the spring is activated to produce a much heavier force, cell-free areas requiring undermining resorption will be created around the canine. Canine movement will be greatly impeded temporarily by the cell-free areas, while the heavier force will now bring large periodontal membrane areas around the molar and premolar to levels that facilitate tooth movement. In this situation, the canine will not move as well as it did in the previous example, although the "anchor" teeth will tend to move freely.

It is possible to take advantage of this phenomenon in some situations, but it is rare that heavy force against a tooth should be used deliberately to temporarily increase its anchorage value. It is much more likely that anchorage values will be exceeded and anchor teeth inadvertently moved because too much force has been used. Differential force, in short, is often brought into play through error; it leads to undesirable types of tooth movement.

Single Versus Two-Point Contact

As was pointed out earlier, when a force is placed against the crown of a tooth with a single point of contact, the tooth tends to tip, rotating around an axis between the crown and the root apex. In this sort of tipping movement, the crown of the tooth moves in the direction desired by the dentist, but the apex of the tooth tends to move in the opposite direction. In order to control movement of the apex of the tooth, or in order to move the tooth bodily, it is necessary to apply force to the crown of the tooth at more than one point simultaneously. This requires either two-point or multiple-point (area) contact.

When removable appliances are used, it may be desirable to design springs so that more than one point on the tooth surface is contacted. Even when this is done, it is difficult to produce anything but tipping movements with such appliances. When orthodontic bands are placed on teeth, attachments that allow area contact and, with it, more precise control over root movements, may be used. It may be accepted as a general rule that removable appliances are adequate for tipping movements but that fixed appliances, which allow more precise delivery of forces to teeth, are essential for root movements.

Retention

At its best, orthodontic tooth movement causes widening of the periodontal membrane space, slight looseness of the teeth, and a degree of disruption of the periodontal membrane fibers. It is thus necessary after moving a tooth orthodontically to retain it in its new position for a period of time until rearragement of periodontal fibers and remodeling changes in the alveolar process can be completed.

Retention of some type is indicated at the completion of tooth movement in every case. There must be something to hold a tooth in its new position until a degree of stability can be developed (Fig. 7–31). It is not always necessary to use an appliance, however. After correction of a crossbite, the tooth is stabilized in its new position by occlusal forces, so that no retention appliance is usually needed.

How long retention will be required is determined by several factors. One of these is the type of tooth movement that has occurred. Reitan has shown that periodontal membrane fibers require 3 to 4 months to complete their reorientation. Gingival elastic fibers tend to be stretched during tooth movement, and these rearrange much more slowly. Teeth that have been rotated are notoriously difficult to keep in a corrected position, probably because of the great degree of stretching of gingival fibers that occurs during rotation.

A major advance in retention of orthodontically rotated teeth was the development of the "circumferential supracrestal fiberotomy" (CSF) procedure by Edwards and independently by other workers. This simple surgical procedure is used to sever the supracrestal gingival fibers following rotation, so that the major cause of rotational relapse is eliminated. A number of reports in the literature now document that CSF enhances stability following correction of rotations. Since there are few hazards to the procedure if it is performed carefully, it has obtained wide acceptance during the past 10 years. Typically, a tooth is rotated and held in its rotated position for several months, until periodontal ligament remodeling is essentially complete. Either at the time of band removal or just prior to it, the gingival tissues are anesthetized, and an incision is made through the gingival crevice to the alveolar crest. Alternatively, vertical incisions can be made adjacent to the interdental papilla. In either case, the object is to sever the supracrestal fibers so that their elastic components relax and reattach in a relaxed position (Fig. 7–32). There is minimal discomfort following the procedure. Periodontal dressings are not required, and complete healing occurs in a short time.

Teeth may also move, after the completion of orthodontic tooth movement, in response to tongue and lip pressures. If a tooth is moved too far labially or buccally,

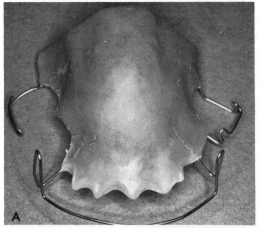

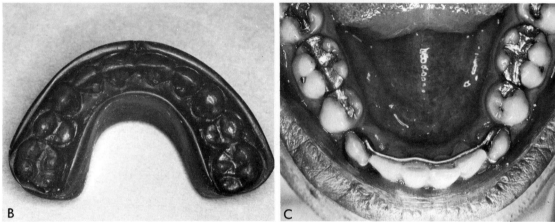

FIGURE 7–31 Shown here are several common appliances used during the retention phase of orthodontics. **A,** The Hawley retainer. This view shows the anterior bow and a clasp. **B,** The positioner. This is a rubber or soft acrylic appliance, similar to an upper and lower mouth guard fused together, which is usually constructed from a model on which the teeth have been repositioned slightly. **C,** The canine-to-canine lingual splint, constructed by soldering a lingual bar to the lower canine bands. This mechanism decreases the chance of recurring lower anterior crowding after a case of severe crowding has been treated. Such a fixed splint is often left in place for 1 to 2 years after completion of orthodontic treatment.

the constant pressure applied by the lip or tongue will move it back to a position of better balance. Teeth cannot be stabilized outside the region of muscular equilibrium without the use of permanent retaining appliances. It is rarely good judgment to move a tooth into a position where permanent retention will be required.

Tooth Movement: A Function of Appliance Design

There are two purposes for the discussion of orthodontic techniques. The first is to describe in detail relatively simple treatment procedures for specific orthodontic problems. These procedures may be carried out readily by a general practitioner who has satisfied himself that the overall treatment of a patient's malocclusion is within his capabilities. They will be useful for common problems in general practice.

The second purpose is to outline in general terms treatment approaches toward complex problems, particularly skeletal discrepancies and severe crowding requiring extraction of teeth. Treatment of such problems falls outside the scope of most general practices. Nevertheless, knowledge of these treatment techniques is valuable for any general practitioner so that he may communicate better with patients, parents, and orthodontists.

Many techniques and many orthodontic

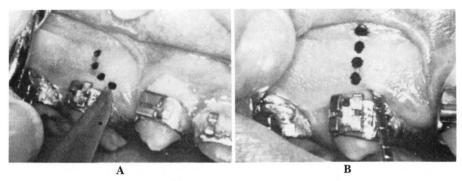

A   B

FIGURE 7–32 *A,* Notice the stretched and distorted tattoo marks following tooth rotation but prior to severing of the supracrestal fibers. *B,* The postoperative tattoo is vertically aligned and demonstrates the relaxed gingival fibers similar to the configuration of the teeth before their movement. (From Edwards, J. G.: A surgical procedure to eliminate rotational relapse. Am. J. Orthodont. 57(1):40, 1970.)

appliances can be used to move teeth. The most important considerations in selecting orthodontic appliances are the type of tooth movement that is needed and the anchorage that is required for that movement. Esthetic values, ease of construction, and other appliance characteristics are secondary. These should be considered only when the anchorage and tooth movement requirements have been satisfied.

Removable Appliances

Any removable appliance whose purpose is the repositioning of teeth consists of three basic components: (1) a rigid framework, (2) clasps or retentive elements, and (3) springs that contact selected teeth to produce the tooth movement. (Some removable appliances, the functional appliance group, have as their principal purpose altering the growth of the jaws, and these have differently designed features. These appliances are discussed later under treatment of skeletal problems.) Removable appliances are designed to be removed by the patient during treatment. They were originally made of gold wrought wire intricately soldered to form a frame, clasps, and spring devices. Crozat appliances of gold are still used occasionally, but these have been made obsolete by the development of more suitable materials. The usual contemporary removable appliance has a plastic (acrylic) framework and uses stainless steel wire for the clasps and springs (Fig. 7–33). The general principles of tooth movement are similar with all removable appliances, whatever the

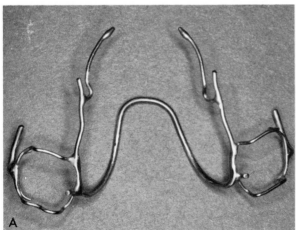
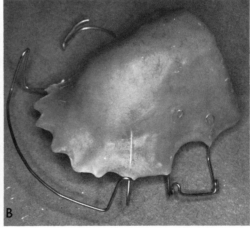

FIGURE 7–33 Two approaches to removable appliance frameworks include *(A)* Crozat appliances with a gold framework and *(B)* Hawley appliances that have an acrylic framework. Both appliances can be effective when used to achieve tipping movements.

material used for any of their components. The effectiveness of the removable appliance is directly related to the skill of the dentist and the cooperation of the patient in wearing it.

Removable appliances are quite effective in aligning teeth where tipping and arch expansion are indicated. Certain types of tooth movement, such as bodily movement or root paralleling following extraction of teeth and most rotational movements, are extremely difficult to produce with removable appliances. For practical purposes, removable appliances are restricted to relatively straightforward tipping movements in situations not involving extraction.

Framework. Modern plastics offer great advantages over wrought metal frameworks in ease of fabrication and reductions in cost and for these reasons have almost totally replaced the older designs. There are two modern approaches toward fabrication of the framework: (1) The framework may be made conveniently from commercial self-curing acrylic resins. It should be nonporous, preferably cured in a pressure cooker under 30 lb of pressure for about one-half hour. If a pressure cooker is not available, porosity can be reduced by allowing the acrylic to cure under warm water (providing the model is thoroughly soaked first to prevent air bubbles from distorting the acrylic). The acrylic should be relatively thin (2 to 3 mm thickness), particularly in the area lingual to the maxillary incisors, where excessive thickness will cause difficulty with speech and overbite. (2) Satisfactory frameworks also can be made from thermoplastic materials, which are heated until pliable and then molded under pressure to the contours of the dental casts. In this technique, a prepared blank of thermoplastic material of the desired thickness is heated and molded to the dental casts using a special machine (for example, the Biostar* unit). The thermoplastic materials have the great advantage that they produce a framework of uniform thickness and contour and can be produced faster and easier for routine applications. The palate portion of an upper removable appliance particularly lends itself to being formed in this way. More complex frame-

*Available through Great Lakes Orthodontics, Buffalo, New York. Manufactured by Scheu Dental, Letmathe, West Germany.

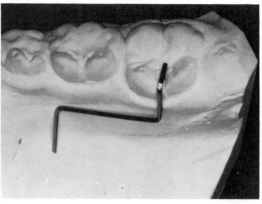

FIGURE 7–34 The occlusal rest is the simplest of clasps. It is fabricated so as to rest on the occlusal surface of a mandibular molar, thus resisting downward displacement of the appliance.

works, such as those that would be used for lower removable appliances, are somewhat harder to form with thermoplastics, but essentially all types of removable frameworks can be made in this way. Most commercially fabricated removable frameworks are now formed using thermoplastic resins rather than self-curing acrylics.

Clasps. A removable appliance is no better than its retentive clasps. If the retentive elements do not fix the removable appliance firmly in place, its springs will be ineffective in producing the desired tooth movement. Four basic clasp designs are commonly used in acrylic removable appliances:

Occlusal Rest. The occlusal rest is a wire extending onto the occlusal surface of a lower molar tooth through the lingual groove. It is a resting type of device designed to prevent the distal portion of the appliance from tipping toward the floor of the mouth (Fig. 7–34).

Circumferential Clasp. This is essentially a round wire clasp similar to those used in partial dentures. It is bent to follow the contours of the tooth, taking advantage of the mesiobuccal or distobuccal undercuts (Fig. 7–35).

Ball Clasp. If there is little or no undercut available for clasping, a simple ball clasp is often effective (Fig. 7–36). This clasp consists of a piece of orthodontic wire with a polished ball of solder on its end. It is bent into the interproximal embrasures and offers fairly good retention, particularly with primary molars.

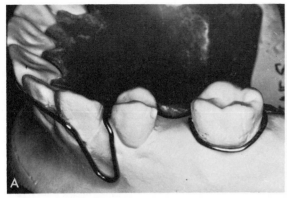
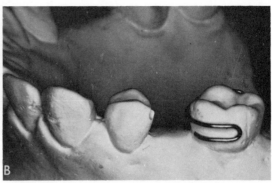

FIGURE 7–35 A circumferential clasp may be of two designs. *A,* The simple circumferential clasp rests below the crest of contour of the retainer tooth, usually at the junction of the gingiva with the crown of the tooth. *B,* The recurved circumferential clasp starts above the crest of contour of the tooth and recurves gingivally below the crest of contour. The lower arm of the clasp gently engages the undercut area. If this arm is activated too strongly, it will tend to extrude the retainer tooth.

Adams Clasp.   The grasping points of this clasp are bent to fit tightly into the mesiolingual and mesiobuccal undercuts of the clasped tooth. The clasp is made by bending a piece of 0.028-inch steel wire as shown in Figure 7–37. Although the Adams clasp is one of the most difficult clasps to bend, it offers the best retention and the least likelihood of breakage and distortion of all the clasps described. Modern removal appliance techniques are based largely on the superior retentive characteristics of the Adams clasp. Interestingly, the Adams clasp is similar in design principles to the Crozat clasp, which was the basis of that family of gold removable appliances of 75 years ago, and may well be the first significant improvement over the Crozat design.

Tooth-Moving Springs.   In considering the design of springs, a few basic mechanical principles must be discussed. These principles are valid for springs contained within fixed and removable appliances.

As wire becomes larger in diameter, its stiffness, or resistance to deflection, increases faster than its strength (Fig. 7–38). From the point of view of appliance design, this means simply that small-diameter, light wire will be most useful in orthodontic treatment.

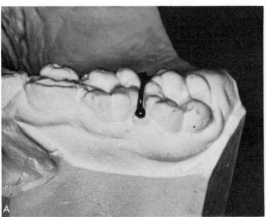
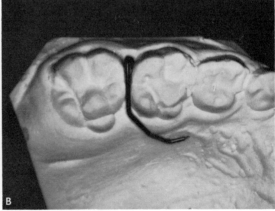

FIGURE 7–36 When a ball clasp is to be used, the interdental papilla in the retentive area is cut from the plaster cast if the clinical crown is short, as is usually the case when primary teeth are clasped. The ball end of the wire is then bent to fit snugly in this undercut area *(A)*. The wire running across the occlusal surface is then bent to conform tightly to the interproximal area between the marginal ridges of the teeth *(B)*.

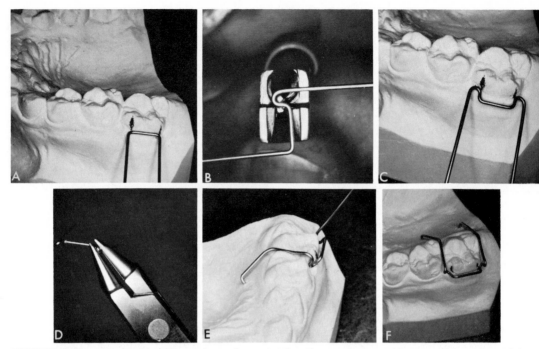

FIGURE 7–37 Fabrication of an Adams clasp. *A,* The distance between the grasping points of the clasp is established by bending the wire as shown. Since the points will fit into mesiobuccal and distobuccal undercuts, the distance between them must be 2 to 3 mm less than the mesiodistal width of the tooth. *B,* Grasping points are created by bending the wire around the beak of the No. 139 pliers. *C,* The fit of the grasping points is checked against the tooth. The points should now fit into the undercuts at the mesiobuccal and distobuccal corners of the tooth. *D,* Grasping points are bent inward approximately 45 degrees, so that they will follow the curvature of the tooth in the undercut area. *E,* The ends of the wire are bent from the grasping points over the contact areas and contoured to extend into the acrylic. *F,* Buccal view of the completed clasp.

As the unsupported length of a piece of wire increases, its springiness increases faster than its strength decreases. This means that if heavier wire is needed for strength in design of an orthodontic appliance, the desired springiness can be obtained by increasing the effective length of the wire used in the spring. The problem of fitting a long wire into a relatively small appliance can be solved either by recurving the wire or by bending a circular loop (helix) into the wire. In making a helix, it is wise to make a relatively large-diameter circle of wire, since this will put less stress on the wire at the complex area of bending and will thus decrease the possibility of breakage.

Supporting a wire at both ends rather than at one end greatly increases both strength and stiffness. This means that in many cases it will be desirable to support springs at only one end in order to produce the appropriate springiness in the wire. It also means that where a long span of wire is to be used, as in a wire bow running around the entire incisor segment, adequate strength and stability can be obtained by supporting the wire at both ends rather than at only one end.

Illustrations of several types of springs that can be used in conjunction with removable appliances are included in the section on correction of specific problems (see pp. 295 to 319).

Fixed Appliances

Appliances using bands are really more semifixed than fixed, since the appliance itself is removable and only the attachments on the teeth are fixed in place. Until the last decade, fixed appliances routinely employed bands cemented around the teeth to hold the attachments. At present, attachments for anterior teeth almost routinely are bonded directly to the enamel, while bands continue

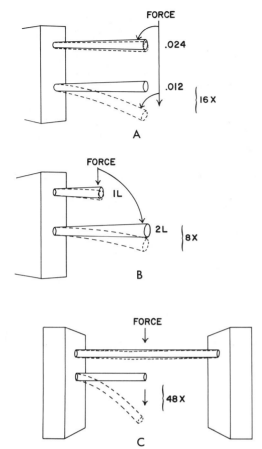

FIGURE 7–38 These diagrams illustrate mechanical principles used in the design of springs for removable or fixed applicances. *A,* If a constant force is exerted, a wire that is one-half the diameter of another will bend 16 times as far. (Springiness of a wire under constant load varies inversely with the fourth power of the diameter.) *B,* When a wire serves as a cantilever beam, doubling its length will cause it to deflect 8 times as far under the same load. (Cantilever beam deflection varies with the third power of the length.) *C,* A beam (wire) supported at both ends is 48 times as resistant to bending as a cantilever beam one half the length of the supported beam.

to be used more often for molars and premolars.

Fabrication and Use of Orthodontic Bands. Orthodontic bands are preferred for molars and some premolar teeth for two reasons: (1) A well-fitted band can withstand greater occlusal or other forces without being dislodged, so that posterior banded attachments are more secure than their bonded equivalents, and (2) the higher soft tissue contours around posterior teeth, particularly in children, may preclude proper placement

of bonded premolar and molar attachments. An orthodontic band can slightly displace gingival tissue. A bonded attachment cannot.

The first consideration in fabricating an orthodontic band is obtaining adequate separation. In most cases it is necessary to separate posterior teeth before bands can be fitted. Band material must slip past the contact points as bands are being made. If the band binds in the proximal areas, it is impossible to obtain good buccal and lingual adaptation, bands are deformed during seating, and the patient finds the procedure painful.

Effective separation for posterior teeth can be obtained by use of soft brass wire twisted tightly around the contact points and left for 3 to 7 days (Fig. 7–39). Posterior separation also can be accomplished by placing small elastomeric rings around the contact point (Fig. 7–40), although if the contacts are extremely tight, it may be very difficult to insert the elastomeric rings. Separation is usually not necessary if only one or two anterior teeth are to be banded, and of course separation is not required when bonded attachments are employed.

Bands for posterior or anterior teeth may be fabricated from strips of stainless steel band material, or they can be purchased preformed in graduated sizes from orthodontic suppliers. Band fabrication using steel strip band material is illustrated in Figure 7–41. Precontoured stainless steel strips, which are supplied in several anatomic variations (Fig. 7–42), can be useful in making bands for canines, premolars, and molars that have extreme contours. The precontoured strips are pinched to fit individual teeth in the same manner as strips of straight band material, except that much less use of contouring pliers is required.

An easier method, although one requiring a larger inventory, is the use of preformed stainless steel bands (Fig. 7–43). These bands are available through several orthodontic suppliers in two styles. They may be purchased as "general purpose" bands that will fit molar, premolar, canine, or incisor teeth on both the right and the left sides of the mouth and in both dental arches. Individualized bands, designed for each tooth in the arch and incorporating right and left side variations, are also available. There is usually little advantage to use of this latter type of band in the general practice office because of the relatively low volume of or-

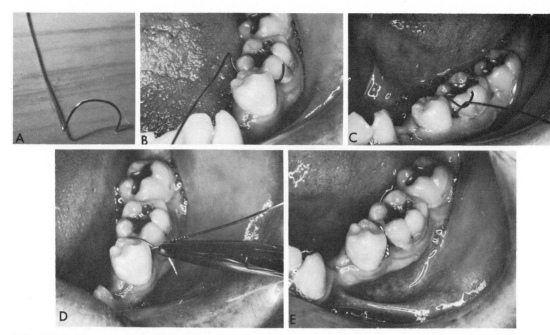

FIGURE 7–39 Separation of posterior teeth prior to banding may be accomplished by use of brass wire. *A,* Soft brass wire, .020 in diameter, is inserted under the contact area from the buccal or lingual side. *B,* The hook shape allows the wire to be passed around the contact. *C,* The end of the wire is brought back over the contact and twisted on the buccal side. *D,* The pigtail is twisted tight, using a needle holder or Howe pliers. *E,* The cut pigtail is burnished against the gingival margin of the tooth. Separating wire of this type should be left in place for 3 to 7 days.

thodontic patients. The individualized bands save little time until the operator becomes thoroughly familiar with their characteristics.

A general practitioner with any interest in orthodontics, even if this involves nothing more than space maintenance for selected child patients, would find it advantageous to maintain an inventory of general purpose molar bands in his office. Molar bands are difficult to pinch from band material and

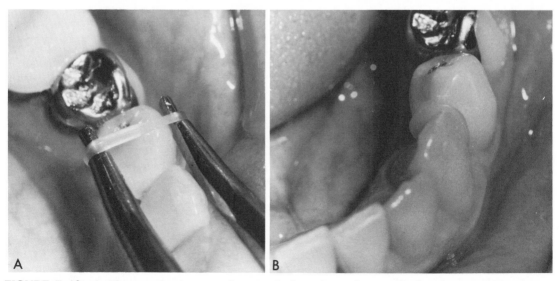

FIGURE 7–40 *A,* Elastomeric rings can be stretched as shown here and placed around the contact point of adjacent teeth. *B,* When the separator is in place, the teeth move apart as the ring contracts to regain its original form.

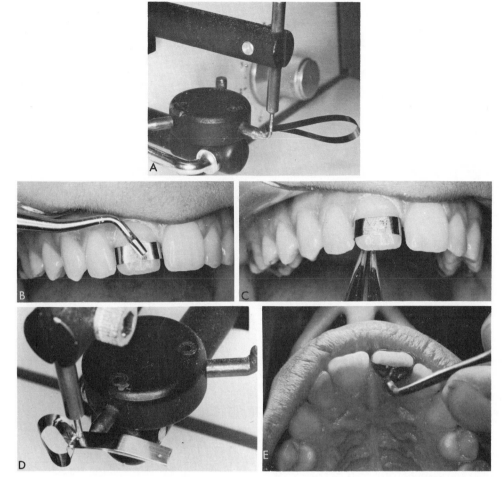

FIGURE 7–41 Fabrication of a pinched band. *A,* The ends of the strip band material are welded together to prevent slipping and distortion of the band while it is pinched, and the strip is seated around the tooth. The .003 band material is best for incisor teeth; .004 is preferred for canines and premolars; .005 or .006 is used for molars. *B,* The band is carefully burnished to fit the tooth's anatomy on the labial surface, with excess band material being pulled to the lingual. *C,* While the band material is held tightly on the labial, the band is pinched with band-pinching pliers or Howe pliers tightly along its lingual surface. *D,* The pinched seam is now welded. *E,* The tab is cut off, the band is reseated on the tooth, and the tab is burnished flat against the lingual contours of the tooth.

are used more frequently than bands for other teeth. The preformed molar bands can be easily adapted to normally shaped teeth or modified by cutting, overlapping, and rewelding for molars with abnormal morphology. Most practitioners will find that bands for other teeth can be pinched from straight or contoured band material as they are needed.

After a satisfactory band has been fitted, brackets or tubes may be attached to hold the desired appliance. Use of precious metal bands requires soldered attachments; either welding or soldering may be used with steel

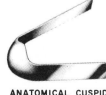

ANATOMICAL CUSPID
BLANKS

BICUSPID BLANKS

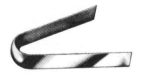

MOLAR BLANKS

FIGURE 7–42 Precontoured band material comes in varying sizes and shapes. (Redrawn by permission of the Unitek Corporation.)

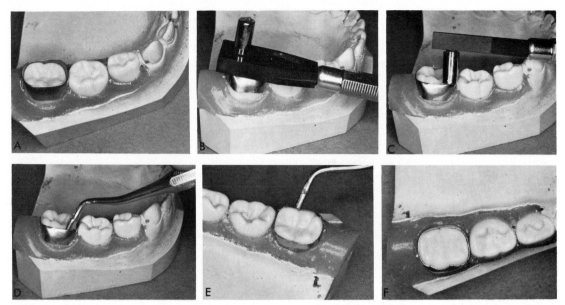

FIGURE 7–43 *A,* A preformed band should snugly fit the tooth. *B,* Its initial seating may be accomplished by finger pressure or by having the patient bite on a flat object such as a band seater or tongue blade. *C,* Final seating is done with pressure from a band seater on the most convex band surface. *D,* Pressure to seat the band should be applied on both mesial and distal corners of the convex surface (lingual of maxillary molar, buccal of mandibular molar). After it is seated, the band should not move under heavy biting pressure. *E,* Final adaptation to the groove of the tooth is accomplished by burnishing. *F,* This is a view of a well-adapted preformed band.

bands, but welding is preferred. A wide range of attachments are offered by orthodontic supply houses, with variations that can be significant in a specialty practice in which a large volume of complex cases are being treated. For orthodontics in general practice, simplicity and versatility of attachments should be the major criteria. For al-

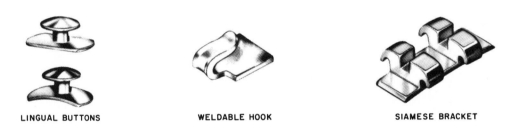

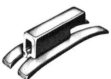

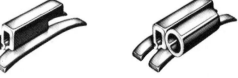

LINGUAL BUTTONS   WELDABLE HOOK   SIAMESE BRACKET

LINGUAL SHEATHS   BUCCAL TUBES

FIGURE 7–44   Some of the most common band attachments are shown in this illustration. (Redrawn by permission of the Unitek Corporation.)

most all purposes, the following should be adequate: rectangular buccal tubes, lingual sheaths for lingual arches, twin (Siamese) edgewise brackets, weldable hooks, and weldable lingual buttons (Fig. 7–44). Use of specific attachments is illustrated in the section on treatment.

If several teeth are to be banded, it is important that all attachments be placed at the same occlusogingival level on the clinical crowns of the teeth, so that a straight arch wire will result in correct vertical position of the teeth. After the bands are seated and adapted, but prior to cementing, an arbitrary height for the attachments should be established that will be satisfactory for all teeth. This height will generally be at the middle third of the clinical crowns, with slight deviations from tooth to tooth depending on cusp height. Maxillary lateral brackets are offset 1 mm toward the incisal edge. The bracket or tube height is scribed into each band with dividers (Fig. 7–45). A second, vertical mark indicating the mesiodistal position of the bracket is then made to complete a cross-etching on the band. These marks serve as a guide during welding of attachments.

Teeth are prepared for band cementation by thorough cleaning. Bands should be cemented with a zinc phosphate dental cement. The cement mix should be slightly thicker than the mix for cementing a crown or inlay. The inside of the band should be coated with cement so that, as the band is seated, cement will fill all voids. If an anterior or lower premolar band is being cemented, it is advisable to place an additional small amount of cement over the labial or convex surface of the tooth before placing the band. This decreases the chance of creating a void in the cement because of tooth morphology. The area should be kept dry until the cement hardens. Excess cement can be removed with a scaler or ultrasonic unit.

Bonded Attachments. Acid etch–composite resin technique for direct attachment of resins to enamel surfaces is the basis for orthodontic bonding of attachments. The technique for bonding an orthodontic attachment is basically similar to applying composite resin for any other purpose. If a plastic orthodontic bracket is employed, the resin can bond chemically to the bracket base. Unfortunately, plastic brackets for orthodontic fixed appliances to date have proved unsatisfactory because of breakage over a period of time. Metal brackets can be bonded satisfactorily if a retentive mesh for mechanical adherence to the resin is provided. Experience has demonstrated that a relatively small mesh size provides adequate retention, and the overall size of bracket bases for bonding to enamel surfaces has been greatly reduced in recent years as the advantages of small bases and small mesh sizes have been appreciated.

The technology of bonding remains in rapid flux, and it is likely that the precise techniques used in the future will not be the same as those in current use. At the time of this writing, there are two basic approaches for direct bonding. The first, which has proven highly satisfactory, uses the same filled resins employed for restorative purposes, with the material mixed to provide a very quick setting time. An individual mix of a small amount of resin is prepared for each bracket. This technique is illustrated in Figure 7–46.

The other approach for direct bonding, which also can be adapted for indirect bonding of a number of brackets at the same time, is based on the use of a two-part resin system. One part is placed on the prepared tooth surface, the other part on the back of the bracket to be bonded. The chemical reaction between the two materials then does not begin until the bracket is placed against the prepared and coated tooth surface, allowing excellent working time up to that point with a quick curing time thereafter.

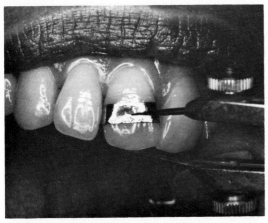

FIGURE 7–45 Location of attachments is marked by scratching the correct height and mesiodistal position on the band with the sharp point of a divider or similar measuring instrument.

With both bonding methods, bond strengths equivalent to the strengths of typical orthodontic bands can be obtained, and bonding now is preferable to banding for most anterior and some posterior teeth.

For the purposes of the generalist who wishes to do some fixed-appliance orthodontics, the best current advice would be to plan to band molar teeth routinely, to bond incisors and canines routinely, and to band or bond premolars depending on the ease of access to these teeth. Bonding premolars in adults after the gingival attachment has receded to the cementoenamel junction is considerably easier than bonding the same teeth during adolescence.

In addition to the instruments and supplies routinely found in dental offices, several other items are needed for limited orthodontic treatment. A list of minimum

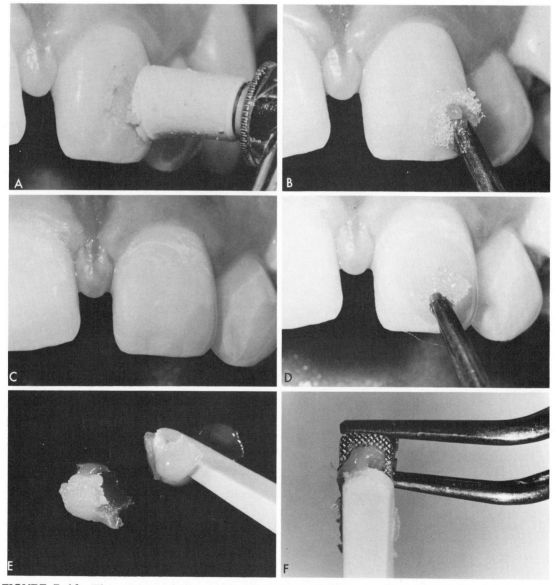

FIGURE 7–46   The steps needed to apply bonded attachments are illustrated in the following sequence. *A,* The tooth is cleaned with a pumice or abrasive cleaning paste using a rubber cup or brush and *(B)* acid etched and washed to obtain *(C)* a well-etched chalky surface that is ready for bonding. *D,* An unfilled resin is applied to the etched surface. *E,* Next, a well-mixed filled resin is *(F)* coated on the back of the attachment.

Illustration continued on opposite page

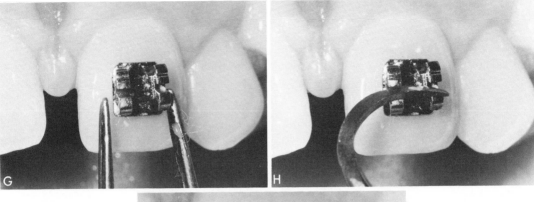

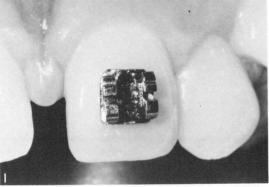

FIGURE 7–46 *Continued G,* The attachment is then placed on the tooth surface and preliminarily positioned. *H,* The bracket is finally oriented and held in position under pressure until the resin has polymerized. *I,* The bracket should be in intimate contact with the tooth and have no excess resin flash or voids. The bracket is now ready for arch wire placement.

instruments and supplies is shown in Table 7–4.

Removable Versus Fixed Appliances: A Comparison

Fixed appliances have two distinct advantages over removables: They offer better control over tooth movement because there is broader and firmer contact of the appliance with the teeth, and since the patient cannot remove a fixed appliance himself, its effectiveness depends less on cooperation and it is less likely to be distorted.

If the required tooth movements are at all complex, the first advantage can become a compelling reason for using fixed appliances. Removable appliances tip teeth quite satisfactorily. Rotation, bodily movement, and intrusion of teeth are extremely difficult to accomplish with a removable appliance, but can be done with fixed appliances. The cooperation factor expresses itself most clearly in the amount of time required to accom-

plish a given tooth movement. Almost invariably, it takes longer to do the same thing with a removable than with a fixed appliance, simply because the patient tends not to wear a removable appliance full-time, and because the force systems developed by the removable appliance often are less effective than could be achieved with a fixed appliance even when the removable one is worn consistently.

In the past, the main advantages of removable appliances were that they were thought to be more acceptable to the patient, since they could be made less conspicuous and removed on special occasions, and that they were easier for the dentist to fabricate and manage. The advantage in patient acceptance has been considerably blunted by the rapid acceptance of fixed-appliance therapy for adults and the widespread availability of orthodontic treatment for adolescents. Now that a sizeable percentage of children in the junior high school age group receive comprehensive orthodontic treatment, wearing a fixed appliance does not set a child

TABLE 7–4   Minimal Required Instruments and Supplies*

Item	Purpose
Instruments	
Welder, light duty	Appliance fabrication
Bird beak pliers (No. 139)	Wire bending
Howe or Weingart pliers	Intraoral appliance manipulation
Wire cutter	Appliance fabrication
Ligature cutter	Cutting ligatures intraorally (only)
Contouring pliers	Band construction
Posterior band remover	Band construction and removal
Mathieu needle holder	Tying ligatures and separating wire
Band driver ("Band biter")	Band seating
Serrated tip amalgam plugger	Band seating
Bow divider	Tooth measurement and band scribing
Sharp Boley gauge	Tooth measurement
Heavy scaler	Cement removal
Supplies	
Maxillary/mandibular preformed molar bands	Fixed appliances
.022″ × .028″ mesh back brackets	Incisor and canine bonding
Straight band material .004″ × .160″	Canine and premolar bands
.022″ × .028″ molar tubes	Attachment for last molar
.045″ molar tubes	Attachment for Kloehn headgear
.022″ × .028″ twin edgewise brackets, medium width	Attachments for canines and premolars
.030″ or .036″ horizontal lingual sheaths	Lingual arch attachments
Weldable or bondable hooks	Cross elastics
Weldable or bondable buttons	Cross elastics
1/4″ medium and heavy latex elastics	Cross elastics
1/2″ light latex elastics	Retraction of anterior teeth
.020″ soft brass wire	Separating wire
.018″ stainless steel wire	Arch wire
.019″ × .025″ stainless steel wire	Molar uprighting spring
.025″, .028″ stainless steel wire	Appliance fabrication
.030″, .036″ stainless steel wire	Lingual arch and W-arch
.038″ stainless steel wire	Quad helix
.010″ ligature wire	Ligation of teeth or arch wire
.009″ × .030″ open coil spring	Molar uprighting
Cold cure acrylic	Appliance fabrication

*Major orthodontic suppliers who offer detailed catalogs are Unitek Corporation, 950 Royal Oaks Drive, Monrovia, California 91016; Rocky Mountain Dental Products Company, P.O. Box 1887, Galapago Street, Denver, Colorado 80201; and Ormco Corporation, 1332 South Lone Hill Road, Glendora, California 91740.

apart and may even have a positive rather than a negative effect as a status symbol. To a large extent, the same now is true for adults, because so many individuals are wearing fixed appliances that social acceptability is not the problem it once was. From the dentist's point of view, it still is easier to take an impression and have a removable appliance fabricated in the laboratory than to prepare a fixed appliance at the chair. The greater effectiveness of the fixed appliance if it is used properly, however, can outweigh this consideration in many instances. Three longer appointments with a fixed appliance may produce the same result as six or eight shorter ones with a removable appliance, with less total time spent in the dental chair and considerably greater efficiency.

Although it is fair to say that the recent improvements in fixed appliances have increased their advantage over removable ones, there is still a place for removable appliances. In our view, modern removable appliances are best suited for producing tipping tooth movements in the maxillary arch. Good fit and good retention can be obtained routinely on maxillary removables, and if complex tooth movement is not required, removable appliances can be employed efficiently. Mandibular removables are inherently less stable because of their horseshoe design and also are less well tolerated by patients even for simple tooth movements. More complex movements, such as those required in uprighting a lower molar, all but require a modern fixed appliance.

Role of Commerical Laboratories

Many commercial laboratories are capable of making excellent-quality orthodontic appliances, fixed or removable, from a prescription design. Indirect bonding techniques allow the fabrication of a fixed appliance with precise placement of attachments, and it also is possible for a laboratory to fabricate satisfactory bands indirectly. The busy practitioner has much to gain from having appliances contructed by a reputable laboratory. Unfortunately, some laboratories suggest that if a set of dental casts is sent to them, they will design an appliance to treat the malocclusion. Such a procedure eliminates orthodontic diagnosis, for even if the technician involved were capable of diagnosis (a doubtful assumption), he would not have adequate information. Asking the technician to design an appliance is analogous to sending the druggist a list of symptoms and having the druggist, without ever having seen the patient, prescribe the medication. The patient in both instances is unlikely to benefit from his encounter with the practitioner.

As a rule, laboratories that serve orthodontic specialists are most likely to perform satisfactory work on a prescription basis. A conversation with a local orthodontist, or a review of advertisements in specialty journals, will allow any practitioner to locate such a laboratory. A carefully prepared prescription should be sent to the laboratory when contruction of an orthodontic appliance is requested.

ILLUSTRATIVE TECHNIQUES FOR TREATMENT OF NONSKELETAL PROBLEMS IN CHILDREN

Arch Circumference (Length) Problems

Space Management for Premature Loss of Primary Teeth

When primary teeth are lost as a result of caries, ectopic eruption, or trauma, the occlusion must be assessed carefully to determine if space maintenance is necessary. Patients with superimposed profile (protrusive or retrusive) and skeletal problems (Class II and III occlusions) on the space maintenance equation demand more than reflexive space maintenance. It may or may not be advantageous to control space if these problems are present. Reasonable judgments regarding space maintenance, whether or not to use it, and which technique to use if space maintenance is appropriate must be made on an individual basis. Data collected from cephalometric radiographs, casts, and intraoral measurements have revealed the following interesting, although limited, information regarding space changes.

Posterior Space Change. The longer a primary tooth has been missing, the greater the incidence and amount of space closure. Closure is more rapid during the first 6 months following tooth loss in either arch and occurs more rapidly in the maxillary arch than in the mandibular arch. Posterior space closure has been noted before and after eruption of first permanent molars. Although space closure is multidirectional, it occurs predominantly from the posterior aspect in the maxillary arch and predominantly from the anterior aspect in the mandibular arch.

Anterior Space Change. The small amount of evidence available indicates that little space loss occurs in the anterior region. Commonly, there is a redistribution of space in the anterior segment following primary tooth loss and, in the case of mandibular canine loss, lingual movement of the anterior teeth has been noted. The site in the arch of the missing tooth or teeth is therefore important.

The need for space maintenance in the anterior segment has not been clearly resolved. Space maintenance in the maxillary anterior segment and the mandibular incisor area is not generally necessary. The mandibular canine area merits space maintenance.

The time of eruption is another factor to weigh in the space maintenance decision. A primary molar lost prior to 8 years of age may delay the eruption of the permanent premolars. Primary molar loss at a later time may accelerate eruption of the premolar teeth. Only by attention to the individual case can one make reasonable judgments.

Patients with Adequate Space: Space Maintenance

Generally, it can be concluded that space maintenance is appropriate when Class I skeletal and dental relationships are present, when adequate space as determined by a

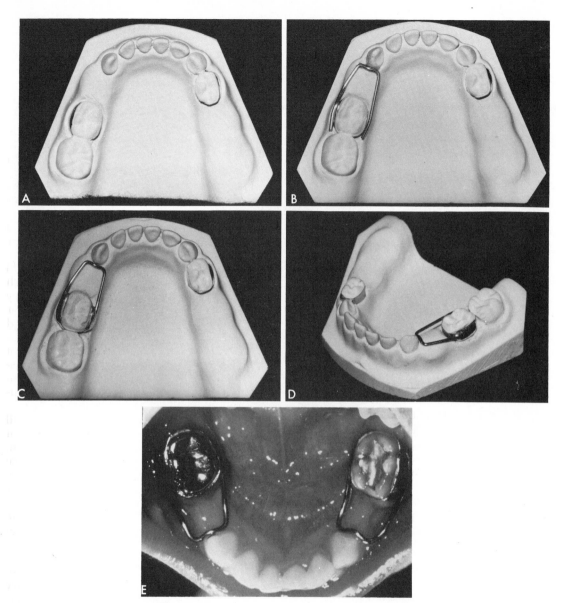

FIGURE 7–47 This cast of the mandibular dentition demonstrates an ideal indication for a band-and-loop space maintainer from the primary left second molar to the canine. As previously described, a band is fit and an impression is made. The band is seated in the impression and stabilized with pins, and *(A)* the impression is poured in stone. *B,* A .030-inch stainless steel wire is bent into a loop to contact the distal surface of the canine at the height of contour. The loop is stabilized prior to soldering. Note that the contour of the wire adjacent to the canine has very little concavity. This allows the canine to move laterally during incisor eruption. *C,* There is adequate faciolingual width of the loop to accommodate premolar eruption. *D,* This view illustrates that the wire is soldered in the center of the band on the facial surface and that the wire is 1.5 mm off the tissue. *E,* The band can be cemented to the crown of a tooth or to a stainless steel crown. The band and loop can be more easily removed and modified or replaced than a crown-and-loop space maintainer.

space analysis is available, and when the facial profile is well balanced, with appropriate lip posture. Even in the presence of these qualifications, poor patient cooperation and

poor oral hygiene may ultimately contraindicate space maintenance.

Appliances for Space Maintenance. The band and loop may be used for anterior or posterior space maintenance (Fig. 7–47). Although the appliance is fixed and therefore requires no manipulation by the patient, the patient's cooperation is necessary to maintain oral hygiene. This appliance should be designed with growth and development of the dental arches and the eruption of succedaneous teeth in mind. This means that the

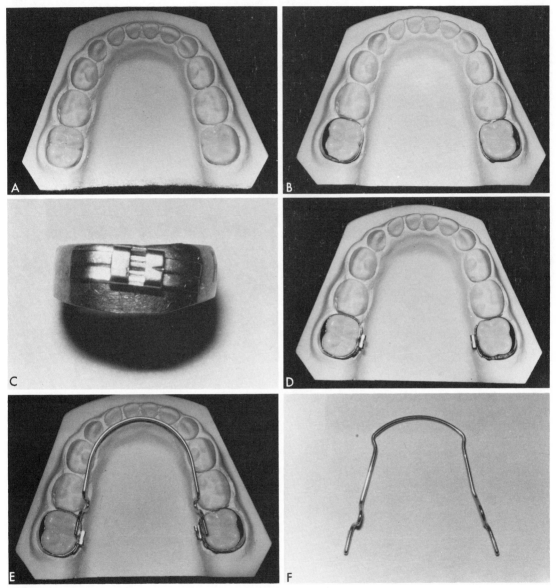

FIGURE 7–48 This series of photographs illustrates the steps in the construction of a fixed removable mandibular lingual holding arch placed on the permanent first molars, although the primary second molars can be used. **A,** The mandibular cast. **B,** The bands are fitted and contoured. **C,** The bands are removed and a lingual attachment is tack-welded in place so that the lock (V-shaped indentation) is positioned distally and the attachment is inclined anterosuperiorly to aid in insertion and removal. **D,** The bands are refitted and recontoured. The placement of the attachment is checked and permanently spotwelded. **E,** At this point an impression can be made so that remaining procedures can be completed in the laboratory or the arch can be completed at the chairside. An appropriate-sized preformed .036-inch lingual arch with adjustment loops mesial to the abutment teeth is recommended. **F,** The final form rests passively on the cingula of the incisors and canines and steps lingually away from the erupting premolars.

Illustration continued on following page

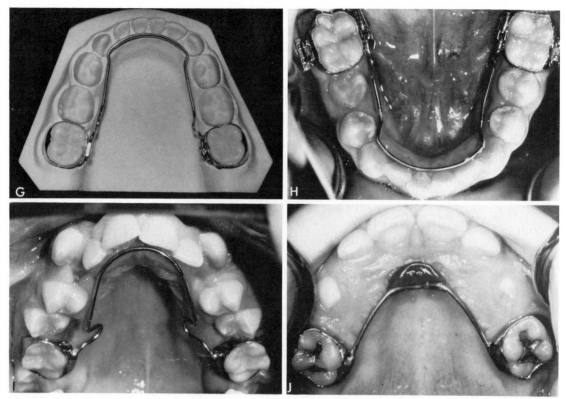

FIGURE 7–48 *Continued **G**,* The finished arch is passive and remains 1.5 mm from the soft tissue. ***H**,* An example of a well-formed .036-inch lingual arch with vertical insertion attachment. ***I**,* A maxillary soldered .036-inch lingual arch is illustrated. This type of appliance can be used when the overbite is limited. Soldered lingual arches are recommended when no adjustments are anticipated. ***J**,* The Nance appliance is constructed using a soldered .036-inch palatal wire and an acrylic button abutted to the palatal tissue to hold the molars in place. Tissue irritation adjacent to the button must be monitored. (Parts H and J are from Machen, J. B., Fields, H. W., and McIver, F. T.: Pedodontics. *In* Review of Basic Science and Clinical Dentistry, Volume II., J. E. Wells, M. V. Reed, and V. M. Coury, eds. Hagerstown, Md., Harper & Row, 1980.)

primary canines should not have their lateral movement restricted. Careful study of the eruption sequence is necessary, and a replacement or modified appliance may be needed at a later date.

The lingual arch appliance may be used in either the maxillary or the mandibular arch and offers anterior, posterior, unilateral, or bilateral solutions to space maintenance (Fig. 7–48). Since permanent incisor tooth buds are positioned lingual to the primary tooth, a lingual arch placed prior to eruption of these incisors could cause problems. This is a fixed appliance and little manipulation by the patient is required, but, again, good oral hygiene is a necessity. Long-term use of the

FIGURE 7–49 This series illustrates the steps in fabrication of the removable partial denture for a child who is missing both anterior and posterior teeth. ***A**,* Initial cast. ***B**,* Adams clasps are bent for as many molars as can reasonably be clasped, the anterior teeth are set, and a labial flange is waxed in place. ***C**,* A stone core is poured over the teeth and the labial flange. ***D**,* The Adams clasps are stabilized and the wax is removed. The stone core holds the teeth in position. ***E**,* Cold-cure acrylic is applied by the "salt and pepper" method, the stone core is replaced and held with a rubber band, and the acrylic is allowed to polymerize. ***F**,* The finished partial denture after trimming and polishing. ***G**,* As an alternative, canines may be clasped with Adams clasps or C-clasps as demonstrated in this appliance.

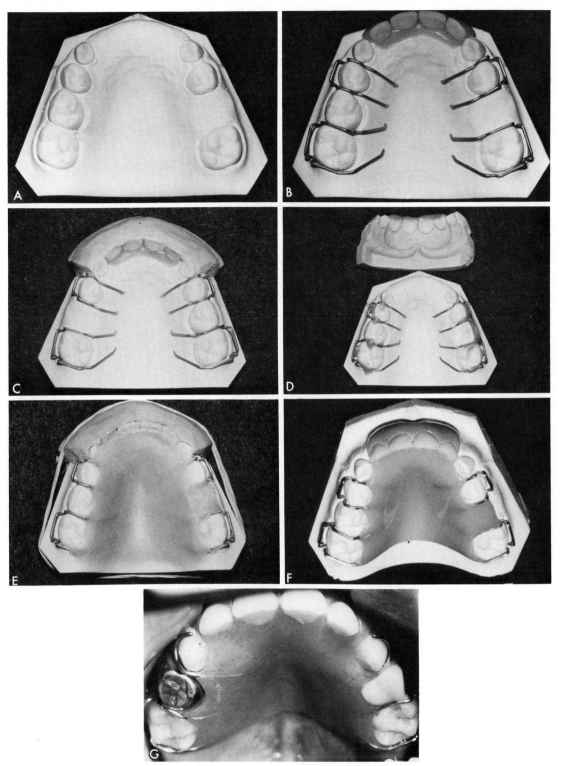

FIGURE 7–49   *See legend on opposite page*

lingual arch may lead to decalcification of the abutment teeth. Therefore, it may be advisable to consider banding primary molars instead of permanent molars.

Acrylic partial dentures are extremely versatile. They may be used for space maintenance in either the maxilla or the mandible, either anteriorly or posteriorly, and either unilaterally or bilaterally (Fig. 7–49). These appliances may be constructed so that they replace occlusal function and are esthetically quite pleasing. Since they are removable, they do demand patient cooperation, but their removable nature also facilitates tooth

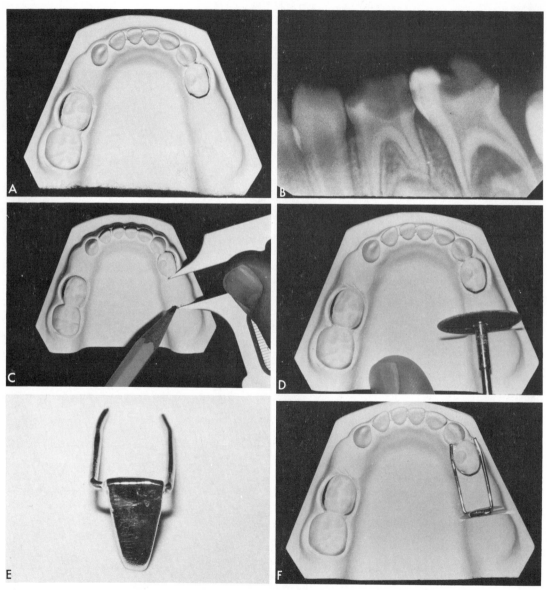

FIGURE 7–50 The technique used to make a distal shoe is illustrated with this cast with a missing primary second molar and an unerupted permanent first molar. **A,** The band is fitted on the primary first molar and an impression obtained. The band is removed from the tooth, stabilized in the impression, and poured in stone. **B,** Measuring from a previous radiograph, the distance from the distal surface of the primary first molar to the uninterrupted permanent molar is determined, taking radiographic magnification into account. **C,** The distance is marked on the cast, and **(D)** a groove is cut for the intra-alveolar blade. **E,** The stainless steel blade is soldered to a .030-inch wire loop, which is **(F)** positioned in the groove.

Illustration continued on opposite page

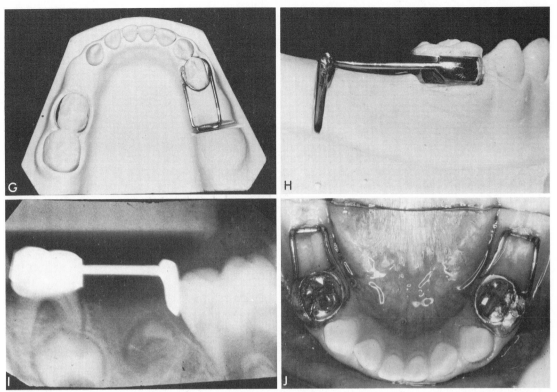

FIGURE 7–50 *Continued G,* The loop is then soldered and polished. *H,* Note that the loop is 1.5 mm off the tissue. *I,* This radiograph shows the distal shoe in place with the proper relationship to the erupting molar. *J,* The intraoral view reveals bilateral distal shoes cemented to stainless steel crowns. These will be easy to remove when the permanent molars have erupted. The blade portion can be incorporated into a removable partial denture if appropriate abutment teeth for a fixed appliance are missing.

and appliance cleaning. Care must be taken when clasping primary canines for retention, since their lateral adjustment during incisor eruption is critical. The eruption of permanent teeth may call for a modification in design.

The distal shoe is usually the appliance of choice when primary second molars are lost owing to caries or ectopic eruption prior to the eruption of the first permanent molar (Fig. 7–50). The orientation of the alveolar portion of the appliance may be used to maintain or slightly increase arch length. The distal shoe may be constructed as a fixed or removable appliance; it may provide occlusal function depending upon both the appliance design and the material of construction. Because it uses a band and not a crown, the appliance can be removed and replaced easily. This appliance is probably contraindicated in patients who are at risk

for debilitation by bacteremia, since complete epithelialization of the tissue surrounding the intra-alveolar portion has not been demonstrated.

Moderate Generalized Space Discrepancy: Space Management and Selective Removal of Primary Teeth

It is a common occurrence to encounter an 8- or 9-year-old child with crowding of the lower permanent incisors, a lesser tendency toward crowding in the upper arch, and a space discrepancy of 2 to 3 mm in each arch. The patient in this category has an overall space shortage of 4 mm or less in one arch and never had enough arch length to accommodate the teeth. In such cases, slight expansion of the arches, coupled with careful timing in removal or disking of primary incisors, canines, and molars, can allow

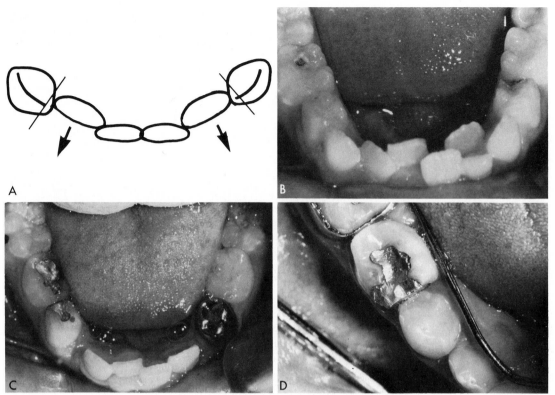

FIGURE 7–51   *A,* Disking the enamel on the mesial surface of the primary canine as illustrated will allow the primary lateral incisiors that are lingually positioned to move facially. In some cases, extraction of the primary canine may be necessary owing to the extent of the space discrepancy. *B,* This patient has lower incisor faciolingual irregularity, a space discrepancy, and a retained primary left lateral incisor. *C,* Two months after extraction of the primary teeth the faciolingual irregularity has resolved and only slight rotational problems remain. *D,* Disking can be used in the posterior segments to allow succedaneous teeth to erupt into limited space. Enamel and a portion of the old restoration were removed in this case.

a child who otherwise would have had moderate crowding throughout life to have an essentially perfect arrangement of teeth.

Disking or selective removal of primary incisors, canines, and molars will help reduce faciolingual irregularity if space is available and will allow the teeth to erupt over the alveolus and through keratinized tissue (Fig. 7–51). On the other hand, rotational changes are not as successfully resolved by selective removal of primary teeth (Fig. 7–52). When the incisors are correctly aligned but the primary canines are tucked lingually, there is a temptation to remove the primary canines and to watch the arch form change. In this instance, the incisors usually develop spacing and fail to develop alignment improvement (Fig. 7–53). Primary teeth should be removed symmetrically, or, if a primary tooth is lost on one side of the arch, the similar tooth on the opposing side should also be extracted (Fig. 7–54). This will encourage symmetry and discourage midline shifts. The key to treatment in cases of moderate space discrepancy is the lower arch, and the appliance of choice is the adjustable loop–lingual arch (Fig. 7–48).

In treatment of a moderate generalized discrepancy, space to alleviate incisor crowding may be obtained from two sources: First, the "leeway space," representing the difference in size between the permanent premolars and primary molars, may be used to prevent mesial migration of the first permanent molar. A lingual arch resting against the cingula of the lower incisors will serve to maintain arch length. The lingual arch is particularly important to maintain the incisor position if primary canines are removed prematurely. Second, space may be gained

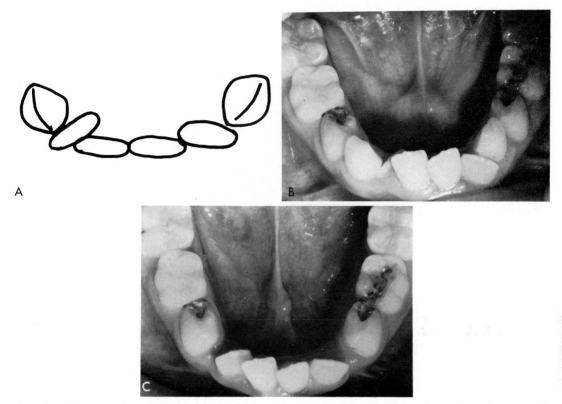

FIGURE 7–52 *A,* When rotational irregularity exists during the transition from the primary to the permanent dentition, disking or extraction of primary canines will usually not resolve the rotational problems. The rotational irregularities of the central and erupting lateral incisors *(B)* before and *(C)* approximately 2 months after extraction of the primary canines. Although the space is available, spontaneous derotation did not occur.

by slight expansion of the arches, achieved by repeated slight widening of the loop in the adjustable lingual arch. This expansion results in tipping the incisors forward. The expansion must be minimal to avoid placing the permanent teeth in an unstable position, but 1 to 2 mm may be readily gained in this fashion; often this is all that is required.

If the lower first permanent molar is prevented from coming forward when the second primary molar is lost in order to alleviate crowding, proper interdigitation of the first molars and other teeth in the buccal segments may not be achieved. Thus, in addition to placing the lower lingual arch, it may be necessary to use an appliance that will tip the upper molar distally into a proper occlusal relationship with the lower molar. Tipping the upper molar back will, of course, also increase arch length in the upper arch and reduce the possibility of crowding there.

Two types of appliances may be used if it is necessary to tip the upper molar back slightly. The first of these is the Kloehn type of face-bow, which uses extraoral force to tip the upper molars back (see Fig. 7–30). This appliance can be quite effective in a short time. Because it has undesirable side effects (especially in elongating the upper molars), it should not be used for more than 3 to 4 months for this purpose. Extraoral force can be quite beneficial in many cases, but its application in limited orthodontics is risky unless it is used with light force and only for short periods of time.

A variety of removable appliances, using finger springs against the molars, also have been advocated for tipping molars back. The general design is similar to that of the helical-spring space-regaining appliance (Fig. 7–55). These appliances use the incisors as anchorage for the bilateral movement of first molars, an arrangement that is likely to

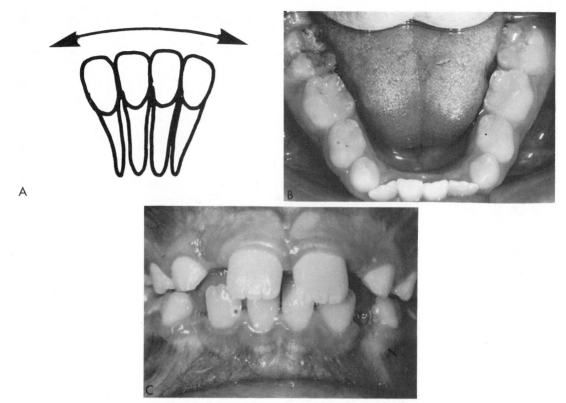

FIGURE 7–53 *A,* When the permanent incisors are positioned with the root apices close together, and *B,* the incisor crowns are aligned but facial to the lingually positioned primary canines, *C,* removal of the primary canines will not improve the arch form but usually leads to spacing of the incisors.

result in protrusion of the incisors rather than backward movement of the molars. The face-bow is a better choice in most cases.

Moderate Localized Discrepancy: Space Regaining

When less than 4 mm of space loss is restricted to one quadrant, the aim of treatment is to reposition the tipped teeth. Repositioning of molar teeth that have tipped forward may be accomplished with a variety of appliances. In the upper arch, the molar teeth show a particular tendency to rotate around the lingual root as they drift forward, so that regaining space may be largely a task of derotating the molars.

The appliance that is the most reliable and controllable for limited space regaining in the maxillary arch is the Hawley appliance incorporating a helical spring and adequate retention. In the mandibular arch either a similar Hawley appliance or an active lingual arch can be used depending upon the teeth

present and the anchorage requirements. Both of these appliances have the liability of moving mandibular incisors anteriorly instead of molars posteriorly. Therefore, these appliances need careful monitoring during

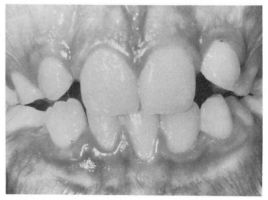

FIGURE 7–54 Loss or extraction of one primary canine usually leads to a midline shift. The mandibular right canine was lost and the midline spontaneously moved to the right in this case.

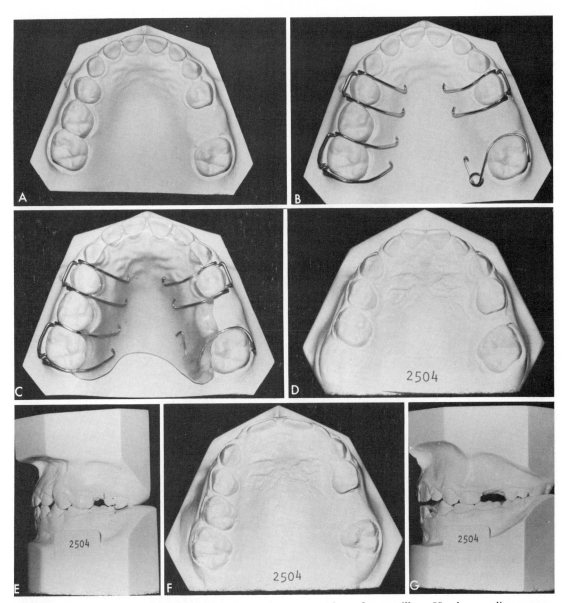

FIGURE 7–55 This series highlights the steps in construction of a maxillary Hawley appliance to retain space lost owing to the mesial tipping of a permanent first molar. *A,* Initial cast. *B,* Adams clasps are fabricated for several teeth to provide good bilateral retention. A labial bow provides very little retention in the mixed dentition. The helical spring is bent from .028-inch wire with the helix over the root apex of the teeth. Wax is used to relieve the helix and free end of the spring in order to prevent embedding in the acrylic. *C,* Cold cure acrylic is applied, polymerized, trimmed, and finished. *D* and *E,* These pretreatment casts show the mesial tipping and rotation of the permanent first molar with resultant space loss. *F* and *G,* These posttreatment casts show distal movement of the permanent first molar, derotation, and space regaining. The final molar relationship is now Class I.

treatment. After the lost space is regained, there should be Class I skeletal and dental relationships, adequate space, and a good facial profile; otherwise, space regaining is probably not the appropriate treatment. If bodily movement of the maxillary first permanent molars has occurred or if the amount of space loss due to tipping is 3 to 4 mm, the use of extraoral force with a Kloehn type of face-bow may be indicated. For most purposes, however, the removable appliances are probably the best choice for space regaining in children. If these appliances are unable to create adequate space, it is likely that the discrepancy is too severe to be handled by routine space-regaining procedures.

Severe Crowding: Comprehensive Orthodontic Treatment

If a space discrepancy greater than 4 to 5 mm exists in either arch, comprehensive or-

thodontic treatment will be required if normal occlusion is to be obtained. Such cases are normally the province of an orthodontist. If a child who also has severe crowding loses a primary tooth prematurely so that a space maintainer or space regainer might otherwise be indicated, it is better to obtain consultation with an orthodontist before proceeding. With a severe space discrepancy, extraction of permanent teeth and use

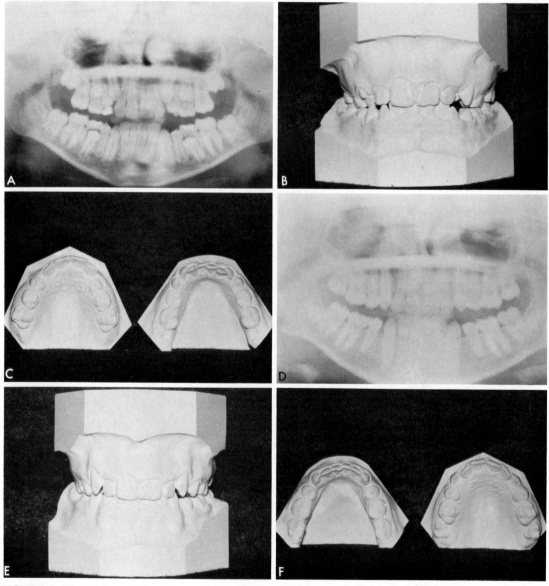

FIGURE 7–56   This case illustrates serial extraction treatment. **A,** This radiograph shows first premolar eruption and impaction of the permanent canines. **B** and **C,** These casts show the corresponding pretreatment irregularity and severe space discrepancy. **D,** This radiograph demonstrates canine eruption, and **E** and **F,** spontaneous improvement of alignment and space closure approximately 1½ years after the extraction of the permanent premolars are illustrated in the posttreatment casts.

Illustration continued on opposite page

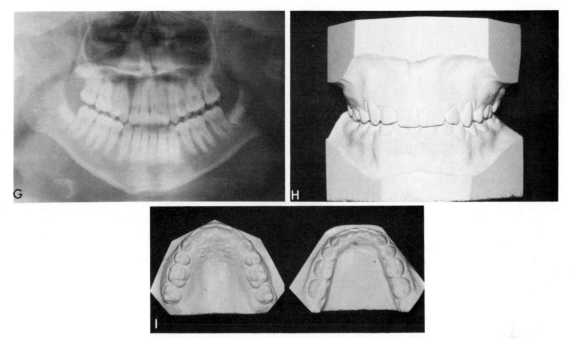

FIGURE 7–56 *Continued G,* This radiograph illustrates the finished case following fixed appliance therapy. *H* and *I,* Since little tooth movement was needed, the active treatment phase required less than 1 year's time.

of full-banded orthodontic applicances to close extraction spaces and parallel the roots of the teeth adjacent to the extraction sites will probably be required. Simple or interceptive orthodontic treatment will not be adequate when a severe discrepancy exists. Space-maintenance, space-regaining, or space-management procedures are of little benefit in such cases.

If a child with a severe discrepancy is seen early, and if there is no skeletal contribution to the malocclusion, the ultimate correction of the malocclusion may be made easier by serial extraction of primary teeth and the subsequent extraction of selected permanent premolars when they erupt. This procedure has the effect of transferring early anterior crowding around to the premolar segment. The extraction of the premolar then relieves the crowding.

At its best, serial extraction can make the necessary follow-up orthodontic treatment easier and quicker and can maintain the integrity of the supporting structures. But serial extraction does not eliminate the necessity for placement of a full-banded orthodontic appliance to close remaining extraction space and to parallel roots of adjacent teeth (Fig. 7–56).

Serial extraction should not be initiated in severe discrepancy cases (discrepancy of 4 to 10 mm) without prior arrangements being made for full-banded treatment later. If no treatment is available, these patients will experience crowding. If the only treatment performed is serial extraction, the end result for the patients could be a mutilated dentition and other occlusal problems as bad or worse for the future health of the dentition than crowding would have been. The general practitioner must recognize that, in some cases, no treatment is the best approach to patient management.

Very Severe Discrepancy (Greater Than 10 mm): Extraction

If a child with a very severe discrepancy is seen, it may be presumed that extractions will be necessary. In such patients an ideal occlusion can be obtained in most instances only if full orthodontic therapy follows extractions. If no orthodontic treatment is available, and if the space discrepancy is greater than 10 mm, there will probably be a net benefit to the patient from serial extraction procedures alone. Only in patients with discrepancy of this magnitude is a den-

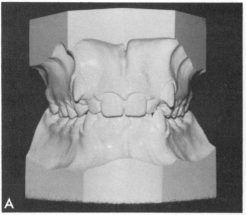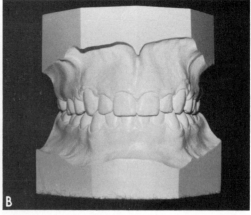

FIGURE 7–57 *A,* This case is very similar to the one described in Figure 7–56 except that the permanent teeth were not extracted until the canines had erupted. This led to compromised periodontal attachment and required 2 years of active orthodontic treatment since more tooth movement was required to obtain a good result *(B).*

tist justified in beginning serial extraction without being sure that full orthodontic therapy is available as a follow-up. Consultation with an orthodontist should be sought whenever possible.

The goal of serial extraction is to eliminate crowding by removing primary teeth as necessary to provide space for alignment of permanent teeth. In a typical patient with very severe crowding, it may be necessary to remove primary canines when the permanent laterals erupt. Again, this procedure will allow the permanent teeth to erupt over the alveolus and in the keratinized tissue. If one primary lateral or canine is lost owing to ectopic eruption of a permanent incisor, the antimere should also be removed to eliminate midline shifts. The procedure culminates with removal of four first premolars prior to the eruption of the permanent canines and second premolars.

In serial extraction cases it is advantageous for the first premolar to erupt ahead of the canine. The normal eruption sequence in the maxilla is for the first premolar to erupt prior to the canine and second premolar, so that usually little difficulty is experienced. In the lower arch, however, the canine and first premolar often erupt almost simultaneously. The eruption of the first premolar may be hastened by removal of the first primary molar 6 to 12 months before this tooth would otherwise be lost. Careful timing of the extraction of the first primary molar will often allow easy removal of the first premolar just as it emerges from the alveolar bone.

In the lower arch, if the canine erupts well ahead of the first premolar, it may be necessary to expose and enucleate the developing first premolar surgically to prevent a more difficult impaction later. In cases of very severe crowding, the permanent canines never should be allowed to erupt before the first premolars have been removed (Fig. 7–57). A summary of serial extraction procedures is shown in Table 7–5.

Related Arch Circumference (Length) Problems

Irregular Spacing of Incisors. Spacing is often observed in the maxillary anterior segment during eruption of the permanent incisors and canines. Many times this condition is eliminated when the canines have completely erupted and no longer place a mesial force on the lateral incisor roots. Therefore, treatment of maxillary anterior spacing should be delayed until eruption of

TABLE 7–5 Serial Extraction Procedure

Extract	Time
Primary central and lateral incisors	Permanent centrals erupting
Primary canines	Permanent laterals erupting
Primary first molars	Six to twelve months before normal exfoliation
Permanent first premolars	Before canine and second premolar erupt

the canines is completed. If spacing persists, however, and if hard or soft tissue anomalies and the occlusion can be eliminated as etiologic agents, the spaces may be closed.

Sometimes flaring is the result of a past thumb-sucking habit. This condition will frequently correct itself when the habit is stopped (see "Anterior Open Bite" later in this chapter), but it may be desirable to tip the teeth back together and close the space with an orthodontic appliance. The removable Hawley appliance is ideal for both of these conditions. The traditional appliance uses a wire bow across the anterior teeth (Fig. 7–58). Acrylic must be cut away on the lingual of the incisors so that these teeth and the gingiva will be free to move lingually. The acrylic should be left fitting closely around posterior teeth, which should not move.

A removable Hawley appliance can be used to bring incisors lingually only if there is adequate vertical clearance. Since the teeth are tipping, the amount of overbite will also increase. This approach to treatment should not be used when there is a Class II skeletal pattern accompanied by the typical deep anterior overbite. Although space closure in these cases may be relatively easy, maintaining the correction is often a problem. Many times a fixed retaining appliance must be used.

Ectopic Eruption. Eruption is ectopic when a permanent tooth causes resorption of a primary tooth other than the one it is to replace, or in the case of the erupting permanent molars, resorption of the adjacent primary teeth. Ectopic eruption of the first permanent molars presents a most interesting problem. This painless and often undiagnosed condition occurs more often in the maxilla than in the mandible. The lack of timely intervention may cause tooth loss and simultaneous space loss. Because of the frequent self-correction of this condition, a period of watchful waiting is probably indicated when small amounts of resorption are observed.

Several methods of intervention are available if they are needed. When a first permanent molar is erupting ectopically, brass ligature wire (.020 in.) may be looped around the contact between the first permanent molar and the second primary molar (Fig. 7–59). By tightening the ligature, pressure can be transmitted to the ectopically erupting permanent molar, which causes it to move distally and allows it to erupt freely. Alternatively, when the occlusal surface of the erupting first permanent molar is accessible, a fixed appliance may be fabricated to apply a distal force to the permanent molar (Fig. 7–60). In patients exhibiting gross resorption of the primary second molar, removal of the tooth may be the treatment of choice. Extraction should be followed by placement of a distal shoe guiding the erupting first permanent molar to a more distal position, or the permanent molar can be allowed to erupt and then be repositioned.

Anteroposterior Problems

The anterior crossbite is probably the most often encountered minor anteroposterior problem in the developing dentition. If the etiology of the anterior crossbite is dental and if space is available, this condition should be corrected.

Common dental etiologies of anterior crossbite include arch length deficiencies, aberrant tooth bud position, ectopic eruption, and retained primary or supernumerary teeth. Before beginning treatment procedures to correct an anterior crossbite, it is necessary to determine that there is enough space to accommodate the teeth if they are moved out of crossbite relationship. A space analysis should be done if there is any doubt as to the availability of adequate space.

If the anterior crossbite is due to a skeletal problem, however, its correction may not be advisable because of the amount of dental compensation required and the probability of recurrence. Class III skeletal problems should be either identified during the profile analysis or suspected by the presence of an anterior *and* posterior crossbite. A skeletal problem should be evaluated carefully by someone prepared to deal with continued abnormal skeletal growth. Uncorrected anterior crossbites often lead to continued functional shifts, tooth abrasion, alveolar warpage, or gingival stripping of mandibular incisors.

As previously described, an anterior crossbite and a Class III molar and canine relationship are present in a pseudo–Class III malocclusion not because of a skeletal problem but as the result of an edge-to-edge incisor relationship that causes an interference in centric relation and an anterior positioning of the mandible to centric occlusion (see Fig. 7–21). By tipping the maxillary incisors

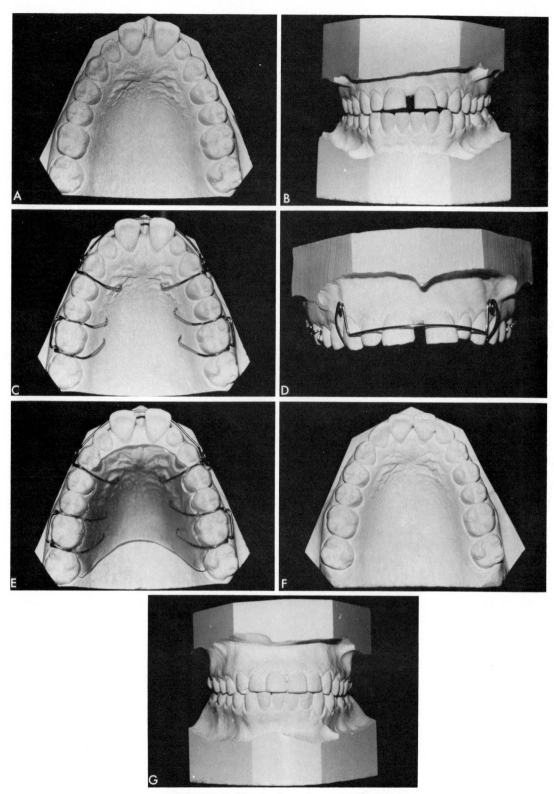

FIGURE 7–58   *See legend on opposite page*

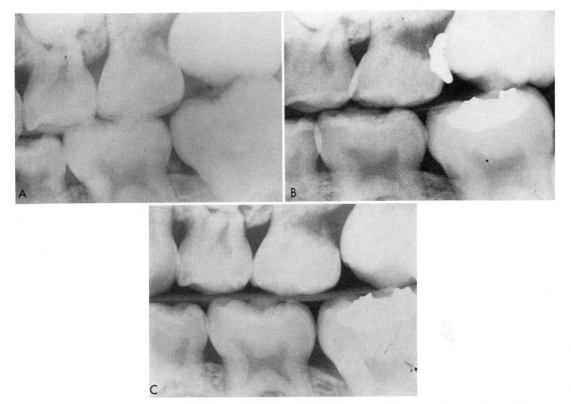

FIGURE 7–59 *A,* An ectopically erupting permanent maxillary first molar caused resorption of the second primary molar roots. *B,* A .020-inch dead soft brass wire is ligated around the contact point and tightened. *C,* After the ligature has been tightened at three 1-week intervals, the first permanent molar is dislodged and erupts into occlusion.

forward and thereby changing their axial inclination, the incisor interference is removed and the anterior positioning of the mandible and the anterior crossbite are eliminated.

Anterior crossbites due to arch length deficiencies can be intercepted by timely extraction of the adjacent primary teeth, which will allow erupting teeth to align in a normal position (Fig. 7–61). A method of correcting an existing single tooth anterior crossbite is through the use of an inclined plane. A tongue blade is one kind of inclined plane and is best used when minimal tooth movement is required and when the tooth in crossbite is already mobile (Fig. 7–62). Adequate overbite to retain the correction is necessary. By applying moderate, continuous force with the tongue blade to the offending tooth, the correction should be effected within 30 to 45 minutes. Single tooth anterior crossbite correction should be done preferably in the office, because this allows

FIGURE 7–58 This case illustrates the use of a Hawley appliance to close excess space in the maxillary arch by lingual tipping of the maxillary central and lateral incisors (*A* and *B*). This is acceptable, since the increased overbite that results from this type of tipping movement will close the open bite. *C,* Adams clasps are fabricated for the permanent first molars and a .025-inch labial bow with helices is used to retract the teeth. *D,* Note that the labial bow rests in the middle third of the teeth and that the wire is approximately 1.5 mm off the soft tissue. *E,* The completed appliance has approximately 2 mm of acrylic removed from the area lingual to the maxillary incisors to allow for incisor movement and soft tissue displacement. *F* and *G,* The space is closed, and the form of the lateral incisors is modified with resin to make their size consistent with the central incisors.

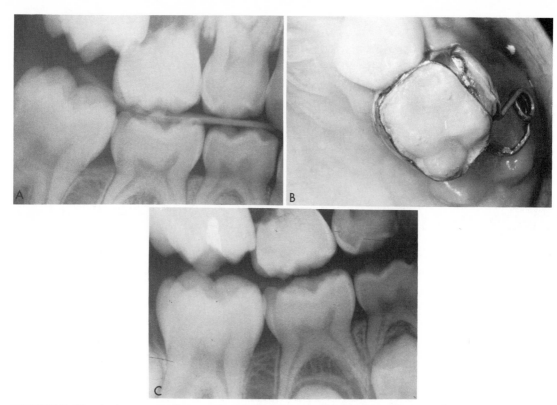

FIGURE 7–60 *A,* An ectopically erupting permanent maxillary first molar caused extensive resorption of the second primary molar. *B,* Owing to the large amount of movement necessary to dislodge the permanent tooth, a band and helical spring appliance (.028-inch wire) is used to tip the permanent molar distally. A small preparation is made in the occlusal surface of the permanent first molar in which to engage the spring. *C,* When the permanent molar moves distally, the appliance is removed and the preparation deepened and restored. The permanent molar continues to erupt and the primary molar remains intact.

the dentist to monitor the tooth movement and reinforce the child's behavior. The discomfort can be withstood easily by some children and cannot by others.

When one or two teeth are in crossbite, a Hawley appliance with finger springs may be used to correct anterior axial inclinations. The major considerations are simplicity, ad-

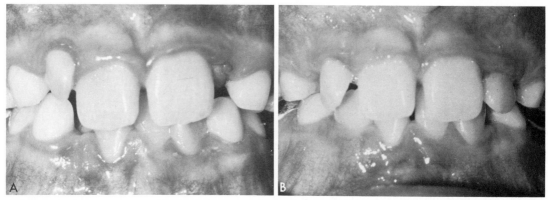

FIGURE 7–61 *A,* This patient exhibits a developing anterior crossbite of the permanent maxillary left lateral incisor due to a lack of space. *B,* Timely extractions of the primary canines allow the lateral incisors to erupt out of crossbite without the need for appliance therapy and thus avoid a shift of the midline.

312

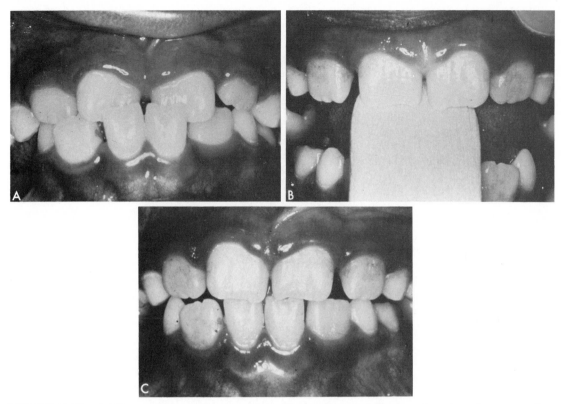

FIGURE 7–62 *A,* The position of the central incisors in this patient caused an interference and an anterior shift to an anterior crossbite in centric occlusion. *B,* Since the teeth are mobile, the patient is instructed to use a tongue blade to apply pressure to the teeth and tip them out of crossbite. *C,* This therapy corrects the crossbite and reduces the anterior shift during closing. (Courtesy of T. R. Oldenburg.)

equate retention, and desired force and range of the finger springs. An effective design incorporates a helical spring for tooth movement combined with Adams clasps for retention (Fig. 7–63). If the overbite exceeds 2.0 mm, a posterior bite plate may be necessary to open the bite and to allow the tooth in crossbite to be moved labially without interference from the occlusion. If a bite plate is used, occlusal contact should be maintained on all the posterior teeth to prevent extrusion.

Transverse Problems

The transverse problem most commonly encountered in developing dentitions is the posterior crossbite. This problem may have a skeletal or a dental component or both. Generally, transverse problems need to be corrected early in the developing dentition since they may cause unwanted growth mod-

ifications or confuse the diagnosis of other conditions.

When only the dental structures are at fault, the constriction may be unilateral or bilateral. In a true unilateral crossbite the constriction affects only one side of the occlusion. A bilateral constriction affects both sides of the occlusion, although the degree of constriction on each side may not be equal. A careful clinical examination combined with correctly trimmed study casts is a necessity for the final diagnosis of a crossbite. Since the transverse problem may be caused by true skeletal asymmetry, the profile analysis is necessary. Occasionally a posteroanterior cephalometric head film can also provide useful information in this diagnosis. Treatment of skeletal transverse problems is discussed later in the appropriate section.

Dental crossbites usually involve teeth with axial inclinations that are not consistent with the rest of the dentition. Crossbites in the

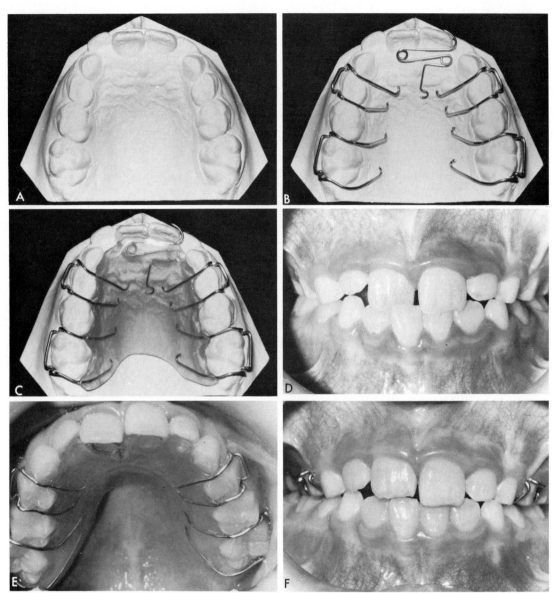

FIGURE 7–63 *A,* This cast demonstrates a situation in which the maxillary central incisors need to be tipped facially to correct an anterior crossbite. *B,* Adams clasps are bent for the posterior teeth to provide good retention, and a double cantilever helical spring is fabricated with .025 stainless steel wire to move the teeth. The helices and the free end are blocked out with wax to prevent acrylic from flowing around them during polymerization. *C,* The finished appliance ready for delivery. Note that the free end of the spring is facial to the incisors and can be used to aid in seating the spring. *D,* A patient with the permanent maxillary right central incisor in crossbite. *E,* In place, a Hawley appliance that incorporates four Adams clasps and a helical spring to move the incisor. *F,* The position at the end of the active tooth movement. Note that the tipping has reduced the overbite; therefore, the appliance will be continued in a passive state until tooth eruption has occurred and the overbite is increased.

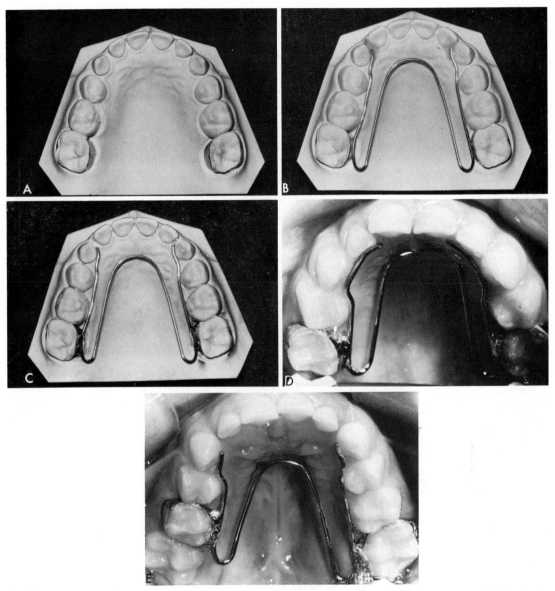

FIGURE 7–64 This cast will be used to demonstrate the steps in W-arch fabrication. *A,* The bands are fitted on the permanent maxillary first molars, and an impression is made. The bands are stabilized and an impression is poured in stone. *B,* A .036-inch stainless steel wire is adapted to contact the lingual surfaces of the teeth that are to be moved facially, but the wire remains 1.5 mm from the palatal soft tissue. *C,* The finished appliance prior to cementation. Note that the wire extends less than 2 mm distal to the permanent molar, which reduces posterior palatal soft tissue irritation. *D,* A W-arch cemented on the second primary molars and contacting all the teeth mesial to and including the lateral incisors. *E,* An unequal W-arch designed to correct a true unilateral crossbite by differentially moving the primary right molars and canine more than the anchorage segment, which also includes a permanent first molar. This appliance should be used until the occlusion is slightly overcorrected and then should be retained.

primary and mixed dentitions are best treated when they are discovered. This will reduce dental alveolar warpage, possibly result in better permanent tooth positions, and eliminate potentially harmful functional patterns. However, when succedaneous teeth or first permanent molars will erupt within 1 year and may also be in crossbite, it is usually best to delay treatment. In a few cases abnormal primary canine morphology causes the patient to occlude in crossbite in order to eliminate an interference. In select cases simple equilibration of the canines rectifies this situation.

There are several reliable appliances to correct posterior dental crossbites. The cemented W arch, which is a fixed appliance, offers reliable correction of the crossbite with little patient cooperation. When used with lingual arms of equivalent length, this appliance is very useful in correcting bilateral constrictions. Alternatively, the lingual arms may be of unequal length (Fig. 7–64), thereby making it possible to control the anchorage of the posterior segment and allowing differential or, in some cases, unilateral movement of the teeth. Three months of retention is usually adequate to maintain the correction.

A quad helix appliance can be used in similar circumstances. This appliance has somewhat greater range and is useful when the constriction is more severe (Fig. 7–65). It also is useful if a thumb-sucking habit is present when a posterior crossbite is to be corrected. The additional bulk of wire in the palate will serve as a reminder and will interrupt the habit as well.

Cross elastics may be used to correct posterior crossbites when alteration of both

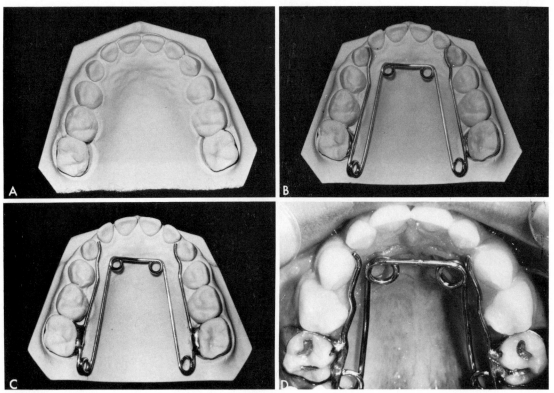

FIGURE 7–65 This appliance will be used to illustrate the steps in quad helix construction. The bands are fitted on the permanent maxillary first molars and an impression made *(A)*. The bands are stabilized and the impression poured in stone. *B,* A .038-inch stainless steel wire is adapted to contact the lingual surfaces of the teeth that are to be moved facially but remains 1.5 mm from the palatal soft tissue. *C,* The finished appliance prior to cementation. Note that the helices adjacent to the permanent molars are approximately 3 mm in diameter and do not extend more than 2 mm distal to the permanent molars in order to reduce palatal soft tissue irritation. *D,* A quad helix seated prior to cementation. By placing the anterior helices close to the incisors, a beneficial side effect may be gained: Finger habits can often be eliminated during crossbite correction.

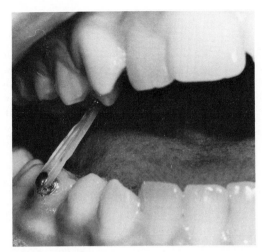

FIGURE 7–66 A cross elastic that will move the maxillary premolar facially and the mandibular premolar lingually is shown in place. This treatment should continue until the two teeth are slightly over-corrected. In this case buttons are bonded to the teeth instead of using bands. Note that although the directional pull is the opposite of that shown in Figure 7–67, both situations have a vertical component of force that can extrude teeth.

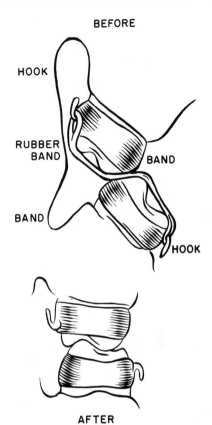

FIGURE 7–67 Effective correction of a single tooth crossbite can be accomplished with a "through-the-bite" elastic mechanism. The teeth in crossbite are banded and hooks are soldered or welded in the direction of the crossbite. A 4- to 6-oz elastic is attached to these hooks and crosses the occlusal plane. The force is reciprocal on both opposing teeth and should tip them into correct alignment.

maxillary and mandibular tooth axial relations is indicated (Figs. 7–66 and 7–67). Since heavy cross elastics must be worn full time by the patient to effect the necessary change, this method demands cooperation by the patient. It may cause extrusion of the teeth owing to the horizontal and vertical direction of force and should be used for rapid, limited treatment. Retention provided by the occlusion should be adequate to maintain the correction.

Vertical Problems

Ankylosed Teeth

It is reasonable to maintain an ankylosed tooth unless teeth distal to the ankylosed tooth begin to tip mesially with resultant loss of arch length or unless the ankylosed tooth is submerged to the point that it causes a periodontal and alveolar bone defect (see Fig. 7–24). In some cases an oversized stainless-steel crown may maintain occlusal contact and prevent distal teeth from tipping mesially. If it becomes necessary to remove an ankylosed tooth, routine extraction procedures usually prove successful. Rarely is

bony dissection necessary. Following the extraction, space maintenance is usually indicated.

Anterior Open Bite and Habit Problems

Almost all children engage in some sort of nonnutritive sucking of a thumb, finger, or other object. Sucking habits of this type are normal in the preschool years. If the sucking habit is prolonged, it is likely that the developing dentition will begin to be affected, and the dentist should become concerned if a child is still sucking his or her thumb at 5 years of age or later. There now are clear data from the United States Public Health Service (USPHS) studies of malocclusion to indicate that prolonged thumb-sucking can

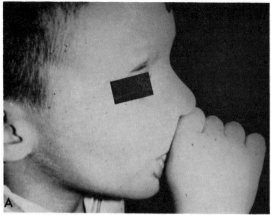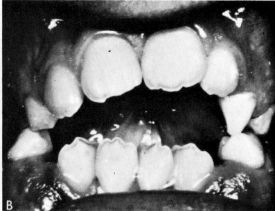

FIGURE 7–68 *A* and *B,* A chronic thumbsucker can produce a severe anterior open bite, with irregular protrusion of the upper anterior teeth and lingual tipping of lower anteriors. Correction of the malocclusion depends on control of the habit. (Courtesy of Dr. M. I. Cohen.)

have a deleterious effect. In their survey of children aged 6 to 11, the USPHS investigators asked about thumbsucking and reported that approximately 15 per cent of all children continue to suck their thumb at the time they begin school, with the percentage declining to about half that at age 11. The incidence of anterior open bite in the children who reported thumb-sucking both day and night was 80 per cent, and two thirds also had some protrusion of maxillary incisors. There is a significant relationship between thumb-sucking and both open bite and incisor protrusion.

It would be desirable to terminate a finger habit as early as possible (Fig. 7–68). A more reasonable approach is to eliminate the habit at least prior to the eruption of the permanent incisors. In any case, habit therapy is not indicated if a child does not want to quit regardless of the dental deformity. Concern and explanation from the dentist are often enough to interrupt the habit. During the time that the dentist is dealing with treatment, it is wise to have the parents refrain from reprimands or punishment. As a next step a reward system based upon praise or a homemade calendar on which stickers are placed to mark days when the habit is not practiced is often helpful. Sometimes a larger tangible reward needs to be negotiated between the child and parent. A reminder such as a Band-aid or a glove can be placed on the offending finger to disrupt the habit. This type of therapy is most successful if the patient is a passive finger sucker during sleep or television viewing.

If all the previously mentioned methods fail, a cemented reminder appliance with a metal framework lingual to the maxillary incisors that does not interfere with the occlusion is helpful (Fig. 7–69). It is necessary to explain the purpose of these appliances to the patient and to stress the fact that the appliance is a reminder and not punishment. Therefore, sharp spurs or a "rake" are not indicated. It is also not realistic to use a removable appliance, since noncompliance is the source of the original problem. Usually a 2- to 3-month period of appliance wear after the habit is extinguished is sufficient to ensure successful treatment.

If there is an anterior open bite, the child will certainly place the tongue tip in the

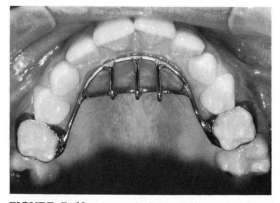

FIGURE 7–69 A reminder appliance made of .038-inch stainless steel wire cemented to the primary molars. This makes the appliance less flexible. This appliance will usually interrupt a finger habit when children want to break the habit.

space between the incisor teeth, thus displaying a "tongue-thrust swallow." During the 1950s and 1960s, much attention was paid to this type of swallow as a cause of open bite. Research findings in the past decade indicate that teeth do not respond to intermittent pressures such as those created during swallowing (or chewing). It therefore seems unlikely that the tongue-thrust swallow is a cause of the open bite. Instead, it is an effect of the open bite. A child must obtain an anterior seal when swallowing in order to keep material from escaping from the front of the mouth. Placing the tongue in an anterior space is an effective way to do this. If thumb-sucking stops, an anterior open bite usually corrects itself spontaneously, and no special therapy aimed at swallowing is indicated. Despite the vogue for "myofunctional therapy" aimed at correcting swallowing patterns, which occurred some years ago, no evidence was ever presented to indicate that this therapy did any good. If a child has good vertical skeletal jaw relationships, an anterior open bite is quite likely to close spontaneously. If there is a vertical growth problem, the open bite may persist, but in this instance it is unrelated to the position of the tongue tip during swallowing, and therapy aimed at swallowing accomplishes nothing.

Although intermittent tongue pressure during swallowing has little or no effect on the teeth, the resting pressures from a tongue that is positioned forward all the time could have an effect. Some children may adopt a forward tongue posture that interferes with closure of an open bite. Before attempting to alter tongue posture, the practitioner should investigate the reason for this. If a child has very large tonsils, for instance, he or she will have no choice but to carry the tongue forward, and attempts to change tongue posture in such a child will fail. In most instances, if the open bite is corrected by moving the teeth into position with an orthodontic appliance, a change in tongue posture will be produced.

Prolonged sucking habits can produce a narrowing of the maxillary arch. If there is a tendency toward bilateral posterior crossbite, which often accompanies an anterior open bite, maxillary expansion may be very helpful in treatment. As previously mentioned, anterior open bites tend to correct spontaneously, but posterior crossbites do not. The dentist should not be so concerned with the anterior open bite that all his attention is focused on that, while a posterior narrowing is overlooked. In fact, correcting the posterior crossbite may totally resolve the transverse and vertical problems.

It is true that the longer an anterior open bite persists, the more difficult it is to correct and the more likely that there is a significant skeletal component. The anterior open bites, which have a good chance for spontaneous correction or correction with simple treatment, such as mild maxillary expansion, usually resolve by 10 years of age. It is probably good judgment to refer patients with open bite who are older than 10 years of age to an orthodontist, since a difficult problem of malocclusion probably exists.

APPLIANCE ADJUSTMENT AND MAINTENANCE

When the time arrives to insert an appliance, careful manipulation of the appliance and interaction with the patient and parent will markedly improve the success rate for orthodontic treatment. Minor misunderstandings can ruin appliances or inhibit treatment progress.

The appliance should be checked at the chairside to ensure that it has been constructed in accordance with the prescription. Obvious problems should be corrected prior to try-in; for example, acrylic projections on the tissue side of the appliance and acrylic flash can be trimmed immediately. When the appliance is first checked intraorally, the fit around the hard and soft tissues will identify sources of irritation and determine if the impression was distorted.

Next, all retentive elements should be adjusted to achieve maximal yet comfortable retention of the appliance. In this regard, crimping the gingival portion of the bands and adjusting clasps are very important. One can attempt to dislodge the clasps and bands with a fingernail or scaler to evaluate the retention.

Finally, the passivity or activation of the appliance should be appraised and adjusted. A passive appliance should rest adjacent to the soft and hard tissue and exert no force when seated. If an appliance is to be active, the dentist should make certain that acrylic and clasp wires are not in the path of de-

TABLE 7–6 Guidelines for Appliance Activation

Appliance	Activation	Expected Movement
Labial bow for incisor retraction	2 mm	1 mm per month
Helical spring to tip incisors or molar	2 mm	1 mm per month
W-arch	4–6 mm	2–4 mm per month
Quad helix	4–8 mm	2–4 mm per month
Cross elastics	4–6 oz 3/16″ or 1/4″ elastics changed 2 times per day	1–2 mm per month

sired tooth movement. Now the appliance is ready for activation. Table 7–6 lists the amount of activation recommended for the appliances discussed in this chapter.

After the appliance has been activated and inserted, the retention is again evaluated. If the retention is less than optimal, either less activation or more retention is necessary. This is also the point at which to record and verify all occlusal relationships relative to the study casts. This information will be necessary in the future to evaluate what progress (the type, direction, and amount of movement) is occurring. Without this information, no valid judgments concerning treatment progress can be made.

Communicating to the patient how to care for and manipulate the appliance is critical to the success of treatment. Often a card stating important elements of appliance wear is helpful to patients, since they forget the information given during the chairside presentation. The following facts should be mentioned to the patient at the appliance insertion appointment.

1. Reiterate the problem being treated and the reason for treatment. This is often forgotten after the initial case presentation.
2. Teeth may be sore from active appliances, but this will pass in about 3 days. Analgesics may be necessary for some patients.
3. Sore soft tissue is reason for concern, and the patient or parent should contact you immediately.
4. Wear the appliance all the time. If the patient can eat with the appliance in place, fewer appliances are lost.
5. Clean the appliance after meals with a toothbrush and toothpaste. This will eliminate mouth and appliance odor.
6. Never lay the appliance down when it is out of the mouth. If this rule is followed loss of appliances will be decreased.
7. Avoid hard and sticky food. This will eliminate appliance breakage.

8. Appliance wear is the patient's and the parents' responsibility. You will encourage wear, but cooperation is their responsibility.
9. If the appliance is broken, lost, or loose, the patient should contact the dentist immediately. If the patient waits until the next appointment, time and tooth movement already accomplished are lost.
10. If the appliance is out of the mouth because of discomfort, store in room-temperature water or in a moist plastic bag. This will reduce distortion.
11. The patient should be told not to play with the appliance. This will distort and fatigue the components.
12. Initially speech may be impaired for 2 to 3 days, but normal speech will return.
13. The dentist will answer any questions.

At the recall appointment the dentist should have the original casts available and attempt to evaluate the treatment objectively. The following steps will provide a guide to the recall appointment.

1. Find out if the patient has any complaints or problems.
2. Let the patient tell you in his own words how much he wears the appliance.
3. Evaluate the oral hygiene. If it is poor, reinforce good hygiene.
4. Check the retention and integrity of the appliance.
5. There should be no soft tissue irritation, caries, or decalcification.
6. Loose bands and bands with cement washout should be recemented.
7. Check for evidence of appliance wear such as mobile teeth or a depression line on the soft tissue from the acrylic.
8. Evaluate the present relationships and record them. By checking these against the pretreatment casts, progress will be evident. At this point, reactivate the appliance.
9. No teeth should be erupting under

TABLE 7–7 Recommended Recall Periods

Appliance	Active	Passive	Retention Period
W-arch or quad helix	3–4 weeks	6 weeks	3 months
Lingual holding arch		3 months	
Band and loop		4–6 months	
Distal shoe		3–4 months	
Hawley retainer	3–4 weeks	3–6 months	2 months
Partial denture		3–6 months	
Cross elastics	3–4 weeks		Bands remain on for 2 months

the appliance. A radiograph may be necessary to avoid inadvertent impaction.

10. Answer any questions.

The recall and retention periods listed in Table 7–7 are recommended for the respective appliances. A systematic approach to appliance monitoring will accelerate treatment and identify problem cases much earlier than would otherwise be possible. This should lead to more treatment successes.

TECHNIQUES FOR TREATMENT OF SKELETAL PROBLEMS IN CHILDREN

Selection of Patients

The most important diagnostic decision in evaluating a child with malocclusion is the determination of whether there is a skeletal contribution to the malocclusion. This decision cannot be made from merely looking at the teeth or casts of the teeth. It must be made from evaluating the facial proportions of the individual, either radiographically or from a study of the facial profile (see diagnosis section). It is axiomatic that children with skeletal malocclusions are much more difficult to treat than children whose problems are limited to the dentition. For this reason, it is wise to consider referring all children with definite skeletal malocclusions to an orthodontist.

Treatment of Class II and Class III malocclusions (which are nearly always due to some degree of skeletal malrelationship) is attempted from a somewhat different frame of reference than is the treatment of Class I malocclusions. It should be possible for a thoughtful and careful practitioner to obtain ideal occlusion for children having Class I malocclusion with moderate discrepancies. This should be the goal of treatment in every Class I case. The treatment of skeletal malocclusions outlined below may fail despite thought and care by the practitioner during treatment, for in these cases success depends in large part on a favorable growth response by the patient. Also, even if a favorable growth response occurs during initial treatment, a period of comprehensive orthodontic treatment may be needed to obtain ideal occlusion.

Despite these warnings, it is recognized that some children with severe malocclusions will be seen for whom prolonged care by a specialist is not available. In these cases the procedures outlined subsequently may be helpful.

Treatment of Transverse and Vertical Problems

By far the most common type of transverse skeletal problem is a narrow maxilla. A bilateral posterior crossbite can be corrected by tipping the maxillary teeth outward, which is appropriate treatment if the problem is a dental malposition, or can be approached by opening the maxillary midpalatal suture (which does not fuse until early adulthood) if the problem is a skeletally narrow maxilla. Until recently, expansion of the maxilla by opening the midpalatal suture was routinely referred to as rapid maxillary expansion or more graphically as "palate splitting." The technique called for placing a jackscrew appliance fitted firmly to the teeth, separating the two halves of the maxilla at a rate of 0.5 to 1.0 mm per day, and then holding the expansion for 8 to 12 weeks while the open suture fills in with new bones (Fig. 7–70). The result initially was a relatively large amount of movement of the two maxillary segments and a relatively small amount of tooth movement. After the desired expansion was obtained, however, some relapse of the bony segments always occurred even though the teeth were held tightly. In other words, tooth movement oc-

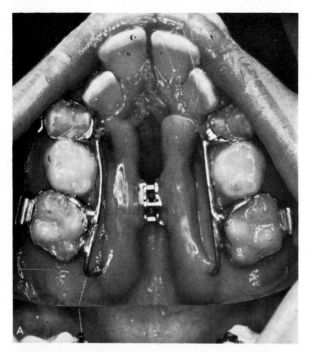

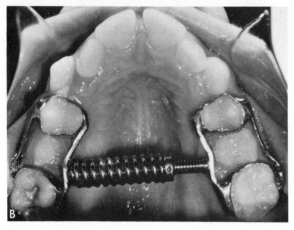

FIGURE 7–70 *A,* This maxillary jack screw expansion appliance has acrylic palatal pads but is fixed to the teeth with bands. *B,* This cemented appliance delivers its force by compression of the large spring. The amount of force can be determined by measuring the amount of spring compression for a given spring size. Since both appliances are fixed, they permit maximum efficiency when suture opening is desired.

curred during the period of fixation and healing following opening of the suture, which served to mask skeletal relapse going on at the same time. The final result of rapid maxillary expansion was approximately equal parts of tooth movement and lateral repositioning of the maxillary segments.

Theoretically, a suture under tension could respond by laying down new bone at a rate of about 1 mm per week. Recent work at the University of Washington has demonstrated that if a moderately heavy spring across the palate is activated to provide a constant 2 to 4 lb force, expansion of the suture will occur at approximately the theoretically maximal

rate. The constant force also produces tooth movement, and after a few weeks, a 50:50 ratio of dental to skeletal effects can be observed. This type of maxillary expansion, in other words, may provide good dental changes and more stable skeletal changes, although no long-term data are available. Because a bilateral crossbite with a severe skeletal constriction in the mixed dentition usually occurs in conjunction with crowding and other occlusal problems, cases of this type are probably best handled by referral.

Both open bite and deep bite vertical skeletal dysplasias have long been considered to be perhaps the most difficult of all orthodontic problems to manage. With the development of modern orthognathic surgery techniques, long-face and short-face problems can be treated in adults. Controlling these growth patterns in children requires controlling jaw position and the eruption of teeth. Extraoral force in a vertical direction, bite blocks to impede eruption in long-face patients, and early surgical intervention to facilitate nasal respiration all have received some emphasis in recent years. In the more severe problems, the prognosis for all these approaches is extremely guarded. Early referral of children who are developing skeletal vertical problems, coupled with a recognition that jaw surgery ultimately may be required, is at present the best approach for these patients.

Treatment of Class II Malocclusion

General Principles

Skeletal Class II malocclusions are characterized by a posterior position of the mandible relative to the maxilla. In some patients, the fault is overdevelopment of the maxilla; in the majority, there is a component of mandibular underdevelopment. The major goal of orthodontic therapy is, of course, to correct the relative posterior position of the mandible. This can occur only if the mandible can be persuaded to grow forward relative to the maxilla. Two basic approaches are possible: An attempt can be made to stimulate mandibular growth, or an attempt can be made to inhibit the growth of the maxilla without affecting the mandible, so that the mandible, growing at its own rate, can catch up with the maxilla. Both approaches have ardent advocates and both succeed—part of the time.

Outright stimulation of growth is clinically unproved, but it is not unreasonable to think that appliances that attempt to stimulate growth may at least serve to remove inhibitory influences and thus facilitate growth. It is well known that many influences can inhibit or at least alter the direction of growth, so that, theoretically, restraining maxillary growth is feasible.

Whenever treatment of a skeletal problem is undertaken, it is imperative that cephalometric films be taken to monitor the growth response. It is easy to be fooled about what is happening by only examining the patient and checking the occlusion. Problems and complications can be far advanced before they are noted in clinical examination alone.

Extraoral Force: Inhibition of the Maxilla

Extraoral force for correction of Class II malocclusion may be delivered by many types of head strap or neck strap arrangements, but for the purpose of the nonspecialist, the Kloehn type of face-bow offers maximum simplicity and versatility. This appliance attaches to bands placed on maxillary first molar teeth (see Fig. 7–30). The inner bow, which inserts into tubes on the molar bands, should not contact any other teeth, and no further banding is required. A cervical neck strap (fitted over a cushioning pad) is commonly used to provide a force of 16 to 20 ounces against the outer bow. In order to be effective, this appliance must be worn 12 to 14 hours every day. It is not enough for the child to wear the appliance just during sleeping hours, but neither is it necessary that it be worn full time; a consistent pattern of use is the critical factor.

In addition to exerting distal pressure against the maxillary molars, which seems to influence the entire maxilla, the Kloehn type of face-bow tends to extrude the maxillary molars. In some deep-bite patients, this can be a desirable side effect, for the extrusion tends to assist in opening the bite anteriorly. If the growth response is poor, however, molar extrusion and consequent downward positioning of the mandible may serve to accentuate rather than to improve the Class II relationship. The cervical neck strap face-bow should never be used initially in patients with an open bite. Even in deep-bite patients, it is essential that the response to the cervical face-bow be watched carefully and that the appliance be discontinued unless a favorable response is noted relatively quickly (in less than 3 months). If the response is good, the face-bow may be used for a year or more.

Retraction of flared maxillary incisors may be done after sufficient vertical clearance has been obtained. Incisors are retracted most easily by a light elastic running across the incisor teeth from hooks on the inner bow of the face-bow (Fig. 7–71). In some instances it may be desirable to band the maxillary central and lateral incisors and to use

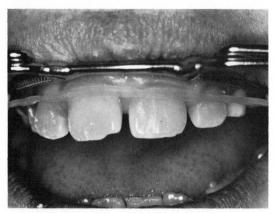

FIGURE 7–71 A light latex elastic may be suspended from small hooks on the inner bow of a face-bow (headgear) to correct anterior flaring, while the outer bow exerts distal force against upper molar teeth. Adequate anterior vertical dimension is required.

TABLE 7–8 Types of Functional Appliances

Passive tooth-borne
  Activator (Monobloc), Bionator
Active tooth-borne
  Bimler, propulsor, Kinetor, Modified activator, Modified Bionator
Passive tissue-borne
  Frankel

a wire retraction loop running from these teeth to a second tube on the first molar bands. Retraction of flared incisors should be deferred until an excellent response has been obtained in correction of molar relationship and in correction of the deep overbite.

The treatment procedure outlined above, calling for use of a cervical face-bow and (perhaps) incisor banding, is deceptively simple, for a great deal of judgment is required to evaluate progress and adjust treatment procedures accordingly. In some cases no other treatment will be necessary, but in most instances other treatment procedures are likely to be needed.

Functional Appliance Treatment: Facilitating Mandibular Growth

An alternate approach to treatment of Class II malocclusion, which is more popular in Europe than in the United States, is the use of appliances that employ a guide plane to ensure that the mandible is held forward at rest in the position desired at the end of the treatment.

Although there are a myriad of functional appliances, they can be divided conveniently into three major groups: (1) tooth-supported passive appliances, (2) tooth-supported active appliances, and (3) tissue-supported passive appliances (Table 7–8). The active appliances incorporate springs to produce tooth

movement, whereas the passive ones rely solely on repositioning the jaw or guiding the teeth as they erupt. Since the major purpose of any functional appliance is to guide growth, tooth movement at the same time is not necessarily advantageous and, in fact, can be detrimental to the desired skeletal effect. Moving the lower teeth forward to correct a skeletal Class II malocclusion is a very different thing from persuading the mandible to grow forward. If the appliance causes tooth movement, this can lead to a correction of the Class II malocclusion without the desired skeletal effect having occurred. For this reason, the passive appliances, which have no springs to cause tooth movement, are more likely to produce skeletal changes than are the active ones, which tip teeth in an active fashion.

The activator appliances incorporate a plastic guide plane into which the patient bites, holding the mandible forward. It should be noted that a distal force is transmitted to the maxillary teeth, as these teeth serve as anchorage to hold the mandible forward. The "activator" also serves as a bite plate and ordinarily incorporates a wire bow across the maxillary anterior teeth to retract and align protruding maxillary incisors (Fig. 7–72). The activator appliances attempt to increase the activity of the masticatory muscles, thereby increasing the distal pull against the maxilla.

The Frankel appliance is the sole representative of the passive, tissue-borne, functional appliance (Fig. 7–73). It uses shields in the buccal vestibules to hold the lips and cheeks away from the dentition, thus promoting arch expansion by changing the balance of resting pressures on the teeth. At the same time, it incorporates a forward position of the mandible, encouraging forward mandibular growth in the same way as do other functional appliances, but with minimal reaction forces against the teeth. For this reason, the Frankel system appears to be potentially the most effective of the func-

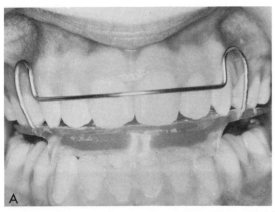
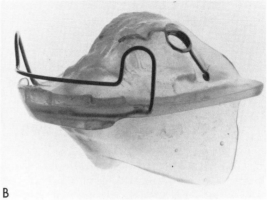

FIGURE 7–72 *A,* This type of activator is used with Class II patients to position the mandible forward and allows the mandibular posterior teeth to erupt. *B,* This view of the activator demonstrates the posterior occlusal stops that control maxillary molar eruption and the lower lingual acrylic extension that guides the mandible into a forward position.

tional appliances in altering skeletal growth. In clinical practice, results with tooth-borne appliances and Frankel appliances tend to be similar.

There is no question that activator, modified activator, or Frankel therapy can be successful. Face-bow therapy is effective also, and the results can be surprisingly similar to those achieved with functional appliances, but it must be emphasized that neither approach always succeeds. A major disadvantage of functional appliance therapy is the possibility of creating a centric occlusion position that differs markedly from centric relation, thus leading to a "dual bite." This may well happen if a good growth response does not occur. From a practical point of view, it may also be significant that with the complex activator appliances it is more difficult for practitioners with minimal experience to make the adjustments necessary to attain successful results.

If a poor growth response occurs, or if the growth period has ended, it may be necessary to reposition teeth to accommodate to the skeletal discrepancy. Surgical repositioning of the maxilla or mandible may be required in severe cases. Patients with such problems require the attention of a specialist.

Crowding of teeth due to arch length discrepancy may occur simultaneously with skeletal malocclusion. Under no circumstances should serial extraction procedures be initiated for patients with Class II or

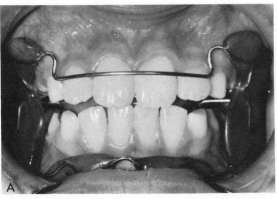
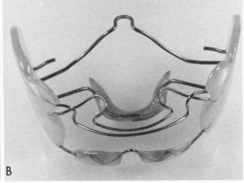

FIGURE 7–73 *A,* This Frankel appliance also positions the mandible forward in the Class II patient. The mandibular posterior teeth are allowed to erupt, and the buccal soft tissue is held away from the dentition by the buccal shields. *B,* This view demonstrates the lingual pad of acrylic that forces the mandible to be positioned forward and the buccal shields and the wire spurs that control maxillary molar eruption.

Class III malocclusion. Orthodontic correction of combined skeletal and arch length problems is difficult, requiring careful anchorage control. Uncontrolled serial extraction may make successful treatment impossible.

Treatment of Class III Malocclusion

It would seem that treatment of Class III malocclusion should be the reverse of that for Class II, but in fact little success has been obtained with attempts to inhibit mandibular growth and very modest success with stimulation of maxillary growth. Fortunately, Class III malocclusion is a much less common problem.

Some authors advocate use of a chin cup connected to a head cap to restrain mandibular growth in children with developing Class III malocclusion (Fig. 7–74). This approach is helpful to some specialists, but it cannot be recommended for other practitioners. A lower incisor should not be removed in a child with a Class III tendency—this will only add dental problems to the skeletal discrepancy.

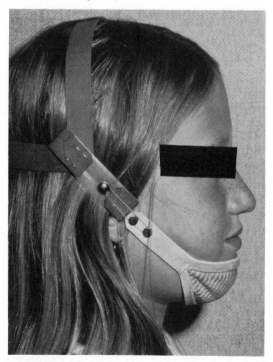

FIGURE 7–74 This chin-cup appliance attached to a head cap places an upward and backward force against the mandible. The appliance illustrated pulls at a 45-degree angle. The angle of pull varies with the requirements of the case.

TECHNIQUES FOR TREATMENT OF ADULTS

Goals of Therapy

The principles of tooth movement are exactly the same for adult patients as for children. The difference is that growth is no longer possible, so that changes in both the horizontal and the vertical dimensions must be made within the existing skeletal configuration. Contrary to the belief of many adult patients and dentists, one is never too old for orthodontics. Although gratifying results may be obtained in adult orthodontics, treating adults does present additional problems beyond those encountered in orthodontic treatment for children. The lack of any assistance in treatment from growth is the major difficulty, but treatment for an adult also generally takes a bit longer than similar treatment for a child and seems to cause greater discomfort for the patient. Adult patients must be highly motivated toward treatment before orthodontic therapy is undertaken.

The goal of orthodontic therapy for children is usually ideal occlusion, or as close to ideal occlusion as can be achieved, with treatment being directed at the whole dentition in order to achieve such occlusion. Adult orthodontics is often undertaken with less comprehensive goals and frequently plays an important role as an adjunct to periodontal treatment and restoration of missing teeth. In these instances orthodontic treatment is directed toward improving some specific aspects of a malocclusion. The only difficulty with limited treatment goals is that they sometimes lead to limited occlusal examination, so that both possibilities and potential difficulties in tooth movement may be overlooked. Compromise treatment is acceptable; a compromise diagnosis is a waste of time.

Uprighting Tipped Molar Teeth

The most valuable use of adult orthodontics as an adjunct to other dental treatment probably lies in uprighting molar teeth prior to placement of fixed restorations. Not only does uprighting the posterior abutment make it easier to construct a good bridge, but this also distributes occlusal stresses on the abutment teeth in a more desirable fashion and may thus contribute to longevity of the restoration. In addition, it has been noted recently that tipped teeth with infrabony pockets may show significant reduction in pocket depth if orthodontic therapy is carried out in conjunction with careful root planing and with home care.

The removable appliances that are effective for regaining space in children when a molar tooth has drifted forward may also be used for molar uprighting in adults (see Fig. 7–55). These appliances are most effective where only a small amount of uprighting is necessary. They are poorly tolerated by patients, particularly in the mandibular arch, and are subject to breakage and distortion. Molar teeth may be uprighted from a severely tipped position most efficiently by use of a fixed appliance banding teeth in the quadrant where uprighting is desired.

A typical situation is one in which the mandibular first molar has been lost some time previously and the second molar has tipped mesially into the first molar space. If the third molar is present, its removal should be considered unless it has a functional antagonist and is vitally needed. It is much more difficult to upright two molars than one.

If the tooth to be uprighted is the last tooth in the arch, and is severely tipped, it is most effectively uprighted by use of an aux-

iliary uprighting spring. For this appliance, the canine and premolars in the quadrant where the uprighting is to be done are banded and stabilized with a relatively stiff passive wire ligated to brackets on these teeth. A segment of rectangular wire is then formed into an uprighting spring (as shown in Figure 7–75) by bending a helical coil into the wire, so that the coil is compressed when the anterior arm of the spring is straightened. This spring delivers a force that tends to depress the stabilized canine-premolar anchor unit and upright the molar. It is important that the molar band carry a rectangular tube and that a rectangular wire be used for the auxiliary spring. Otherwise, the molar can roll buccally or lingually as force is applied. Occlusal reduction to take the molar being uprighted out of occlusion is necessary.

If the distal molar tooth is not badly tipped, or has been nearly uprighted by the use of the auxiliary spring just described, it may be possible to upright the tooth fully by inserting a flexible round (0.018-inch) arch wire, which is tied to the bands on the anchor teeth and allowed to run distally through the buccal tube of the molar. A coil spring (0.009-inch wire is suggested) is then compressed between the molar tooth and the premolar mesial to it (Fig. 7–76). The coil spring should not be completely compressed, for in this situation too much force

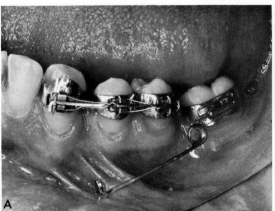 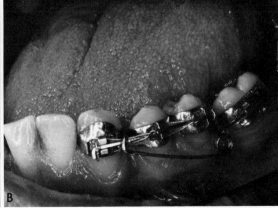

FIGURE 7–75 Uprighting molars in adults: *A,* A molar uprighting spring before activation. The premolar teeth and canine are stabilized by a .019 × .025 arch wire that fits passively into brackets on these teeth. The uprighting spring must be made of rectangular wire to prevent lingual rolling of the molar (.019 × .025 is recommended). The loop in the uprighting spring is bent gingivally to prevent it from being disturbed by the occlusion. A small hook is bent into the mesial end of the wire. *B,* The spring is activated by lifting this hook across the stabilized buccal segment. Care should be taken that the hook rests between teeth so that as the molar is uprighted, the spring may slide distally along the stabilized segment of the arch wire.

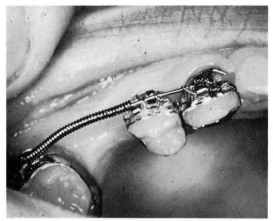

FIGURE 7–76   A condensed coil spring may be used to upright a tipped molar into a final vertical position. A segment of .019 × .025 arch wire is inserted into the molar tube and fitted to the premolar and canine. A coil spring (.009/.030 lumen) is then compressed between the buccal tube of the molar and the bracket of the premolar. The coil spring should be compressed approximately 2 mm, depending on its length. Rotation of the premolar must be prevented by use of a twin bracket, antirotation bracket arm, or staple.

may be exerted. A twin (Siamese) bracket (or a Lewis bracket that incorporates an antirotation arm) must be used on the premolar to prevent mesiolingual rotation.

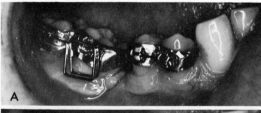

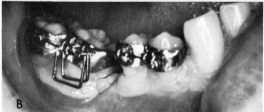

FIGURE 7–77   **A,** If a third molar is to be retained and the second molar is to be uprighted, the box loop is a useful mechanism. A .017 × .025 wire is bent with a rectangular loop opposite the second molar bracket, which places an uprighting force on the molar tooth. **B,** Note how the box loop distorts as the tooth is engaged and the loop is activated.

Where it can be used, the coil spring segment is very effective. Most patients are best treated by using the auxiliary spring initially, then changing to the compressed coil spring after some uprighting has occurred.

If it seems absolutely necessary to upright a second molar and retain the third molar behind it, another appliance using the segmented banding approach may be employed. In this case the most distal molar is banded and carries the buccal tube. The molar band mesial to it has a wide Siamese edgewise bracket welded to its buccal surface. The canine and premolars are banded and carry twin edgewise brackets as before. A rectangular wire (0.019 × 0.025 inch is recommended) is then fabricated with a box loop bent into the wire to provide a gentle uprighting force on the mesially located tipped molar (Fig. 7–77). The horizontal portion of the loop should be in alignment with both the mesial and the distal segments of the rectangular wire so that it fits passively into the rectangular brackets.

The box-loop mechanism allows the skilled operator a great deal of control and enables the tipped molar to be partially rotated if necessary. It is quite difficult to fabricate, however, and its use is recommended only in unusual circumstances. In most instances it is much better to extract the third molar before beginning the uprighting of the second molar.

Three to 6 months should be allotted to accomplish the uprighting of a severely tipped molar. It must be realized that molar teeth have broad root surfaces and that movement of these teeth requires a great deal of patience on the part of both the dentist and the patient. It is important to relieve occlusal interferences in order to get a molar tooth to tip back properly.

Other Orthodontic Procedures

The localized nature of most orthodontic procedures for adults means that these procedures may often be better accomplished with a small number of banded or bonded teeth, although it might appear that a removable appliance would work equally well. Through-the-bite elastics are particularly effective in correction of posterior crossbites in adults (see Fig. 7–66). If it is necessary to move a tooth in one arch more than the teeth in the other arch, this may be done by banding several teeth where minimal movement is required and by grouping these teeth together as an anchor unit. Removable appliances are much less effective for crossbite correction.

For malaligned or protruded teeth in the anterior region, a Hawley type of appliance may be employed (see Fig. 7–58) but only if there is adequate vertical clearance so that lower incisor teeth do not strike the palatal portion of the appliance. Banding molars and bonding anterior teeth and using a light resilient arch wire to produce alignment offer the greatest efficiency in treatment.

Banding teeth also offers a more effective way of overcoming problems produced by deep overbite, which can be quite frustrating to try to correct in adults. Overbite correction requires changes in anterior vertical dimension, but since no further vertical growth is available, overall changes must be kept within the rather small limits determined by the patient's tolerance. A bite plate may be used with an adult, but the appliance does not work so readily as with a child. With patience, a great deal of bite opening can be accomplished. In order to maintain the correction, it may be necessary to have the patient wear a bite plate indefinitely at least part of the time.

The difficulty to be expected in retaining teeth in a new position in an adult should always be considered. After uprighting of a molar, the fixed restoration serves as a permanent retainer. Occlusal forces tend to maintain the tooth that has been moved from crossbite into a normal relationship. If flared incisors are retracted, however, it is unlikely that there will be any effective force, except an orthodontic retainer, to oppose the force that led to the protrusion in the first place. Consequently, prolonged need for the orthodontic appliance can be expected. The same is true, and perhaps even more so, after increase in vertical dimension in order to correct a deep overbite. There will be a tendency for the former vertical dimension to return, and with it, the overbite. The practitioner must remember that moving the teeth is one thing; retaining them in the new position is something else.

Orthognathic Surgery

Orthognathic surgery, that is, repositioning the jaws or the segments of the dental alveolus or both to correct severe malocclusion, has become a relatively frequent procedure in the past decade. In the 1960s, the great majority of surgical procedures on the jaws were mandibular osteotomies to correct excessive growth of the mandible. By 1980, surgical procedures had been developed to allow correction of essentially any type of se-

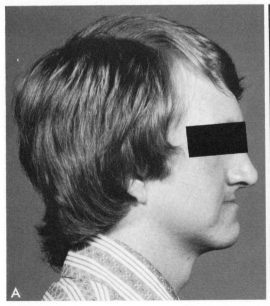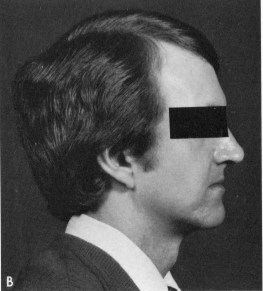

FIGURE 7–78 Skeletal maxillary deficiency treated by Lefort I osteotomy to advance maxilla. *(A)* before treatment and *(B)* after treatment.

vere malocclusion, and surgical procedures on the maxilla were as frequent as those on the mandible (Figs. 7–78 and 7–79).

The advances in surgical orthodontics have enabled the treatment of patients in the last decade who previously were untreat-able, with great benefit to these severely handicapped individuals. Carefully coordinated orthodontics and surgery are required for optimal results—neither the orthodontist nor the surgeon can treat such problems alone. Although an in-depth discussion of

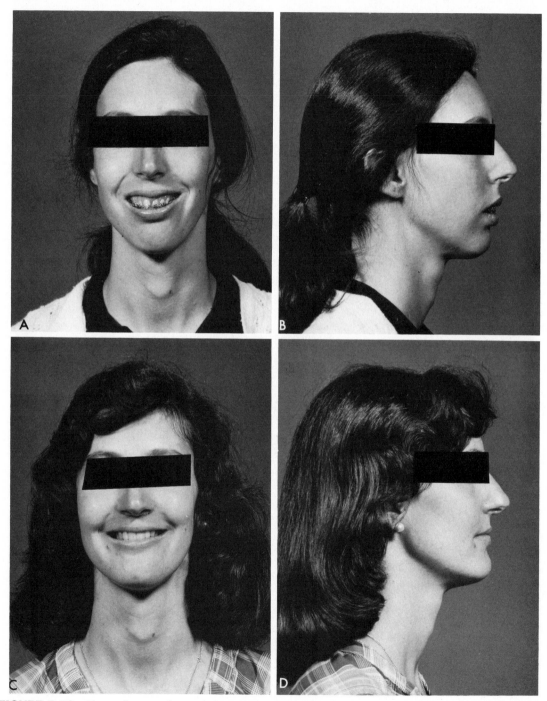

FIGURE 7–79   "Long face syndrome" treated by surgical intrusion of the maxilla. *(A)* and *(B)*, before treatment and *(C)* and *(D)*, after treatment.

surgical orthodontics is beyond the scope of this chapter, current practitioners should be aware that severe open bite, mandibular deficiency, crossbite, maxillary protrusion, and a host of other problems now can be corrected by surgical procedures on the maxilla, mandible, and chin. In most areas, there now is a referral center at which patients who would benefit from this treatment can be evaluated.

COMPLICATIONS OF ORTHODONTIC TREATMENT

Two types of complications may occur in orthodontic treatment: problems of increased susceptibility to other types of dental disease as a result of orthodontic treatment and problems due to orthodontic tooth movement itself. Of the two, problems relating to caries and gingival inflammation occurring during orthodontic treatment are much more common.

Orthodontic appliances of any type trap food, debris, and plaque and thus, by their presence, increase susceptibility to decalcification, decay, and gingival inflammation. This means that a high standard of oral hygiene is an absolute necessity if orthodontic treatment is to be performed successfully. All carious lesions should be restored before orthodontic therapy is begun, and periodic checks for caries must continue during treatment.

Areas of particular susceptibility to decay when removable appliances are used are at the linguogingival margins of maxillary posterior teeth and around clasps. With fixed appliances, bucco- and linguogingival margins of bands and the periphery of bonded attachments are potential sites for caries and decalcification. Decay does not occur under properly formed and cemented orthodontic bands (though decay will occur if cement has washed out from under a poorly fitting band). The gingival margin of even the best band forms a ledge on which debris may be maintained, and this area, particularly on canines and premolars, will be susceptible to decalcification unless good oral hygiene is maintained.

The presence of orthodontic appliances also predisposes to gingival inflammation, with the orthodontic appliances serving as a source of chronic irritation. Gingival response to removable appliances varies greatly with the fit of these appliances and the type of tooth movement being attempted. Some degree of gingival response may be expected when bands are fitted subgingivally, as they often must be to obtain a good fit on posterior teeth. In most cases gingival inflammation clears promptly when orthodontic appliances are removed. Gingival problems rarely become severe enough to require specific treatment during orthodontic tooth movement. Severe inflammation is usually related to poor oral hygiene and may result in a permanent reduction in the height of the supporting attachment. Occasionally, particularly when severely crowded anterior teeth have been aligned by orthodontic tooth movement, gingivoplasty will be required to produce proper gingival contours after appliances are removed.

Although idiopathic root resorption is seen in individuals who never had orthodontic treatment, it now seems clear that orthodontic treatment does increase the risk of apical root resorption. There is some evidence to indicate that the use of unusually heavy orthodontic forces predisposes to root resorption. It is undeniably true, however, that some degree of root resorption may occur in association with any type of orthodontic tooth movement, no matter how light the forces used. A reasonable view is that orthodontic treatment enhances any innate tendencies for root resorption but that orthodontic forces of ordinary magnitude cause little or no root resorption in persons who are not otherwise susceptible to this phenomenon.

It is possible to apply orthodontic forces so brutally that permanent periodontal membrane damage, leading to ankylosis or devitalization of the involved tooth, occurs. Complications of this type are exceedingly rare.

A more subtle complication of orthodontic tooth movement itself may occur if teeth are moved so that maximal occlusion of the teeth and centric jaw relation no longer coincide. The resulting shift of the jaw into maximal occlusion may go undetected unless occlusal relationships are carefully checked. Creation of such a "dual bite" is particularly likely to happen in treatment of Class II malocclusion. Many patients will consciously or unconsciously hold the mandible forward as Class II treatment proceeds, giving a false impression of progress.

QUESTIONS

1. Describe the two groups of orthodontic patients who can best be treated in a general practice.

2. What proportion of young patients can be aided by preventive and interceptive orthodontic treatment?

3. During adolescence, is there relatively more maxillary or mandibular growth? What are the orthodontic implications of this relationship?

4. What postadolescent changes can be expected in facial soft tissue contours?

5. When performing a profile analysis, what types of patients are most difficult to evaluate?

6. What assumptions underlie a space analysis completed during the mixed-dentition period?

7. How is dentoskeletal protrusion related to crowding?

8. Describe the relationships between root length, primary tooth extraction timing, and the time of eruption of permanent teeth.

9. What two major variables determine the response of a tooth to orthodontic force? How can they be controlled?

10. Differentiate between anchorage and retention as they relate to appliance design.

11. How does posterior space change when a primary tooth is lost prematurely in the primary or mixed dentitions?

12. What conditions are most appropriate for the implementation of serial extraction procedures?

13. What type of alignment problems are most reliably remedied by selective removal of primary teeth?

14. With regard to diagnosis and treatment, differentiate between posterior, skeletal, and dental crossbites.

15. When is treatment indicated for an anterior open bite?

16. Contrast the treatment approaches for a maxillary skeletal excess (protrusion) and a mandibular skeletal deficiency (retrusion) in the growing Class II patient.

17. What distinguishes an adult's orthodontic treatment from that of a child?

18. Describe the steps involved in uprighting a mesially tipped permanent molar in an adult patient.

19. For what problems is orthognathic surgery the best treatment approach?

20. Name the two types of complications most often encountered during orthodontic treatment.

See answers in Appendix.

REFERENCES

1. Ackerman, J. L., and Proffit, W. R.: The characteristics of malocclusion: A modern approach to classification and diagnosis. Am. J. Orthod., 56:443–454, 1969.
2. Ackerman, J. L., and Proffit, W. R.: Preventive and interceptive orthodontics: A strong theory proves weak in practice. Angle Orthod., 50:75–87, 1980.
3. Bien, S. N.: Hydrodynamic damping of tooth movement. J. Dent. Res., 45:907–914, 1966.
4. Bolton, W. A.: Disharmony in tooth size and its relation to the analysis and treatment of malocclusion. Angle Orthod., 28:113–130, 1958.

5. Edwards, J. G.: Surgical procedure to eliminate rotational relapse. Am. J. Orthod., 57:35–45, 1970.
6. Enlow, D. H.: Handbook of Facial Growth, 2nd ed. Philadelphia, W. B. Saunders Company, 1982.
7. Graber, T. M.: Orthodontics: Principles and Practice, 3rd ed. Philadelphia, W. B. Saunders Company, 1972.
8. Haryett, R. D., Hansen, R. C., Davidson, P. O., and Sandilands, M. L.: Chronic thumbsucking: The psychological effects and the relative effectiveness of the various methods of treatment. Am. J. Orthod., 53:559–85, 1967.
9. Hixon, E. H., and Oldfather, R. E.: Estimation of the sizes of unerupted cuspid and bicuspid teeth. Angle Orthod., 28:236–240, 1958.
10. Kelly, J. E., and Harvey, C. R.: An assessment of

the occlusion of the teeth of youths 12–17 years. Rockville, Md., National Center for Health Statistics, DHEW Pub. No. (HRA) 77–1644, 1977.

11. Kelly, J. E., Sanchez, M., and Van Kirk, L. E.: An assessment of the occlusion of the teeth of children. Rockville, Md., National Center for Health Statistics, DHEW Pub. No. (HRA) 74–1612, 1973.

12. Moorrees, C. F. A.: The Dentition of the Growing Child: A Longitudinal Study of Dental Development Between 3 and 18 Years of Age. Cambridge, Harvard University Press, 1959.

13. Moyers, R. E.: Handbook of Orthodontics, 3rd ed. Chicago, Year Book Medical Publishers, Inc., 1973.

14. Norton, L. A., and Proffit, W. R.: Molar uprighting as an adjunct to fixed prosthesis. J. Am. Dent. Assoc., 76:312–316, 1968.

15. Owen, D. G.: The incidence and nature of space closure following the premature extraction of deciduous teeth: A literature survey. Am. J. Orthod., 59:37–49, 1971.

16. Popovich, F., and Thompson, G. W.: Evaluation of preventive and interceptive orthodontic treatment between three and eighteen years of age. *In* Cook, J. T. (ed.): Transactions of the Third International Orthodontic Congress. St. Louis, C. V. Mosby Company, 1975, Chapter 26.

17. Proffit, W. R., and Bennett, I. C.: Space maintenance, serial extraction, and the general practitioner. J. Am. Dent. Assoc., 74:411–419, 1967.

18. Reitan, K.: Tissue behavior during orthodontic movement. Am. J. Orthod., 46:881–900, 1960.

19. Salzmann, J. A.: Practice of Orthodontics. Philadelphia, J. B. Lippincott Company, 1966.

20. Tanaka, M. M., and Johnston, L. E.: The prediction of the size of unerupted canines and premolars in a contemporary orthodontic population. J. Am. Dent. Assoc., 88:798–801, 1974.

21. Vig, P. S., and Cohen, A. M.: Vertical growth of the lips: a serial cephalometric study. Am. J. Orthod., 75:405–415, 1979.

22. Vig, P. S., and Fields, H. W.: Occlusal development: Predictive problems and clinical implications. *In* Stewart, R. E., Barber, T. K., Trontman, K. C., and Wei, S. H. Y. (Eds.): Pediatric Dentistry: Scientific Foundations and Clinical Practice. St. Louis, C. V. Mosby Company, 1982, Chapter 18.

DANIEL P. CASULLO

OCCLUSION IN GENERAL PRACTICE

Section I: Theory

INTRODUCTION

For the generalist, the practice of dentistry is anything but routine. Unlike the specialist who manages a fixed set of dental problems circumscribed by his or her discipline, the general dentist treats a heterogeneous patient population. Each patient presents with a unique and often complex combination of conditions and aberrations in occlusal form and function. General practitioners not only must be able to diagnose disease entities and recognize occlusal abnormalities but also must understand the significance and implications of the ongoing interplay between unpredictable local environmental factors and individual host resistance. This understanding requires knowledge of all the dental disciplines, especially occlusion, which is an integral part of all dental therapeutics.

This chapter is organized into two sections. The first section covers theoretical material—the physiologic, pathologic, and therapeutic occlusions; the etiology of occlusal disease; the effects of disease on occlusal form and function; and the principles of occlusal form and function. The second section presents practical material—the treatment of a variety of cases. The intention is to present a broad enough spectrum of permutations in the selected cases to make clear the significance of occlusion in dental therapeutics. Because classification of patients according to case type is impossible—no consistent, rational organizing principle could

be identified—cases are ordered by the severity of disease, the extent of the deformity created, and the amount of treatment required to resolve the problem.

Objectives

The objective of this chapter is to present a rationale for the management of disease directly caused by occlusal activity (severe wear, pulpal involvement, occlusal traumatism, extracapsular temporomandibular joint dysfunction) and disease (dental caries, inflammatory periodontal disease) that involves occlusal form and function. The clinician should be able to (1) recognize health in spite of its deviation from a preconceived idea of what is normal, (2) recognize and organize disease directly caused by occlusal problems, (3) establish a rationale for occlusal therapy based upon the recognition of disease and etiologic factors, (4) understand the principles of occlusal form and function and their relevance to dental treatment, and (5) understand the management of dental disease and its implications for occlusal form and function.

The role of occlusion in general practice can be extremely complex and demanding depending upon the individual practitioner's desires. This chapter is intended to set forth guidelines for recognition of occlusal problems in general practice and a rationale for the management of these problems.

OCCLUSAL DISEASES

Occlusal diseases—excessive or severe wear, pulpal involvement, occlusal traumatism, and

The author would like to thank Drs. Morton Amsterdam, Leonard Abrams, Arnold Weisgold, and Robert Vanarsdall for their contributions to this chapter.

extracapsular temporomandibular joint dysfunction—are defined as injuries resulting primarily from the individual patient's response to excessive, abnormal forces. Other diseases—dental caries, gingivitis, periodontitis, and pulpal involvement—are defined as injuries resulting from the destructive byproducts of microbial plaque.

Occlusal form and function are defined as the static relationship and the morphology of tooth cusps, occlusal surfaces, and dental arches and the dynamic movements of the mandible produced by the collective function of the structures of the masticatory system: the teeth (including the pulp), the periodontium, the temporomandibular joint and its associated structures, and the lip, cheek, and tongue system.

Occlusal form and function are an important consideration in *all* therapeutics because any aberration has the potential to initiate or accelerate a disease process. The basis for treatment then becomes the thorough understanding of physiologic, pathologic, and therapeutic occlusions.

PHYSIOLOGIC, PATHOLOGIC, AND THERAPEUTIC OCCLUSIONS

A *physiologic occlusion* is characterized by health. Quite simply, at the time of evaluation there are no positive clinical findings, no objective signs or subjective symptoms of disease, and no patient complaints, despite the fact that obvious occlusal abnormalities may be present (Fig. 8–1). The patient is comfortable, has no complaints about masticatory ability, phonetics, or the cosmetic arrangement of his or her teeth, and requires no treatment.

A *pathologic occlusion* is one that requires treatment as a result of breakdown of the tissues of the masticatory system, as manifested by signs or symptoms of a disease process or as a result of patient complaints.

A *therapeutic occlusion* is one that the dentist establishes in his or her correction of a pathologic occlusion. The goal of treatment is to set up an occlusion that is physiologic, conducive to health, and acceptable to the

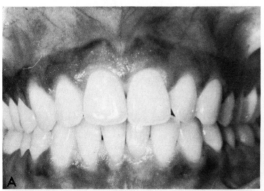
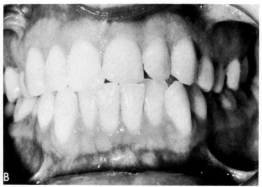
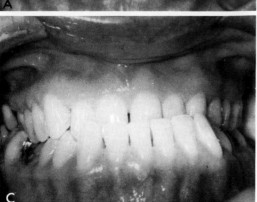

FIGURE 8–1 Physiologic Occlusion. *A,* Occlusal form and function are normal in this 23-year-old patient. ***B,*** The facial view of this 37-year-old patient demonstrates excessive posterior cuspal prominences relative to anterior tooth relations, resulting in minimal overbite, no overjet, and ineffectual anterior guidance. Although there are interferences in all tooth-contacting movements, there are no signs of disease and no patient complaints. At this time, the patient requires only maintenance therapy. ***C,*** Facial view of a 49-year-old patient with Class III malocclusion reveals severe malocclusion and aberration in form and function, yet the tissues are healthy. The patient is comfortable, has no complaints concerning appearance, phonetics, and mastication and requires only maintenance therapy.

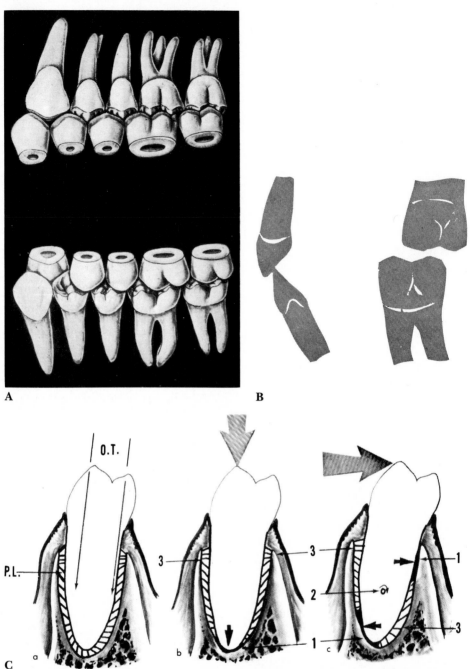

FIGURE 8–2 Ideal Function of Posterior and Anterior Teeth. The form and functional capabilities of the posterior and anterior teeth are in harmony with the mechanical Class III lever system. One of the primary functions of the posterior teeth is to support the occlusal vertical dimension. An extremely important function of the anterior teeth is to disarticulate the posterior teeth in all protrusive and lateral-protrusive contacting movements. As such, anterior and posterior teeth sustain a mutually protective relationship. This relationship becomes important in the etiology of all occlusal disease and in therapy. *A,* Ideal posterior tooth relations to support occlusal vertical dimension in the maximum intercuspal position. (From Abrams, L., and Coslet, J. G.: Occlusal Adjustment. *In* Goldman, H. M., and Cohen, D. W.: Periodontal Therapy, 6th ed. C. V. Mosby, Saint Louis, 1980, p. 569.) *B,* Anterior teeth separate posterior teeth in protrusive contacting movements. (From Abrams, L., and Coslet, J. G.: Occlusal Adjustment. *In* Goldman, H. M., and Cohen, D. W.: Periodontal Therapy, 6th ed. C. V. Mosby Co., Saint Louis, 1980, p. 571.) *C,* Since 80 per cent or more of the principal fibers of the periodontal ligament are oblique fibers, vertical forces are best tolerated by the periodontal attachment apparatus. Horizontal and torsional forces tend to be more destructive. (Courtesy of Leonard Abrams and Morton Amsterdam.)

336

patient. The elimination of all disease and patient complaints and the establishment of occlusal form and function, based on the knowledge of what causes occlusal disease, will maintain health in the future. The therapeutic occlusion is discussed in detail on pages 360 to 363.

Generally, the make-up of occlusal contacts in this corrected occlusion includes the support of the occlusal vertical dimension by the posterior teeth and the support of all lateral contacting movements by the anterior teeth. Freedom of mandibular movement is provided by the anterior teeth separating the posterior teeth in all protrusive and lateral-protrusive contacting movements (Fig. 8–2).

ETIOLOGY OF OCCLUSAL DISEASE

Regardless of the etiology of occlusal disease, host resistance—the adaptive capacity of the patient to withstand insult to the tissues—is the most important factor in the initiation and progression of occlusal disease.

Parafunctional Habits

The normal functions of the masticatory system include cosmetic effect, mastication, phonetics, and swallowing. Abnormal functions or parafunctions include tooth-to-tooth habits, such as clenching and grinding; musculature-to-tooth habits, such as lip-cheek biting; and object-to-tooth habits, such as chewing on the stem of a pipe. The precise mechanism that influences the initiation of such habits is unknown but is thought to be triggered by psychogenic factors (i.e., anxiety) or occlusal factors.

The forces exerted during parafunction far exceed the forces of normal function in magnitude, frequency, and duration, and the amount of tooth contact involved during parafunctional activity is far greater than that during normal masticatory function. During normal mastication, chewing occurs on the working side, and function of the masticatory system in all movements should occur according to the principles of a Class III lever system (Fig. 8–3). This mechanical design provides for optimal dissipation of occlusal forces delivered to the teeth.

Habits may or may not be pathogenic.

The destructive potential of parafunctional activity depends on the particular physiologic tissue limits of the host; on the presence and severity of inflammation; on occlusal aberrations in form and function; and on the type of habit, the duration of tooth contact, the strength of musculature, and the inclination, magnitude, and frequency of the force.

Occlusal Interferences

Interferences are aberrations in occlusal morphology that prevent or impede freedom of mandibular movement into or from occlusal contacting positions (Figs. 8–4 and 8–5). Such occlusal aberrations may be present developmentally, caused by physiologic or pathologic tooth migration, or induced iatrogenically. Common causes of interferences include: (1) lack of harmony between anterior guidance and posterior cuspal form, the plane of occlusion, and the curve of Spee and transverse curve; (2) wear of the palatal aspect of maxillary anterior teeth and the labial and incisal aspects of mandibular anterior teeth; (3) wear of the guiding inclines of maxillary posterior teeth and supporting cusps of mandibular anterior teeth (working side); (4) tilting, drifting, or extrusion of teeth (Fig. 8–6) resulting from a severe loss of tooth structure or from one or more missing teeth; (5) iatrogenic problems—restorations with excessive cusp height, overcarved restorations (Fig. 8–7), overgrinding of the anterior teeth on the working side (Fig. 8–8), and inadequately restored supporting cusps or guiding inclines on the working side.

Occlusal interferences may be loosely grouped into three categories by the direction of associated mandibular movement: (1) lateral-protrusive (working and nonworking), (2) protrusive, and (3) retrusive.

A *lateral-protrusive* interference is a posterior tooth contact that prevents anterior tooth guidance in a lateral-protrusive movement. It may occur on the working side (the side to which the mandible is directed in lateral-protrusive movements) or on the nonworking side (the side opposite the working side). The nonworking interference, which is often implicated in the initiation of occlusal traumatism and myofascial pain dysfunction syndrome, is the most destructive of all interferences.

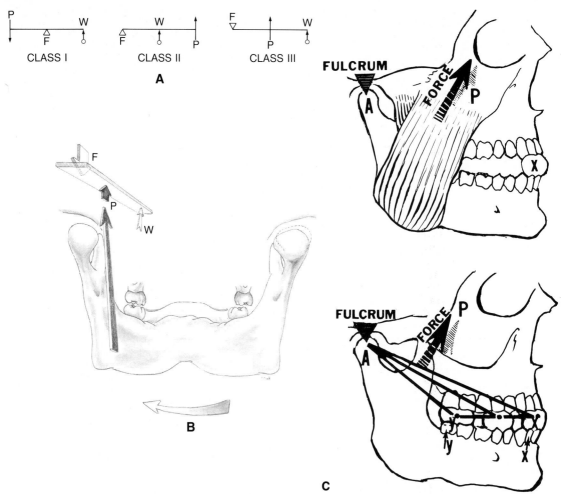

FIGURE 8–3 Leverage and Mechanical Design Influential in Force Distribution. *A,* Levers are classified as Class I, II, or III according to the variable relationship of the component factors: the fulcrum (F), the power or force (P), and the work or weight (W). A Class I lever is the most efficient; it exerts the greatest force at the work area with the least applied force or power. The Class II lever is less efficient, and the Class III is the least efficient of the three. (Adapted from Huffman, R. W., and Regonos, J. W.: Principles of Occlusion. Columbus, Ohio, H and R Press, 1980.) *B,* Normal masticatory function in a Class III lever system. Normal masticatory function (chewing) occurs on the working side and involves minimal, if any, tooth contacts. When the principles of a Class III lever system are applied to normal masticatory function, the working condyle is seated in the fossa and acts as the fulcrum (F), the muscles of mastication act as the power source (P), and the teeth act as the work area (W). Increasing the distance of the work area from the power source (muscles of mastication) and fulcrum (condyle) decreases force and stress in all areas. *C,* This buccal view demonstrates the ideal Class III lever system. In all functional and parafunctional mandibular movements, this mechanical design provides the most benign force distribution to all areas of the masticatory system (the teeth, periodontium, TMJ, and associated structures). Increasing the distance of the work area (Y to X) from the power source (muscles of mastication) and the fulcrum (condyle) also decreases force and stress in all areas. (From Krause, B., Jordan, R., and Abrams, L.: Dental Anatomy of Occlusion. Baltimore, The Williams & Wilkins Co., 1969, p. 204.)

A *protrusive interference* is a posterior tooth contact that prevents anterior guidance in a protrusive movement. It may occur on the right or left side or on both sides simultaneously.

A *retrusive interference* is a tooth contact that prevents maximum intercuspation when the mandible moves along the terminal hinge arc of closure. This deflective movement is not necessarily pathologic. If a dis-

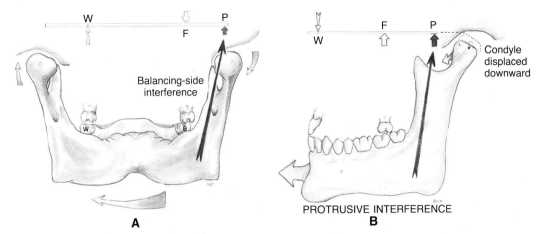

A

B

PROTRUSIVE INTERFERENCE

FIGURE 8–4 Leverage and Mechanical Design of Nonworking (Lateral-Protrusive) and Protrusive Interferences. Hypothetical relations between severe protrusive and lateral-protrusive interferences causing excessive force deliverance to the teeth and periodontium.

Severe nonworking (lateral-protrusive) interferences *(A)* can prevent the seating of the working condyle in the fossa; severe protrusive interferences *(B)* can prevent fulcrum stability of either condyle. This means that the normal site of the fulcrum—the condyle—is transferred to the tooth associated with the interference.

The proximity of the tooth (fulcrum) to the muscles of mastication (power source) can create a mechanically advantageous Class I lever system. Excessive occlusal forces are created as a result of the relocation of the fulcrum to a tooth level. During parafunction, force magnitude is even greater, and duration of force application is increased. Moreover, because tooth contacts occur on an incline, force deliverance is horizontal (off-axis). The cumulative effect of all these circumstances is excessive force, which may cause injury to the teeth, the muscles of mastication, or the periodontium.

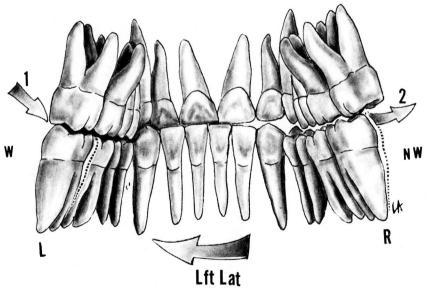

Lft Lat

FIGURE 8–5 Destructive Ability of Nonworking Interferences on the Lower Posterior Teeth. During left lateral contacting movement, working contact (W) of posterior teeth (arrow 1) tends to condense the teeth in their normal "splinted" arrangement in the arch. On the nonworking side (NW), the lower tooth tends to be "lifted" out of its splinted arrangements in the arch with great leverage (arrow 2) and is subject to the effects of maximal destructive horizontal forces. (From Abrams, L.: Occlusal Adjustment of the Natural Dentition. Cont. Dent. Ed., Vol. 1, No. 11, Philadelphia, Univ. of Pa., 1978.)

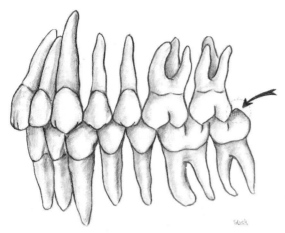

FIGURE 8–6 Protrusive and Lateral-Protrusive (Nonworking Side) Interference Caused by Extruded Cusp or Tooth. The unopposed, unworn distobuccal cusp of the mandibular terminal molar (arrow) is a common finding in Class II posterior tooth alignment or when maxillary teeth have been lost. This cusp often is involved as a posterior interference in protrusive and lateroprotrusive (nonworking side) movements. Single selective grinding of this nonfunctional area (shaded) removes the interference without changing the stability of the tooth in the maximum intercuspal position. (From Abrams, L.: Occlusal Adjustment of the Natural Dentition. Cont. Dent. Ed., Vol. 1, No. 11, Philadelphia, Univ. of Pa., 1978.)

ease process is active, however, a retrusive interference may become a contributing etiologic factor. Consequently, it is important that mandibular movement and deflection be assessed in both vertical and horizontal directions.

The mechanically disadvantageous location of anterior teeth relative to the condylar centers of rotation (fulcrum) and the muscles of mastication (a Class III lever) means that force application during anterior guidance is minimal and therefore benign. In contrast, the proximity of posterior teeth to the fulcrum (condyle) and to the muscles of mastication creates a mechanical advantage (a Class II lever), so that posterior interferences that generate forces perpendicular to the long axis of teeth have considerable destructive capability. At first, wear of the guiding inclines on the working side can actually be therapeutic, diminishing the locking effects on working interferences. However, as wear progresses, it creates nonworking contacts that become nonworking interferences. Eventually, the nonworking interferences are broadened with wear, in-

creasing the magnitude of the force exerted and the duration of the contact. In this case, the nonworking interference can become a fulcrum, thus causing even greater force generation to the tooth.

In summary, interferences may or may not be pathogenic. The destructive potential of an interference depends on the particular physiologic tissue limits of the host; the presence and severity of inflammation and mechanical aberrations; the direction, frequency, and magnitude of the force (proximity of the force to the muscles of mastication); the presence of parafunctional activity (the forces generated by interferences during parafunction, which have a greater destructive capability than during normal function); and the capability of the force to precipitate or exacerbate a parafunctional habit.

EFFECTS OF DISEASE ON OCCLUSAL FORM AND FUNCTION

The Teeth and Pulp

Pulpal Involvement and Wear

Excessive occlusal forces can compromise the blood supply to the teeth, eliciting a pulpal response (hyperemia) that can result in pulpitis and necrosis. A more common sequela of abnormal forces at the tooth level, however, is excessive and severe wear.

Wear itself is not pathologic and does not represent an indication for therapy. Signs of minimal, isolated wear such as flattened occlusal surfaces, incisal edges, and interproximal contacts are common. Wear is a normal, physiologic phenomenon that occurs during the aging process. Thus, the clinical significance of wear must be measured in relation to the patient's age; what is considered normal for a person of 50 years of age may be excessive for a person of 25 years (Figs. 8–9 and 8–10).

Because wear is progressive and creates broad occlusal contacts, the magnitude and duration of forces increase over time. This increase in force results in further wear, which often becomes more and more severe and generalized, as evidenced by the creation and exacerbation of occlusal surface deformities, the continued loss of tooth struc-

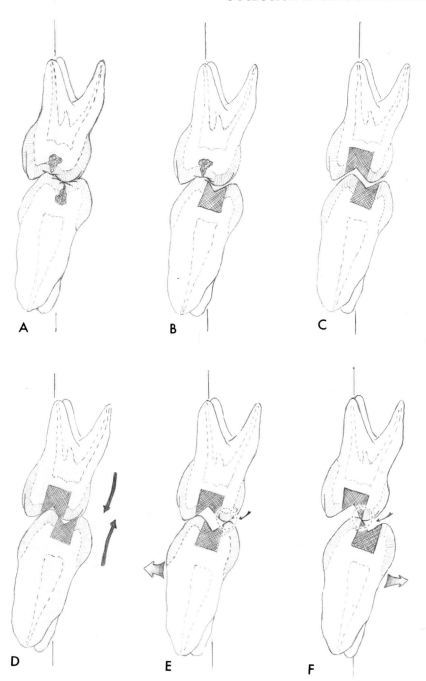

FIGURE 8–7   Nonworking Interferences Resulting From Faulty Amalgam Restorations. *A,* Simple restorative treatment is indicated to manage carious lesions on the occlusal surfaces of these properly occluding first molars. *B,* The amalgam restoration on the mandibular molar was overcarved, resulting in the disarticulation of the maxillary supporting (palatal) cusp. *C,* The amalgam restoration on the maxillary molar was also overcarved, resulting in the disarticulation of the mandibular supporting (buccal) cusp. *D,* The subsequent extrusion of these inadequately restored teeth creates a deeper fossa and a steeper cuspal form. *E,* The increased cuspal prominences caused excessive working contacts (here the lingual cusp) in lateral-protrusive movements. *F,* The increased cuspal prominences also caused nonworking interferences in lateral-protrusive movements (here the contact of the lingual aspect of the lower buccal cusp with the buccal aspect of the upper palatal cusp).

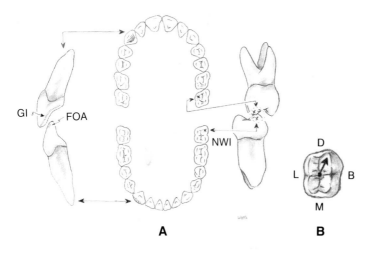

GI — FOA

NWI

A

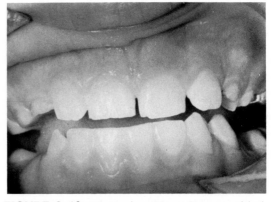

D

L — B

M

B

FIGURE 8–8 Nonworking Interferences Resulting From Lack of Contacts on the Working Side. *A,* Nonworking interferences can be caused by a lack of tooth contacts on the working side, which can result from drifting, severe wear, or inadequate restorations. GI, Guiding incline; FOA, Functional outer aspect; NWI, Nonworking interference. *B,* The arrow on the occlusal surface of the mandibular second molar shows the direction of movement of the maxillary palatal cusp.

ture approaching the dentin, and tooth and root fractures. Ultimately, wear can lead to reverse curve of Spee and transverse curve, pulpal involvement (hyperemia followed by pulpitis and eventual necrosis), pulp exposure, and loss of normal function.

Wear becomes pathologic when the normal function or the survival of a tooth or the dentition is jeopardized. The diagnosis becomes one of clinical judgment, based on an assessment and correlation of the amount and extent of wear, the patient's age, the development of patient symptoms (usually sensitivity to hot and cold, indicating pulpal involvement), and the presence and destructive

capability of forces generated by parafunctional habits or occlusal interferences (Fig. 8–11).

Dental Caries

When caries destroys tooth structure and becomes a contributing etiologic factor in an occlusal or periodontal disease process, destruction of the periodontal tissues is usually isolated. However, severely broken-down, carious teeth can create open contacts, poor embrasure form, and plunger cusps. All of these conditions promote food impaction and the accumulation of microbial plaque, which lead to soft tissue inflammation and enlargement. Advanced caries is often responsible for tooth loss, especially the loss of lower first molars. Missing and decayed teeth can also lead to the drifting and tilting

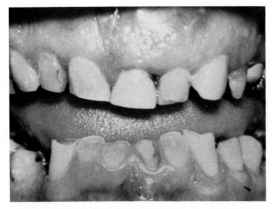

FIGURE 8–9 Severe Wear. The severe wear of the teeth is a result of excessive forces generated during tooth-to-tooth parafunction (clenching and grinding). It is more than likely that the initiation of the frequent parafunctional activity was a result of extreme and long-term occupational stress. The patient is a laborer employed in the construction of high-rise buildings.

FIGURE 8–10 Excessive Wear. Because this is the dentition of a 10-year-old child, the wear on the anterior (permanent) teeth is considered excessive and severe.

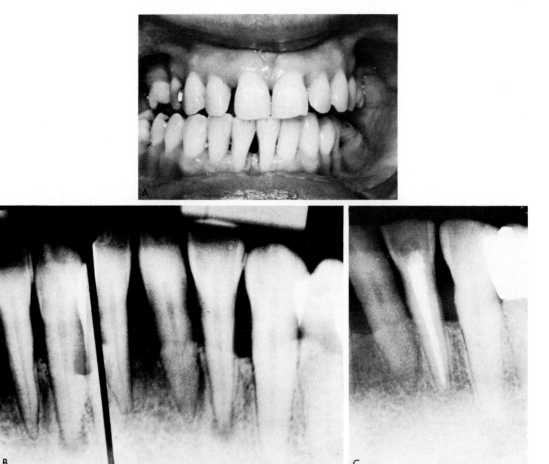

FIGURE 8–11 Pulpal Disease. *A,* Excessive, off-axis force application resulted in the flaring of the maxillary anterior teeth and pulpal necrosis of the mandibular lateral incisor. These forces were caused by contact of the maxillary and mandibular lateral incisors occurring during parafunctional activity associated with a protrusive habit pattern. *B,* The nonvital status of the mandibular lateral incisors is manifested by the periapical radiolucency. (The diagnosis of pulpal necrosis was substantiated clinically by a negative response to the electric pulp test.) Root canal therapy was instituted. *C,* Healing of the periapical lesion is confirmed in this 1-year postoperative radiograph.

of contiguous teeth and the extrusion of opposing teeth. Loss of arch integrity causes increased cuspal prominences and aberrations in the plane of occlusion and the curve of Spee, resulting in protrusive, lateral-protrusive, and retrusive interferences. Concurrent periodontal disease and excessive, abnormal force application accelerate the rate of destruction and lead to the loss of support of the occlusal vertical dimension. This loss destroys the symbiotic relationship between the anterior and posterior teeth. Generalized mobility and fremitus of the maxillary anterior teeth result from excessive off-axis forces generated by the mandibular anterior teeth. A dentition so afflicted is said to be in the early stage of posterior bite collapse.

Left unattended, early posterior bite collapse usually results in (1) pathologic migration and flaring of the maxillary anterior teeth, contributing to the loss of effective anterior tooth guidance; (2) progressive posterior tooth loss; (3) tongue-thrusting habits associated with spacing and open contacts; (4) advanced periodontal disease with secondary occlusal traumatism; and (5) possible flaring of the mandibular incisors.

The Periodontium

The periodontium has a great capacity to adapt to excessive forces through repair and regeneration, commonly evidenced by radiographic signs of hyperfunction—increased opacity of lamina dura around the periodontal ligament (PDL) space (Fig. 8–12). But repeated excessive force application by occlusal interferences and parafunctional habits can lead to the *dystrophic* destruction of the attachment apparatus. This destruction is known as occlusal traumatism, sometimes referred to as the lesion of occlusal trauma. (Because occlusal traumatism is a dystrophic disease process, it does not cause epithelial migration and resultant pocket formation.)

Injury to the periodontal support results in qualitative and quantitative changes in the tissue, which may be seen histologically as hemorrhage; thrombosis of the blood vessels; necrosis and hyalinization of the connective tissue of the periodontal ligament; and resorption of the bony wall of the alveolus.

Radiographic evidence of occlusal traumatism in the attachment apparatus includes a widened PDL space, loss of continuity of the lamina dura, loss of definition of the PDL space, root fractures, and root and osseous resorption. Clinical manifestations of occlusal traumatism are increasing mobility, visible tooth movement, fremitus (palpable tooth movement), and tooth migration. Symptoms are usually limited to tenderness, sensitivity, or pain.

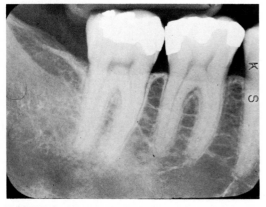

FIGURE 8–12 Hyperfunction. The adaptive capacity of the attachment apparatus to excessive forces is demonstrated by the thickened lamina dura and yet a widened PDL space around the second molar. This condition is associated with an overcarved amalgam restoration and a nonworking interference.

When an adequate quantity of periodontal support remains to withstand the normal forces of occlusion, yet excessive parafunctional forces exceed the adaptive capacity of the attachment apparatus, the disease process is referred to as primary occlusal traumatism. Inflammation is usually concomitant with primary occlusal traumatism (Fig. 8–13A). Initially, the two disease processes exist as discrete entities, with gingivitis involving the gingival unit and primary occlusal traumatism involving the attachment apparatus. If the gingivitis goes untreated, it can evolve into a periodontitis, seen radiographically as dissolution of the crestal lamina dura and the marginal bone at its most coronal level.

Since periodontitis is a progressive disease, it will ultimately extend so far apically into the attachment apparatus that the inflammatory and occlusal disease processes merge and become a single entity in which the inflammation acts to enhance the destructive capacity of the occlusal forces, accelerating the breakdown of the attachment apparatus and exacerbating mobility and fremitus. When the quantity of the remaining intact attachment apparatus has been compromised by periodontal disease and cannot withstand the normal forces of occlusion, the disease process is referred to as secondary occlusal traumatism (Fig. 8–13B).

The Temporomandibular Joint and Associated Structures

Disorders of the TMJ and associated structures may be an intracapsular or an extracapsular dysfunction. Intracapsular TMJ dysfunction involves the joint proper and is usually associated with a systemic disorder, such as arthritis. Extracapsular TMJ dysfunction, also known as myofascial pain dysfunction syndrome (MPDS), is of dental origin and involves the muscles of mastication.

Differential diagnosis is difficult. Patients with intracapsular and extracapsular TMJ disorders may share many key symptoms such as pain, clicking, crepitus, mandibular deviation, and limited opening or may suffer from both disorders. Establishing a correct diagnosis is further complicated by the fact that MPDS is manifested almost entirely by unreliable, subjective patient symptoms.

Nevertheless, patients with extracapsular TMJ dysfunction do present with certain classic signs and symptoms. MPDS patients

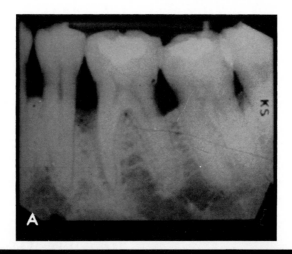

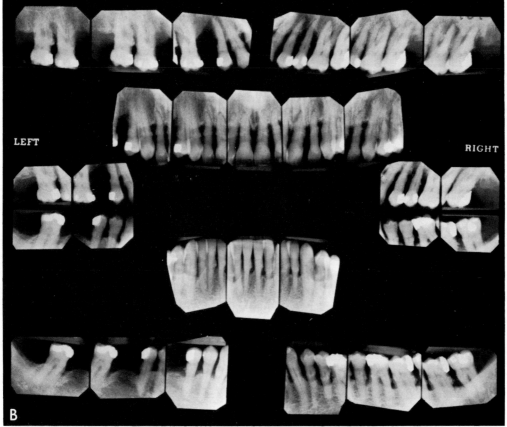

FIGURE 8–13 Radiographic Signs of Occlusal Traumatism. *A,* Primary occlusal traumatism is manifested on this mandibular first molar by a widened periodontal ligament space, loss of continuity, and definition of the lamina dura. ***B,*** This full set of radiographs is of the mouth of a patient with secondary occlusal traumatism. Like primary occlusal traumatism, it is manifested by a widened periodontal ligament space and loss of continuity and definition of the lamina dura. However, bone loss is much more extensive and the supporting structures are unable to sustain normal forces.

are usually young (19 to 28) and female (60 to 70 per cent). The disorder is characterized by anxiety and by a lack of radiographic evidence of injury. The pain associated with MPDS is located in the region of the muscles of mastication. It is dull, of long duration, and most noticeable to patients in the morning on waking and during stressful events.

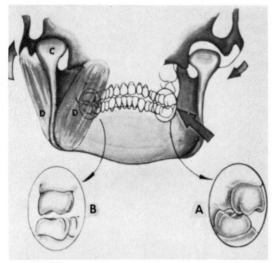

FIGURE 8–14 Nonworking Interference Causing Muscle Spasm and Pain on the Working Side. Hypothetical relation between interference on nonworking side and muscular spasm and pain on working side. Nonworking interference *(A)* (large diagonal arrow) prevents teeth from contacting on functional working side; as patient attempts to bring working teeth into occlusion *(B)*, there is a tendency for working condyle *(C)* to be displaced superiorly (vertical arrow). So-called splinting reflex tends to limit condylar displacement, with possible joint and ligament injury by means of spasm in working side musculature. (From Abrams, L., and Coslet, J. G.: Occlusal Adjustment. *In* Goldman, H. M., and Cohen, D. W.: Periodontal Therapy, 6th ed. C. V. Mosby, Saint Louis, 1980, p. 587, and courtesy of Morton Amsterdam, Philadelphia, Pa.)

Finally, patients with MPDS have a negative history of rheumatoid or osteodegenerative arthritis, recent dental treatment, parotid gland disease, sinus problems, neuromuscular disease, neurovascular disease, and tic douloureux.

MPDS is usually caused by excessive force application at a tooth level. Such forces are generated by all types of parafunctional habits and occlusal interferences, most often the nonworking interference, that cause a muscle spasm on the working side (Fig. 8–14). Abnormal forces exceed the adaptive capacity of the tissues of the muscles of mastication, resulting in spasm and injury.

The Lip, Cheek, and Tongue System

Parafunctional habits associated with the structures of the lip, cheek, and tongue have the potential to create aberrations in occlusal form and function (which can cause occlusal interferences), to induce tooth-to-tooth parafunction, and to lead to the breakdown of the attachment apparatus. Lip habits can cause flaring of the anterior teeth. Tongue habits, acquired as an adult or retained from infancy, can create an imbalance between the forces generated by the tongue and the forces generated by the lips and cheeks. This imbalance can alter tooth position and result in tooth mobility. Cheek-biting, lip-biting, and tongue habits can produce anterior and posterior open bite by disarticulating some teeth and causing the eruption of others.

THE PRINCIPLES OF OCCLUSAL FORM AND FUNCTION

The form and function of the individual components of the masticatory system in its ideal condition present a mutually protective system. Individual deviation from what is ideal or normal in the form and function of this system is not the primary criterion for treatment. The examination process must determine disease, patient complaints, and all etiologies. The need for and extent of treatment are dictated by the recognition of the patient's response to disease and the presence of etiologic factors that may be exacerbated by a deviation in ideal form and function. Therefore, the assessment of the mechanical aspects of the maxillomandibular positions and movements and the articulation of teeth within the dental arch and between dental arches becomes most important. This section defines terminology,* discusses the basic components of mandibular positions and movements, and describes the complex relations between these components and individual teeth and groups of teeth.

Mandibular Positions

There are three fundamental positions associated with occlusion: maximum intercuspal position (MIP), retruded contact position on the terminal hinge arc of closure (RCP), and postural position (PP). These positions are used as reference points for all other mandibular positions and movements and for therapeutics. Their clinical relevance will

---

*This terminology and its organization are important in the examination process (see Fig. 8–24).

become apparent during the examination and the diagnosis process, during the treatment-planning phase, and during the determination of the appropriate criteria for the therapeutic occlusion.

Maximum Intercuspal Position

The maximum intercuspal position (MIP, also known as habitual occlusion and centric occlusion) is a tooth to tooth relationship that represents the most closed position of the mandible to the maxilla. In the examination process, it is the position in which all mandibular movements begin and terminate. The MIP is used to assess fremitus patterns and interarch landmark relations in the sagittal, transverse, and vertical planes.

Because the MIP is maintained by proprioception, it changes as a result of parafunctional activity, restorative therapy, physiologic tooth migration, and disease. Consequently, the MIP is not reliably reproducible—an important consideration in clinical practice.

Retruded Contact Position

The terminal hinge arc of closure is the path the mandible follows when the condyles are in the most posterior, superior position in the glenoid fossa. The retruded contact position (RCP) is the first tooth contact along the terminal hinge arc of closure and prevents movement of the mandible into the MIP. Centric relation is the term used to refer to the mandibular position in which the MIP and RCP coincide. Although this position has been found to occur naturally in only about 10 per cent of young healthy individuals, centric relation is usually the therapeutic position established during treatment.

Postural Position

The postural or rest position is the jaw-to-jaw relationship assumed when the head is in an upright position; it is usually located 3 to 5 mm inferior to the MIP. The postural position is free of tooth contacts and is maintained by the muscles of mastication as they work only to counteract the forces of gravity. The rest position is highly variable, changing in response to pathology and to alterations in posture, muscle tone, age, and occlusal relations. Neither the postural posi-

tion nor the movement from the postural position to the MIP is reliably reproducible.

Mandibular Movements and the Envelope of Motion

Posselt's envelope of motion (Fig. 8–15) graphically depicts the path of the mandibular incisor on a median plane throughout the range of mandibular movement. It identifies the relative locations of mandibular positions. The superior border represents a retrusive protrusive movement, determined by tooth-to-tooth relations and by the structure of the TMJ (condylar path). Five occlusal positions, including the RCP and the MIP, occur along the superior border of the envelope of motion. The direction of movement from the RCP to the MIP is upward and forward; the distance between these positions, known as the RC-IC discrepancy, ranges from 1 to 2 mm in most persons and is not, in itself, pathologic.

The posterior border represents two movements. The first, called the terminal hinge movement, is the path between the RCP and the point at which the external

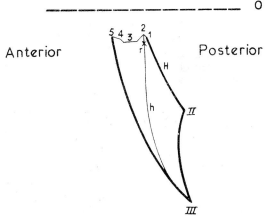

FIGURE 8–15 Envelope of Motion. The sagittal or median view of the envelope of motion, which demonstrates the relative locations of specific positions and movements. *Key:* 1, Retruded contact position; 2, Maximum intercuspal position; 3, Edge-to-edge occlusion; 4, Anterior biting to a reverse overlap; 5, Protruded contact position; H, Terminal hinge movement; h, Habitual closing movement; II, Transition from terminal hinge to further posterior opening; III, Maximum opening; r, Postural position; O, Line parallel to occlusal plane. (From Posselt, U.: The Physiology of Occlusion and Rehabilitation, London, Blackwell Publications, 1962, p. 44.)

pterygoid muscles induce the forward translation of the mandible. The second movement is the path between the translation point and the point of maximal mandibular opening. These borders are determined by ligaments, which are protected by the muscles of mastication.

The anterior border opening movement begins at maximal protrusion and ends at maximal opening. This movement is of little practical value.

Guidance

Guidance refers to the influence of the form of the dentition and joint activity on mandibular movements. An intimate relationship exists between condylar guidance and anterior tooth guidance, which act in harmony to disarticulate the posterior teeth. There is also a complex interplay between anterior teeth and condylar guidance and the occlusal factors that affect posterior cuspal effectiveness, namely, the plane of occlusion, the curves of Spee and Wilson, tooth positioning, and landmark relations as well as the cuspal heights themselves.

Anterior Tooth Guidance

Anterior tooth guidance is the relationship of the labial and incisal aspects of mandibular anterior teeth to the palatal and incisal aspects of maxillary anterior teeth in protrusive and lateral-protrusive movements. The two components of anterior guidance—overbite and overjet—are evaluated in both the MIP and the RCP. Overbite is the vertical overlap of teeth. It is the vertical distance from the incisal edge of the maxillary incisors to the incisal edge of the mandibular incisors. Overjet is the horizontal overlap of teeth. It is the horizontal distance from the incisal edge of the mandibular incisors to the lingual surface of the maxillary incisors.

The anterior and posterior teeth are mutually protective. The anterior teeth protect the posterior teeth by supporting protrusive and lateral-protrusive movements, which prevents posterior tooth contacts. Lateral protrusive movements can be supported by the canines (canine guidance) or by the canines along with the supporting cusps of mandibular posterior teeth (functional outer aspect, or FOA) and the guiding inclines of maxillary posterior teeth (group function).

Protrusive movements are supported by the incisors, at times in combination with the canines.

The posterior teeth protect the anterior teeth by supporting the occlusal vertical dimension. This protection is accomplished by the cradling action of supporting cusps, mandibular buccal cusps, and the maxillary lingual cusps in the opposing central fossa area.

If the function of either the anterior or the posterior group of teeth is lost, the function of the other group as well as their symbiotic relationship is jeopardized.

Condylar Guidance

Condylar guidance is the effect of the anterior eminence and medial wall of the glenoid fossa on the condyle in protrusive and lateral-protrusive movements. The capacity of condylar guidance to provide for disarticulation of posterior teeth is related to the inclination of the eminence in the fossa. The steeper the eminence, the more effective the condylar guidance. Clinically, any alteration in anterior tooth guidance requires an assessment of condylar guidance.

Two other important considerations in condylar guidance are the Christensen phenomenon and the Bennett movement. When the mandible is protruded and the condyle has descended the anterior eminence, it influences the disarticulation of the posterior teeth. The space created in the molar region is a result of the Christensen phenomenon (Fig. 8–16). When the mandible is moved laterally, the immediate side shift of the working side condyle is known as the Bennett movement. Clinically, the side shift must be analyzed in all advanced restorative and selective grinding procedures. It can affect the mesial distal placement and selective grinding procedure of the buccal cusp and the maxillary guiding inclines on the working side.

Arch Rhythmicity

Arch rhythmicity refers to an intra-arch *skeletal* form, which is described as square, round, or pointed. It also refers to the intra-arch and interarch *dental* form, which is characterized by a gradual decrease in cusp height and width from the anterior to the posterior part of the mouth (Fig. 8–17). Posterior cuspal form must be in harmony with

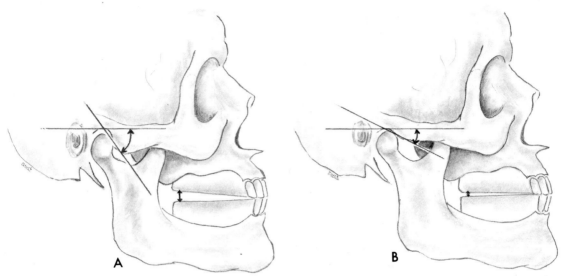

FIGURE 8–16   Condylar Guidance. Condylar guidance has a direct effect on posterior tooth clearance in protrusive movements. When anterior tooth guidance is held constant, posterior clearance increases as the angle of the eminence increases. This is demonstrated by the limited clearance associated with a shallow angle *(B)* and by the greater clearance associated with a steeper angle *(A)*. This positive correlation between the angle of the eminence and the degree of posterior tooth clearance is known as the Christensen phenomenon.

anterior tooth form and condylar guidance. As dentists, we would like maximal posterior cuspal form in order to enhance esthetic appearance and function, yet not to the extent that excessive forces are generated by pos-

terior tooth contacts in mandibular movements. If all guidance factors, tooth and condylar, remained constant and we varied the planes and curves of occlusion, we could change posterior cuspal effectiveness (that

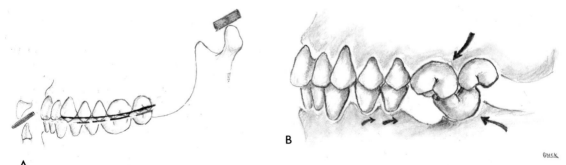

FIGURE 8–17   Dental Arch Rhythmicity and Disruption of Arch Rhythmicity and Continuity. *A,* Arch rhythmicity is the flowing arc established by anterior tooth relations and posterior cuspal heights that diminish gradually from the anterior to the posterior part of the mouth. It includes an evaluation of the planes of occlusion, curve of Spee, and transverse curve as well as the anterior overbite/overjet relations and posterior cuspal form. When arch rhythmicity is compromised by aberrant posterior cuspal form and incisal relations, harmony between the two groups of teeth is lost and can result in interferences and excessive forces. ***B,*** Loss of the mandibular first molar typically results in mesial drifting of the second molar, distal tilting of the bicuspids, and extrusion of the maxillary first molars. The aberrant plane of occlusion and curve of Spee caused by the malpositioned teeth results in retrusive, lateral-protrusive, and protrusive interferences. While this situation is in itself not necessarily pathologic, if it is to be corrected, the curve of Spee and plane of occlusion must be corrected in order to avoid iatrogenically causing or propagating the interferences, excessive forces, and periodontal disease.

is, a cusp's ability to contact in horizontal mandibular movements). These are important considerations in all orthodontic, restorative, and occlusal therapies. This skeletal and dental form and function are influenced by the slope of the plane of occlusion and the shapes of the curve of Spee and the transverse curve (curve of Wilson).

Plane of Occlusion

The plane of occlusion is the surface formed by connecting the two distobuccal cusp tips of the most terminal molars and the two cusp tips of the canines (Fig. 8–18). The anteroposterior dimension may be visualized as the chord of the circle of which the curve of Spee is an arc. The anterior boundary of the plane is the imaginary line perpendicular to the long axes of the canines. If the plane were rotated on the canine-to-canine axis, its slope would change. This slope is used to describe the occlusal plane, which can be elevated, normal, or depressed.

The clinical importance of the slope of the plane of occlusion and its relative elevation is its influence in determining the effectiveness of posterior cusps, which is significant for optimal occlusal function. This is because the greater the cuspal effectiveness, the greater the capacity of the cusp to contact during function, which can result in an interference in a protrusive or lateral-protrusive movement.

In short, depressing the plane of occlusion decreases cuspal effectiveness; elevating the plane of occlusion increases cuspal effectiveness. However, it must be recognized that a depressed or extruded tooth is discounted when establishing the plane of occlusion. Consequently, the tooth "deviates" in function, that is, its cuspal effectiveness is not in accordance with the plane of occlusion. To plan and execute treatment properly, "secondary" planes of occlusion, as dictated by any depressed or extruded teeth, must be visualized and assessed in conjunction with the "primary" plane of occlusion.

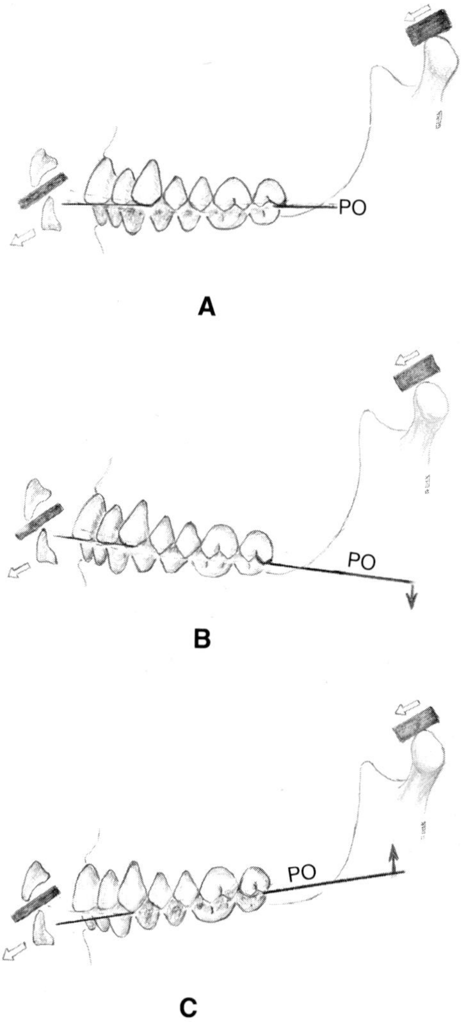

Curve of Spee

The curve of Spee (Fig. 8–19) is an anteroposterior curve that connects the buccal cusp tips of the teeth in a quadrant, ex-

A

B

C

FIGURE 8–18 Plane of Occlusion. *A,* The plane of occlusion (PO) must be visualized as an imaginary line that connects the cusp tip of the canine and distobuccal cusp of the terminal molar in each quadrant. The elevation or depression of the plane of occlusion is influential in cuspal effectiveness, that is, the capacity for a given cuspal height to contact. *B,* The depressed plane of occlusion functionally decreases cuspal height so that relatively steep prominences can be tolerated or established therapeutically to enhance appearance or function. *C,* The elevated plane of occlusion functionally increases cuspal height so that posterior tooth interferences are more likely to occur in protrusive and lateral-protrusive movements.

tending from the most terminal molar to the canine. The plane of occlusion can be considered as the chord of the circle of which the curve of Spee is an arc. The curve of

FIGURE 8–19 **Curve of Spee.** *A,* Moderate or normal curve of Spee is composed of individual planes of occlusion of the posterior teeth (broken line). *B,* Exaggerated curve of Spee is composed of individual planes of occlusion of the posterior teeth (broken line). Arrow shows position where the plane of occlusion changes from depressed in the premolar region to elevated in the molar area. When the curve of Spee is exaggerated, the molars exhibit severe elevation of their individual planes of occlusion and the premolars exhibit depression of their individual planes of occlusion. Thus, we can see that the elevated plane of occlusion associated with the exaggerated curve of Spee requires shallow cuspal form to avoid posterior tooth contacts. The depressed plane of occlusion associated with premolars allows steeper cusp form because the actual cuspal effectiveness of the premolars is decreased. *C,* The flat or reverse curve of Spee is associated with a depressed plane of occlusion in the molar region, functionally decreasing molar cuspal height, and an elevated plane of occlusion in the premolar region, functionally increasing cuspal height. Discrepancies between apparent and functional cuspal height are not problematic in this case, since they do not have the potential to jeopardize or interfere with normal occlusal function.

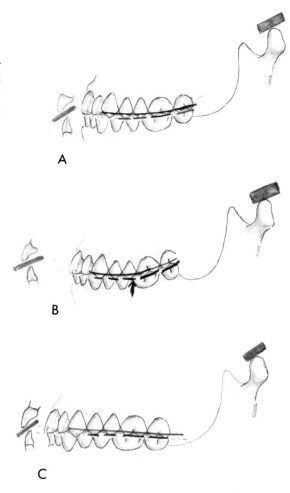

A

B

C

Spee can be described as moderate (Fig. 8–19*A*), exaggerated (Fig. 8–19*B*), or flat or reversed (Fig. 8–19*C*). In visualizing these curves (from a lateral view) and extending their arc, the moderate curve would create a large circle and the exaggerated curve would create a small circle. Clinically, the curve of Spee can be viewed as a compilation of individual (or groups of) planes of occlusion of all the teeth. These planes must be assessed individually and then related to the posterior cuspal height and form. In the exaggerated curve of Spee, the plane of occlusion in the molar region is elevated, whereas the plane of occlusion in the premolar region is depressed. Therefore, cuspal height can be greater in the premolar region (decreased cuspal effectiveness due to depressed plane of occlusion) than in the molar region (increased cuspal effectiveness associated with elevated plane of occlusion).

Transverse Curve

The transverse curve, or curve of Wilson (Fig. 8–20), is a mediolateral curve that connects the cusp tips of a posterior tooth to the cusp tips of its counterpart in the opposite quadrant of the same arch. The transverse curve is referred to as exaggerated, moderate, normal, or flat. Like the plane of occlusion and associated curve of Spee, the transverse curve also affects posterior cuspal effectiveness. The usual alignment of the mandibular posterior teeth is one of lingual version or pitch, thus placing the buccal cusp more cranial than the lingual cusp. This creates a transverse curve that is concave above and convex below. The exaggerated transverse curve is the arc of a small circle, and the moderate or normal curve is the arc of a large circle.

Clinically, one must visualize the transverse curve on one side of the mouth at a

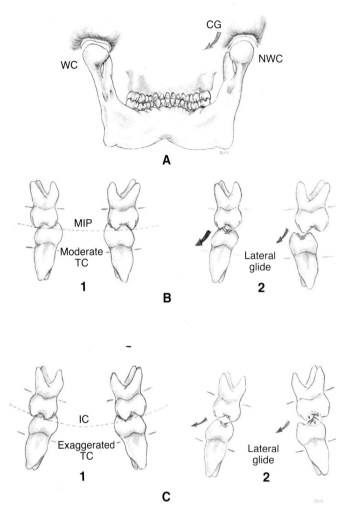

FIGURE 8–20 Transverse Curve. A, The arc of the transverse curve can affect the ability of a given cusp to interfere in protrusive and lateral-protrusive movements. In both *A* and *B,* the cuspal forms are identical. The condylar guidance (CG) and nonworking condyle (NWC) incisal guidance have the same relationship. *B* (1) The moderate transverse curve (TC) is associated with a normal plane of occlusion. MIP, Maximum intercuspal position. (2) Consequently, in the lateral-protrusive movements, there is no discrepancy between apparent and functional posterior cuspal height. There is guidance on the working side and disarticulation on the nonworking side. *C* (1) The exaggerated transverse curve (TC) is associated with an elevated plane of occlusion, thereby functionally increasing molar cuspal height on the nonworking side. IC, Intercuspal closure. (2) In the lateral-protrusive movement, the nonworking interference is present.

given time in order to assess cuspal effectiveness. An exaggerated transverse curve has the same effect as raising the plane of occlusion. In other words, a posterior tooth in severe lingual version will have greater capacity for cuspal contact in protrusive and lateral-protrusive movements than if the same tooth had a normal or moderate transverse curve. Therefore, teeth with a pronounced transverse curve will have a greater capacity to create a nonworking interference. It must be understood in this discussion that we have assumed that incisal guidance, cuspal guidance (on the working side), and condylar guidance (on the nonworking side) have the same angle. Changing tooth position by creating different curves and planes can influence posterior cuspal effectiveness, that is, the ability of a posterior cusp to contact in protrusive and lateral-protrusive movements.

The form of posterior teeth in both an anteroposterior and a mediolateral direction must allow anterior tooth and condylar guidance. The patient's occlusal function and appearance are improved when the cusp form is as steep as possible without interfering in protrusive and lateral-protrusive movements.

Arch Continuity

Dental arch continuity is an intra-arch and interarch form that is characterized by even marginal ridges, proper axial inclination, and continuous buccolingual, linguo-occlusal, and central fossa lines; in other words, the absence of open contacts, plunger cusps, and missing, fractured, mobile, and malposed teeth.

Buccolingual and Mesiodistal Landmark Relations

Normal buccolingual landmarks are marked by the following relationships: The

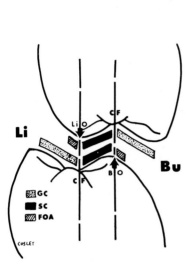

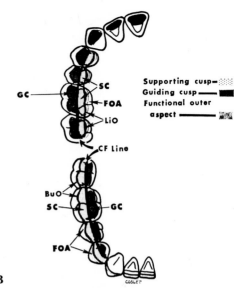

FIGURE 8–21 Occlusal Landmark Relations. *A,* Buccolingual landmark relations. Li, Lingual, Bu, Buccal. Note the following: BO, Bucco-occlusal line angle of lower posterior tooth; CF, Central fossa line of upper posterior tooth and lower posterior tooth; LiO, Linguo-occlusal line of upper tooth; GI, Guiding incline of upper posterior tooth and lower posterior tooth; SC, Supporting cusp of upper tooth and lower tooth; FOA, functional outer aspect of upper or lower teeth. (From Goldman, H. M., and Cohen, D. W.: Periodontal Therapy, 5th ed. C. V. Mosby, Saint Louis, 1973, p. 568, and courtesy of Morton Amsterdam, Philadelphia, Pa.) *B,* Cuspal groups include supporting cusps, guiding inclines (note that this includes lingual surface of upper anterior teeth), and FOA (note that this includes incisal edges of lower anterior teeth). Landmarks of teeth include bucco-occlusal line, central fossa line, and linguo-occlusal line. (From Abrams, L., and Coslet, J. G.: Occlusal Adjustment. *In* Goldman, H. M., and Cohen, D. W.: Periodontal Therapy, 6th ed. C. V. Mosby, Saint Louis, 1980, p. 568, and courtesy of Morton Amsterdam, Philadelphia, Pa.)

bucco-occlusal line of the lower arch articulates with the central fossa line of the upper arch, and the linguo-occlusal line of the upper arch articulates with the central fossa line of the lower arch (Fig. 8–21*A*).

In normal or ideal mesiodistal landmark relations, the supporting cusp tips articulate with the marginal ridge area, except for the mesiolingual cusp of the maxillary first molar and the distobuccal cusp of the mandibular first molar, which occlude with the central fossa area (Fig. 8–21*B*).

Landmark relations are evaluated in the sagittal (mesiodistal), transverse (buccolingual), and vertical dimensions. Because tooth relations may vary according to mandibular positions, especially with malocclusions, they are assessed at the maximum intercuspal position (MIP), the retruded contact position (RCP), and the postural position.

Buccolingual landmarks are essential for occlusal stability. It is not unusual to find that as the mandible moves along the terminal hinge arc of closure to the RCP, the buccal cusps of the mandibular teeth relate lingually to the opposing central fossa area.

This occurs because the narrower part of the mandible relates to the wider part of the maxilla when the mandible is retruded. The extent of this disparity is an important consideration in determining the type and amount of occlusal therapy (Fig. 8–22).

Mesiodistal landmarks can also change when the mandible is retruded, with mandibular cusps relating distal to the marginal ridge of the opposing teeth. This change in mesiodistal posterior landmark relations is generally not critical. The anterior tooth relations are the most important to evaluate, since retruding the mandible causes an increase in overjet and a decrease in overbite. This can compromise the anterior tooth guidance required of the anterior teeth.

Malocclusions

Although malocclusions per se are not pathologic, orthodontic correction is sometimes indicated to manage disease, treat patient complaints, and satisfy the requirements of a therapeutic occlusion. Orthodontic

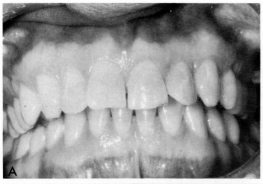
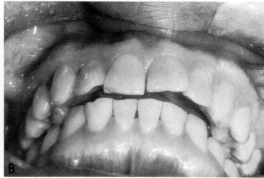
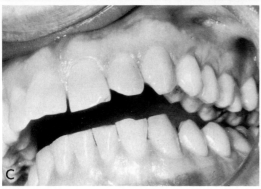

FIGURE 8–22 Disparity in Landmark Relations as the Mandible Moves From the Maximum Intercuspal Position to the Retruded Contact Position. *A,* This labial view of the maximum intercuspal position demonstrates a healthy periodontium and what appears to be normal occlusal form and relations. The chief complaints of this 24-year-old patient are nocturnal bruxism, wear of the lower incisors, and episodic temporomandibular joint pain. *B,* At the maximum intercuspal position, there is a 3 to 4 mm overjet of the anterior teeth and poor buccolingual landmark relations of the premolars. *C,* The buccolingual landmark relations at the retruded contact position are severe. The mandibular teeth are completely palatal to the maxillary teeth. The vertical dimension is so increased at this position that it does not allow for adequate freeway space. It is impossible to execute selective grinding or restorative dentistry at this position owing to the severe landmark relation of the teeth and the severe skeletal discrepancy.

correction is necessary because the functional inadequacy of malocclusions has the potential to initiate or accelerate disease and to interfere with the execution of treatment. Familiarity with the Angle system of classification of the various types of malocclusion is helpful in the diagnosis and treatment of disease. This classification is based on the sagittal relationship between the mandibular and maxillary first molars. Canine-to-canine relations are used if the molars are missing or malposed. Functional problems inherent in the various malocclusions will be described.

The determination of malocclusions should be made at the RCP as well as at the MIP because of the potential for a severe discrepancy in landmark relations. Discrepancies can occur with Class I malocclusions, which can exhibit Class II tooth relations in the retruded contact position, and with the Class II malocclusions, which can exhibit more extreme and deviant buccolingual tooth relations, possibly total crossbite, in the retruded contact position.

In normal occlusion all teeth are properly aligned. The mesiobuccal cusp of the maxillary first molar occludes with the mesiobuccal groove of the mandibular first molar; the mandibular canine occludes with the distal half of the maxillary lateral incisor and the mesial incline of the maxillary canine.

The Class I malocclusion has normal occlusion except for malposed teeth, such as crowding crossbites and rotations (Fig. 8–23A). In the Class II malocclusion the buccal groove of the mandibular first molar is distal to the mesiobuccal cusp of the maxillary first molar and the mandibular canine is distal to the maxillary lateral incisor. A malocclusion can be the result of a dental disparity or a combination of a dental and a skeletal disparity. When the malocclusion is a result of a skeletal disparity, the size of the mandible is inadequate relative to the size of the maxilla. This can be caused by an underdeveloped mandible, an overdeveloped maxilla, or both.

The Class II, Division I malocclusion is

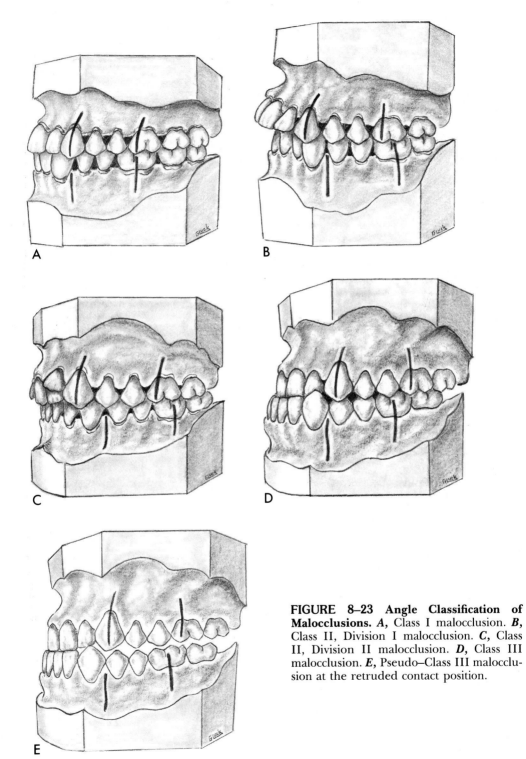

FIGURE 8–23 Angle Classification of Malocclusions. *A,* Class I malocclusion. *B,* Class II, Division I malocclusion. *C,* Class II, Division II malocclusion. *D,* Class III malocclusion. *E,* Pseudo–Class III malocclusion at the retruded contact position.

characterized by excessive overjet (Fig. 8–23B). Overbite can range from an open bite to a deep bite. Protrusion of the maxillary incisors and malposition of the canines result in ineffective anterior tooth guidance. Impaired anterior guidance causes protrusive and lateral-protrusive interferences involving the posterior teeth. Because the anterior tooth position prevents normal function, patients can develop abnormal swallowing patterns, tongue thrusts, and lip habits. These parafunctional activities act to perpetuate or exacerbate the functional deformity associated with the malocclusion and can accelerate the disease process.

In an attempt to compensate for an aberrant facial profile, patients often have a tendency to move the mandible forward. This parafunction results in posterior tooth contacts and an increase in the duration and frequency of protrusive interferences. The sequelae can exacerbate myofascial pain dysfunction syndrome and wear of or occlusal traumatism of the posterior and anterior teeth.

It is not uncommon to find advanced periodontal disease and secondary occlusal traumatism with associated posterior tooth loss. Local environmental conditions in the Class II, Division I malocclusion with an open bite are hardly conducive to health; in fact, they are the most likely to break down. Nevertheless, highly resistant patients can maintain a physiologically healthy occlusion, so prophylactic therapy is still contraindicated.

The Class II, Division II malocclusion (Fig. 8–23C) is characterized by a deep overbite, no overjet, crowding of the anterior teeth, excessive anterior guidance, and a dual plane of occlusion with depressed posterior teeth and overerupted anterior teeth. This relationship prevents the posterior teeth from receiving the forces of excessive bruxism. The anterior teeth, on the other hand, receive excessive forces because of the deep overbite and the strong musculature often associated with the Class II, Division I malocclusion. These forces can result in fractures, occlusal traumatism, and severe wear of the anterior teeth. The deep overbite is also responsible for the infringement of the mandibular anterior teeth or the soft tissues around the palatal aspect of the maxillary incisors. The deep overbite along with crowding of the anterior teeth can also lead to food impaction between the palatal aspect of the maxillary anterior teeth and the labial aspect of the mandibular anterior teeth and, eventually, to periodontal disease.

In the Class III malocclusion (Fig. 8–23D) the mandibular arch is mesial to a normal arch. It results from a skeletal deformity in which the size of the mandible is excessive relative to the size of the maxilla. This can be caused by an overdeveloped mandible, an underdeveloped maxilla, or both. It can also be the result of a dental disparity or a combination of a dental and skeletal disparity.

The malocclusion may be characterized by anterior crossbite, which does not permit anterior guidance. At times, the posterior teeth are also in crossbite, so that the entire maxilla falls within the confines of the mandible. Because of the locked-in occlusal scheme, no lateral or lateral-protrusive movements are possible, and bruxism does not usually develop. Protrusive movements, which would exacerbate the aberrant facial profile, are avoided by the patient.

Because the lower anterior teeth are lingually pitched, retrusive movements traumatize the upper anterior teeth, which could initiate occlusal traumatism. In addition, deviant anterior tooth relations can lead to food impaction and dental caries in the upper anterior teeth.

The pseudo–Class III malocclusion (Fig. 8–23E) is distinguished from the true Class III malocclusion in that the mandible can be moved along the terminal hinge axis to establish an edge-to-edge relationship.

Section II: Treatment

OCCLUSAL HISTORY AND EXAMINATION

Treatment of occlusal disease is based on a thorough history and an examination in order to establish a correct diagnosis, isolate the causes of disease, and investigate patient complaints. The actual examination of the occlusion must be executed in conjunction with study models, with a thorough clinical examination of all structures of the masticatory system, and with appropriate radiographic examination. The use of an appropriate chart facilitates the gathering of necessary data. Figure 8–24 provides an example of a chart containing a logical sequence of requisite examination procedures; its use will increase the efficiency and completeness of the examination process. Upon completion of the examination, the clinician should be able to establish whether or not an occlusion is physiologic or pathologic and should be able to determine the required therapy.

The examination of the occlusion is divided into six parts: (1) subjective symptoms; (2) examination of dental and skeletal forms and relations; (3) examination of the three basic mandibular positions (maximum intercuspal position, postural position, and retruded contact position); (4) examination for parafunctional habits; (5) radiographic signs of occlusal disease; and (6) signs of related disease. All parts of the examination chart must be completed and correlated with each other in order to make appropriate treatment decisions. The clinician must evaluate the subjective symptoms of the patient to ascertain whether function is adequate, appearance is esthetically acceptable, and the present dental arrangement is comfortable.

Dental and skeletal forms and relations correlate interarch and intra-arch skeletal and dental forms. If severe problems exist in any area at this time, the study models must be mounted to the retruded contact position on a semiadjustable articulator. The various components of dental arch continuity and rhythmicity must be visualized to assess their functional interarch relations.

The examination of the three basic mandibular positions is done in both static and dynamic aspects. It is executed with mounted study casts and direct visual examination of the mouth. It includes guided and unguided functional movements. The free way space is analyzed at all three positions and is measured in millimeters. Although the free way space may seem adequate when measured from the maximum intercuspal position, it may be inadequate when measured from the retruded contact position because of a severely extruded tooth.

Maximal mandibular opening ranges from 35 to 50 mm. Evaluation of maximal opening and any deviation helps in assessing the health of the muscles of mastication. Parafunctional and normal functional patterns must be analyzed to assess aberrant tooth positions and tooth contacts that may be influential in a disease process.

Although the chart should be self-explanatory, several points should be made. First, it is critical to understand that patient symptoms are, by definition, subjective. The rationale for a treatment plan must not rely exclusively or primarily on the dentist's clinical judgment and experience or on inferences and assumptions made about the patient's dental problems. This would involve minimizing or denying the importance of the individual patient's desires. If the patient's opinions and sentiments are not actively elicited and genuinely respected, the dentist could "treat" a functionally healthy physiologic occlusion. For example, the clinician may suggest tooth replacement in a patient who has adapted to a missing tooth and who reports no impairment in normal function and no complaints or dissatisfaction with appearance, phonetics, or mastication. The clinician must recognize that not all patients need a full complement of teeth for health, function, and comfort.

Second, the clinician should not expect patients to report parafunctional habits. This is because habits are initiated at an unconscious level so that patients are often unaware of engaging in parafunctional activity. However, other symptoms associated with parafunction, such as tension or head, neck, and TMJ pain, will usually be reported if habits are pathogenic.

Third, a clinical assessment of the muscles of mastication via visual and tactile examination is made to determine tone and

OCCLUSAL HISTORY AND EXAMINATION CHART

Name _____ Age _____ Occupation _____

SUBJECTIVE SYMPTOMS OF OCCLUSAL DISEASE

Esthetics _____   Phonetics _____
Positive occlusal sense _____   Mastication _____
Tooth sensitivity _____   Food impaction _____
TMJ pain _____   Clicking _____
Crepitus _____   Limited movement _____
Anxiety _____   Parafunctional habits _____
Head and neck pain _____   Muscle sensitivity _____

EXAMINATION OF DENTAL AND SKELETAL FORMS AND RELATIONS

Skeletal Arch Form:
Maxillary _____   Mandibular _____
Interarch discrepancy _____

Dental Arch Continuity:

Open contacts _____   Wear patterns _____
Uneven marginal ridge _____ Plunger cusps _____
Malposed teeth _____   Tooth fractures _____
Mobility patterns _____
Missing Teeth: Location   Reason   Duration
    Maxillary   _____
    Mandibular   _____

Dental Arch Rhythmicity:

Plane of occlusion: Curve of Spee:

	Depressed	Normal	Elevated			Flat	Moderate	Exaggerated
Rt. Max./Mand.	_____	_____	_____	Rt. Max./Mand.		_____	_____	_____
Left Max./Mand.	_____	_____	_____	Left Max./Mand.		_____	_____	_____

Transverse curve: Flat _____   Normal _____   Exaggerated _____
Posterior tooth (cusp) form _____   Anterior tooth form _____

EXAMINATION AT THE MAXIMUM INTERCUSPAL POSITION

Angle classification _____
Anterior guidance: Overbite (mm) _____   Overjet (mm) _____
Landmark relations: Mesiodistal _____
                      Buccolingual _____
Fremitus on closing into MIP (location) _____
Fremitus in lateral-protrusive movement (location) _____
Fremitus in protrusive movement (location) _____
Interferences: Right   Left
    Lateral-protrusive, working   _____   _____
    Lateral-protrusive, nonworking   _____   _____
    Protrusive   _____   _____

FIGURE 8–24 Occlusal History and Examination Chart. The occlusal history and examination chart follows a sequence convenient for the general practitioner. All occlusal findings must be correlated with the presence of disease or patient complaints in order to organize the sequence and to integrate therapy.

Illustration continued on opposite page

EXAMINATION AT THE POSTURAL POSITION AND VERTICAL DIMENSION

Choose two reference positions (intraorally or extraorally) to measure vertical dimension, e.g., the marginal gingiva of the canines.

Vertical dimension of the postural position (mm) _____

Vertical dimension of occlusion at RCP (mm) _____

Vertical dimension of occlusion MIP (mm) _____

Free way space of RCP (VD of PP–VD of RCP) (mm) _____

Free way space of MIP (VD of PP–VD of MIP) (mm) _____

Maximum opening: (mm) _____ Deviation _____

EXAMINATION AT THE RETRUDED CONTACT POSITION

Initial contact (retrusive interference) _____

Mandibular deflect of the MIP: Vertical distance (mm) _____

                                      Horizontal distance (mm) _____

                                      Direction _____

Landmark relations: Mesiodistal _____ Buccolingual _____

Angle classification _____

EXAMINATION FOR PARAFUNCTIONAL HABITS

Musculature: Lips _____ Cheeks _____

                 Tongue _____ Muscles of mastication _____

Swallowing: Adult tongue thrust _____

              Infantile retained tongue thrust _____

Type of habit: Tooth-to-tooth _____

              Tooth-to-musculature _____

              Tooth-to-object _____

RADIOGRAPHIC SIGNS OF OCCLUSAL DISEASE

Widened PDL space _____ Root fracture _____

Loss of continuity of lamina dura _____

Loss of definition of PDL space _____

Periapical radiolucency (associated with wear) _____

Root and osseous resorption _____

SIGNS OF RELATED DISEASES

Dental caries _____

Inflammatory periodontal disease _____

Pulpal disease _____

FIGURE 8–24 *Continued*

Illustration continued on following page

Symptoms of Occlusal Disease	Signs of Occlusal Disease	Signs and Symptoms of Related Inflammatory Disease	Aberrations in Occlusal Form and Relations

Diagnoses _____

_____

_____

_____

_____

_____

_____

_____

Occlusal and Concomitant Treatment Required _____

_____

_____

_____

_____

_____

_____

_____

FIGURE 8–24 *Continued*

strength, both of which are positively correlated with the magnitude and destructive capabilities of forces associated with occlusal interferences and parafunctional habits. The tone and strength of the tongue also have a positive correlation with the capacity of a habit to result in an open bite. A scalloped lateral border is an indication that the patient unconsciously presses the tongue against the teeth.

Fourth, a space is provided at the end of the form for the integration and correlation of all significant findings: signs and symptoms of occlusal disease and related inflammatory disease, and relevant aberrations in occlusal form and function. Pertinent data from other sources, such as past dental history, medical history, caries and periodontal records, radiographs, and study models, are included. This composite is a valuable aid in developing the diagnosis.

THE THERAPEUTIC OCCLUSION

Criteria

The goal of occlusal treatment is not to establish an ideal Class I occlusion but to set up an occlusion that is physiologic and conducive to health in relation to the form and function of the individual patient's masticatory system.

Although it would be impossible to compile a list of all definitive criteria that the ideal occlusion should satisfy for all patients, it is possible to develop a consensus on key characteristics considered to be conducive to a healthy local environment. These are:

1. a stable, intercuspal position at the retruded contact position along the terminal hinge arc of closure, supported bilaterally on the posterior teeth and allowing for an

adequate free way space;

2. unrestrained protrusive and lateral-protrusive movement from centric relation;

3. optimal axial inclination of teeth to diminish destructive horizontal or off-axis forces;

4. proper coronal forms and proximal relationships to provide maximal protection for the attachment apparatus;

5. support of occlusal vertical dimension by the posterior teeth;

6. disarticulation of the posterior teeth by the anterior teeth in all protrusive and lateral-protrusive movements; and

7. satisfaction of all subjective patient needs.

Determining the extent and type of therapy required to establish a therapeutic occlusion is a complicated and challenging process, involving the evaluation and correlation of the relevant data. This includes an accurate assessment of (1) the presence and destructive potential of disease entities, (2) the presence and destructive potential of occlusal aberrations, (3) the extent and severity of destruction caused by disease and occlusal aberrations, (4) the desires and symptoms of the patient, (5) the patient's age, (6) the adaptive capacity of the tissues, (7) the capability of a particular treatment to reverse a disease process or correct an occlusal deformity, and (8) the amount and complexity of treatment required to reverse a disease process or correct an occlusal deformity.

Maximum Intercuspal Position Versus Centric Relation

The clinician must decide whether it is appropriate to work to the maximum intercuspal position (MIP) or to re-establish it at the retruded contact position along the terminal arc of closure. Thus, the first decision to be reached is whether the MIP is to be maintained or re-established on the terminal hinge axis.

Centric relation is a therapeutic position in which (1) MIP and RCP are coincident; (2) all muscles and ligaments on both sides of the TMJ are balanced; (3) the condyles are on the terminal arc of closure; and (4) the free way space is adequate. These factors make centric relation reliably reproducible, optimally stable, and physiologically acceptable. Moreover, because stability is not a function of proprioception, alterations in oc-clusal form resulting from disease and therapy do not have the potential to induce occlusal awareness, making the patient conscious of occlusal function, which normally involves reflexive activity. It is therefore preferable to establish centric relation in the therapeutic occlusion.

To make this decision, it is necessary to evaluate the severity of occlusal deformity, the extent of disease, the amount of therapy required, the degree of host resistance, and the subjective needs of the patient. The MIP is indicated for cases requiring minimal therapy, such as isolated caries in an otherwise healthy mouth or incipient inflammatory periodontal disease. The MIP is also used when the amount of therapy necessary to achieve a therapeutic occlusion is excessive in relation to the deformity or is contraindicated because the patient does not have the desire or the requisite funds or emotional stability. The centric relation position is used in patients lacking occlusal stability or requiring a significant change in the occlusal scheme, including (1) occlusal disease, such as severe wear, occlusal traumatism, and extracapsular TMJ dysfunction; (2) multiple missing teeth requiring advanced restorative dentistry; (3) rampant caries; and (4) an edentulous arch.

Articulators

Diagnostic casts, mountings, and wax-ups are essential to determine the effectiveness and adequacy of proposed modalities of treatment and to estimate the extent and type of therapy required. For these purposes, the semiadjustable articulator, such as the Hanau, Whip-Mix, or Denar articulator, is more appropriate for use in general practice than either the nonadjustable or the fully adjustable articulator. The semiadjustable articulator is simple to use, durable, and accurate for diagnosis and treatment planning and for the fabrication of fixed and removable prostheses. More important than the choice of articulator, however, is the accuracy of the casts and the registration and transfer of records. In the fabrication of the final restoration, it is absolutely essential to have a centric relation record at an acceptable occlusal vertical dimension. This requires setting up all the requirements of a therapeutic occlusion in the provisional restoration, assessing the occlusal scheme in the mouth (especially in the periodontally involved case); checking all protrusive and lateral-protrusive movements for mobility and fremitus patterns; and executing occlusal adjustment by selective grinding to alleviate any remaining problems. Such adjustments cannot be made on the articulator whether it is fully adjustable or not.

This careful and methodical planning of treatment allows easy recording and transfer to the articulator. If an alteration in occlusal vertical dimension is required on the articulator, a new centric relation record must be taken and the casts remounted on the articulator. All other information recorded and transferred to the articulator is arbitrary, including (1) face-bow mounting, (2) intercon-

dylar distance, and (3) protrusive and lateral-protrusive check-bites, which should be taken no more than 3 to 5 mm from the centric relation position.

Occlusal Appliances

The occlusal appliances most frequently used as adjuncts in therapy are the modified Hawley appliance (Hawley bite plane) and the nightguard (Fig. 8–25). The bite plane is an active device, whereas the nightguard is passive. Indications for their use are therefore quite different.

The maxillary Hawley bite plane is a useful diagnostic and therapeutic device em-

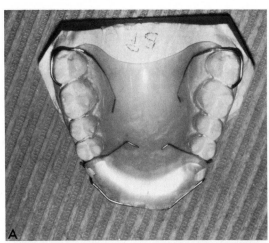
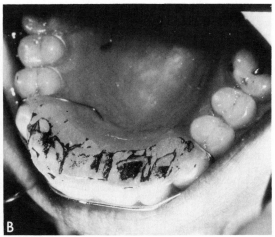
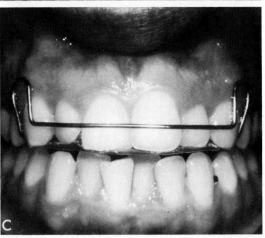

FIGURE 8–25 Modified Maxillary Hawley Bite Plane. A, Modified Hawley bite plane with labial bow and full palatal coverage extending above the length of contour of the palatal aspect of the maxillary posterior teeth. The labial bow and position of the acrylic of the palatal aspect of the posterior teeth provide for maxillary tooth stability. **B,** Hawley bite plane placed in a patient with temporomandibular joint pain. The lower incisors are left malaligned and not adjusted in this type of patient. **C** (1) The Hawley bite plane is adjusted to a flat plane on the lingual aspects of the maxillary anterior teeth. The adjustment of the platform allows for even and simultaneous contact of the mandibular anterior teeth at an acceptable occlusal vertical dimension. (2) The posterior teeth are disarticulated 1 mm in the premolar region and do not contact in any movements or positions. Protrusive and lateral-protrusive movements are supported by the occlusal vertical dimension as well as the palatal platform of the bite plane. (3) The condyle is on the terminal hinge axis at the same time the anterior teeth are occluding maximally with the bite plane. This provides bilateral, simultaneous neuromuscular contraction of the internal pterygoid, masseter, and temporalis muscles.

ployed for occlusal, periodontal, restorative, orthodontic, and myofascial pain dysfunction syndrome treatment (MPDS). The bite plane acts immediately to redirect occlusal forces to the anterior teeth, to stabilize maxillary posterior teeth, and to disarticulate the posterior teeth. Disarticulation of the posterior teeth serves to:

1.   eliminate posterior tooth contacts or interferences;
2.   eliminate retrusive interferences;
3.   control excessive forces associated with parafunctional activity;
4.   allow for movement of the mandible to the terminal hinge axis;
5.   allow for the evaluation of landmark relations;
6.   facilitate occlusal adjustment;
7.   confirm differential diagnoses (e.g., MPDS);
8.   break up proprioception;
9.   allow for posterior eruption; and
10.   allow for rest of the attachment apparatus.

The greatest advantage of the bite plane is also its greatest liability, namely, disarticulation of the posterior teeth and the consequent posterior eruption.

The clinician must assess the amount of anterior overbite and overjet present. If the patient has minimal overbite or excessive overjet and thus very little anterior guidance, posterior eruption could cause an increase in occlusal vertical dimension, resulting in decreased effectual anterior guidance and increased posterior tooth contacts in protrusive and lateral-protrusive movements.

The nightguard is a maxillary appliance that contains the teeth in the maxillary arch, induces maximum and even distribution of all tooth contacts, and allows freedom in all protrusive and lateral-protrusive movements. This results in the elimination of interferences and the control of parafunctional activity.

OCCLUSAL ADJUSTMENT BY SELECTIVE GRINDING

Adjustment of the occlusion by selective grinding is instituted (1) to eliminate or control the excessive forces associated with interferences and parafunctions in order to protect the tissues of the masticatory system and promote healing; (2) to establish tooth relations that afford optimal function and comfort to the patient; and (3) to set up an occlusion that is harmonious and stable for restorative therapy. Occlusal adjustment is never indicated for prophylactic reasons.

Altering tooth relations can make patients conscious of occlusal function and the presence of their teeth, creating an occlusal awareness or positive occlusal sense. This problem is often extremely difficult to resolve.

While selective grinding is an excellent adjunct to all therapy, it must be approached with caution. Prior to adjusting the occlusion, the clinician must do a complete occlusal examination and a diagnostic mounting and selective grinding on the articulator in order to determine if the RCP can be made coincidental with the MIP. Landmark relations may be poor and preclude occlusal adjustment. For example, the Class II, Division I malocclusion, which gets worse as the retruded contact position is approached, may not be managed by selective grinding alone and may require full orthodontic correction. Selective grinding may not be indicated in a dentition characterized by severely worn and flat posterior teeth or when a significant vertical and horizontal discrepancy exists between the RCP and the MIP. In this case, an insufficient amount of tooth structure may preclude the possibility of doing occlusal adjustment. Full orthodontic correction, occlusal therapy, and advanced restorative dentistry could be required.

Technique

The technique of occlusal adjustment by selective grinding to the retruded contact position is divided into four steps. The first step involves major changes in the occlusal scheme. Retrusive interferences, usually the lingual incline of mandibular supporting cusps and buccal incline of maxillary supporting cusps, are eliminated in a systematic and conservative fashion so that maximal contact can be established without infringing on the free way space or altering the capacity of the occlusal vertical dimension to provide effective anterior guidance. Supporting cusps are modified so that they relate to the opposing central fossa area and are in a position that will allow contact with the inner incline of buccal cusps of the maxillary teeth

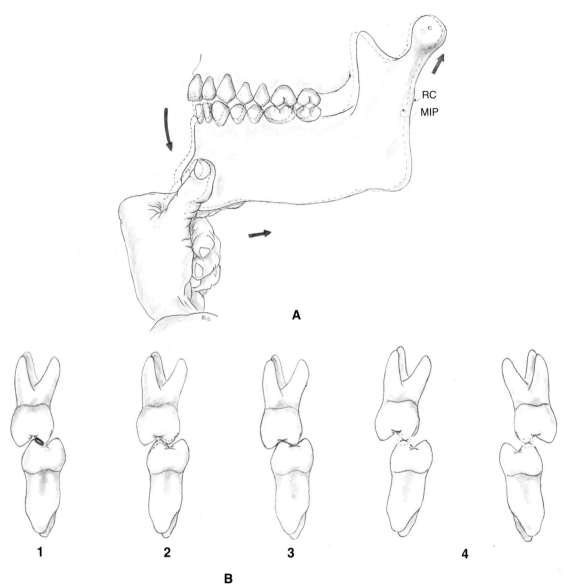

FIGURE 8–26 Occlusal Adjustment by Selective Grinding to Correct Landmark Relations. *A,* Moving the mandible from the maximum intercuspal position (MIP), indicated by the dotted line, to the retruded contact (RC) position on the terminal hinge axis, indicated by the solid line, increases the occlusal vertical dimension and changes mesiodistal landmarks. ***B*** (1) In the initial tooth contact on the terminal hinge axis, the buccal incline of the maxillary palatal cusp articulates with the lingual incline of the mandibular buccal cusp. (2) Selective grinding is implemented to eliminate retrusive interferences and to widen the maxillary palatal cusp and mandibular buccal cusp to correct buccolingual landmark relations. Additional selective grinding is then executed to define the functional outer aspect (FOA), which helps compensate for the widened occlusal table. (3) Occlusal adjustment by selective grinding has successfully corrected landmark relations, which are shown at the retruded contact position. (4) In this case, the severity of the buccolingual landmark relations, shown at the retruded contact position, precludes correction by selective grinding alone. Tooth movement via adjunctive orthodontics is required.

in lateral and lateral-protrusive movements (Fig. 8–26). Occlusal deformities that disrupt arch continuity and rhythmicity are corrected at this time. This correction includes adjusting open contacts, leveling marginal ridges, and shortening excessively prominent cusps and plunger cusps that can cause protrusive and lateral-protrusive interferences. If Class I mesiodistal landmarks cannot be established, the maxillary guiding incline may be modified with a platform to provide a contact area for the supporting cusps. At the end of this first step the supporting cusp should be in the opposing central fossa in preparation for cuspal modification to provide freedom of mandibular movement in all excursive movements.

The second step in treatment is to modify the most coronal millimeter of tooth surface on the buccal and labial surfaces (functional outer aspect, or FOA) of all mandibular teeth in the arch. This creates a smooth, continuous band that enhances the capability of the fossa to cradle the supporting cusps. Once established, the FOA is not altered—all further changes are made in the maxillary arch.

The third step is to refine the palatal and guiding inclines of the maxillary teeth so that the mandible can move freely in protru-sive and lateral-protrusive directions. At this time it must be determined whether or not additional tooth contacts are needed. This decision is based on the periodontal support of teeth, ascertained by testing for fremitus and mobility at the centric relation position and in protrusive and lateral-protrusive movements.

To support protrusive movement, occlusal adjustment of the maxillary anterior teeth should be aimed at maximizing the number of tooth contacts between the palatal aspects and incisal edges of the upper teeth and the labial aspects and incisal edges of the lower teeth (Fig. 8–27A). If fremitus and mobility persist, the slope of the inclination of the palatal surfaces of the upper anterior teeth is made more shallow to gain maximal tooth contact and to alleviate and distribute horizontal forces. This phase of selective grind-

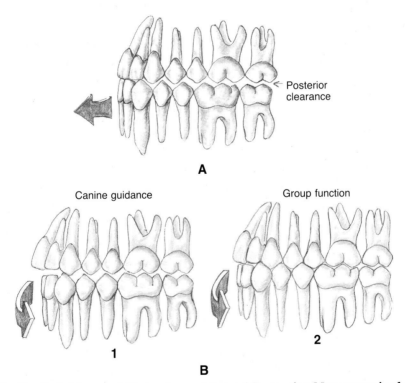

FIGURE 8–27   Tooth Guidance of Protrusive and Lateral-Protrusive Movements in the Adjusted or Restored Occlusion. *A,* In a direct protrusive movement, the labial and incisal surfaces of the mandibular anterior teeth contact the palatal aspects of the maxillary anterior teeth to disarticulate the posterior teeth. *B,* Support of lateral-protrusive movements occurs on the working side and usually presents with two alternatives: (1) canine guidance, which disarticulates all posterior teeth on the working and nonworking sides; and (2) group function (on the working side), which provides for disarticulation of the posterior teeth on the nonworking side and establishes tooth contacts on the working side that gradually diminish from the anterior to the posterior part of the mouth. This includes the anterior teeth and guiding cusp of the posterior teeth on the working side.

Illustration continued on following page

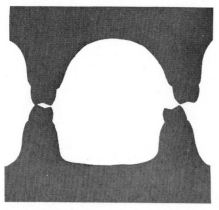
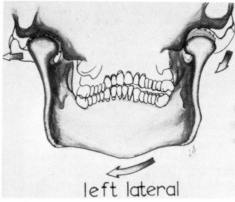

C

FIGURE 8–27 *Continued C,* In a left lateral-protrusive movement, although either canine guidance or group function may occur, there are neither cross-tooth nor cross-arch balancing contacts. (From Goldman, H. M., and Cohen, D. W.: Periodontal Therapy, 5th ed. C. V. Mosby, Saint Louis, 1973, p. 570, and courtesy of Morton Amsterdam, Philadelphia, Pa.)

ing is done conservatively and is constantly monitored to avoid creating posterior tooth contacts or interferences.

Lateral-protrusive movements may be supported by canine guidance or group function (Fig. 8–27B). When canine guidance is adequate, no adjustments are necessary. However, when the canines are weak, exhibiting fremitus and mobility, it is necessary to establish group function by modifying the maxillary canines. This is accomplished through a reduction in the slope of the palatal aspect of the canines, which provides for posterior tooth contacts on the working side between the FOA of lower teeth and the guiding inclines of upper teeth (Fig. 8–27C). Subsequent adjustment of the guiding incline is made in a judicious manner to establish contacts that decrease gradually in number and inclination from the anterior to the posterior part of the mouth.

To prevent the initiation of parafunctional habits or positive occlusal awareness, all ground tooth surfaces are polished at the end of each visit. In addition, occlusal relations must be monitored because of the potential for retrusive interferences to develop as a result of changes in tooth position.

The fourth and final step in occlusal adjustment involves a re-evaluation. Occlusal adjustment by selective grinding may have induced or failed to correct nonworking interferences. These interferences must be eliminated. However, because the cusp associated with the nonworking interference

supports the occlusal vertical dimension, management of this occlusal aberration requires a considerable degree of clinical judgment. The following procedures may be used: (1) reducing the depth of the opposing mandibular central fossa, (2) establishing a groove or track in the mandibular buccal cusp to accommodate the movement of the maxillary supporting cusp, and (3) doing restorative dentistry either to increase the slope of the upper canine palatal incline or build up the FOA of the lower canine, whichever is the more conservative procedure for the individual patient.

It may also be found during the re-evaluation stage that the weakened posterior teeth cannot support the occlusal vertical dimension adequately or that lateral-protrusive movements are supported only by the guiding inclines of posterior teeth. In such cases, restorative dentistry may be necessary to modify the palatal aspect of the maxillary canines with a platform to aid in supporting and stabilizing the occlusion. Upon completion of occlusal adjustment, a nightguard is often used to control nocturnal parafunctional activity.

MANAGEMENT OF DENTAL CARIES

The placement of a single restoration in the treatment of an isolated carious tooth in an otherwise healthy mouth is one of the most common procedures in general practice. But, before proceeding with this simple operative technique, the clinician must first assess occlusal morphology and relations to ascertain the presence of any signs of incipient disease or occlusal aberrations that might complicate or compromise restorative therapy.

In the restoration of a single carious lesion, it is not unusual to find isolated occlusal abnormalities or pathologic tooth migration associated with the decayed tooth. In such cases, the correction of these deformities would be indicated, since occlusal aberrations have the potential to decrease the longevity of the restoration. Occlusal adjust-

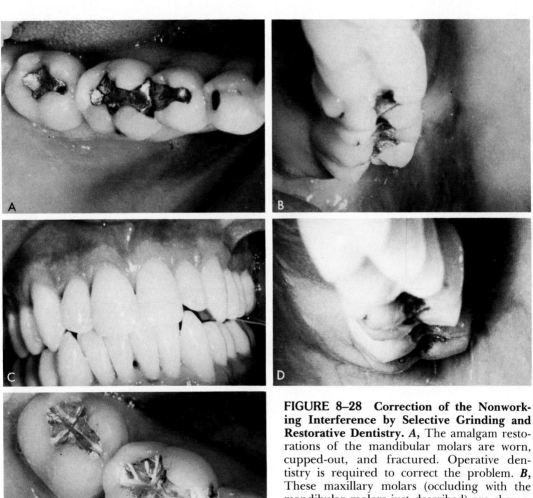

FIGURE 8–28 Correction of the Nonworking Interference by Selective Grinding and Restorative Dentistry. *A,* The amalgam restorations of the mandibular molars are worn, cupped-out, and fractured. Operative dentistry is required to correct the problem. *B,* These maxillary molars (occluding with the mandibular molars just described) are characterized by steep, hanging palatal cusps and are associated with interferences. *C,* Dental floss is manipulated to confirm the presence of a right nonworking interference. The replacement of the amalgam restorations presented the opportunity to correct the nonworking interferences. The rationale for occlusal adjustment in this case is to correct a problem possibly created by wear and breakdown of the amalgam restorations and treatment being executed primarily for control of dental caries. Occlusal adjustment is done to enhance the longevity of the restoration and create favorable occlusal forces. *D,* Selective grinding was employed to reshape and shorten the palatal cusps. The new palatal forms are tested for clearance in lateral-protrusive movements. Once freedom of movement is established, the inadequate mandibular amalgam restorations are replaced. *E,* The central fossa areas of the new amalgams have been shallowed out to support the palatal cusp in the maximum intercuspal position (MIP). (Because the scope of the problem was limited and the extent of requisite therapy minimal, all treatment was done at the MIP.)

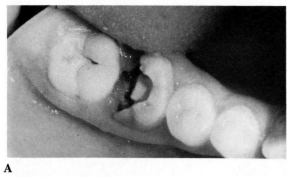

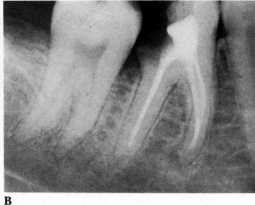

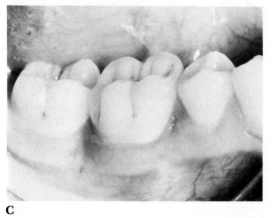

FIGURE 8–29 Caries and Localized Sequelae
A, In this preoperative radiograph, severe, long standing caries has destroyed the entire dista half of this (endodontically treated, nonvital mandibular first molar, resulting in mesial drif of the second molar and the encroachment on the broken-down tooth and embrasure space. *B* Subsequent food impaction and plaque and cal culus accumulation caused soft tissue inflamma tion, edema, and enlargement. Since the localized disease and occlusal problem caused by the carie occurred in an otherwise healthy mouth, treatment was done at the MIP. Treatment consisted of per odontal therapy, adjunctive orthodontics, occlusal adjustment, and restorative dentistry. *C,* The fina restoration is in place. The disease processes have been reversed, the deformities eliminated, and arc continuity restored. (See Chapter 12, Figure 12–3, for complete treatment.)

ment by selective grinding is a concomitant to the primary restorative treatment that is aimed at the elimination of decay (Fig. 8–28). For example, in the treatment of a single decayed tooth associated with an isolated protrusive or nonworking interference, the interfering supporting cusp is reduced and the depth of the central fossa of the restoration is deliberately shallowed.

In addition to interferences, other minor occlusal abnormalities often associated with a broken-down tooth require adjustment. Examples of such abnormalities include plunger cusps, open contacts, uneven marginal ridges, and sharp edges of tooth structure that are conducive to fractures. When it appears likely that minor occlusal adjustments in the opposing arch will be required in addition to the operative procedure, it is highly advisable that the patient be so informed before restorative therapy is initiated. This engenders a sense of trust on the part of the patient and prevents any misunderstanding. Since the extent of destruction caused by the caries is isolated and minimal

and the therapy required is simple, isolated occlusal adjustments are done in the MIP.

Caries often destroys tooth contacting sur faces, resulting in the drifting and migration of contiguous teeth and extrusion of oppos ing teeth into the decayed tooth area. The changes in tooth position may compromise or destroy embrasure spaces and lead to open contacts, loss of occlusal contacts, food impaction, and soft tissue inflammation This situation would require caries contro with an amalgam restoration as a temporar measure (if needed) and management of soft tissue inflammation followed by adjunc tive orthodontics to regain normal embra sure spaces, correct the axial inclination of teeth, and close open contacts. Occlusal ad justment by selective grinding would be ex ecuted to level the opposing extruded teeth and correct the plane of occlusion, alleviat ing any nonworking or protrusive interfer ences that may have developed. The fina restoration required of this tooth is usuall an onlay or a full crown to replace the los tooth structure, maintain arch integrity, and

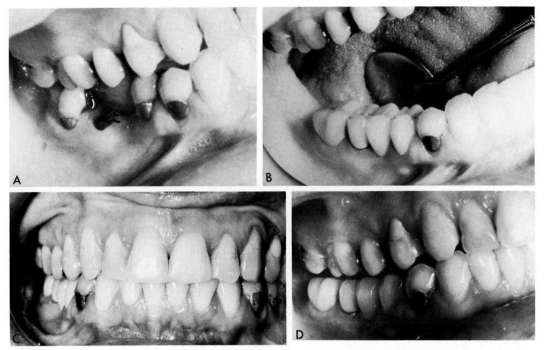

FIGURE 8–30   Restorative Therapy via Fixed Prosthesis in the MIP. A, The mandibular right second molar and the distal root of the first molar are decayed. (The mesial root was previously extracted as a result of caries.) There were no other signs or symptoms of disease, and the occlusion was stable in this 57-year-old patient. **B,** Treatment consisted of a fixed bridge, in place in the mandibular arch, with concomitant occlusal adjustment by selective grinding to eliminate occlusal aberrations in the opposing arch. Because of the isolated nature of the problem, the maximum intercuspal position was used in therapy. **C,** The final restoration is in place at the MIP. **D,** Canine guidance has been maintained supporting the right working movement and disarticulating all posterior teeth.

re-establish adequate occlusal and proximal tooth contacts (Fig. 8–29). Because the problem occurs in an otherwise healthy mouth and is isolated in nature (that is, the restorative dentistry involves only one or two teeth), treatment may be done at the MIP, although a clinical judgment must be made for each individual patient (Fig. 8–30).

MANAGEMENT OF OCCLUSAL TRAUMATISM WITH INFLAMMATORY PERIODONTAL DISEASE

Occlusal traumatism—the injury to or the destruction of the attachment apparatus by abnormal excessive forces—is usually accompanied by inflammatory periodontal disease and is associated with aberrations in occlusal form and function. Control of inflammatory periodontal disease is a key consideration in

the treatment of occlusal traumatism. The destructive capability of abnormal occlusal forces is virtually neutralized when local environmental conditions are conducive to health and signs of inflammatory disease are absent.

Primary Occlusal Traumatism With Gingivitis

In cases of primary occlusal traumatism with gingivitis, the requisite treatment is simple and conservative. This is because both disease processes are incipient and separate, so injury to the periodontal structures is minimal. Both disease processes and associated clinical signs are readily reversible with minor therapy. Treatment usually requires simultaneous implementation of periodontal and occlusal therapies. Periodontal therapy involves scaling and root planing to control the inflammation; occlusal therapy involves

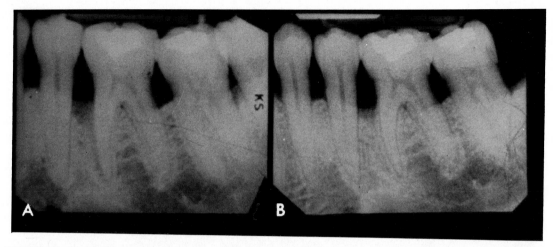

FIGURE 8–31 Primary Occlusal Traumatism. *A,* Radiographic signs of primary occlusal traumatism include a widened periodontal ligament (PDL) space, loss of continuity, and loss of definition of the lamina dura (alveolar wall). In the more advanced stages of primary occlusal traumatism, radiographic manifestations are more extensive and severe. Note the severe widened PDL space and bone loss on the mesial aspect of the first molar. *B,* Reversal of the disease process is confirmed by an absence of radiographic signs.

selective grinding to eliminate interferences and the use of a nightguard to control nocturnal parafunctional activity.

Primary Occlusal Traumatism With Periodontitis

If gingivitis goes untreated, it will progress and ultimately extend into the attachment apparatus as periodontitis. In the case of primary occlusal traumatism with periodontitis, the two disease processes may or may not remain discrete entities (Fig. 8–31). In general, signs of periodontitis and occlusal disease are more pronounced and more widespread than signs of gingivitis, yet the quantity of periodontal support is still sufficient to withstand the forces delivered during normal function. Although the patient's adaptive capability may still be operative, so that damaged or injured tissues are likely to respond well to treatment, the presence of disease should be of concern to the clinician because of the progressive nature of the disease process, the susceptibility of the patient, and the possibility that loss of the attachment apparatus may have been so extensive that damage to the tissues is not reversible.

Primary Occlusal Traumatism and Tooth Mobility

Mobility may be associated with any one or a combination of the following: (1) in-

flammatory disease: gingivitis, incipient or moderate periodontitis, or pulpitis; (2) a readily identifiable occlusal etiology: an interference or a parafunction; (3) thin osseous and soft tissue complex and short, underdeveloped roots; and (4) temporary hormonal imbalance, especially during pregnancy and menstruation. To determine the requisite treatment and the sequence of therapy, all of these factors must be assessed and clinical judgment rendered. This may be simple or quite involved.

Control of soft tissue inflammation is executed routinely in conjunction with occlusal therapy, if needed. However, if no occlusal problem is evident and the mobility is generalized and associated with inflammatory periodontal disease, the approach to treatment is more conservative, involving soft tissue management only, followed by a period of healing and re-evaluation. If mobility diminishes, no further treatment is required. But, if mobility persists or becomes more severe, the occlusion is carefully re-examined for the presence of interferences that may have resulted from changes in tooth position induced by the periodontal disease. If no interferences are discovered, undetectable nocturnal bruxism may be occurring and nightguard therapy should be instituted.

When a tooth contact or an interference causes visible tooth movement in a protrusive or lateral-protrusive movement, isolated occlusal adjustment by selective grinding is indicated to eliminate destructive occlusal forces. When a patient presents with signs (wear or widened PDL space) or symptoms (pain or impaired function) of a tooth-to-tooth parafunction associated with mobility, a nightguard to control excessive forces is the treatment of choice. When mobility is associated with missing teeth, restoration of arch continuity and stability with a fixed prosthesis is implemented whenever possible.

Secondary Occlusal Traumatism and Periodontitis

Combined secondary occlusal traumatism with periodontitis represents one of the most challenging conditions the general practitioner will ever treat. The associated destruction requires extensive restorative treatment and clinically exacting procedures (Fig. 8–32).

The quantity of the attachment apparatus is so diminished that the teeth can no longer sustain forces delivered during normal function. Concurrent occlusal and periodontal treatment is instituted immediately. Definitive and frequent scaling and root planing along with patient instruction in oral hygiene procedures is done to control inflammation. Hawley bite-plane therapy to protect the teeth from destructive force application is used continuously throughout treatment.

The next phase of treatment involves further occlusal therapy. First, all teeth in secondary traumatism must be stabilized. This may be difficult because of extreme mobility; excessive clinical crown length; loss of arch continuity; egregious aberrations in occlusal form, such as a Class II, Division I malocclusion; and severely distorted occlusal planes and curves. Hawley bite-plane therapy, initiated in the first phase of treatment, is used to help re-establish arch integrity, stabilize the maxillary teeth, redirect occlusal forces to maxillary and mandibular anterior teeth, disarticulate the posterior teeth, provide occlusal rests for all posterior teeth,

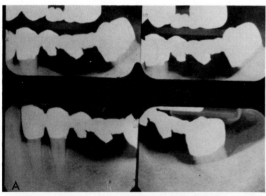
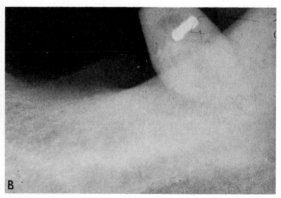
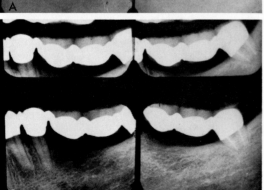

FIGURE 8–32 Secondary Occlusal Traumatism. *A,* In cases of secondary occlusal traumatism all radiographic signs of primary occlusal traumatism are present, but bone loss is much more extensive. This mandibular second molar, restored in an extruded position, destroyed arch rhythmicity, resulting in interferences in protrusive and lateral-protrusive movements. In addition to the excessive occlusal forces associated with the interference, horizontal forces were generated by parafunctional activity. To control occlusal forces, Hawley bite plane therapy and selective grinding were instituted, in conjunction with periodontal therapy. *B,* This 6-month postoperative radiograph demonstrates healing of the attachment apparatus. Intentional endodontic therapy was necessary to correct the elevated plane of occlusion and exaggerated curve of Spee and transverse curve, thus eliminating the interference. *C,* The final restoration is in place, 2 years after treatment was initiated.

control parafunction, eliminate interferences, evaluate landmarks, facilitate all occlusal adjustments, and aid in locating the true terminal hinge axis (Fig. 8–33).

Patients with secondary occlusal traumatism with advanced periodontitis often require advanced periodontal therapy: (1) strategic extraction, regenerative procedures (curettage of two- or three-walled infrabon defects), and root resection for maxim healing of the attachment apparatus; (2) ad vanced surgical procedures for pocket elim ination and correction of deformities cre ated by periodontal disease; and (3) splintin for periodontal stabilization.

Splinting is a useful adjunct in the trea

Text continued on page 38

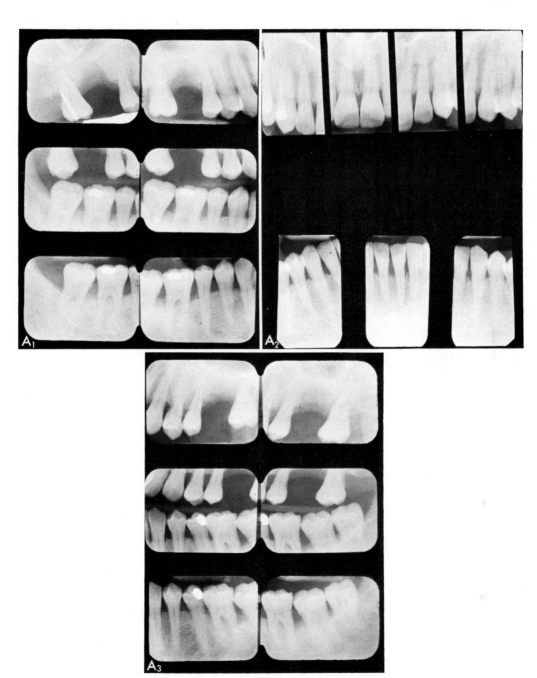

FIGURE 8–33 *See legend on opposite page*

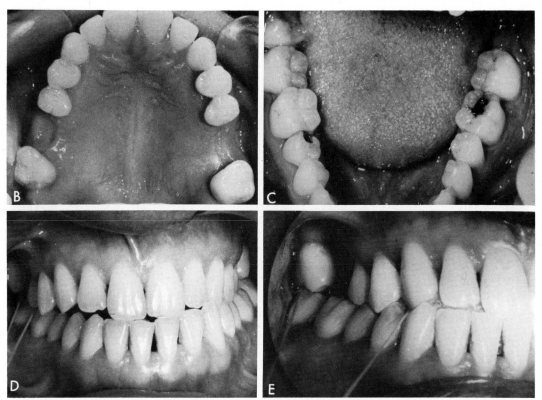

FIGURE 8–33 Severe Occlusal Deformities and Combined Disease Processes. *A,* This set of radiographs of a 38-year-old patient illustrates a dentition with combined inflammatory and occlusal periodontal disease. In addition to malposed mandibular teeth and missing maxillary first molars, the molars are in secondary occlusal traumatism, and the anterior teeth and premolars are in primary occlusal traumatism and exhibit radiographic signs of periodontitis. (The severe periodontal defects were corroborated clinically by 8 to 10 mm pocket probings.) *1,* This radiograph of the left side demonstrates the advanced bone loss around the maxillary second molar and the mandibular second molar, especially the distal aspect of each terminal molar. The mandibular molars have Class II furcation involvements. *2,* Radiograph of the anterior teeth displays generalized calculus formation and bone loss, especially around the mandibular incisors. *3,* The radiographs of the right posterior sections show the advanced bone loss around the maxillary second premolar and second molar. The distal aspect of the mandibular first molar has a severe infrabony defect and Class II furcation involvement. The second and third molars have secondary occlusal traumatism. *B,* The maxillary occlusal view demonstrates the unworn occlusal surfaces of the posterior teeth. The maxillary first molars were lost as a result of acute periodontal abscesses, disrupting arch continuity. (This was the patient's only complaint.) *C,* Arch rhythmicity has been destroyed. The plane of occlusion on the right side is elevated; the curve of Spee on the right side is exaggerated, and the transverse curve on both sides is severely exaggerated; the marginal ridges are uneven; the molars and premolars are lingually pitched; and the posterior cuspal height is functionally greater than anterior guidance. *D,* In a left lateral-protrusive movement, there is a right nonworking interference between the right maxillary and mandibular molars. This must be correlated with the radiographic findings, mobility, and aberrant occlusal form. *E,* In a right lateral-protrusive movement, there are excessive posterior tooth contacts on this right working side. Wear of the canine, resulting from parafunction, has contributed to the increase in posterior tooth contacts.

Illustration continued on following page

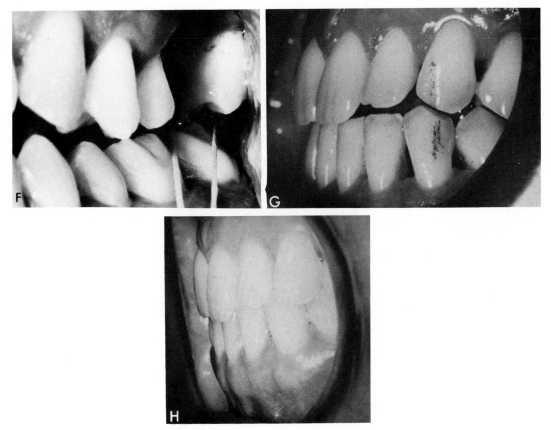

FIGURE 8–33 *Continued F,* Dental floss is manipulated on the left side during the right lateral-protrusive movement to reveal a nonworking interference. Contact is between the buccal incline of the maxillary palatal cusp and the lingual incline of the mandibular buccal cusp. **G,** At the retruded contact position, anterior tooth relations have changed minimally, about 1 mm. Note the wear of the canines. **H,** Anterior tooth relations, as shown in the maximum intercuspal position, are marked by a negative overjet and a minimal overbite, inadequate for posterior cuspal height and the elevated plane of occlusion and exaggerated curves of occlusion (especially the transverse curve).

Illustration continued on opposite page

OCCLUSAL HISTORY AND EXAMINATION CHART

Name _Elsie Smith_   Age _38_   Occupation _Housewife_

SUBJECTIVE SYMPTOMS OF OCCLUSAL DISEASE

Esthetics _Unhappy with missing molars_
Positive occlusal sense _Negative_
Tooth sensitivity _Molar areas_
TMJ pain _Negative_
Crepitus _Negative_
Anxiety _Patient concerned about recent tooth loss_
Head and neck pain _Negative_

Phonetics _Negative_
Mastication _Negative_
Food impaction _Negative_
Clicking _Negative_
Limited movement _Negative_
Parafunctional habits _Nocturnal bruxism_
Muscle sensitivity _Negative_

EXAMINATION OF DENTAL AND SKELETAL FORMS AND RELATIONS

Skeletal Arch Form:
Maxillary _Normal_   Mandibular _Class III tendency_
Interarch discrepancy _Angle Class III tendency_

Dental Arch Continuity:

Open contacts _None_
Uneven marginal ridge _Generalized_
Malposed teeth _18, 30, 31, 32_
Mobility patterns _Generalized moderate_

Wear patterns _Minimal (anterior teeth)_
Plunger cusps _None_
Tooth fractures _None_

Missing Teeth:	Location	Reason	Duration
Maxillary	1, 3, 14, 16	3 & 14 advanced periodontitis	6 months
Mandibular	17	Wisdom tooth	10 years

Dental Arch Rhythmicity:

Plane of occlusion:

	Depressed	Normal	Elevated
Rt. Max.		×	
Rt. Mand.			×
Left Max.		×	
Left Mand.		×	

Curve of Spee:

	Flat	Moderate	Exaggerated
Rt. Max.		×	
Rt. Mand.			×
Left Max.		×	
Left Mand.		×	

Transverse curve: Flat _____   Normal _____   Exaggerated __×__
Posterior tooth (cusp) form _Excessive_   Anterior tooth form _Inadequate_

EXAMINATION AT THE MAXIMUM INTERCUSPAL POSITION

Angle classification _Class I_
Anterior guidance: Overbite (mm) _1_   Overjet (mm) _0_
Landmark relations: Mesiodistal _Normal_
                     Buccolingual _Normal_
Fremitus on closing into MIP (location) _7 & 8_
Fremitus in lateral-protrusive movement (location) _5 & 6, 12 & 13_
Fremitus in protrusive movement (location) _Negative_

Interferences:	Right		Left
Lateral-protrusive, working	3/31	5/28	12/20
Lateral-protrusive, nonworking	3/31		14/18
Protrusive	3/32		

FIGURE 8–33 *Continued I,* Completed occlusal history and examination chart.

Illustration continued on following page

EXAMINATION AT THE POSTURAL POSITION AND VERTICAL DIMENSION

Choose two reference positions (intraorally or extraorally) to measure vertical
dimension, e.g., the marginal gingiva of the canines.

Vertical dimension of the postural position (mm) _(Free way space) 21___ Cervical mand. rt. canine to max. rt. canine____
Vertical dimension of occlusion at RCP (mm)_____ 20_____
Vertical dimension of occlusion MIP (mm)_____ 18_____
Free way space of RCP (VD of PP–VD of RCP) (mm) _____ 2_____
Free way space of MIP (VD of PP–VD of MIP) (mm)_____ 3_____
Maximum opening: (mm) _42_____ Deviation _None_____

EXAMINATION AT THE RETRUDED CONTACT POSITION

Initial contact (retrusive interference) _3/32_____
Mandibular deflect of the MIP: Vertical distance (mm) _1_____
                                Horizontal distance (mm) _1_____
                                Direction _To the right_____
Landmark relations: Mesiodistal _Good_____ Buccolingual _Good_____
Angle classification _No significant change_____

EXAMINATION FOR PARAFUNCTIONAL HABITS

Musculature: Lips _Negative_____   Cheeks _Negative_____
              Tongue _Scalloped border_____ Muscles of mastication _Normal_____
Swallowing: Adult tongue thrust _Negative_____
             Infantile retained tongue thrust _Negative_____
Type of habit: Tooth-to-tooth _Bruxism_____
                Tooth-to-musculature _Negative_____
                Tooth-to-object _Negative_____

RADIOGRAPHIC SIGNS OF OCCLUSAL DISEASE

Widened PDL space _All molars_____   Root fracture _____
Loss of continuity of lamina dura _All molars_____
Loss of definition of PDL space _All molars_____
Periapical radiolucency (associated with wear) _None_____
Root and osseous resorption _None_____

SIGNS OF RELATED DISEASES

Dental caries _Negative_____
Inflammatory periodontal disease _Generalized periodontitis more severe at all molars_____
Pulpal disease _Negative_____

FIGURE 8–33 *I Continued*

Illustration continued on opposite pag

Symptoms of Occlusal Disease	Signs of Occlusal Disease	Signs and Symptoms of Related Inflammatory Disease	Aberrations in Occlusal Form and Relations
Bruxism	Mobility on molar region Widened PDL spaces Thinning lamina dura	Generalized plaque, especially on palatal and lingual surfaces of all posterior teeth	Poor dental rhythmicity Exaggerated transverse curve Inadequate overbite and overjet of anterior teeth for posterior cuspal form

Diagnoses _Generalized periodontitis with localized secondary occlusal traumatism in all molars_

Occlusal and Concomitant Treatment Required _1. Scaling and curettage and root planing_
2. Hawley bite plane
3. Occlusal adjustment by selective grinding
4. Correct transverse curve
5. Re-evaluation
6. Maxillary fixed bridges (questionable owing to finances)
7. Nightguard

FIGURE 8–33 *I Continued*

Illustration continued on following page

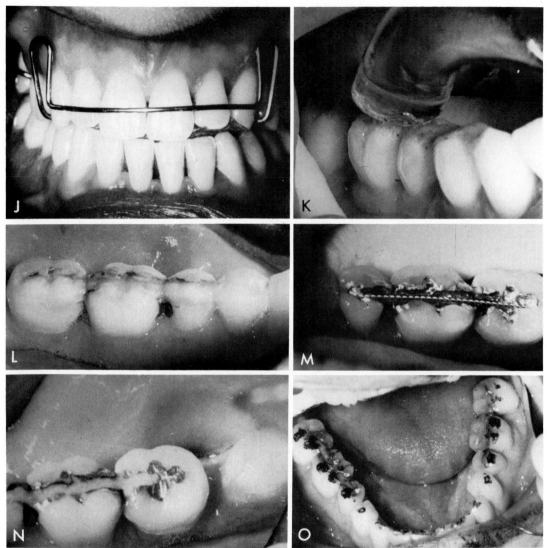

FIGURE 8–33 *Continued J,* The initial treatment plan was limited to occlusal and periodontal therapy owing to patient financial and emotional considerations. Because of the extensive nature of the deformities and requisite treatment, the retruded contact position was used to establish the therapeutic occlusion. A Hawley bite plane is in place in the mouth. Bite plane therapy, which was continued throughout treatment, was used to facilitate occlusal adjustment, provide rest for the attachment apparatus, and relieve excessive occlusal forces associated with interferences and parafunction. This was done in conjunction with scaling, root planing, and open-flap curettage, which effectively reversed the periodontitis, promoting healing of the attachment apparatus. *K,* Occlusal adjustment via selective grinding successfully eliminated the retrusive interferences, but could not eliminate the nonworking interferences that involved the same cusps, nor correct the severely aberrant plane and curves of occlusion that required restorative dentistry on both sides of the mouth. On the right side, Nuva materials were used to shallow out the central fossa area of the mandibular molars and to build up the lingual aspect of these teeth, thus correcting the transverse curve on the mandibular right quadrant. *L,* Lingual aspect built up in Nuva to correct the transverse curve. *M,* Restoration of occlusal form on the left side of the mouth also required shallowing out of the central fossa area of the mandibular molars by selective grinding. Restorative dentistry involved placement of amalgams and an A-splint. The channels are prepared in amalgam; .016 dead soft twisted wire is in place. *N,* Amalgam, acrylic, and wire A-splint shallows out the central fossa of the mandibular teeth, and then the palatal cusp of the maxillary molar is adjusted to eliminate the nonworking interference. *O,* The occlusal view of the mandibular arch shows the correction of arch rhythmicity and form.

Illustration continued on opposite page

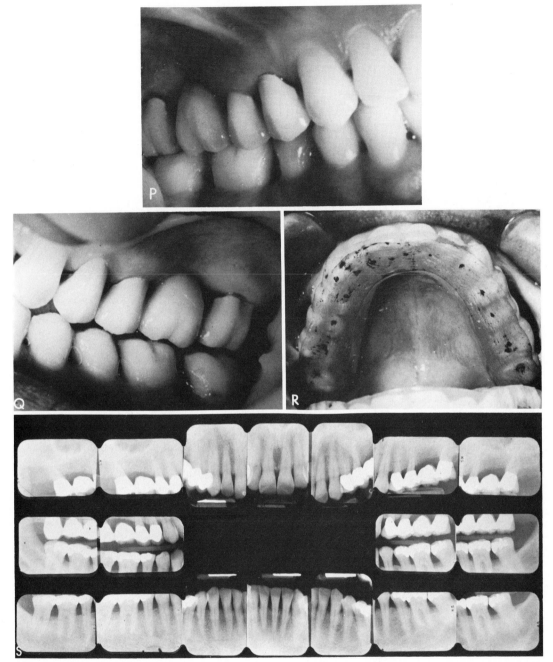

FIGURE 8–33 *Continued* **P,** One year after periodontal and occlusal therapy, the patient decided to have the maxillary molars replaced with fixed bridges. The occlusal form and function established in Phase I therapy simplified the advanced restorative treatment. Harmony between anterior tooth relations and posterior cuspal height has been restored as displayed at the right maximum intercuspal position. **Q,** Effectual anterior guidance has been established via group function (canines and premolars). Freedom of movement and posterior tooth clearance are shown here in a left lateral-protrusive movement. Note support of this movement by the canines and first premolars. **R,** A nightguard was placed to control nocturnal parafunction. The smooth tooth-contacting surface of the appliance provides for optimal force distribution and freedom in all protrusive and lateral-protrusive movements. **S,** These 6-year postoperative radiographs show healing of the periodontal tissues and confirm the arrest of all disease processes.

ment of excessively mobile teeth in secondary occlusal traumatism. It is used in conjunction with correction of the occlusal scheme, not as a substitute for poor occlusal relations. Splinting can help stabilize weak teeth by increasing the number of abutments so that forces are more favorably received and optimally distributed; maintain tooth position and relations after orthodontic therapy; prevent the eruption of unopposed teeth without the use of a partial denture; and prevent open contacts and resulting food impaction.

Re-establishing arch continuity with a fixed prosthesis is important to help stabilize the occlusal scheme, distribute and alleviate excessive forces, and set up a therapeutic occlusion. Thus, adjunctive orthodontics may be required to correct axial inclinations so that forces will be delivered vertically along the long axes of the teeth.

Occlusal traumatism and inflammatory periodontal disease can be identified and monitored with objective clinical and radiographic signs. This objectivity enhances the ability of the practitioner to evaluate the progress of therapy accurately and substantiate the reversal of the disease process. Successful treatment of occlusal traumatism is evidenced clinically by a decrease in mobility and fremitus, and radiographically by a thinner, more distinct PDL space and by a more continuous and distinct lamina dura. These changes occur because the actual injury to the attachment apparatus, caused by both primary and secondary occlusal traumatism, is reversible when treated.

RESTORATION OF ARCH CONTINUITY

Fixed Prosthesis

Maintenance of arch integrity is essential for masticatory efficiency, maximal distribution of force and stress, and optimal occlusal stability and function. Thus, when a tooth is extracted as a result of advanced caries, periodontal disease, or endodontic failure, immediate replacement with a three-unit fixed prosthesis is indicated to preserve arch continuity and integrity. However, when a patient has had a tooth missing for many years with no signs of disease and no complaints, tooth replacement is not necessarily indicated. This is because the patient has

successfully adapted to the anomaly; replacing the tooth would require intervening in physiologic occlusion.

When a fixed prosthesis is used as a multiple tooth restoration, the clinician can work to the MIP only if conditions are optimal; that is, if the occlusion is physiologic, if minimal or no tooth migration has occurred, an adequate number of anterior tooth contacts are present, if a posterior molar contact exists, and if the opposing arch has stable occlusal contacts. When working to the MIP, careful clinical judgment must be exercised; otherwise, the practitioner could be building a condition into a dentition that is not conducive to health, resulting in the perpetuation or exacerbation of occlusal disease. Occlusal adjustment is executed along with the restorative therapy to eliminate aberration associated with the restoration in an attempt to create an environment conducive to the survival of the prosthesis.

Another situation that warrants the use of the MIP is the severe malocclusion, such as the Class II, Division I or the Class III, which cannot be selectively adjusted to the RCP, although it would be unquestionably ameliorated by a stable therapeutic occlusion such as advanced therapy might provide. If the local conditions necessitate working to the RCP, or if the RCP can be achieved with minimal effort, the clinician should take advantage of the situation and gain a stable occlusion by making the MIP coincident with the RCP while attempting to fulfill the other criteria of a therapeutic occlusion with the restoration and with selective grinding.

When tooth loss results in malpositioning–overeruption of an opposing tooth or drifting or tilting of contiguous teeth—restorative treatment cannot be initiated until adjunctive orthodontics and selective grinding with Hawley bite-plane therapy have been completed. The use of the bite plane is indicated to disarticulate the posterior teeth to alleviate excessive occlusal forces; to allow for analysis of landmark relations in the RCP; and to facilitate tooth movement and selective grinding procedures. All therapy is done at the RCP. This is because nearly one half of the posterior occlusion is involved, because adjunctive orthodontic treatment is employed, and especially because it is necessary to gain the mechanical advantages of centric relation and the therapeutic occlusion (Fig. 8–34). Upon completion of therapy, all buccolingual landmark relations

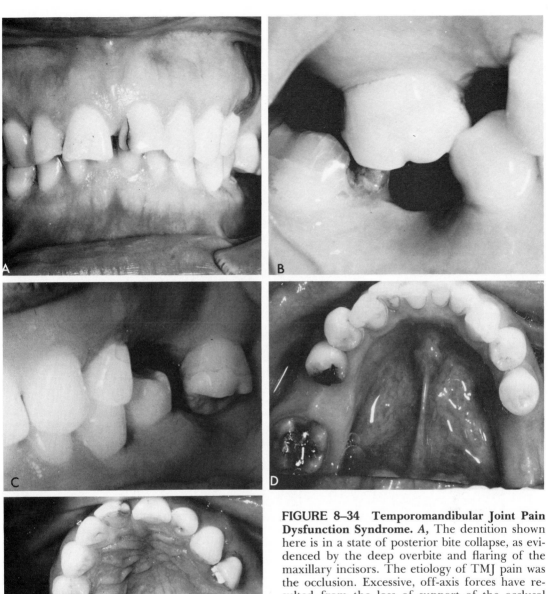

FIGURE 8–34 Temporomandibular Joint Pain Dysfunction Syndrome. *A,* The dentition shown here is in a state of posterior bite collapse, as evidenced by the deep overbite and flaring of the maxillary incisors. The etiology of TMJ pain was the occlusion. Excessive, off-axis forces have resulted from the loss of support of the occlusal vertical dimension, extreme occlusal deformities, and parafunctional habits. Patient complaints include TMJ symptoms, occlusal awareness (bruxism), and dissatisfaction with appearance and masticatory function. However, the periodontium is healthy despite the excessive forces. *B,* Tooth loss has led to the extrusion of the maxillary molars and the mesial drifting of the lower molars, resulting in a deformed plane of occlusion, curve of Spee, and transverse curve. The posterior teeth do not occlude, but interdigitate. *C,* Tooth loss is more extensive on the left side of the mouth. The maxillary molar and mandibular premolar are severely extruded. *D,* This occlusal view of the mandibular arch reveals the crowding of the incisors, mesial inclination of the left molar, buccal inclination of the premolars, and poor premolar contacting relations. *E,* The maxillary dentition shows signs of severe wear. The premolar cusp is fractured and the incisors are flared.

Illustration continued on following page

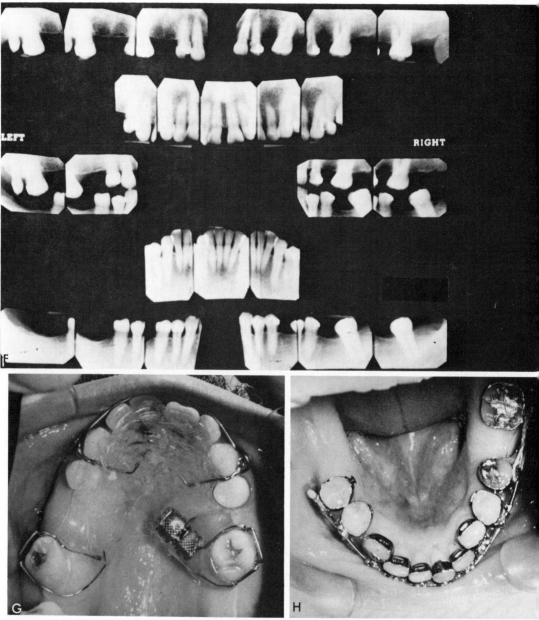

FIGURE 8–34 *Continued F,* Radiographs demonstrate that the attachment apparatus has remained i tact, confirming periodontal health. The patient is highly resistant to periodontal disease. *G,* Treatme consisted of occlusal therapy, adjunctive orthodontics, and restorative dentistry, which were executed the retruded contact position. Hawley bite plane therapy was instituted first, to confirm the suspecte occlusal etiology of the TMJ problem. The patient's symptoms were relieved, a definitive diagnosis extracapsular TMJ dysfunction was made, and therapy was begun. *H,* Adjunctive orthodontics trea ment was implemented in the mandibular arch to level and align the posterior teeth and to correct th plane of occlusion, curve of Spee, and transverse curve. Hawley bite plane therapy was used as an a junct to facilitate tooth-movement procedures.

Illustration continued on opposite pag

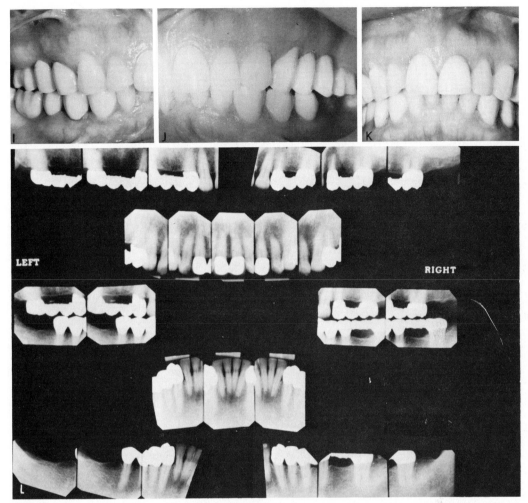

FIGURE 8–34 *Continued I,* Occlusal form and function have been restored, as seen from a right buccal perspective. *J,* Corrected occlusal relations are shown from a left buccal view. *K,* A frontal view of the therapeutic occlusion is shown. *L,* Occlusal relations and tooth position have remained stable, as demonstrated by these 6-year postoperative radiographs.

open contacts, and the plane of occlusion, curve of Spee, and transverse curve should have been corrected so that harmony with condylar and anterior tooth guidance is optimal.

The dentition characterized by more than one tooth-bordered edentulous span is usually in a state of posterior bite collapse. The support of the vertical dimension of occlusion is lost or compromised, and the mutually protective relationship between the posterior and anterior teeth is lost. Treatment begins with control of all soft tissue inflammation and, if necessary, with correction of flared mandibular anterior teeth by adjunctive orthodontics followed by stabili-

zation with an acid-etch composite resin or with 0.010 dead soft wire. This sets up the lower anterior teeth for Hawley bite-plane therapy, which is employed to test and to reestablish the occlusal vertical dimension, to disarticulate the posterior teeth, to provide occlusal rests for the periodontal ligament, and to facilitate further adjunctive orthodontics.

Once malposed posterior teeth have been corrected by orthodontics and occlusal therapy, a posterior provisional restoration is fabricated to replace missing teeth, maintain tooth relations, and support the occlusal vertical dimension. The maxillary teeth are then retracted to regain effective anterior guidance.

Before the final restoration is fabricated, the results of all therapeutics, especially periodontal and occlusal therapy, are re-evaluated clinically and radiographically. Problems may remain. Interferences, mobility, or fremitus require correction of the occlusal schemes. An inadequate amount of attachment apparatus means the restoration must be extended to include more teeth. When a healthy local environment is established, all requirements of the therapeutic occlusion are satisfied, and the patient's subjective requirements are met, the final res-

toration may be fabricated using the provisional restoration as a template.

Removable Prosthesis

When a terminal abutment is lost and a tooth- and tissue-borne distal extension removable partial denture (unilateral or bilateral) is required for the replacement of multiple posterior teeth, the occlusal vertical dimension and all protrusive and lateral-protrusive movements must be supported by the remaining natural dentition—not by the

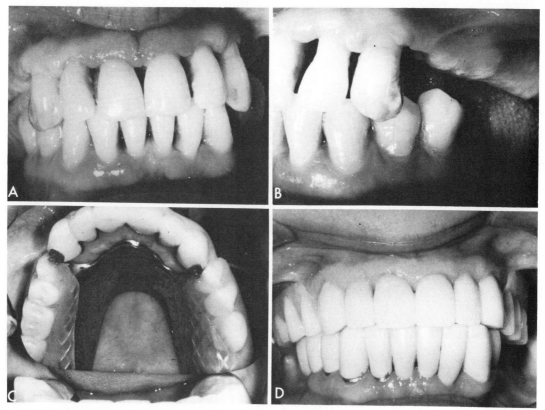

FIGURE 8–35 Support of the Occlusal Vertical Dimension by a Modified Maxillary Fixed Prosthesis. *A,* All maxillary posterior teeth have been lost, resulting in posterior bite collapse and excessive, off-axis force deliverance to the remaining maxillary teeth. Those anterior teeth are in secondary occlusal traumatism and exhibit severe flaring, fremitus, and mobility. The mandibular teeth are also periodontally involved and mobile. *B,* Total absence of posterior teeth leads to loss of support of the occlusal vertical dimension as seen on the left side. Both fixed and removable prostheses are required. The maxillary arch will be restored with a canine-to-canine fixed bridge and a bilateral distal extension removable partial denture; the mandibular arch will be restored with a fixed splint. *C,* The fixed and removable maxillary prostheses are in place. The palatal form of the anterior fixed bridge has been modified to redirect forces along the long axes of the teeth to support the occlusal vertical dimension and to support all protrusive and lateral-protrusive movements. *D,* The maxillary and mandibular fixed bridges and the maxillary distal extension removable denture are in place. The occlusal vertical dimension is supported by the modified maxillary anterior bridge and the splinted mandibular anterior teeth, not by the maxillary removable prosthesis.

removable prosthesis and underlying edentulous ridge. Unlike the alveolus, which is protected from vertical occlusal forces by the periodontal ligament, the residual ridge has no such protective mechanism and is highly susceptible to resorption.

When the periodontal support of the remaining dentition is adequate, the clinician may proceed with establishing the criteria for a therapeutic occlusion. However, when the remaining posterior teeth are weak, the occlusal vertical dimension and protrusive and lateral-protrusive movements may need to be supported by the maxillary canines, which are adjusted with a palatal platform that provides for contact with the mandibular canine or first premolar. This modification is made by selective grinding, with an acid-etch composite, or with a cast restoration.

When the posterior teeth are missing and the maxillary anterior teeth are flared and periodontally weak as a result of secondary occlusal traumatism, an adjunctive orthodontic procedure is used to reposition the teeth over basal bone and to redirect forces along the long axis of the teeth (Fig. 8–35). The anterior teeth are then splinted with a fixed prosthesis with modified palatal forms, similar to those of the Hawley bite plane, to support the occlusal vertical dimension, redirect the forces vertically along the long axes of the teeth, and support all protrusive and lateral-protrusive movements. The platform provides a smooth, even movement and minimizes the vertical component of these excursions to help alleviate excessive horizontal forces (Fig. 8–36). When the mandibular incisors as well as the posterior teeth are missing but the canines remain, tooth replacement with a fixed prosthesis is recommended. This recommendation is made because with a removable prosthesis the abutment tooth is straddled by two edentulous spans and acts as a center of rotation during function. Thus, during protrusive and lateral-protrusive movements, the prosthesis produces torque and transmits off-axis forces to the abutment tooth.

In the final stage of posterior bite collapse, any remaining mandibular posterior teeth and all maxillary teeth are lost. Management of this situation involves a maxillary complete denture opposing a mandibular bilateral distal extension removable partial denture, which requires establishing and maintaining a bilaterally balanced occlusion. Because natural anterior teeth remain in the lower arch, resorption of the maxillary anterior edentulous ridge will occur at an accelerated rate. The full denture settles, disturbing the bilaterally balanced occlusion. This causes interferences in all protrusive and lateral-protrusive movements as well as in the centric relation position, which generates excessive, off-axis forces, eventually resulting in resorption of the mandibular residual ridge. The consequent instability of the lower partial denture induces torque in the abutment teeth with the possible breakdown of their periodontal support. To help prevent denture instability and resorption, the maxillary denture canines are modified with a lingual platform, thus redirecting forces vertically and distributing stress optimally.

Cases involving a maxillary complete denture opposing a bilateral distal extension denture must be monitored constantly for changes in occlusal relations. The denture should be rebased, remounted, and adjusted whenever necessary.

MANAGEMENT OF EXCESSIVE AND SEVERE WEAR

In cases of severe or excessive wear, the goal of treatment is to prevent further destruction by controlling parafunctional forces. This is routinely accomplished with night-guard therapy or Hawley bite plane. When restorative therapy is required, it should be as simple as possible.

Occlusal adjustment by selective grinding to eliminate interferences associated with the restoration of a tooth may be indicated to alleviate excessive occlusal forces and to obviate the potential of inducing an interference that could cause destructive parafunctional activity (Figs. 8–37 and 8–38).

Wear can be so severe and generalized that advanced restorative therapy is necessary. The treatment of such cases does not necessarily require an alteration in the vertical dimension of occlusion (VDO), which has the potential to cause or accelerate bruxism. An increase of the VDO can result in an increase in the frequency and magnitude of force application during parafunctional activity and can interfere with the freedom of the mandible to move in a lateral or lateral-protrusive direction. An attempt should therefore be made to maintain the VDO. Passive eruption can usually help preserve

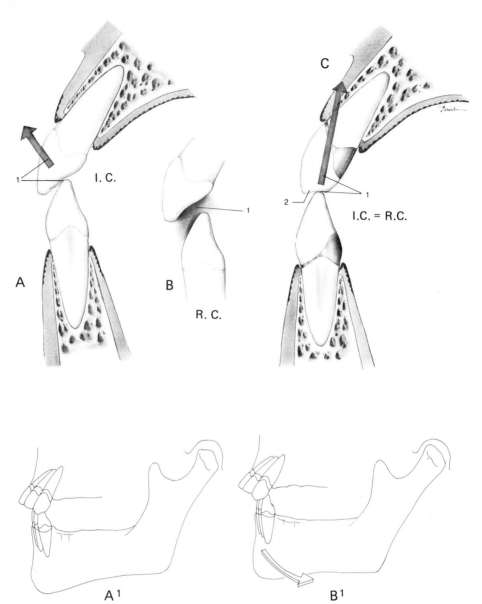

FIGURE 8–36   Modification of Palatal Surface of Maxillary Anterior Teeth to Support Occlusal Vertical Dimensions. In treating the patient with total loss of the posterior teeth or their functional capacity to support the occlusal vertical dimension or both, Amsterdam has presented the modified palatal surface. It is based on the principles of the Hawley bite plane and redirects force and stress along the long axis of the remaining anterior teeth. *A,* Intercuspal closure (IC). Arrow indicates the horizontal component of force, which is unfavorably dissipated. *A¹,* The maximum closure position, representing the most closed position the mandible may achieve in relation to the maxilla when teeth are present. *B,* Mandible moving in the retruded arc of closure (RC). (1) The space created as the mandible moves downward and distally in its terminal arc of closure results in a decrease in vertical overbite and an increase in horizontal overjet. *B¹.* The terminal arc of closure. Where the terminal arc of rotation is distal to the IC position, the mandible moves more distally and normally results in an increase in horizontal overjet and a decrease in vertical overbite. Actually, any increase in occlusal vertical dimension will result in an increase in overjet and a decrease in overbite. This phenomenon is accentuated, however, when IC is anterior to RC. Conversely, any decrease in the occlusal vertical dimension will decrease the overjet and increase the overbite. *C,* (1) The modified lingual form creates a vertical stop which provides for a more favorable force direction and dissipation (arrow). (2) The provision for proper anterior guidance in coordination with the mediolateral condylar path. (From Amsterdam, M., and Ingber, J.: The Distal Extension Case—Tooth-Tissue Borne Removable Appliance. Cont. Dent. Ed., Philadelphia, Univ. of Pa., Vol. 1, No. 9, 1978.)

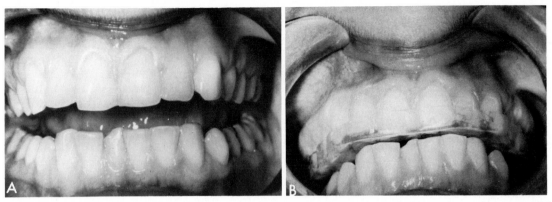

FIGURE 8–37 **Excessive Wear.** *A,* These wear patterns are excessive relative to the patient's age (22 years). The patient reported nocturnal grinding and had developed a positive occlusal awareness. *B,* A maxillary nightguard was the treatment of choice to stop the accelerated wear, control nocturnal bruxism habits, and eliminate the patient's positive occlusal awareness.

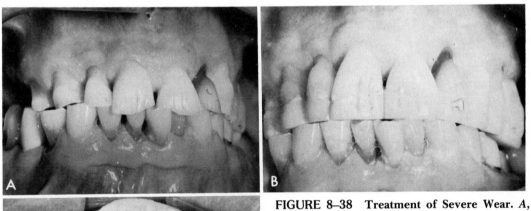

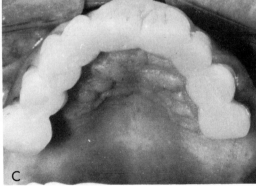

FIGURE 8–38 **Treatment of Severe Wear.** *A,* Wear of this dentition was due to constant clenching and grinding reported by this 62-year-old patient. The progression of wear was so advanced that cast restorations for optimal protection of the destroyed teeth were indiciated. *B,* Because the treatment of choice was prohibitively expensive, parafunctional activity was controlled with occlusal appliances—a nightguard and a dayguard. The dayguard is the functional equivalent of a nightguard but is fabricated with tooth-colored acrylic. *C,* Occlusal view of dayguard. Note the smooth occlusal surface.

the VDO. If an alteration in the VDO is deemed necessary for restorative therapy, the change should be kept to a minimum.

MANAGEMENT OF MYOFASCIAL PAIN DYSFUNCTION SYNDROME (MPDS)

It is not unusual to discover that a patient who presents with symptoms suggestive of MPDS has endured pain for some time and has been the unfortunate victim of any amount of ineffective treatment. It is ironic that the anxiety produced by successive treatment failures and unfulfilled expectations exacerbates the pain, which in turn reinforces the anxiety. So it should not be surprising that the MPDS patients exhibit a negative attitude as a natural manifestation of their lack of faith in the dental (and medical) profession, whose efforts to resolve their problem have not been successful.

The importance of interpersonal relations in the management of MPDS patients is readily apparent. In fact, the doctor-patient relationship could be considered the sine qua non of successful treatment. The clinician should try to establish a relaxed and amiable relationship with the patient. He should be understanding, show sincere concern and empathy, listen attentively, and explain patiently the probable psychogenic etiology of the dysfunction. Available modalities of treatment should be explained carefully to the patient. This approach should foster a sense of confidence, hope, and trust in the patient, should help alleviate anxiety, and should enhance the likelihood of patient cooperation in therapy, a crucial factor in successful treatment.

Because the differential diagnosis of MPDS is so complicated, the clinician must rely on a tentative diagnosis in the early stages of therapy, proceeding under the assumption that the TMJ disorder is extracapsular with origins in the masticatory system. The working diagnosis can be continued only after treatment is initiated and patient symptoms have been ameliorated.

Since the clinician is compelled to depend on an unreliable diagnosis, it is essential for treatment to progress slowly and to be approached cautiously and conservatively. This conservatism precludes immediate occlusal or restorative therapy. In the early phase of treatment, when no definitive diagnosis has been established, irreversible procedures are contraindicated because if it is later determined that the diagnosis was *not* correct, any alterations made in the occlusal scheme could exacerbate or induce symptoms, complicate subsequent treatment, and jeopardize the prognosis.

Initial treatment (concurrent physiotherapy and pharmacotherapy) is directed at a muscular level. Tranquilizers relax the muscles and are indicated to alleviate acute symptoms, which are often precipitated by stressful events. Physiotherapy can be accomplished with a variety of techniques: (1) moist heat provides immediate, short-term relief of pain, and (1) moist heat application relaxes the muscles and controls spasm, (2) ethyl chloride spray provides immediate, short-term relief of pain, and (3) stretching exercises control clicking and facilitate the movement of the mandible into an open position. But the nocturnal use of the Hawley bite-plane therapy is the most important form of treatment. It eliminates proprioception, inducing bilateral relaxation of the musculature; controls spasms; eliminates all posterior tooth contacts, enabling freedom of mandibular movements; and allows the condyles to move to their most posterior and comfortable position. However, the use of Hawley bite-plane therapy is limited and must be monitored closely to prevent the eruption of the posterior teeth, which would exacerbate the problem. Because the bite plane acts as an occlusal negating device, it establishes whether or not the occlusion is a cause of the TMJ disorder.

Once the patient's symptoms have been significantly alleviated, the clinician may proceed with any necessary occlusal or restorative therapy. All treatment should be executed over a period of time to give the clinician the opportunity to monitor the patient's response to therapy. This helps minimize the amount and complexity of treatment. It also helps minimize any alterations in the treatment that become necessary.

MANAGEMENT OF DISEASE ASSOCIATED WITH MALOCCLUSIONS

The treatment of advanced occlusal or periodontal disease is greatly complicated by a malocclusion. In general practice the Class

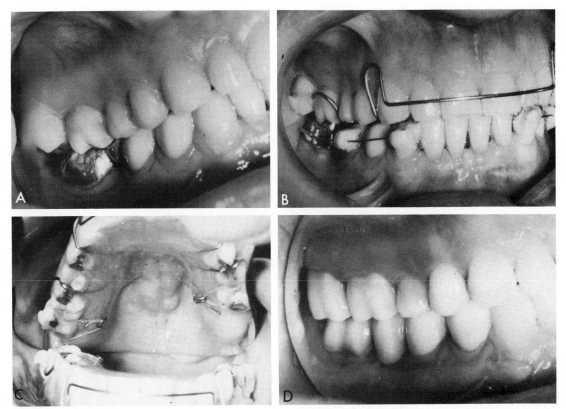

FIGURE 8–39   Correcting Landmark Relations in a Class I Malocclusion. A, Malalignment of the posterior teeth has disturbed arch continuity and occlusal function. The buccally inclined maxillary second molar is totally out of contact with the mesially inclined mandibular first molar. **B,** The Hawley bite plane with palatal cleats, used here in conjunction with elastic bands, served as an active appliance, moving the maxillary second molar palatally to correct buccolingual landmark relations. In addition, by disarticulating the posterior teeth, the bite plane facilitated tooth-movement procedures aimed at uprighting the lower first molar. **C,** Occlusal view of Hawley bite plane with palatal cleats and elastics to move the maxillary second molars palatally. **D,** The final restorations are in place. Correction of landmark relations increased occlusal surface contacts, so optimal force distribution was achieved.

I malocclusion, characterized by malposed teeth resulting from physiologic or pathologic migration or crowding, is the most common form of malocclusion. Orthodontic treatment to resolve subjective patient complaints, usually concerning appearance, or to reverse a disease process and correct deformities brought on by disease includes correcting the buccolingual landmark (crossbite), closing mesial and distal space, uprighting molars, correcting rotated teeth, and inducing eruption (Fig. 8–39).

When the arch form or the arch-to-arch relations associated with a skeletal dysplasia require treatment, management by the orthodontist is usually indicated. It is the responsibility of all therapists involved in the care of any patient to monitor and control inflammation.

Class II, Division I Malocclusion

In the Class II, Division I malocclusion, treatment should be aimed at establishing effective anterior guidance to disarticulate the posterior teeth. The factors in effective treatment procedures include the degree of open bite and the presence and severity of disease and occlusal abnormalities, especially missing teeth, which accelerate breakdown (Fig. 8–40).

When the open bite is less than 4 mm, selective grinding along with restorative therapy can sometimes provide for anterior guidance. When present, the maxillary canines can be modified with a lingual platform using a cast restoration or can be modified simply by using composite resin with the acid-etch technique. This will redirect forces vertically on the canines and facilitate pro-

Text continued on page 394

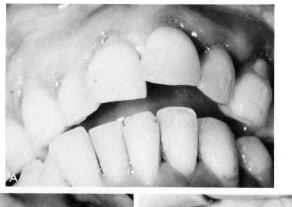

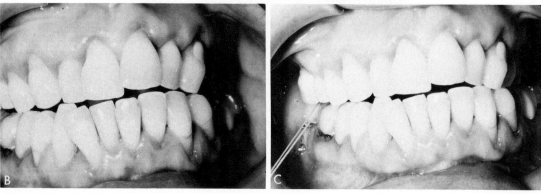

FIGURE 8–40 Managing Disease and Occlusal Deformities in the Class II, Division I Malocclusion.
A, Aberrant occlusal relations and accelerated breakdown mark this Class II, Division I malocclusion, shown here in the maximum intercuspal position. The deformed occlusal scheme and excessive posterior tooth interferences, in addition to inadequate restorations and the accumulation of plaque and calculus, have led to secondary occlusal traumatism as well as the loss of the maxillary second molars. It can be seen here that the maxillary left canine is out of contact with the mandibular incisors. There is a 4-mm overjet and a negative overbite, causing the excessive posterior tooth interferences. *B,* No anterior tooth contact is possible in lateral-protrusive movements. *C,* Dental floss is manipulated to confirm a right nonworking interference in a left lateral working movement.

Illustration continued on opposite page

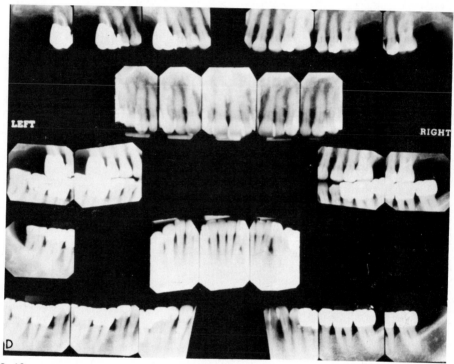

FIGURE 8–40 *Continued* ***D,*** The radiographs manifest extensive bone loss, severe osseous defects, including Class III furcation involvement, a widened periodontal ligament space, loss of continuity, and loss of definition of the lamina dura. This radiographic evidence of secondary occlusal traumatism was substantiated by 5- to 7-mm pocket probings, through-and-through furcation probings, and extensive mobility patterns. Treatment will include occlusal adjustment, advanced periodontal therapy, and restorative dentistry. The retruded contact position is indicated for such extensive therapy.

Illustration continued on following page

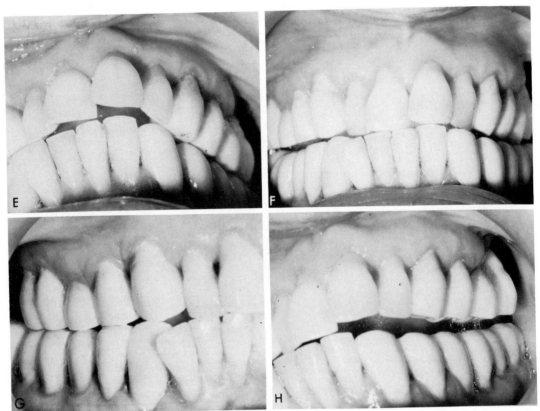

FIGURE 8–40 *Continued* **E,** Selective grinding was instituted to eliminate all posterior tooth interferences and to decrease overjet and increase overbite. To establish effective anterior guidance, an alteration in the occlusal vertical dimension was necessary. The maxillary anterior fixed prosthesis, shown here in place at the centric relation position, was fabricated with a modified palatal form to help support the occlusal vertical dimension and all protrusive and lateral-protrusive movements. Scaling and root planing were unable to eliminate the periodontal problems. Surgery was required for pocket elimination. **F,** Anterior tooth contacts provide for the disarticulation of all posterior teeth in protrusive movements. **G,** Owing to the periodontally weakened anterior teeth, it was necessary to establish group function—in this case, involving the canines and all posterior teeth—for effective anterior guidance. Group function is shown here supporting a right working movement. **H,** At the same time, the posterior teeth are disarticulated on the left nonworking side.

Illustration continued on opposite page

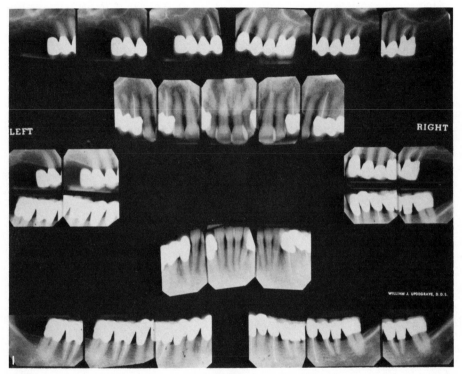

FIGURE 8–40 *Continued I,* These 2-year postoperative radiographs show the healing of the attachment apparatus, the osseous defects, and the lamina dura.

trusive movements by disarticulating the posterior teeth for 1 to 2 mm until the incisors can be engaged. Conventional use of the Hawley bite plane is contraindicated because it would induce posterior eruption, which would exacerbate the open bite. However, if the bite plane is placed with the posterior teeth in contact, it can provide for anterior guidance and control parafunctional activity.

When the open bite exceeds 4 mm, treatment becomes more difficult and more complex and often involves periodontal, myofunctional, occlusal, orthodontic, and restorative therapy. Most cases, however, can be managed without orthognathic surgery. The final result is visualized, and treatment is carefully planned and coordinated with all participating specialists.

Class II, Division II Malocclusion

When advanced restorative or occlusal therapy is required for the Class II, Division II malocclusion, the problem that must be alleviated is the dual plane of occlusion with excessive overbite and no overjet (Fig. 8–41). Hawley bite-plane therapy is instituted to induce posterior eruption, to redirect off-axis forces to protect the maxillary anterior teeth, to level the plane of occlusion, to maintain the position of lower incisors, and to control

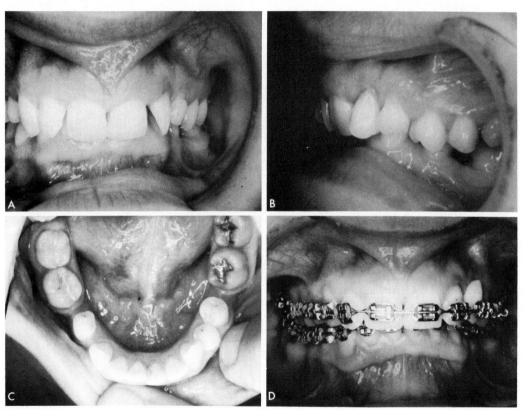

FIGURE 8–41 Managing Disease and Occlusal Deformities in the Class II, Division II Malocclusion. A, This Class II, Division II malocclusion is in posterior bite collapse and exhibits aberrant anterior tooth relations: deep overbite and rotated and labially inclined maxillary left incisors. Owing to the posterior bite collapse, the anterior teeth are in primary occlusal traumatism and the mandibular incisors impinge on the palatal soft tissues, causing periodontal involvement and pain on mastication. **B,** Landmark relations are abnormal: The maxillary first premolar is buccally inclined, the maxillary central incisors lingually inclined, and the maxillary lateral incisors labially inclined. A maxillary deciduous canine is present. **C,** In the mandibular arch, tooth loss and malpositioning are extensive. The posterior teeth are depressed and the anterior teeth extruded, creating an aberrant dual plane of occlusion. Full orthodontic correction will be required to set up the occlusion for restorative therapy. **D,** Orthodontic treatment is in progress.

Illustration continued on opposite page

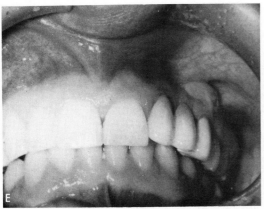 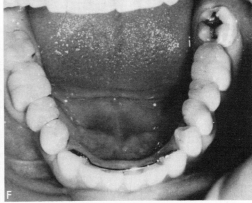

FIGURE 8–41 *Continued E,* Arch continuity and rhythmicity have been restored. *F,* Correction of the overbite, dual plane of occlusion, landmark relations, and poor esthetics has been achieved with combined orthodontic and restorative therapy. (Orthodontic therapy performed by R. L. Vanarsdall, Philadelphia, Pa.)

nocturnal parafunctional activity (see Fig. 8–33). The maxillary and mandibular incisors are leveled and shortened to control destructive occlusal forces and to help correct the duel plane of occlusion. At times, restoration of the canines is indicated to alleviate excessive force application on the incisors and to help support the vertical dimension of occlusion. Although the posterior teeth are protected from horizontal forces by excessive anterior guidance (excessive overbite and a little overjet), the anterior teeth can be severely traumatized in all lateral-protrusive movements.

Class III Malocclusion or Pseudo–Class III Malocclusion

The most important consideration in treating disease associated with Class III or pseudo–Class III malocclusion is to establish correct incisor relations to provide effective anterior guidance. This minimally requires correcting anterior tooth relations to place the maxillary incisors labial to the mandibular incisors. The corrected anterior tooth position usually has minimal overbite and overjet, resulting in excessive posterior cuspal form as compared with the anterior tooth relations. Extensive selective grinding and occlusal adjustment are required to correct the posterior cuspal form and other abnormalities in occlusal morphology. If restorative dentistry is required, it must be in concert with the anterior guidance factors, e.g., modified posterior cuspal form (Fig. 8–42).

Oftentimes, owing to the extreme dental or skeletal discrepancy, the Class III or pseudo–Class III malocclusion requires total orthodontic therapy to correct not only the anterior tooth position but also the severe posterior tooth relations and the severe posterior open bite when the anterior teeth are related edge to edge on the terminal hinge axis.

SUMMARY

This chapter on occlusion helps the general practitioner organize the myriad factors involved in the complex patient population he or she treats. The first half of the chapter provides a rationale for treatment based upon the criteria of a physiologic occlusion. The criteria for disease and patient complaints directly attributable to occlusal problems are presented as well as dental disease that requires occlusal consideration. In the section on examining and treating the pathologic occlusion, the fundamentals of occlusal form and function are discussed.

The second half of this chapter presents treatment of problems that illustrate the principles described earlier, with demonstration of case types often seen in private practice. We have not limited this section to any criteria specifying what constitutes occlusion in general practice. The general practitioner must be aware of and become conversant with the complex occlusal factors seen in both general and specialty practice. The general practitioner has a primary role

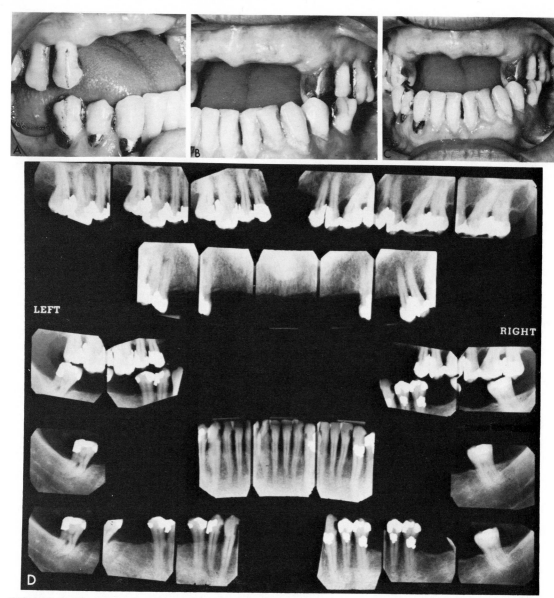

FIGURE 8–42   Managing Extensive Disease and Severe Occlusal Deformities in the Class III Malocclusion. *A,* This 48-year-old patient with a Class III malocclusion has lost all his anterior teeth because of extensive caries. In this maximum intercuspal position, the posterior tooth landmarks are edge to edge and in crossbite. There are multiple etiologic factors: plaque, calculus, the severe malocclusion, and extensive tooth loss. ***B,*** The left buccal view displays the severe buccolingual landmark relations. ***C,*** The right buccal view demonstrates a 2-mm vertical IC–RC discrepancy. ***D,*** The radiographs manifest multiple tooth loss, poor restorative dentistry, extensive bone loss, and signs of occlusal traumatism. Treatment included initial periodontal therapy and caries excavation to control all active disease. The lower anterior teeth were stripped and retracted to lessen the Class III tooth position. The molars were uprighted and the occlusion was set up in provisional restorations.

Illustration continued on opposite page

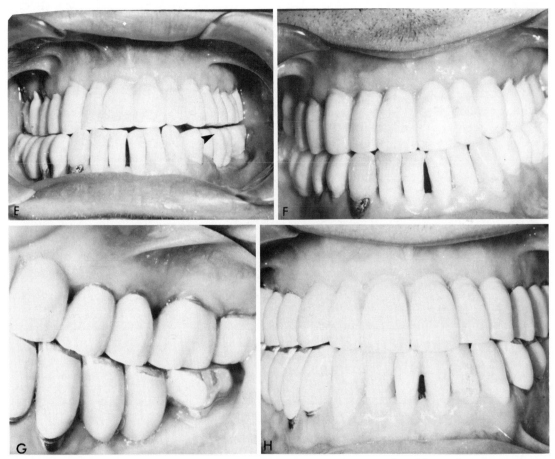

FIGURE 8–42 *Continued* **E,** Full maxillary provisional restoration was placed in conjunction with mandibular posterior bridges. The final occlusal scheme required edge-to-edge anterior tooth relations, which provided for disarticulation of all posterior tooth contacts in protrusive and lateral-protrusive movements. Note the modified posterior cuspal form required for the corrected anterior Class III tooth relations. **F,** This view of right lateral-protrusive movement displays the group function on the working side and disarticulation of the nonworking side. This occlusal scheme must be established in the provisional restoration to ensure the establishment of a therapeutic occlusion in the final restoration. **G,** Direct view of final case. Note anterior tooth relations. **H,** Buccal view of correct posterior buccolingual landmark relations and modified posterior cuspal form.

Illustration continued on following page

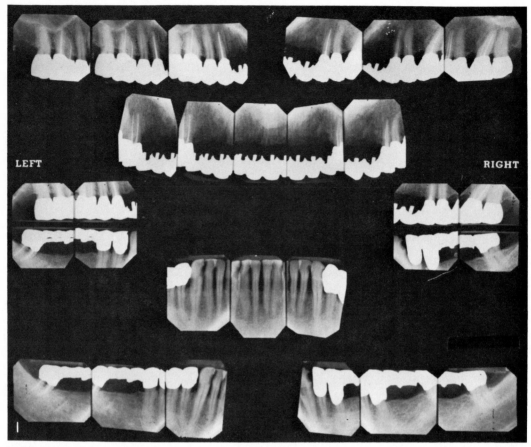

FIGURE 8–42 *Continued I,* These 3-year postoperative radiographs show the final restoration in place and the healing of the attachment apparatus and osseous defects.

in identifying problems, referring patients to a specialist, and treating patients in conjunction with the specialist.

The general practitioner must recognize problems early and base his or her practice on sound principles of preventive dentistry in order to avoid the complex and debilitating problems associated with advanced oc-

clusal and related disease. It is important to note that with impeccable plaque control the two diseases (periodontal disease and dental caries) most influential in occlusal problems can be controlled, preventing the hopeless situation created by the cumulative effect of multiple disease processes acting in concert with excessive forces.

QUESTIONS

1. A physiologic occlusion
   a. always has canine guidance or group function in lateral-protrusive movements
   b. is a healthy dentition that requires no treatment
   c. has dental disease that must be corrected
   d. is an occlusion that requires only occlusal adjustment by selective grinding
2. The posterior group of teeth function to
   a. disarticulate the anterior teeth in protrusive movement
   b. disarticulate the anterior teeth in lateral-protrusive movement
   c. support occlusal vertical dimension
   d. support all clenching and grinding movements

3. The forces generated at tooth level during normal function are greater than during parafunction. True or false?

4. Common causes of occlusal interferences are
    a. lack of harmony between anterior guidance and posterior cuspal form
    b. tilting, drifting, or extrusion of teeth
    c. wear
    d. all of the above

5. The interference most often implicated in the initiation and progression of occlusal traumatism and myofascial pain dysfunction syndrome is
    a. the working side interference
    b. the nonworking side interference
    c. the protrusive interference
    d. all of the above

6. All nonworking interferences are pathologic. True or false?

7. Any and all wear of teeth is pathologic and must be treated. True or false?

8. Posterior bite collapse is
    a. an etiology of occlusal disease causing advanced periodontal breakdown
    b. caused by an interference and bruxism
    c. a term to describe a number of sequelae caused by the loss of support of the occlusal vertical dimension by the posterior teeth
    d. always present in cases of tooth loss

9. Radiographic evidence of occlusal traumatism can include
    a. a widened periodontal ligament space
    b. a loss of definition of periodontal ligament space
    c. root fractures
    d. all of the above

10. The postural position is
    a. a reproducible position used in all therapy
    b. a reference position for all mandibular movement
    c. highly variable and subject to change
    d. all of the above

11. Although malocclusions per se are not pathologic, orthodontic corrections are executed in adults to
    a. treat disease associated with the malocclusion
    b. satisfy the requirements of a therapeutic occlusion
    c. treat patient complaints associated with the malocclusion
    d. all of the above

12. A therapeutic occlusion is characterized by
    a. Class I molar relation
    b. occlusal relations that are conducive to health:
        (1) a 2 mm IC-RC discrepancy;
        (2) unrestrained protrusive and lateral-protrusive movement from centric relations; and
        (3) support of the occlusal vertical dimension
    c. 2 and 3 of B
    d. 1 and 3 of B

13. Centric relation is a therapeutic position
    a. applicable to complete dentures only
    b. that has the MIP (maximum intercuspal position) and RCP (retruded contact position) coincidental
    c. in which the condyles are displaced 1 mm anterior to the terminal hinge axis
    d. all of the above

14. Centric relation position is used
    a. for single crown restoration

b. in situations requiring an extensive change in the occlusion, such as rampant caries or advanced restorative dentristry
c. all periodontal therapy
d. all of the above

15. The maxillary Hawley bite plane is a useful appliance for
a. periodontal therapy (occlusal traumatism)
b. adjunctive orthodontics
c. myofascial pain dysfunction syndrome
d. all of the above

16. Occlusal traumatism is
a. excessive forces generated to the periodontium
b. the injury to the attachment apparatus caused by abnormal excessive forces
c. severe wear
d. TMJ pain

17. Secondary occlusal traumatism is associated with
a. extensive loss of attachment apparatus
b. severe wear
c. TMJ dysfunction symptoms
d. all of the above

18. The existing MIP (maximum intercuspal position) is used in multiple tooth restorations if
a. the occlusion is otherwise physiologic
b. mobility patterns are minimal
c. periodontal defects are minimal
d. all of the above

19. When removable partial dentures are employed, the occlusal vertical dimension must be supported by the base bone associated with the edentulous ridge. True or false?

20. All temporomandibular joint dysfunction syndrome patients are treated by
a. medication
b. selective grinding
c. analgesics
d. none of the above

See answers in Appendix.

REFERENCES

1. Abrams, L.: Occlusal Adjustment of the Natural Dentition. Cont. Dent. Ed., Philadelphia, Univ. of Pa., Vol. 1, No. 11, 1978.
2. Abrams, L., and Coslet, J. G.: Occlusal adjustment by selective grinding. *In* Periodontal Therapy, 5th ed. H. M. Goldman and D. W. Cohen (eds.) St. Louis, The C. V. Mosby Co., 1973.
3. Ackerman, J. L., and Proffitt, W. R.: The characteristics of malocclusion: A modern approach to classification and diagnosis. Am. J. Orthod. 56:433, 1969.
4. Alderman, M.: Disorders of the temporomandibular joint and related structures. *In* Oral Medicine, L. Burket (ed.) Philadelphia, J. B. Lippincott Co., 1971.
5. Alderman, M.: The Management of the Patient With Myofascial Pain Dysfunction Syndrome. Cont. Dent. Ed., Philadelphia, Univ. of Pa., 1978.
6. Amsterdam, M.: Periodontal prosthesis—twenty-five years in retrospect. Alpha Omegan, Dec. 1974.
7. Amsterdam, M., and Abrams, L.: Periodontal prosthesis. *In* Periodontal Therapy, 5th ed. H.

Goldman and D. W. Cohen (eds.). St. Louis, The C. V. Mosby Co., 1973.
8. Amsterdam, M., and Ingber, J.: The Distal Extension Case—Tooth-Tissue Borne Removable Appliance. Cont. Dent. Ed., Philadelphia, University of Pennsylvania, Vol. 1, No. 9, 1978.
9. Anderson, D. J., and Picton, D. C. A.: Tooth contact during chewing. J. Dent. Res., 36:21, 1957.
10. Angle, E. H.: Classification of malocclusion. Dent. Cosmos, 41:248, 1899.
11. Beaudreau, D.: The role of the posterior fixed bridge in occlusion. Dent. Clin. North Am., March 1965, p. 13.
12. Bilmoria, K. F.: Malocclusion—its role in the causation of periodontal disease—an epidemiological study. J. All India Dent. Assoc., Oct. 1973, p. 293.
13. Cohen, D. W., Keller, G., Feder, M., and Livingston, E.: Effects of excessive occlusal forces on the gingival blood supply. J. Dent. Res., 39:677, 1960.
14. Geering, A. H.: Occlusal interferences and functional disturbances of the masticatory system. J. Clin. Periodontol., 1(2):112, 1974.
15. Geiger, A. M., Wasserman, B., Thompson, R., and Turgeon, L.: Relationship of occlusion and periodontal disease. V. Relation of classification of oc-

clusion to periodontal status and gingival inflammation. J. Periodontol., *43*:554, 1972.

16. Graf, H.: Bruxism. Dent. Clin. North Am., *13*:659, 1969.
17. Hickey, J. C., Lunbeen, H. C., and Bohannan, H. M.: A new articulator for use in teaching and general dentistry. J. Prosth. Dent. *18*:425, 1967.
18. Hirschfeld, I.: The individual missing tooth: A factor in dental and periodontal disease. J. Am. Dent. Assoc., *24*:56, 1937.
19. Huffman, R. W., and Regonos, J. W.: Principles of Occlusion. Columbus, Ohio, H and R Press, 1980.
20. Jankelson, B., Hoffman, G. M., and Hendron, J. A.: The physiology of the stomatognathic system. J. Am. Dent. Assoc., *46*:375, 1953.
21. Kraus, B., Jordon, R., and Abrams, L.: Dental Anatomy and Occlusion: A Study of the Masticatory System. Baltimore, Williams & Wilkins Co., 1969.
22. Leoff, M.: Clamping and grinding habits: Their relation to periodontal disease. J. Am. Dent. Assoc., *31*:184, 1944.
23. McLean, D. W.: Physiologic vs. pathologic occlusion. J. Am. Dent. Assoc., *25*:1593, 1938.
24. Nyman, S., Lindhe, J., and Ericsson, R.: The effects of progressive tooth mobility on obstructive periodontitis in the dog. J. Clin. Periodontol., *5*:213, 1978.
25. Posselt, U.: The Physiology of Occlusion and Rehabilitation, 2nd ed. Philadelphia, F. A. Davis Co., 1968.
26. Posselt, U.: Studies in mobility of the human mandible. Acta Odontol. Scand. (suppl. 10), *10*:3, 1952.
27. Rosenberg, E. S.: Treatment of occlusion as an adjunct to periodontal therapy. S. Afr. Soc. Periodontol., June 1967.
28. Vanarsdall, R. L.: Uprighting the Inclined Mandibular Molar in Preparation for Restorative Treatment. Cont. Dent. Ed., Philadelphia, Univ. of Pa., Vol. 1, No. 2, 1977.
29. Weisgold, A., and Laudenbach, K.: Occlusal etiology and management of disorders of the temporomandibular joint and related structures. Alpha Omegan, Dec., 1976.
30. Weisgold, A., and Rosenberg, E.: Occlusal therapy. *In* Current Therapy in Dentistry, H. Goldman, H. Gilmore, W. Irby, and R. McDonald (eds.). St. Louis, The C. V. Mosby Co., 1977.
31. Yuodelis, R., and Mann, W.: The prevalence and possible role of nonworking contacts in periodontal disease. Periodontics, *3*:219, 1965.
32. Zander, H., and Polson, A.: Present status of occlusion and occlusal therapy in periodontics. J. Periodontol., *48*(9):540, 1977.

9

GORDON J. CHRISTENSEN

RESTORATIVE DENTISTRY IN GENERAL PRACTICE

OBJECTIVES

This chapter is designed to stimulate general practitioners to (1) analyze their current philosophies, abilities, and techniques in restorative dentistry (complex operative dentistry, fixed prosthodontics, and occlusion); (2) determine if changes could improve the service they render their patients in restorative dentistry; and (3) apply information in this chapter to their clinical practices.

After the completion of this chapter, readers should be able to accomplish the following tasks:

1. Improve the management of restorative dentistry patients, including lessening the patient's fear by educational, pharmaceutical, and psychologic means.

2. Implement fundamental principles underlying complex treatment in restorative dentistry, such as improving the quality and longevity of treatment, preventing dental caries after restorative therapy, and providing better diagnostic and treatment-planning services.

3. Build up teeth, using castings, composite resin, or amalgam before final dental rehabilitation procedures.

4. Practice currently endorsed principles for tooth preparation in complex restorative dentistry.

5. Compare types of restorations used in restorative dentistry in relation to optimal location for use, indications, contraindications, and expected longevity.

6. Use new knowledge of the biologic considerations in restorative dentistry, such as maintenance of periodontal health, margin location for restorations, dental pulp considerations, and the significance of occlusion.

7. Apply moderately complex occlusal adjustment procedures to dental practices, affording higher quality restorative dentistry.

8. Accomplish dental rehabilitation restoring one side of the mouth at a time.

9. Accomplish dental rehabilitation restoring all of the posterior teeth at one time.

10. List, discuss, and apply the specific timing, sequences, relationships, and concepts that are inherent in any complex restorative therapy, such as the relationship of periodontal therapy, endodontics, orthodontics, occlusal adjustment, and oral surgery to restorative therapy.

Modern restorative dentistry has broad boundaries. To restore means to put back into the former or the original state, to repair, to renew, to reconstruct, or to return to a healthy state. As applied to clinical dentistry, the term usually means restoration of the natural teeth. In a broader sense, however, it is also used to denote replacement of teeth or restoration of function of the teeth or mouth.

Restorative dentistry, as used in this chapter, implies prevention, diagnosis, and treatment of diseases of the dentition; correction of malformations and of accidental injuries affecting the permanent dentition by restoration of parts of teeth; replacement of missing teeth with fixed restorations, and restoration of function, including occlusal adjustment. *As defined in this chapter, it includes operative dentistry, fixed prosthodontics, and some aspects of occlusion.*

In the United States today most general

The author acknowledges the contributions of Dr. Harry C. Lundeen, University of Florida, to the material contained in this chapter.

dental practice (estimates say 70 per cent or more) is devoted to the repair and restoration of the natural teeth. Because of the great volume of patients the general practitioner treats, the restorative procedures that he performs are limited generally to operative dentistry and some phases of fixed prosthodontics, such as restoration with silver amalgam, composite or microfill resin, cast restorations, porcelain-fused-to-metal crowns, or fixed partial dentures. Most general practitioners do not involve themselves with comprehensive mouth rehabilitation routinely and seldom accomplish compacted gold restorations, porcelain inlays, complex gold or porcelain restorations, or occlusal therapy.

At present there is no recognized specialty called restorative dentistry. Most of the advanced restorative procedures and occlusal therapy are accomplished by (1) board-certified specialists in fixed prosthodontics, and (2) general practitioners who have limited their practice to advanced restorative procedures. There are also some general practitioners who have expanded their knowledge since dental school and who accomplish this phase of dentistry along with many other types of treatment. It is the latter type of practice, the author feels, that should be encouraged and developed to meet the needs of the present and of the future.

The next few decades will bring increased demand for the phases of restorative dentistry that are not usually accomplished by the general practitioner today. Third-party payment plans are making dentistry available to people who could not afford it in the past. Education about dentistry is reaching more patients, and as a result, they are demanding treatment. Periodontics and endodontics are preserving the natural dentition longer, and these retained teeth, often unstable, require restorative treatment. More people have money to spend on dentistry than ever before. People are living longer, and therefore teeth and restorations must last longer. The need for the more complex phases of restorative dentistry is evident. The general practitioner will have to supply the major part of the increased treatment load.

The role of the general practitioner in restorative dentistry can be as little or as great as his motivation, interest, and training dictate. The addition of advanced restorative techniques to general practice requires willingness on the part of the practitioner, additional expense for equipment, and time to learn some fundamental concepts.

This chapter presents the general practitioner with some of the background required for accomplishing more advanced phases of restorative treatment. Particular emphasis has been placed on preventive aspects of restorative dentistry, treatment planning for comprehensive restorative dentistry, and techniques and procedures for accomplishing full-mouth rehabilitation.

MANAGEMENT OF THE RESTORATIVE DENTISTRY PATIENT

Not all patients who are in need of extensive restorative therapy are good candidates for such treatment. Some patients lack knowledge about restorative dentistry and are not prepared emotionally for it. The time required to educate patients adequately before treatment varies considerably, but it is time well spent.

A lay person's understanding of modern dentistry and what it can do for him is based largely on previous experiences in dental offices and knowledge gained from reading or conversations with others. Commercials on radio and television have played an important role in shaping the public's image of dentistry. Therefore, it can be expected that new patients will exhibit a wide variety of levels of understanding about dental treatment. The extremes vary from the well informed to the completely uninformed, and the level of dental knowledge may not be correlated with the individual's intellectual or socioeconomic status. Usually the better informed patient is one who has received high-quality restorative treatment or has been referred by another patient who has benefited from such treatment. At the other extreme, the patient whose past dental experiences include only emergency extractions is usually uninformed and unappreciative. This type of person will probably require significant education before accepting treatment.

Each new patient requiring extensive restorative treatment should be evaluated in terms of his understanding of restorative dentistry. The practitioner must decide at which level communication should begin in order to avoid future problems in management. Methods of educating and managing the uninformed or misinformed patient are considered here.

Patient Education

The successful management of a patient through all phases of extensive restorative treatment requires more than technical proficiency, good staff support, and an efficiently run dental office. Of equal importance is the dentist's skill in overcoming the patient's fears and educating him concerning the nature of the dental problem, the value of treatment for it, and the importance of home care of the teeth.

At an initial appointment with a new patient, one of the first considerations is the recognition and control of the patient's apprehensions, which are based on fear of the pain associated with dental treatment. Fear of pain strongly influences the acceptance or rejection of a treatment plan.

The second consideration in successful management is the avoidance of unfavorable patient reactions that may be due to misinformation concerning dental treatment. Information concerning the projected treatment must be supplied in the depth or the detail required for the specific patient.

Allaying the Patient's Fears

Fear of dental treatment is learned from past personal experience in dental offices and from listening to horrifying tales related by others. Some patients admit their fears during the initial appointment, but in others the fears may not be readily apparent. A very simple test can be used that will reveal many clues about an individual's apprehensions. At the initial appointment, the dentist can deliberately perform a simple dental procedure, such as the excavation of a carious lesion and the placement of a sedative cement or the replacement of a broken amalgam. In a few minutes' time the dentist can learn about the patient's fear of local anesthetic and reaction to dental instrumentation. At the same time, the dentist can begin his re-education program by using a topical anesthetic before injection, by using instru-

ments carefully, and by performing all steps gently. This may be the first time the patient has experienced painless dentistry. No amount of lengthy conversation to dispel a patient's fears is so effective or so convincing as the actual performance of a painless dental procedure. In this manner the dentist has an opportunity to eliminate very strong psychologic blocks in the patient's mind prior to discussing an extensive restorative treatment plan.

At the time alginate impressions are made for diagnostic casts, the dentist has an opportunity to eliminate any apprehensions the patient may have about this procedure. By skillful handling of materials plus a careful explanation of what is being accomplished and why it is necessary, the operator can gain the patient's confidence and also prepare him for similar impressions that must be made during the treatment phases.

Presenting Information to the Patient

An effective method for explaining the patient's dental problems is the use of before-and-after colored slides or photographs of other patients who have received treatment for similar problems. Occasionally patients want to know all the details of the laboratory work. This type of patient should be shown how the restorations are made. Most patients, however, are not interested in the laboratory procedures and are less demanding of the dentist's time.

There are many reasons why an ideal, esthetically pleasing result cannot always be achieved. However, in most instances, patients will accept compromises if they understand the nature of their dental problems and are convinced the dentist is doing the best he can on their behalf. Two examples of subjects requiring explanation are: (1) that restorative materials have limitations in their esthetic properties and (2) that anterior edentulous ridges are often poorly suited for the adaptation of esthetically pleasing pontics, especially if the maxillary canines are missing.

When patients exhibit the following behavior, patient education has failed: (1) cancellation of appointments or tardiness, (2) complaints about lengthy appointments, (3) objection to temporary restorations, and (4) expression of resentment of postoperative thermal pulp sensitivities. Patients who return for treatment appointments with excessive calculus and food debris on their teeth have not been convinced of the importance of home care and should receive further education before continuing treatment.

Drugs Used as Aids in Management

Different patients require different levels of drug therapy for successful restorative dentistry. The dentist can usually recognize the needs and the desires of each patient as the necessary preoperative diagnostic procedures are completed and can estimate the amount and type of drug that will be required during treatment procedures.

Because comprehensive restorative dentistry involves long appointments, sometimes 2 to 3 hours and longer, patients may require special consideration, including the use of analgesic and sedative drugs.

Analgesics

Analgesic drugs lower the perception of pain without producing unconsciousness. Their value may be due partly to the placebo effect. They are indicated at the completion of a long restorative dentistry appointment and are appreciated by most patients. By the time the patient has returned home, the anesthetic has lost its effectiveness, but the analgesic has taken effect. Various combinations of aspirin with phenacetin and caffeine are used commonly. When a stronger analgesic than aspirin is needed, codeine is usually prescribed by the author. Codeine (30 to 60 mg every 4 hours), alone or in combination with aspirin and phenacetin, is a strong analgesic, effective for most pain associated with restorative dentistry.

Use of nitrous oxide has increased in the past decade. Many dentists who perform comprehensive restorative dentistry use this drug to calm patients and to help them accept therapy. Although nitrous oxide provides relaxation for patients, it has limitations as well. Communication with the patient during therapy and the patient's ability to assist the dentist often require a high degree of mental alertness. Nitrous oxide lessens patient response. Also, many appointments for extensive restorative dentistry require 3 to 4 hours, and administration of nitrous oxide for this length of time is a problem. For these reasons, nitrous oxide for extensive restorative dentistry should be used with care.

Sedatives

When sedated, patients have reduced cortical excitability and are relaxed and tranquil. This state is less extreme than the sleeplike condition produced by hypnotic drugs. Apprehensive patients may require sedative or hypnotic drugs prior to and following restorative treatment.

Barbiturates can be prescribed for use the night before the restorative appointment so that preoperative insomnia is avoided. If the patient has a good night's rest, he will be better prepared for the treatment session. Short-acting barbiturates such as pentobarbital sodium or secobarbital sodium (50 to 100 mg) are appropriate drugs for this purpose. However, they should not be used for patients with liver damage or liver disease.

These same drugs may also be used for sedation shortly before the treatment session. Pentobarbital sodium should be taken 1 hour prior to treatment. The shorter acting secobarbital sodium should be administered ½ hour before treatment. Patients under the influence of drugs should not operate their automobiles; they should be accompanied to the treatment session by a responsible person.

When the patient is in pain, barbiturates are not so effective as they would be ordinarily. If used postoperatively, they should be taken in conjunction with an analgesic.

The majority of restorative dentistry patients will not require the use of sedatives. However, when indicated, these drugs are invaluable.

Tranquilizers

Although most drugs produce some amount of "placebo" tranquility or "peace of mind," the term *tranquilizer* is applied to those drugs that exert a central suppressant action. These compounds have not been thoroughly investigated in relation to their use in dentistry. It has been observed, however, that a dentist who demonstrates an air of sympathetic understanding with the patient may create the same effect that tranquilizer drugs produce.

Since many people take these drugs routinely, there is the possibility of duplication of drugs unless a thorough patient medical history is taken. If a patient is taking barbiturates, the use of tranquilizers may produce a deep depression and is definitely contraindicated. There are also a few side effects that would contraindicate their short-term use in restorative dentistry. Dentists should thoroughly review the action of these drugs before prescribing them.

Hypnosis

The trauma of restorative dentistry can be greatly reduced if the patient has been taught simple concepts of self-relaxation. The author uses various levels of hypnosis on many patients undergoing complex restorative dentistry. By this educational process, the patients are helped not only with the immediate problem of restorative dentistry procedures but also with other painful or stressful life situations that arise daily. A course in hypnosis is valuable for those who perform complex restorative therapy.

PRINCIPLES OF RESTORATIVE DENTISTRY

Preventive Restorative Dentistry

Caries Prevention

Principles of preventive dentistry are a basis of restorative dentistry. Theoretically, it is now possible to eliminate dental caries almost entirely in a given population if the individuals participate actively in a program of prevention. However, even though emphasis on patient education has increased and preventive measures are gaining acceptance slowly, the elimination of dental caries has thus far not been attained. Dentists should continually teach preventive dentistry concepts to their patients. The dentist who provides excellent restorative treatment without thoroughly indoctrinating the patient in the importance of keeping his or her mouth healthy has failed to fulfill his total obligation to the patient. The best restorative treatment will degenerate if the dentist and the patient fail to practice prevention.

High-Quality Restorations

Placement of high-quality restorations, regardless of the material used, is one way in which the restorative dentist can practice preventive dentistry. Unfortunately, it becomes necessary to replace far too many restorations because of the operator's failure to accomplish high-quality initial treatment. Studies have estimated that 60 per cent or more of the dental restorations now in patients in the United States should be replaced.

Each restorative material used in dental treatment has an expected longevity. It is within the ability of most dentists to attain the maximal service for restorations through careful application of the materials. Because of busy practices, less than adequate dental education, and financial reasons, many dentists do not produce high-quality restorations. The result is premature breakdown of restorations and recurrent dental caries or periodontal disease. Though initial placement of high-quality restorations may take slightly longer than ordinary treatment and may require a slightly higher fee, in the long run it is far less time-consuming for the dentist and less expensive for the patient than replacement of restorations after they have broken down.

The Mouth as a Functioning Unit

The focus of dentistry has changed from concentration on the restoration of single teeth to a concern for more comprehensive treatment of the patient's mouth as a whole. In the past, single teeth have been restored with little regard for their contribution to the entire occlusion. Recently, there has been much emphasis on the concept of the mouth as a functioning unit of the body, and many dentists are now applying this concept in their practices.

Diagnosis and treatment planning should be based not only on the caries and periodontal status of the mouth but also on the condition of the occlusion. It is well accepted that the dentition of a child is in a constant state of change, but practitioners have been slower to accept the fact that the dentition of the adult also changes and adapts to differences in health, environment, and other factors. Careful consideration of occlusion is necessary prior to any restorative or periodontal treatment to ensure maximal longevity of the treatment.

The dental profession has made great progress in educating patients about prevention of dental disease. High-quality dentistry is now being practiced by some dentists. Occlusion is receiving greater attention than it was given previously in the teaching programs in some dental schools and is being emphasized in continuing education courses. However, the full application of these concepts in dental practice will require interest on the part of the practitioner and time to incorporate them into his or her practice.

Diagnostic Procedures

Use of diagnostic aids in assessing the mouth and in planning treatment has increased significantly over the past few years. Refined radiographic techniques have produced high-kilovoltage radiographs with less contrast and greater diagnostic value. The use of panoramic radiographs has allowed easy and rapid survey of the entire mouth. Many practitioners have now recognized the importance of mounted diagnostic casts for patients experiencing occlusal problems or temporomandibular joint pain or for whom extensive restorative treatment is planned.

The fundamentals of diagnosis for restorative treatment are known to all general practitioners. When a tooth is carious or the restoration in it has broken down, the tooth requires a new restoration. Problems arise when single teeth alone are diagnosed and treated without regard to the remainder of the mouth.

The following section will discuss the basic diagnostic aids to restorative dentistry with emphasis on assessment of the entire mouth, including occlusal analysis.

Radiographic Survey

A complete intraoral radiographic examination is a requirement for all adult patients in need of extensive restorative treatment. To be of maximal benefit, radiographic findings must be correlated with information derived from clinical examination and analysis of casts.

A review of oral radiography is not within the scope of this chapter. Instead, some suggestions are offered concerning the handling of radiographs in the dental office, so that a maximal amount of diagnostic information may be obtained from them.

The mobility of much of the population today, plus the frequency of referrals in current dental practice, often necessitates the transfer of radiographs from one dental office to another. When radiographic films that are outdated, are of poor quality, or are incomplete are received, new radiographs should be taken immediately. If previous radiographs are to be used, it is helpful to the dentist to remount them in the manner familiar to him so that he will avoid misinterpretations.

Radiographs should be regarded not only as valuable for present diagnostic purposes but, equally important, as long-term records useful in comparing and in interpreting changes that may occur following treatment of the patient. The quality of film processing must be monitored constantly by the dentist to ensure that the films will be long-lasting. When inadequately trained auxiliary personnel are assigned the task of developing radiographs, carelessness or ineptness in the processing procedures can result in subsequent film deterioration, rendering the radiographs useless for future reference.

Patients with temporomandibular joint problems should have radiographs of the temporomandibular joints taken as a routine procedure. Negative findings provide valuable diagnostic information, since they may rule out abnormalities and fractures. Many dentists require at least an adequately positioned panoramic x-ray. At present temporomandibular joint radiographs are not commonly made by the general dentist, but the procedure for doing so is not complicated and can be easily accomplished with the regular dental x-ray unit and a small amount of accessory equipment.*

Occlusal Analysis

Functional analysis of occlusion involves the study of the occlusal relationships of the teeth of opposing dental arches during terminal hinge jaw closure and throughout the eccentric range of mandibular movement. The purpose of the analysis is to detect which teeth or parts of teeth, if any, deflect jaw closure, resulting in unfavorable (horizontal or tipping) forces on teeth, trauma due to premature contacts, or interferences that may act as trigger mechanisms for bruxism. After the disharmonies or interferences

---

*Available from Denar Corp., 901 E. Cerritos Ave., Anaheim, CA 92805, or Up Rad Corp., P.O. Box 23770, Fort Lauderdale, FL 33307.

have been recognized, a judgment can be made concerning the possibilities of modification of the occlusal surfaces by restorations or by selective grinding to produce more favorable vertical forces and to help to decrease the trigger areas of bruxism.

Occlusal analysis, as a diagnostic procedure in restorative dentistry, should be accomplished often with the aid of articulator-mounted casts. Evaluation of the natural dentition by direct observation of the patient's mouth without the aid of casts has many limitations when one is planning occlusal or restorative therapy. The cheeks interfere with the buccal view of posterior teeth, and it is impossible to study the dentition from the lingual aspect. If a patient is instructed merely to "chew around" on articulating paper, the resultant markings are too confusing to be of any diagnostic value whatsoever. Also, in such a procedure, the patient may bypass occlusal interferences entirely as a result of the conditioned-reflex avoidance pattern, a natural characteristic of the neuromuscular system. If the dentist does not understand this very important proprioceptive feedback phenomenon, unnecessary grinding may be done on the wrong teeth or the whole procedure may be abandoned because of the difficulty in interpreting the markings.

The two most important types of occlusal disharmonies, associated with bruxism and temporomandibular joint and muscle dysfunction, are the slide from centric relation to centric occlusion and the interferences on the nonworking sides of the mouth. The location of the interferences causing the slide from centric relation to centric occlusion can be identified readily on mounted casts. It is necessary, however, that the operator understand terminal hinge movement of the mandible and be able to make accurate positional records along this arc of closure for the purpose of mounting the mandibular cast. Hand-held casts fitted together into the intercuspal or centric occlusion position reveal no information about this most important type of occlusal disharmony.

When casts are mounted on an acceptable semiadjustable articulator, the interferences on the nonworking sides also can be identified. Accuracy in reproducing mandibular movement is limited, but in many instances the cusp relationships of the casts will be exact enough to indicate where the dentist should look for the interferences in the mouth. Only simple restorative procedures should be undertaken without unmounted or mounted casts.

Oral Examination of Teeth and Supporting Structures

When extensive occlusal reconstruction is planned, several considerations other than the routine inspection and charting of each tooth must be kept in mind. In many instances, the teeth that must receive crowns have been restored several times in the past. Every surface may contain some restorative material in various stages of breakdown. This means that a considerable amount of treatment may be necessary to establish the proper foundation for acceptable coronal preparations. For example, extensive pin-and-amalgam or pin-and-composite cores may be required, and the need for these should be recognized during oral examination. Time must be allotted for these procedures in the treatment plan, and the fee must reflect this additional foundation work. The full extent of the treatment plan and all its implications should be explained to the patient before initiation of treatment.

The need for endodontic therapy during the restorative treatment phase or later should be considered for all teeth with possible pulpal involvement. Overerupted teeth may require intentional extirpation of the vital pulp. Again, the best time to discuss such matters with the patient is before any treatment has begun.

The examination of the supporting structures should follow the steps recommended in this book for careful periodontal probing and charting. Periodontal considerations especially important for restorative dentistry include plans for splinting teeth with weakened support and careful evaluation of the attached gingiva to ensure that the gingival margins of restorations will not terminate in alveolar mucosa.

Treatment Planning

Considering the Whole Patient

The past decade has brought increased interest in more thorough treatment planning for dental patients. Previously, the image of the dentist was that of a practitioner who treated only the obvious dental needs of patients. As a carious lesion appeared, it was restored. In recent years, however, consideration of the patient as a whole has been stressed in treatment planning. The patient's emotional and financial needs as well as his systemic health are now considered extremely important factors in planning dental treatment.

Several approaches have been used for treatment planning: (1) the dentist determines the ideal treatment, and the patient either accepts or refuses to undergo treatment; (2) the dentist suggests several alternative treatment plans to the patient at varying costs, and the patient makes a selection, usually on the basis of cost; and (3) after discussing finances and assessing the patient's level of interest in oral health, the dentist suggests the treatment plan that he feels is best for the patient under the circumstances. He may also present an alternative plan later if the patient cannot afford the suggested plan.

The first method leaves little choice for the patient, and it is unacceptable often because he may be unable to afford the fee involved. Frequently the second approach, which makes the patient decide on treatment, is unsatisfactory because the patient is not qualified to judge what restorations may be optimal in esthetic appearance, function, and longevity. The dentist is the authority on oral health and should be the one to decide whether amalgam, cast gold, or porcelain-fused-to-metal restorations are the best treatment for a particular patient. The dentist should prescribe and carry out the treatment that is most appropriate after considering all the circumstances and thoroughly informing the patient of all the factors relevant to treatment. Thus, it is the third method that is recommended.

No matter which approach to treatment planning is used, the dentist should seriously consider the needs, desires, and capabilities of each patient before discussing the merits of various kinds of restorative treatment. Among the many factors that should be considered in developing a restorative treatment plan are the obvious but often overlooked factors of health, age, sex, occupation, education, past dental experience, and the financial implications of the projected treatment. Also, since the success of comprehensive restorative dentistry depends on the patient's cooperation in oral physiotherapy, it is good practice to plan treatment after the patient has had an opportunity to demonstrate his ability and interest in the maintenance of his oral health.

Planning for Dental Rehabilitation

Many people could benefit from an occlusal rehabilitation by the time they are 30 to 40 years of age, even though they have had "regular" dental care since childhood. There are many reasons why the teeth and occlusion of such individuals are in poor condition. In some instances, most of the teeth may have been restored with extensive amalgam or composite resin restorations because of high caries activity in early life. The occlusion may have been poorly reproduced in restorations placed during adolescence. If extracted teeth have not been replaced, the occlusion will have undergone destructive changes, resulting in tipping, migration, or elongation of teeth. Frequently the proximal contours of amalgam restorations are inadequately reproduced. Margins of the amalgam restorations as well as the enamel of the remaining weakened cusps may be broken. Re-establishing the occlusion and developing the proper external tooth contours for this type of patient could help to prevent tooth fractures, further injury to the periodontium, or future temporomandibular joint and muscle dysfunction.

Although the term *dental rehabilitation* (or reconstruction) is often associated with replacement of all existing restorations at the same time, it may mean the rebuilding of a single tooth or of 32 teeth. The same concepts of occlusion that apply to multiple tooth restorations are also applicable to single-tooth restorations. Each tooth must function in harmony with the entire masticatory system. Therefore, regardless of whether a single tooth or many teeth are to undergo reconstruction, the occlusion must be analyzed, adjusted if necessary, and continually observed during treatment if a satisfactory result is to be obtained.

It is common knowledge that many dental patients cannot afford, or do not require, immediate total mouth rehabilitation. In such cases, single teeth may be rebuilt as individual restorations fail. Full-mouth rehabilitation can be accomplished in one of several different ways: one tooth, one quadrant of the mouth, one half of the mouth, or a full mouth at one time. The result will be slightly different in each situation. However, in the majority of patients, an acceptable clinical result may be obtained by any of these methods. Only in situations of totally mutilated occlusions need the entire mouth be prepared at one time.

The advantages and disadvantages of the various approaches to full-mouth rehabilitation are discussed in the following section.

Classification of Methods for Dental Reconstruction

Rebuilding One Tooth at a Time. When a single-tooth restoration is provided for a patient whose original restorative treatment was of high quality, and whose occlusal relationship is satisfactory, it can be expected to serve for many years. In such instances the replacement of a number of single restorations over a protracted period can produce successful overall rehabilitation. However, if all the original restorative treatment appears to require immediate replacement, single-tooth rebuilding will be time-consuming, painful, and less successful than the more comprehensive forms of treatment. The patient will require many treatment sessions, will have to be anesthetized many times, and will be inconvenienced with temporary restorations over a long period. Furthermore, the eventual occlusal relationship resulting from the single-tooth treatment cannot be determined with accuracy because single, new restorations are placed in opposition to, and adjacent to, teeth that have not been restored to proper anatomic form and function. The result is a dentition that may not function well as a unit. When single-tooth rehabilitation is planned over a period of time, occlusal equilibration should be accomplished before treatment to preclude rebuilding potential problematic occlusal relationships in the new restoration.

Quadrant Treatment. An increasingly popular sequence of treatment is the reconstruction of one quadrant of the mouth at a time. Tooth preparations are usually completed in one appointment, and the restorations are placed at the second appointment. If the opposing arch of teeth and restorations are well formed and will provide a good occlusal relationship for the new restorations, this sequence of treatment will be successful. If the opposing restorations need replacement also, the dentist must adjust the opposing occlusal surfaces so that the new restorations are not constructed to an unacceptable relationship. Occlusal equilibration should be accomplished before restorative therapy is begun.

Full-arch Treatment. The full-arch reconstruction sequence produces the same problems associated with quadrant rehabilitation. The new restorations are limited in their function and anatomy by the previously existing opposing restorations. An additional disadvantage of full-arch rehabilitation is that the original vertical dimension of occlusion may be lost when all the teeth in the arch are prepared.

Reconstruction of One Side of the Mouth at a Time. This method of treatment has several advantages: (1) the basic vertical dimension of occlusion of the patient remains unchanged because the opposite side of the mouth maintains the relationship; (2) the anatomy and function of the rehabilitated side may be adjusted and formed to the best possible relationship, since the only limitations in the development of function are working, nonworking, and protrusive interferences on the remaining teeth (however, these should and can be adjusted carefully before rehabilitation is begun); and (3) the patient has one "normal" side on which to masticate while treatment is under way.

Simultaneous Rehabilitation of All Teeth. This approach allows maximal freedom in the development of a new occlusal relationship. The dentition may be developed into a properly functioning unit. It is usually indicated when all of the teeth in the mouth require occlusal coverage or when the vertical occlusal relationship requires alteration. If several teeth, particularly the anterior teeth, do not need full coverage, and the vertical dimension of occlusion does not require changing, the reconstruction of one side of the mouth at a time may be preferable.

Occlusal rehabilitation of all the teeth at the same time is one of the most complex forms of advanced restorative dentistry. The successful management of the various procedures necessary to provide the patient with the best possible occlusion may require education beyond the traditional dental school program. The restorative dentist must acquire a thorough knowledge of the physiology of mandibular movement and positions as a foundation for understanding occlusal adjustment and must also be familiar with the use of instruments that permit accurate reproduction of jaw movement and positions. He or she must invest the time necessary to learn to prescribe laboratory procedures that will create occlusal form, that will subject the teeth to the least amount of occlusal stress. The dentist must develop clinical proficiency in impression-making techniques and accuracy in mounting casts on the articulator, since these procedures are essential for the laboratory fabrication of restorations.

The procedures used in simultaneous restoration of posterior teeth on both sides of the mouth are described briefly later in this chapter. Since space does not permit a full discussion of all the complexities involved in this form of treatment, only the highlights of this method of rehabilitation are included. The general practitioner with insufficient background should refer cases requiring simultaneous occlusal reconstruction of all teeth to a colleague who has demonstrated competence in this area.

Types of Restorations Used in Dental Reconstruction

Patients requiring dental rehabilitation present a variety of problems. Whether a single tooth or many teeth are to be restored, judgments must be made concerning the type of restoration to be used. The choice may depend on the condition of other restorations in the mouth and their potential for breakdown, occlusal relationships with other teeth, and the method to be used for dental restoration. The expected longevity of the new restoration to be placed must be carefully considered not only in terms of its appropriateness for the individual tooth but also in terms of its functioning relationship with other parts of the mouth over a protracted period of time.

Conservative Restorations for Anterior Teeth. Because of the nature of anterior restorative materials, less than ideal treatment for anterior teeth is often provided for patients for whom nearly ideal treatment is rendered for posterior teeth. A patient who

TABLE 9–1   Types of Restorations Commonly Used in Restorative Dentistry

	Indications	Contraindications	Strengths	Weaknesses	Longevity
Amalgam, silver	Incipient, moderate-sized, and some large lesions	Large intracoronal restorations (cusp replacement), endodontically treated teeth	Good marginal seal, strength, longevity, manipulability, cariostatic qualities	Tarnish, stains, marginal breakdown, color	About 20+ years
Cast gold (inlays, onlays, and crowns)	Large lesions, teeth requiring additional strength, teeth used in rebuilding or changing occlusion	Adolescents, high caries activity, anterior teeth in which metal would show excessively	Reproduces anatomy well; onlays and crowns may increase strength of tooth; longevity	Cement margin, time required for placement, high fee, poor esthetic appearance, thermal sensitivity	Indefinite
Compacted golds (gold foil, powdered gold, mat gold)	Initial Class III and Class V lesions for patients of all ages	Periodontally unstable teeth, teeth in which metal will be visible, high caries activity	Marginal integrity, longevity	Time-consuming, high fee, poor esthetic appearance, difficulty in placement	Indefinite
Porcelain jacket crowns	Anterior teeth requiring extensive coverage	Teeth subject to heavy occlusal forces	Esthetically pleasing	Lack of strength, poor marginal adaptation	About 10+ years
Porcelain inlays	Class V and some Class III areas in which good esthetic result is desired	Preparations that lack retention, high caries activity	Esthetically pleasing	Marginal opening, high fee, difficulty of procedure	About 10+ years
Porcelain-fused-to-metal crowns	Teeth requiring full coverage and subject to heavy occlusal forces	Adolescents (because a great amount of tooth reduction is necessary)	Strength, good marginal seal	Esthetic appearance not as good as porcelain jacket crowns, wears opposing teeth	Estimate 10+ years
Resin, composite (used with acid etch and bond)	Large Class III, Class IV, and Class V lesions	Very large restorations	Esthetically pleasing for a few years, ease of use	Longevity	6 years

has had all his posterior teeth restored with crowns or onlays often receives full-coverage restorations on his anterior teeth as part of the total treatment. In many instances, these full-coverage restorations could have been delayed or eliminated by the more conservative use of compacted gold, porcelain inlays, or composite or microfill resin. At times, resins are the only materials that can be used; the teeth may be too broken down for gold foil yet not sufficiently damaged to require full coverage. However, the restorative dentist should have competence in the use of compacted golds, porcelain inlays, and small inlays or pinlays so that he may provide the proper type of restoration when such treatment is indicated.

Compacted Gold Restorations. The term "compacted gold" covers all forms of pure gold that are placed in cavity preparations and cold-welded into a coherent mass by the use of a compacting force. Although gold foil has been used as a routine treatment procedure for years by a few practitioners, it is seldom used by most dentists. It remains an unexcelled treatment for incipient Class III or Class V carious lesions.

Powdered gold and mat gold have been recommended more recently as acceptable materials, and clinicians report excellent results with their use. One advantage of these other forms of gold is that placement of larger pieces is easier than with gold foil; however, compacting forces must be heavier to effect adequate compaction. The author recommends the placement of powdered gold and mat gold with mechanical compacting devices when these restorations are indicated.

Porcelain Inlays. Although for years these restorations were not used much, they have regained favor since the introduction of direct-firing porcelain inlay investments. Several of these investments make accuracy possible and allow the fabrication of esthetically pleasing, long-lasting restorations.

A summary of the indications, contraindications, strengths, weaknesses, and approximate longevity of various types of anterior and posterior restorations is presented in Table 9–1. The estimates of longevity are based on the assumption that the restorations were of high quality when placed initially.

BIOLOGIC CONSIDERATIONS

Tooth Restoration in Relation to Other Forms of Therapy

Whenever comprehensive rehabilitation of the dentition and occlusion is planned, restorative treatment must be considered in relation to other forms of therapy required. For example, teeth in need of endodontic therapy may have to be treated before restorations are begun. In most situations, periodontal therapy should be completed before restorative treatment. If a harmonious relationship exists between the periodontist and the restorative dentist, the treatment may be accomplished concomitantly, with obvious advantages to both. Old restorations may be replaced with temporary restorations that the periodontist can remove during periodontal procedures.

In determining the sequence for the various types of treatment, the dentist must consider the possible effects of one form of therapy on another. Since restorative dentistry is so closely related to endodontic and periodontal therapy, some of the important areas in which these forms of treatment may overlap or influence each other are discussed here.

Periodontal Considerations

The treatment of periodontal disease has become a routine part of the general practice of dentistry, with the result that practitioners are focusing increased attention on the interrelationship of periodontal and restorative procedures. Not only does the condition of the periodontium influence the success or failure of restorative treatment but the quality of the restorations has an important effect on the periodontal supporting system. It is the responsibility of the dentist to see to it that restorations are formed and placed in such a way that they will enhance periodontal health instead of contributing to periodontal disease. Furthermore, when treated periodontal disease exists, the restorative dentist can aid in maintenance of periodontal health by placement of well-functioning restorations. One of the most common problems in restorative dentistry today is placement of restorations in the presence of periodontal disease.

Choice of Restoration and Tooth Preparation

In some clinical situations, the restorative dentist has little choice as to the type of preparation to be used for a particular tooth. At other times, a decision for or against full coverage may be made. Unfortunately, the decision is often influenced not by consideration of the potential effects of the preparation on the patient's oral health but by the fact that the full-coverage restoration is easier than the partial-coverage restoration. Careful, conservative treatment planning usually results in a decrease in the use of full crowns.

Selection of the type of restoration should be based on the restorative need of each individual tooth and its relationship to the patient's occlusion and periodontium. Adequate retention and strength can be obtained from either partial-coverage or full-coverage restorations. Whenever possible, however, the use of subgingival full crowns should be avoided. The gingival irritation associated with the tooth preparation necessary for these restorations and the problems encountered in maintenance after treatment make the subgingival full-crown restoration less desirable than the supragingival full crown or the partial crown.

Another important periodontal factor to be considered in preparation of teeth is that gingival damage may be caused by careless use of burs and diamond stones. It is practically impossible to determine when the epithelial attachment is being destroyed by these instruments. Careful preoperative use of a periodontal probe around the teeth to be prepared will help the operator to avoid cutting the epithelial attachment. Visualization of how the final preparation will look as well as the careful and judicious use of instruments during tooth preparation will also help to reduce gingival damage.

Location of Margins

Although controversy about the location of margins has existed for decades, most of the existing research supports the view that margins of restorations should be kept supragingival whenever possible. Supragingival margins are desirable because they are easily observed during placement of the restoration, are easily finished, are easily repaired if repair is necessary, are nonirritat-

ing to the periodontium, and are usually on enamel, affording less chance for future caries.

However, whenever one or more of the following situations exists, margins should be placed subgingivally: (1) Esthetic considerations demand subgingival placement on the facial surface (the lingual margin may be supragingival); (2) the tooth is too short for adequate retention of the crown; (3) caries exists subgingivally; (4) untreatable root sensitivity or postperiodontal therapy forces subgingival placement; or (6) the patient's physical or emotional condition will not allow adequate oral hygiene.

Impressions

Gingival tissue may be lacerated during improper impression procedures following tooth preparation. However, judicious use of impression techniques will help to prevent permanent damage to the periodontium.

Gingival retraction, necessary for making impressions, may be obtained by mechanical techniques, chemical compounds, electrosurgical instruments, or a combination of methods. Retracting cords are now used by most dentists for this purpose. Cords for gingival tissue retraction have been advocated for years and can be used with relative safety. Their functions are to separate the free gingiva gently from the surface of the preparation during impression procedures and to stop gingival bleeding, which may accompany or follow crown preparation. The author used cords most of the time, but electrosurgery is used occasionally.

The cord should fill the gingival sulcus, but undue force should not be directed against the epithelial attachment. In areas of the mouth such as the facial surfaces of mandibular canines and premolars or maxillary canines, where there may be little attached gingiva, a gingival tear can be produced easily if tissue-packing cords are not used with caution. If retraction cords are used properly, little gingival trauma will result. Most gingival tissue looks nearly normal 1 or 2 days after careful crown preparation, gingival retraction, and impressions.

Tube impressions are used by some restorative dentists for making impressions of a single tooth preparation. If the tube is adapted well to the preparation and its length is carefully related to the gingival margin and the subjacent epithelial attachment, the impression may be made with little trauma to the gingiva. On the other hand, if excessive force is used on the tube or if the tube is improperly adapted and overextended, these impressions may strip the epithelial attachment from the tooth structure.

When subgingival margins are required, the author uses a two-cord procedure for most complex rehabilitation procedures. The technique follows:

1. *Initial* tooth preparation is accomplished with a large diamond stone using water coolant. This preparation does *not* go below the gingiva.
2. A cord is packed below the gingiva. Regular Gingipak is used normally. This procedure retracts the gingival tissue in direct relation to the epithelial attachment.
3. The preparation is finished with a bur (No. 1171L) using a high-speed handpiece with air coolant alone. Adequate vision is mandatory. The preparation is cut to the level of the cord.
4. A second, smaller cord is placed to gently compress the first cord (one-half strand of Gingipak).
5. The second cord is removed.
6. The impression is made with the first cord *in place*.

Design of Restorations

Contour. One of the most serious faults in restorative treatment is the gross overcontouring of most full-coverage tooth restorations. Gingival problems are more severe in patients with overcontoured rather than with undercontoured crowns.

The porcelain-fused-to-metal restoration is particularly conducive to overcontouring. At least 1.0 to 1.5 mm of facial tooth structure must be removed to allow adequate space for metal and porcelain. The stronger metals require less tooth structure removal. Few restorative dentists provide this space. In the tooth preparation, depth-gauge grooves should be cut in the mesial, distal, facial, and lingual surfaces to the depth of the desired final preparation. The teeth can be reduced easily to optimal depth if the grooves are made before gross tooth reduction. *The final restoration should be no larger than the original tooth.* Adequate tooth reduc-

tion permits proper contour. Without proper reduction, overcontoured crowns are inevitable, and periodontal disease will follow.

Bifurcation and trifurcation areas of teeth exposed by periodontal therapy should not be closed by overcontoured and overextended restorations. They must remain open for proper stimulation and oral hygiene.

Overcontouring creates gingival problems, and it also makes the development of esthetic restorations nearly impossible. The best guide to coronal contour in a mouth with a healthy periodontium and proper occlusion is the contour that nature gave the tooth. When a change must be made in the occlusion or occlusal plane, a departure from the natural contour of the teeth may be necessary in the fabrication of the restorations. In such instances, careful treatment planning with the long-range periodontal health of the patient in mind is certainly indicated.

Surface Characteristics of Teeth. Dentists often discuss the necessity of reproducing occlusal anatomy and grooves in restorations. They support concepts ranging from flat occlusal surfaces without grooves to normal occlusal anatomy with many minute grooves and fissures. Little experimental evidence is available to support either extreme. Nature has not made many mistakes in the formation of the human body. On that basis, the development of the original occlusal grooves, triangular and marginal ridges, and embrasures is sound practice. These anatomic features permit proper interdigitation during occlusion and good occlusal function. If the teeth chew more efficiently and do not occlude with broad flat surfaces, there is less stress applied to them, less stress on the periodontium, and, consequently, a healthier periodontium.

Tooth Splinting. If it is deemed advisable to join teeth together to maintain the periodontium, the method to be used in joining them must be considered carefully. Depending on the method selected, the teeth may become more stable or they may remain as mobile as they were before splinting. Two mobile teeth with buccolingual movement will not necessarily be more stable when joined together than they were individually. In the construction of the splint, one or more sound teeth on either side of the mobile teeth must be included. If all the teeth of a quadrant are mobile, effective immobilization usually requires cross-arch splinting or at least the inclusion of the canine in the quadrant being treated.

Overcontouring of cast splints is common. These crowns should be the same size and contour as the original teeth, or perhaps even smaller. The only necessary deviation from the original contour, aside from whatever occlusal alterations may be indicated, is that required to join the contact areas.

Splinting is invaluable when indicated and properly executed but if abused provides no positive aid and, in fact, may result in deterioration of the periodontium.

Pontic Design. The health of edentulous areas is enhanced by cleanliness. The placement of a fixed partial denture that overlaps the edentulous ridge to a great degree hinders cleaning of that ridge. The resultant gingival irritation, susceptibility of the abutment teeth to caries, and poor esthetic result emphasize the need for an optimal pontic-ridge relationship. Slight contact with the gingival tissue on the facial aspect for proper esthetics, with an open lingual embrasure, is usually advisable. (The reader should consult one of the many texts on fixed prosthodontics for a thorough discussion of pontic design.)

Pulpal Considerations

The pulpal condition of each tooth included in the patient's treatment plan should be known as completely as possible before restorative treatment is begun. Frequently, a tooth that has had endodontic therapy requires coverage of all cusps for strength. Thus, the placement of an intracoronal restoration in a tooth with a questionable pulp is not good treatment planning, inasmuch as subsequent endodontic therapy would necessitate replacement of this restoration with a new, extracoronal restoration. The placement of a restoration in a vital tooth should not result in pulpal death, causing unneeded discomfort and expense for the patient.

Ultrahigh-Speed Handpieces

The literature is filled with contradictory reports concerning the traumatic effects of ultrahigh-speed rotary instruments. When they were introduced, their tremendous speed seemed to suggest that large amounts

of coolant would be necessary for tooth preparation. As practitioners became familiar with these handpieces, various techniques evolved for reducing the heat generated by them. Some favored air-water spray during tooth preparation; others advocated preparation with air coolant alone. Research investigators began to report results that varied widely, depending on what had been evaluated and which clinical techniques had been used. Both clinicians and pathologists have noted histologic changes when cutting is done with air coolant alone, but their interpretations of these changes have differed. They have not agreed as to which histologic criteria are significant clinically.

Although tooth preparation with an air coolant alone may be totally harmless to the dental pulp, the author prefers the use of an air-water spray with ultrahigh-speed instruments. The operating field is kept clean and free of debris when a water spray and a high-velocity suction system are used. Chips of tooth or restorative material are aspirated and are thus prevented from flying into the face of the operator. The odor accompanying tooth reduction and the removal of dental caries is almost entirely eliminated when an air-water spray is used. The author, therefore, advocates the use of an air-water spray coolant for gross tooth-cutting procedures with an ultrahigh-speed handpiece and the use of air coolant alone for better vision in the final finishing of tooth preparations.

Pulp-Desensitizing Agents, Bases, Liners, and Varnishes

The dental pulp is extremely recuperative; it survives many insults, not the least of which is the exposure to desensitizing and sterilizing solutions ranging from caustics to tap water. Little research information has been published on cavity-sterilization agents, and as a result, practitioners' preferences for particular agents are largely empirical. It is doubtful that a tooth preparation can be sterilized or that it is desirable to do so.

Materials used as pulp-desensitizing agents, bases, liners, and varnishes have shown varying results. Although zinc phosphate cement has long been used as a pulp-insulating medium or base, it has been shown to be irritating to the dental pulp and is not recommended in deep tooth preparations unless an additional pulp protective liner is used.

Calcium hydroxide is a reparative dentin stimulator and cavity liner that has been used extensively over the past decade. Preparations such as Dycal, Life, Procal, and Renew, which include other ingredients mixed with calcium hydroxide, are easier to use because they have a creamy consistency and set rapidly. Natural gum varnishes such as copal, resin, or synthetic resins have been accepted by some researchers but are questioned by others, who believe them to be only partially effective in sealing cut tooth walls. The majority of evidence seems to favor the use of these cavity varnishes under amalgam fillings and zinc phosphate cement.

Zinc oxide–eugenol cements are effective temporary restorations. They seal the cavity walls well and have a palliative effect on the pulp. Some practitioners are using EBA*– zinc oxide–eugenol cements as final cementing agents with success.

Steroids have been used on exposed dentin as desensitizing agents. The effect of these anti-inflammatory agents has been reported to be a reduction in postoperative sensitivity associated with newly inserted restorations, and they are recommended for use on very sensitive teeth. Steroids are also recommended if teeth are extremely sensitive when crowns are tried in the mouth without anesthesia. Thymol crystals and myriad other preparations are used by practitioners for desensitizing dentin. Little more than empirical information is available on them.

Pulp capping during comprehensive restorative treatment is a questionable procedure. If it seems advisable to cap a small coronal pulp exposure, the restoration for the tooth should be at least an onlay rather than an intracoronal restoration. In the event that endodontic treatment is required in the future, the restoration will be acceptable in terms of strength. Pulp capping of lateral pulp exposures in rehabilitative cases is not indicated because of the difficulty of any future endodontic therapy.

For tooth cleansing, the author recommends large amounts of tap water, followed by a calcium hydroxide preparation over the deep areas that appear to be close to the pulp. A layer of one of the copal type of cav-

ity varnishes is indicated if amalgam or zinc phosphate cement is to be used.

Pins for Added Retention

Pins have many advantages and have become a mainstay for retention of core build-ups in restorative dentistry. However, it is a lucky or extremely cautious operator who does not expose a pulp occasionally when using this form of retention. If a pulp exposure occurs during preparation of a channel for a stainless-steel pin, it is advisable to coat the area with calcium hydroxide and relocate the pin at another point. The patient should be forewarned that endodontic therapy could become necessary in the future. The author uses 0.021-inch pins most commonly.

Malleting Associated with Compacted Golds

This chapter has advocated the use of compacted golds as restorative materials. A study completed at the University of Washington showed that, over a four-year period, only slightly more than 1 per cent of the teeth in which gold-foil restorations were placed by students required subsequent endodontic therapy. This is a small percentage when one considers the problems associated with a student environment. Nevertheless, as with any other form of dental restoration, there is a chance of damage to the pulp when gold is compacted into a cavity preparation.

Occlusal Considerations

Traditionally, dentists have placed considerable emphasis on the prevention and interception of malocclusion during the growth and development of the child. Much less consideration has been given to the factors causing malposition of the teeth during the adult years. Alterations of the occlusal relationships of teeth, resulting from wear and the placement of restorations, continue throughout life. Migration of teeth can occur whenever the integrity of the dental arch is destroyed by failure to restore proximal contacts properly or by failure to replace extracted teeth.

Some occlusal problems are observed frequently enough to be listed as classic examples. One of these is the overerupted man-

---

*EBA is *o*-ethoxybenzoic acid.

dibular third molar. This tooth can create the primary occlusal interference restricting bilateral movement of the mandible, and secondary occlusal changes that occur on the diagonally opposite side of the mouth. Mandibular movement is possible only to the side of the overerupted third molar. The anterior teeth on the other side, toward which movement is not possible, develop secondary elongation or exhibit an absence of wear, indicating loss of function.

Failure to replace extracted permanent first molars is another common cause of occlusal problems. Loss of the mandibular permanent first molar permits the second and third molars to tip mesially and lingually so that they are subjected to severe nonworking side interferences.

When molar restorations in the form of large amalgams or crowns are overcarved on their occlusal surfaces, the centric supporting contacts may be lost. The teeth may then continue to erupt until centric contacts are again established. The resultant effect on chewing or closure in the centric occlusion position may be inconspicuous, but the newly acquired eccentric interferences may result in an intolerable situation for the patient.

Another occlusal problem is created by the extraction of an overlapped or rotated mandibular incisor, done with the good intention of improving the esthetic appearance of the patient's crowded mandibular anterior teeth. Natural forces will not automatically rearrange these teeth; instead, several unfortunate things may happen. First, as the anterior arch collapses, the teeth may erupt, depending on the anteroposterior relationship of the mandible to the maxilla. The result may be an increase in the anterior vertical overlap, with the mandibular incisors impinging on the palatal tissues. Second, the posterior teeth, perhaps imperceptibly, may be subjected to newly acquired eccentric interferences as the mandibular canines lose their functional contacts with the maxillary canines. A mandibular anterior tooth should be extracted only after careful occlusal and arch-to-arch analysis. Usually, orthodontic guidance must be provided.

Whenever a single tooth demonstrates greater mobility than the other teeth in a quadrant, the occlusion should be studied carefully. Early recognition and correction of occlusal overloading can reverse the pathologic changes. The benefit of such correction will be manifested radiographically by regeneration of bone and clinically by decreased mobility.

A prophylactic occlusal adjustment for every patient in a busy dental practice is neither feasible nor advisable. On the other hand, the dentist should take advantage of the opportunity to examine a patient's occlusion at the time restorative procedures are being rendered. Whenever major resurfacing of posterior segments is planned, occlusal adjustment to eliminate discrepancies must be considered. At the time the diagnostic casts are mounted on an articulator and the occlusal analysis is done, the interferences located between the centric relation and the centric occlusion positions as well as those located on the nonworking side can be identified and corrected.

ILLUSTRATIVE TECHNIQUES AND PROCEDURES FOR ORAL REHABILITATION

In this section, two of the previously mentioned methods of rehabilitation will be described and illustrated: rehabilitation of one side of the mouth at a time and simultaneous rehabilitation of all posterior teeth. The sequence of procedures used in each type of rehabilitation in shown in Table 9–2.

The techniques that are basically the same for both procedures will be described first: occlusal analysis and preliminary adjustment, preliminary amalgam or composite-resin build-up, and designs for tooth preparations for extracoronal restorations. Following the description of these techniques, a clinical case will be used to illustrate the subsequent steps for each method of rehabilitation. The basic principles involved in these two methods may be applied to single tooth, quadrant, or any other type of occlusal rehabilitation.

Types of Casts Used in Reconstruction

Three different types of casts are used in occlusal rehabilitation; each represents a specific phase of treatment.

Diagnostic Casts

Diagnostic casts are used for the occlusal analysis, treatment planning, and recording

TABLE 9–2   Procedures in Dental Rehabilitation

Preliminary Procedures
1. Radiographic survey
2. Fabrication and mounting of diagnostic casts
3. Diagnosis and occlusal analysis
4. Treatment planning
5. Initial adjustment of gross occlusal interferences
6. Preliminary rebuilding of dental structures with amalgam or composite cores
7. Occlusal correction

Rehabilitation of One Side of the Mouth at a Time
1. Preparation of teeth for extracoronal restorations (preferably one quadrant or one side of the mouth at a time)
2. Fabrication of working casts from full-arch impressions
3. Interocclusal records and mounting of casts in a semiadjustable articulator (Whip-Mix or other)
4. Trimming and waxing of dies
5. Fabrication of restorations by the laboratory
6. Try-in of castings for checking of proximal contacts, color, occlusion, contour, and margins
7. Remounting and adjusting of occlusion if necessary
8. Cementation
9. Repetition of procedures for alternate side of the mouth

Simultaneous Rehabilitation of All Posterior Teeth
1. Preparation of teeth for extracoronal restorations (by quadrants or more)
2. Temporary restorations
3. Full-arch working casts mounted in a fully adjustable or a semiadjustable articulator
4. Fabrication of castings from full-mouth occlusion concept
5. Try-in of restorations for checking of proximal contacts, color, occlusion, contour, and margins
6. Fabrication of remount casts with acrylic matrix
7. Occlusal correction of castings on remount casts in the articulator
8. Cementation of finished restorations

---

of the patient's occlusion before treatment. They are made of die stone from impressions made with alginate impression materials. To be useful for diagnostic purposes they must be accurate reproductions of the occlusal surfaces of all the teeth in the arch, showing clearly the facets of wear (Fig. 9–1).

Working Casts

Working casts are also stone casts. They are constructed from impressions made with polysulfide, condensation or addition reaction silicone, polyether, or reversible hydrocolloid materials following tooth preparation. Wax patterns for castings are formed on these casts (Fig. 9–2).

Remount Casts

Remount casts are used in making the final occlusal corrections of the castings. A special technique, using low-fusing metal, may be employed in forming the casts (Fig. 9–3).

Accurate Cast Mounting

Part of the success in indirect fabrication of multiple cast restorations from working casts depends on the care and accuracy with which the casts are mounted in the articulator. Restorations accurately fitted to dies in the laboratory may be useless when placed in the patient's mouth if an error was made in the cast-mounting procedures.

Two types of face-bows are used for mounting maxillary casts in the articulator. For simple restorative procedures, an ear face-bow is used with a semiadjustable articulator (Whip-Mix or other). The ear face-bow is adjusted on the patient by means of arbitrary skull reference points. The external auditory meatus is used for the posterior reference point and the nasion for the anterior reference point. This method is simple, rapid, and sufficiently accurate for restorative procedures that do not require several cast mountings in centric relation (Figs. 9–4 to 9–6).

The hinge-axis face-bow is used during occlusal reconstruction procedures that require the mounting of maxillary casts in a fully adjustable articulator at several stages of treatment. Three reference points may be marked on the skin with tattoo dye at the time of the initial mounting of the diagnostic casts. The two posterior reference marks represent the hinge-axis points. The third, or anterior, reference point is marked on the side of the nose, 2⅛ inches superior to the incisal edges of the maxillary central incisors. The anterior reference point is arbitrarily selected to position the occlusal plane of the maxillary cast conveniently, approximately midway between the upper and lower members of the articulator. The same articulator settings can be used throughout the treatment phases because the reference points, marked with long-lasting tattoo dye, are unchanged for each face-bow transfer (Fig. 9–7).

The mandibular cast is mounted in the articulator by use of an interocclusal centric relation wax record. The wax record is

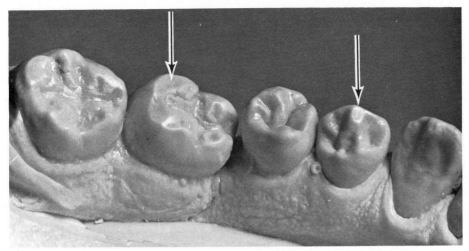

FIGURE 9–1 Abraded areas of the enamel, representing tooth-to-tooth wear, are readily identifiable on the diagnostic stone casts.

formed on the patient; the mandible is guided along the terminal hinge arc of closure in order to obtain cusp imprints in the wax. When the wax record is transferred to the articulator, the terminal hinge axis of the patient and the opening and closing axis of the articulator become the same. When the ear face-bow is used for mounting the maxillary cast, the interocclusal wax record should be made as thin as possible to compensate for discrepancies that may result from the use of arbitrary reference points.

Occlusal Analysis and Adjustment

This section will describe the recognition and correction of occlusal discrepancies, using the most common types of occlusal interferences of the natural dentition to illustrate the procedure. The reader is referred to Ramfjord and Ash's text for an extensive coverage of the objectives, indications, and techniques of occlusal adjustment.

Occlusal adjustment of the natural dentition by grinding is a limited procedure. Cer-

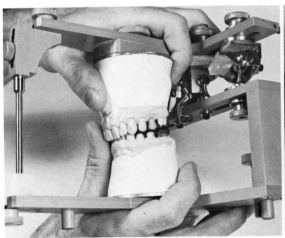

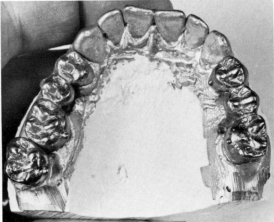

FIGURE 9–2   **FIGURE 9–3**

FIGURE 9–2 The occlusal surfaces are formed in wax on full-arch stone working casts that have been mounted in the articulator.

FIGURE 9–3 Remount casts contain the castings. Refinement of the occlusal surfaces is accomplished after these casts have been mounted in the articulator.

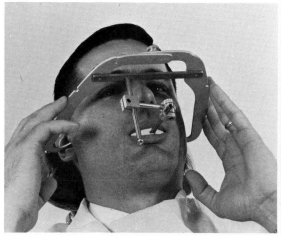 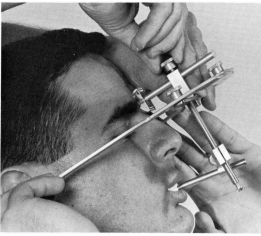

FIGURE 9–4   FIGURE 9–5

FIGURE 9–4   When the ear face-bow is adjusted on the patient, the external auditory meatus is used for the posterior reference point.

FIGURE 9–5   The nasion is used as the anterior reference point, which functions to position the occlusal plane of the maxillary cast approximately midway between the upper and lower members of the articulator.

tain types of occlusal discrepancies cannot be corrected by grinding. Instead, the teeth should be restored, repositioned orthodontically, or, in some instances, extracted.

The recognition and correction of occlusal interferences in the natural dentition are facilitated by an understanding of the physiology of mandibular movement rather than by mastery of a regimented series of grind-

ing rules. The operator (1) must be able to evaluate terminal hinge movement of the mandible readily as well as determine the location and direction of the working and nonworking pathways of the cusps; (2) must understand how pain in the teeth, periodontium, muscles, or the temporomandibular joint affects mandibular movement, making the location of interferences difficult; and

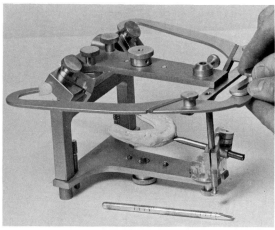 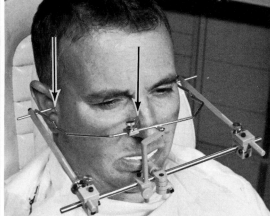

FIGURE 9–6   FIGURE 9–7

FIGURE 9–6   Because of its self-centering design, the ear face-bow is easily assembled on the articulator.

FIGURE 9–7   Hinge-axis face-bows may be aligned to precise reference points marked on the skin with tattoo dye.

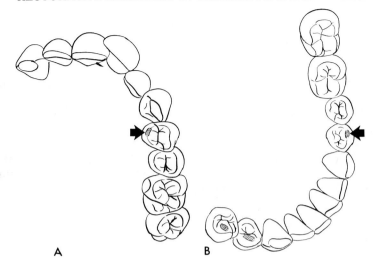

FIGURE 9–8 *A,* A frequent site of cuspal interference in the terminal hinge closure is the mesial inner incline of the lingual cusp of the maxillary first premolar. *B,* Another is the opposing distal inner incline of the buccal cusp of the mandibular first premolar.

A

B

(3) must be able to identify the slide from centric relation to centric occlusion and the contacts on the nonworking sides, which have been shown to be the most important cuspal interferences involved in bruxism and in temporomandibular joint and muscle dysfunction.

An evaluation of terminal hinge closure can be made on an articulator, provided the mandibular cast was mounted with a centric relation record. The articulator-mounted casts can be kept in the operatory when the patient is examined. The casts enhance visualization of the tooth inclines involved in the slide from centric relation to centric occlusion. The interferences observed on the casts are guides for finding prematurities in the mouth.

Interferences causing the mandible to slide forward will be located on distal inclines of lower cusps and on mesial inclines of upper cusps (Fig. 9–8). The decision as to which tooth should be ground is always based on the evaluation of the importance of the involved cusps in maintaining the stability of the centric stops. The median plane graphic tracing provides a method of visualizing the character of the slide and how it will change when the inclines are altered (Fig. 9–9).

Cuspal interferences causing a lateral slide should also be removed (Figs. 9–10 and 9–11). After correction, the patient should be able to exert bilaterally balanced closure forces any place between the centric relation and the centric occlusion positions without striking an incline.

Nonworking-side interferences mainly in-

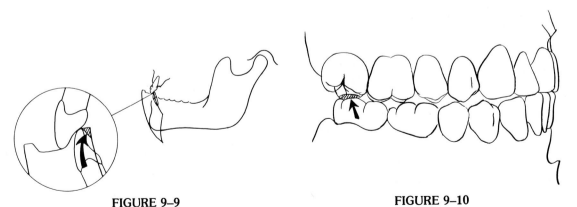

FIGURE 9–9

FIGURE 9–10

FIGURE 9–9 Selective grinding procedures eliminate interferences that act as trigger areas for bruxism, thus providing a more favorable and stable bracing of the mandibular teeth against the maxillary teeth in the retruded position during swallowing.

FIGURE 9–10 Cuspal interferences creating a lateral deviation of mandible during terminal hinge closure may be difficult to detect directly in the mouth because patients often avoid them by reflex.

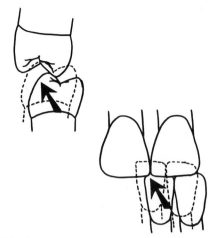

FIGURE 9–11   Full-arch casts accurately mounted in the articulator reveal a lateral shift during terminal hinge closure.

volve the molar teeth. Knowledge of the direction of the cusp pathways on the teeth will facilitate identification of these interferences on the casts and in the mouth. On the lower teeth the nonworking pathways are distobuccal in direction. The upper teeth have opposite, or mesiolingual, nonworking pathways (Figs. 9–12 and 9–13). Bennett movement allows the cusps to pass more mesially on the lower teeth and more distally on the upper teeth (Figs. 9–14 and 9–15). The findings on the articulator-mounted casts may not correspond entirely with those in

the mouth and will depend on the accuracy of the articulator in reproducing the Bennett movement. Only markings in the mouth can provide the final information about where the adjustment is needed.

Nonworking-side interferences are represented by collisions between centric supporting cusps of both arches (Figs. 9–16 to 9–18). The decision concerning where to grind is based on the importance of the involved cusps in maintaining the stability of the centric stops, which is determined by study of the articulator-mounted casts (Fig. 9–19) and the mouth. Correction is made by creating an escapeway—distobuccal grooves in the lower teeth or mesiolingual grooves in the upper. If the lower buccal cusps have no centric contacts, the correction must be made in the lower (Fig. 9–20).

Interferences on the working side are of less significance in functional disturbances. In the natural dentition, no attempt is made to reduce the anterior teeth in order to bring posterior cusps into contact on the working side unless the maxillary canine is mobile or missing. Grinding of the working side can create new interferences on the nonworking side, which must be re-examined immediately.

Cuspal interferences on the posterior teeth in the protrusive or lateral-protrusive glide should be removed to create group function of the anterior teeth (Figs. 9–21 and 9–22).

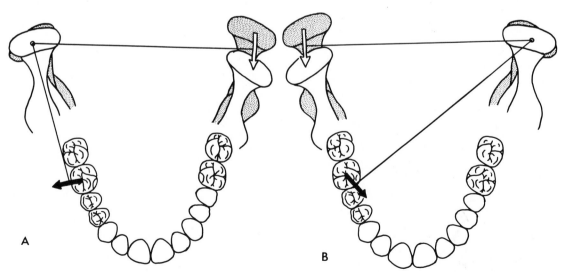

FIGURE 9–12   *A,* With the distobuccal cusp of the mandibular first molar used as an example, this diagram shows that the working pathway is represented by the buccal groove of the maxillary molar. *B,* The nonworking pathway of the maxillary molar takes a mesiolingual direction.

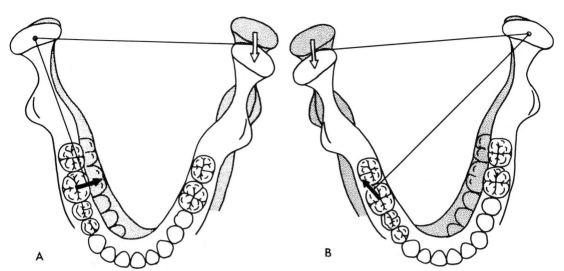

FIGURE 9–13 *A,* With the mesiolingual cusp of the maxillary first molar used as an example, this diagram shows that the working pathway is represented by the lingual groove of the mandibular molar. *B,* The nonworking pathway of the mandibular tooth takes a distobuccal direction.

During the remounting procedure, interferences in eccentric position are corrected before those of the centric position; this sequence helps to prevent overreduction of a casting in centric position. The amount of correction necessary in castings is usually very slight compared with the initial adjustments required for correction of the gross interferences.

Prelimary Rebuilding of Dental Structures with Amalgam

Several years ago the most popular method for rebuilding teeth was the placement of gold onlays or crowns, with cast pins for retention. The pins had to be parallel to one another to allow the restoration to be seated. Broken-down teeth with conical roots did

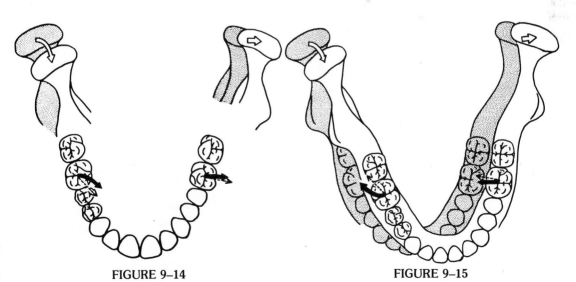

FIGURE 9–14   FIGURE 9–15

FIGURE 9–14   Bennett movement alters the border pathways, permitting the mandibular buccal cusps to reach more distally on the maxillary teeth during lateral movements. (Bennett movement is represented by the dark arrows.)
FIGURE 9–15   The maxillary lingual cusps can reach more mesially on the mandibular teeth. Notice that Bennett movement has a greater influence on the nonworking than on the working side (dark arrows).

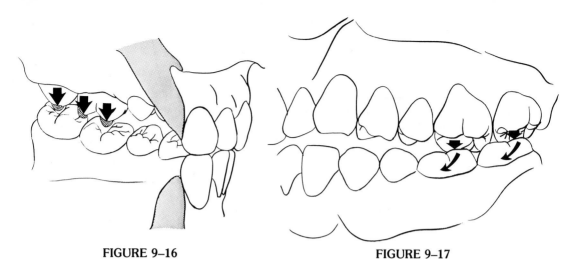

FIGURE 9–16   FIGURE 9–17

FIGURE 9–16   This view cannot be seen by direct observation of patient's mouth because it is obscured by the teeth, lips, cheeks, and tongue. The diagram demonstrates how nonworking side interferences can be inadvertently created by grinding of the canines on the working side.

FIGURE 9–17   This view can be seen only with a mirror or by severe retraction of the lips and cheeks. The opposing interfering inclines are marked with tape or ribbons as the mandible is guided along the border paths of lateral movement.

not provide much tooth structure for placement of the parallel pins. Also, the large amount of metal required for the casting was conducive to postoperative thermal sensitivity in the tooth. In addition, the costs of laboratory work and metal were excessive. The use of stainless steel pins to aid in the retention of silver amalgam restorations or

composite restorations has provided an important solution to the problem of rebuilding broken-down teeth. The amalgam or composite resin is used to restore the teeth to normal contour and anatomy before mouth rehabilitation with cast metal or porcelain-fused-to-metal restorations.

The advantages of building up teeth before preparing them for final restorations are evident. On the completion of the bases, the dentist knows the condition of the teeth. If endodontic therapy is needed, it may be

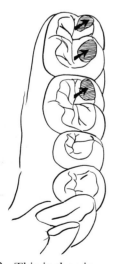

FIGURE 9–18   This is the view commonly seen in the mouth after the interferences have been marked. Now a decision must be made concerning where to grind, because opposing centric cusps are involved.

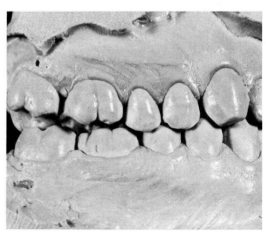

FIGURE 9–19   A close study of the casts will reveal the locations of the centric holding cusps.

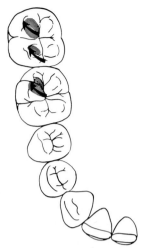

FIGURE 9–20 Corrections for the nonworking side interference can be made on the maxillary or mandibular teeth. In this instance, nonworking side escapeways can be made on the mandibular teeth without jeopardizing the centric stability because the mandibular buccal cusps do not act as centric stops (see Fig. 9–19).

accomplished at this time. The teeth are known to be sound and to be capable of providing retention for castings.

Silver amalgam as a core has the following advantages over composite resin: (1) cariostatic activity, (2) seal of margins, (3) lack of water sorption during service, and (4) less pulpal reaction.

Composite resin as a core has the following advantages over silver amalgam: (1) speed of placement, (2) early strength, and (3) less thermal conductivity.

The author favors silver amalgam as a build-up if one or more of the following conditions are present: (1) history of high caries activity or (2) very little remaining supragingival tooth structure, requiring that the core placement be close to the final margin of the restoration.

The author uses composite resin as a build-up when only a small portion of the coronal portion of the tooth needs rebuilding.

Procedures for Amalgam Build-up

An example of a typical patient requiring preliminary restoration of all posterior teeth before reconstructive procedures is shown in Figure 9–23. In such instances, rebuilding of the teeth may be accomplished with a minimal expenditure of time and minimal discomfort to the patient by use of the following procedures.

Diagnostic Procedures. A definitive treatment plan should be formulated before the amalgam base restorations are begun. Teeth with little coronal tooth structure remaining, for which full-crown restorations are planned, require retentive pins and amalgam build-up. Teeth for which gold onlays are planned may not require amalgam build-up, because the basic cusp structure

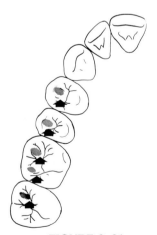

FIGURE 9–21

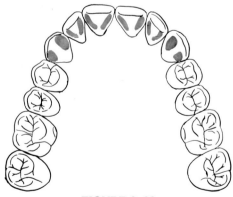

FIGURE 9–22

FIGURE 9–21 Cuspal interferences in the protrusive glide can be detected on the lingual triangular ridges of the maxillary buccal cusps (as shown here) and on the buccal triangular ridges of the mandibular lingual cusps.

FIGURE 9–22 Whenever possible, the adjustments made should limit tooth contacts during eccentric movements to the anterior teeth.

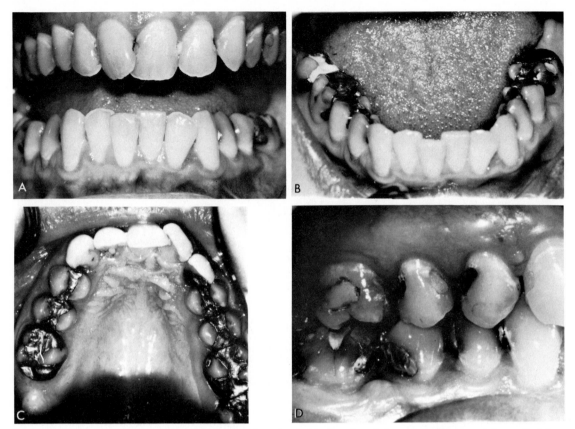

FIGURE 9–23 *A,* Labial view of 30-year-old patient showing breakdown of old restorations. *B,* Mandibular occlusal view showing broken-down amalgams requiring replacement. Note the lack of proper occlusal anatomy and contour on the molar restorations. *C,* Maxillary occlusal view. *D,* Recurrent caries, amalgam breakdown, and silicate cement dissolution are evident in both arches.

will usually retain the onlay, and the onlay itself strengthens the tooth. Teeth requiring slightly more preparation length may be built up with composite resin.

Preoperative full-mouth radiographs are helpful for estimating the pulpal condition of each tooth and the extent of the carious lesions. Bite-wing radiographs are particularly valuable for the determination of the presence of dental caries and the locations to place retentive pins.

Accurately mounted diagnostic casts supplementing an occlusal examination will reveal the areas that need occlusal adjustment. These areas should be adjusted before the amalgam procedures are begun. *The patient's occlusion should be acceptable before any amalgam build-up is started to allow maximal time for temporomandibular joint response, repositioning, and healing.*

A careful, detailed oral examination and the communication of the findings to the pa-tient are necessary preoperative measures. The need for endodontic therapy, possible extractions, and other foreseeable problems should be explained thoroughly. Periodontal therapy may be completed before, or during, the restorative treatment. (The patient whose teeth are shown in Figure 9–23 was treated periodontally prior to restorative treatment.)

Isolation of All Teeth on One Side of the Mouth With an Extra-Heavy Rubber Dam. If a great deal of amalgam build-up is necessary, the treatment may have to be accomplished one quadrant at a time. However, to conserve time, it is preferable that an entire side of the mouth be built up at one time.

The use of a metal abrasive strip on the contact areas of the old restorations facilitates placement of the dam (Fig. 9–24). The time the rubber dam saves in the total operation and the additional safety it provides by

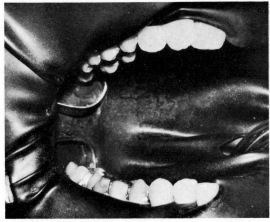

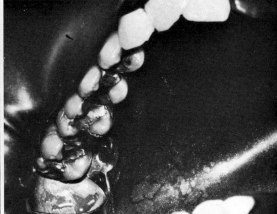

FIGURE 9–24   **FIGURE 9–25**

FIGURE 9–24   Extra-heavy rubber dam, applied to one half of the mouth, retracts the tongue and cheeks as well as the gingival tissue, protects the patient from swallowing or aspirating debris, and keeps saliva and blood from the area.
FIGURE 9–25   Maxillary right quadrant prior to amalgam removal.

its protection of the pharynx and trachea are certainly reasons enough for its use. Since the application of the dam provides an unobstructed operating field, the dentist may work efficiently, using his time and effort to the best advantage. Also, patients usually feel protected and reassured by the placement of the dam.

Removal of Maxillary and Mandibular Amalgam Restorations.   Figure 9–25 shows the preoperative view of one quadrant, which will be illustrated to the completion of the amalgam bases. An ultrahigh-speed handpiece and a suitable bur, such as a No. 56 or 57, allow removal of amalgam restorations in a minimum of time. A water spray and high-velocity suction apparatus are essential adjuncts to this procedure. Cavity preparations should be typical in form, with the exception that retentive areas in dentin should be accentuated. These areas will help to keep the deeper portions of the amalgam in place when the exterior tooth preparation is made later. If any of the existing restorations that are to be replaced do not require amalgam bases, they may be left intact until the teeth are prepared for the final restorations.

Removal of Deep Amalgam and Bases. Questionable areas of deep caries should be left intact until the bulk of the old amalgam has been removed (Fig. 9–26). Removal of all deep areas simultaneously is a more organized, safer, and less time-consuming

method than removal of deep areas one at a time as the bulk of the amalgam is removed (Fig. 9–27). After the old amalgam restorations, including deep areas, have been removed, it should be determined whether any teeth will require endodontic therapy. To allow easy access to the pulp in a tooth that will have to be treated endodontically, a soft base material may be placed in the area over the pulp with the amalgam base surrounding it. Pulp extirpation may then be accomplished after placement of the base amalgam in remaining teeth.

Placement of Pulp Protective Materials. Pulp protective materials were discussed under Biologic Considerations in this chapter.

Many old restorations, particularly amalgams, have very little base material under them. When these restorations are replaced, bases of zinc phosphate or other materials need not be used under the amalgam. The dental pulps have responded already to the depth of the old restoration. A thin layer of calcium hydroxide (about 0.5 mm thick) followed by cavity varnish is recommended for these areas. Since each situation presents different problems, the clinical judgment of the dentist is the final deciding factor in determining whether insulating bases are necessary (Fig. 9–28).

Pin Placement.   Those teeth that require retentive pins may be treated simultaneously. The vast majority of retentive pins used under core build-up materials are of

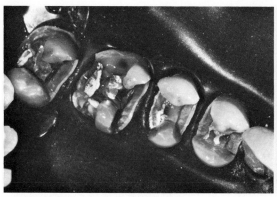

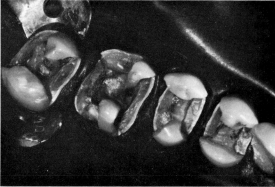

FIGURE 9–26   FIGURE 9–27

FIGURE 9–26 Removal of gross amalgam, with the deepest portions of old restorations and base left intact.

FIGURE 9–27 Removal of all deep areas of old restorations and base at one time is more efficient and safer than removal of single deep areas during excavation of gross amalgam.

the "screw-in" type (Fig. 9–28). The individual dentist's preference will determine the number of pins needed. However, as few pins as possible should be used, since pulp exposure may occur during preparation of the channel for the pin. The pins should extend about 1.5 to 2.0 mm into the tooth and amalgam. Excessive length is unnecessary.

Matrix and Amalgam Placement. The final contouring and carving of the amalgam bases do not require the same attention as that given an amalgam that is to be used as a final restoration. However, proximal contact and coverage of all cavosurface margins are desirable because the restorations will serve for a short time before final tooth preparation.

Two mechanical matrices separated by one tooth may be applied at the same time (Fig. 9–29). After the two amalgams have been placed and carved, the matrices are then transferred to the remaining two teeth, and the amalgam bases are inserted (Fig. 9–30). At times, use of the Caulk Auto Matrix is very desirable for build-up procedures.

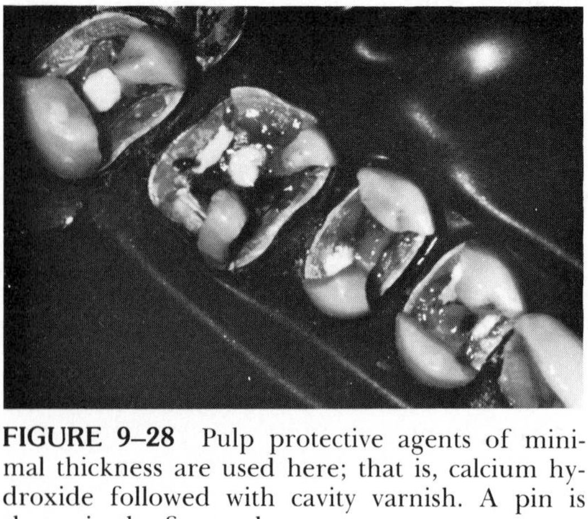

Usually there are enough cusps remaining to allow an approximation of the correct occlusal plane. After placement of all restorations and removal of the rubber dam, additional carving may be necessary.

Occlusal Correction. Since a great amount of tooth structure is replaced when amalgam bases are inserted, a careful postoperative analysis of the occlusion is necessary before the patient is released. Since both the mandibular and the maxillary teeth on one side are anesthetized, adjusting the occlusion may be difficult; nonetheless, the occlusion should be adjusted to remove gross prematurities in all mandibular excursions. (The dentist may want to follow the technique described in the section on occlusal adjustment.) It is desirable to wait at least 1 week before the tooth preparation session to allow recovery from the trauma of the build-up procedure. If occlusal prematurities are not removed, patient discomfort and trauma to the teeth will be severe during that time.

FIGURE 9–28 Pulp protective agents of minimal thickness are used here; that is, calcium hydroxide followed with cavity varnish. A pin is shown in the first molar.

The Acid Etch–Resin Concept in Complex Restorative Dentistry

In past decades, complex rehabilitation implied that all teeth would receive the most long-lasting restorative therapy possible. This

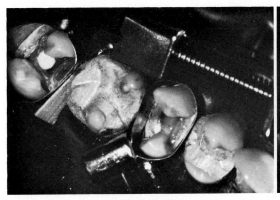
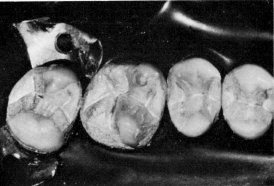

FIGURE 9–29   FIGURE 9–30

FIGURE 9–29   Two circumferential matrices in place. Insertion of restorations alternately rather than consecutively provides maximal access for contact area restoration and ease of manipulation.
FIGURE 9–30   Base amalgams inserted.

included Class III, IV, and V inlays, with various difficult techniques to allow these anterior tooth restorations to be acceptable esthetically. Further, it included porcelain jacket or other crowns on teeth that were only partially destroyed, resulting in the needless cutting away of significant amounts of tooth structure.

The introduction and eventual popularity of the acid etch–resin concept have changed previous beliefs and attitudes significantly. Practitioners are now preserving moderately broken-down or carious anterior teeth with acid etch–resin procedures instead of more extensive and expensive crowns or other cast restorations. These techniques allow esthetically pleasing, relatively simple, easily replaced, inexpensive anterior tooth restorations of intermediate longevity for patients receiving oral rehabilitation. However, patients should be advised that acid etch–resin restorations have an expected esthetic longevity of 3 to 5 years or more and that they may need to be replaced at that time.

Acid Etching of Teeth for Resin Retention

The procedure of acid etching of enamel for retention of resin was introduced into dentistry during the mid-1960s. Various procedures and concepts have been used with varying levels of success since that time. The technique has been practiced commonly in dentistry since the early 1970s, and clinical investigations have shown effective retention of resin over several years.

Currently accepted acid etching procedures follow.

1. *Débridement.* Clean tooth surfaces thoroughly with flour of pumice and water in a soft rubber cup to remove surface debris. Use of fluoride-containing or oil-containing prophylactic pastes should be avoided because they inhibit the acid-etch procedure.

2. *Tooth Structure Removal.* Removal of a few microns of tooth enamel on surfaces on which resin will cover the superficial enamel layers (veneers, and so on) is desirable to remove the fluoride-rich, acid-resistant layer, thus enhancing the action of the acid etchant.

3. *Acid Etch.* Etch with 37 to 50 per cent unbuffered phosphoric acid. Although investigations have used citric, lactic, nitric, and other acids, the preponderance of opinion and scientific research supports the use of phosphoric acid at this time. The etchant may be liquid or gel. Liquids are used more commonly, but gels may be desirable occasionally to control the extent of the etchant more carefully. Liquids have been shown to effect a more homogeneous etch than gels. Whichever mode of delivering acid to the tooth surface is used, the dentist must take care to restrict the acid etchant to the area to be etched, keeping it away from adjacent teeth to avoid unwanted etching. Research has suggested that the etchant be placed on the enamel surface and allowed to etch for 60 seconds for permanent teeth and 120 seconds for primary teeth. Scrubbing the etchant into the tooth is not desirable and overetching should be avoided. Dentin surfaces

do not etch well with phosphoric acid, and acid placement on these surfaces is not necessary or desirable.

4. *Wash.* Etched surfaces should be washed for 15 to 30 seconds with water spray from a typical dental air-water syringe. This time period may seem excessive, but research has shown that there is an increasing bond strength when surfaces are washed for longer periods of time up to 30 seconds. In an area where the water does not contain minerals, washing may continue for up to 30 seconds. If your water is highly mineralized, 15 seconds is adequate, since the etched surfaces will begin to remineralize from the minerals in the water.

5. *Dry.* Etched enamel surfaces should be dried thoroughly with a clean, dry, non-oily air stream. Many air lines in dental offices are contaminated with oil or water. The dentist can determine easily if his line is contaminated by blowing air on a transparent glass or plastic surface. If an oil or water scum appears, the air lines need to be repaired, or an air dryer should be placed on the lines. Use of one of several commercially available drying agents containing ethanol, ether, acetone, or other chemicals will remove the oil scum and debris from etched enamel surfaces, but avoidance of depositing the scum initially is the best solution.

One of the major reasons for failure of acid etch–resin restorations is contamination of the etched enamel surface with oil, dirty water, saliva, blood, debris from the dentist's fingers, or other matter. If such contamination is suspected, the surfaces should be re-etched for 10 seconds, washed, dried, and re-evaluated visually for a clean, even, chalky appearance.

Use of Bonding Agents

Many studies have supported the use of bonding agents (unfilled or slightly filled, nonviscous BIS-GMA [bisphenol A glycidyl methacrylate] resins) before placement of filled, putty resin into or onto etched enamel surfaces. These resins have been shown to improve the seal of the filled resin to the etched tooth surfaces, thereby lessening leakage at a subsequent time. Conversely, some investigators have shown that bonding agents are unnecessary, contending that the filled resin can be placed on the etched surfaces adequately without a bonding agent.

Many tooth restorations are placed in or on relatively inaccessible locations, where it is illogical to assume that mere placement of a putty mass into a preparation will assure physical contact of the putty resin with the etched enamel walls. In fact, it is difficult in some clinical situations to be certain that all of the intricate aspects of the tooth preparation are filled with fluid-bonding resin, much less viscous, puttylike, filled resin.

For the aforementioned reasons, the author suggests strongly the following bonding procedure for allowing the optimal contact of resin with etched enamel walls, the highest achievable level of retention, and the lowest leakage patterns at a later time: (1) After thorough drying of etched surfaces with dry, clean air stream, apply a small amount of a bonding agent. (2) Blow a stream of air onto the bonding agent, driving most of it out of the tooth preparation and leaving only a thin layer of bonding agent present on the acid-etched surface. (3) Place putty directly on the bonding agent, not allowing time for the bonding agent to set. This technique assures the thinnest layer of bonding agent possible, the optimal physical contact of resin with tooth, and the shortest time involvement. It is *not* necessary to polymerize the layer of bonding agent before placing the putty resin.

Acid Etch–Resin Procedures Useful in Complex Restorations

Adding Onto the Contour of Teeth. Frequently patients are encountered who require numerous complex restorations in the posterior of the mouth, who do not desire orthodontics, and who have one or more anterior tooth diastemas. Such spaces between teeth can be closed easily by following the procedures outlined and by adding resin onto enamel tooth surfaces that are unprepared mechanically. Attempts are not made to overlay facial tooth surfaces excessively unless necessitated by discoloration or other factors. The resin "add-on" is placed only to the extent that the contour of the teeth needs to be extended. Such restorations are strong, are esthetically pleasing, and have a longevity of several years. Replacement in future years is accomplished easily and is inexpensive for the patient. Figures 9–31 and 9–32 show the before and after views of a diastema closure using a smooth surface microfill resin.

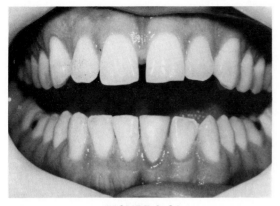

FIGURE 9–31

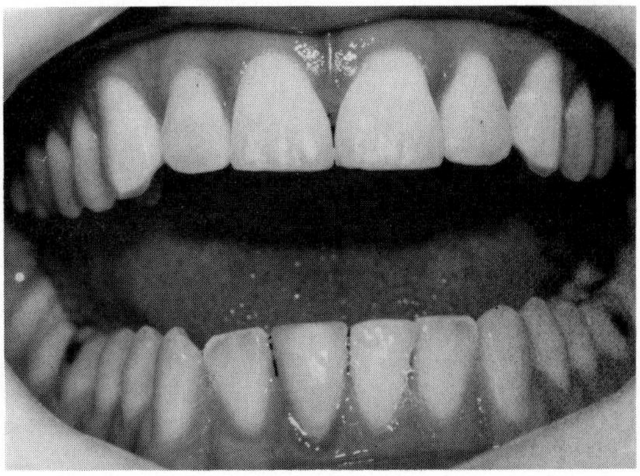

FIGURE 9–32

FIGURE 9–31   Facial view of a patient desiring the closure of a diastema between teeth Nos. 8 and 9 but not desiring more extensive and expensive therapy with crowns or orthodontics.
FIGURE 9–32   Completed view of patient shown in Figure 9–31 demonstrating closure of diastema with a smooth-surfaced microfill resin (Kulzer, Durafill).

Class IV Restorations.   Extensive oral rehabilitations of past years almost demanded replacing Class IV restorations with difficult and often unesthetic cast-gold or gold-foil. Although cast-gold and gold-foil restorations are extremely desirable restorations where indicated, acid etch–resin restorations are reliable, intermediate-longevity substitutes for them in extensive facial display situations. Research has supported the several-year longevity of Class IV acid etch–resin restorations. When the procedures outlined previously are carried out carefully, the restorations are strong and esthetic. However, replacement at a later date must be planned and explained to the patient. Figures 9–33 and 9–34 demonstrate a typical Class IV treatment situation.

Veneering.   Occasionally, discolored, notched, eroded, abraded, or otherwise esthetically unpleasing anterior teeth may be treated by veneering a small amount of resin on the facial surfaces of acid-etched teeth. Such procedures are sometimes desirable for patients in need of extensive oral rehabilitation. The results of such procedures are shown in Figures 9–35 and 9–36.

Other Acid Etch–Resin Uses in Complex Restorative Dentistry.   Typical Class III and Class V restorations have been shown to be better when completed using the acid-etch concept. Greater longevity and less

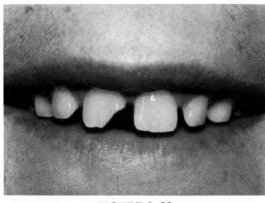

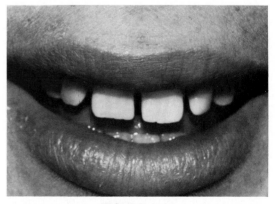

FIGURE 9–33

FIGURE 9–34

FIGURE 9–33   Facial view of tooth requiring Class IV restoration.
FIGURE 9–34   Completed treatment for patient shown in Figure 9–33. A small particle–sized composite resin was used in this situation (L. D. Caulk, Prisma).

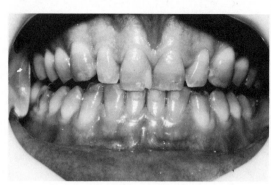

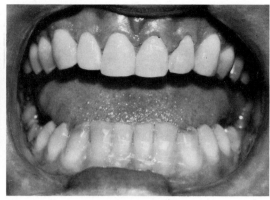

FIGURE 9–35

FIGURE 9–36

FIGURE 9–35 Preoperative photograph of patient for whom acid etch–resin veneers were elected instead of full crown restorations.

FIGURE 9–36 Completed veneer treatment for patient shown in Figure 9–35 (Vivadent, Heliosit).

margin staining should be observed when the acid-etch and bonding procedures are used for all resin restorations.

Splinting of teeth with acid etch–resin procedures is very useful for patients who have mobile teeth but who do not desire to have crowns or onlays for splinting. Simple restorative procedures, accompanied by a piece of orthodontic wire placed lingually and resin placed interproximally and lingually, can create strong, esthetic, long-lasting splints.

Use of the acid etch–resin technique in complex restorative dentistry is an excellent, esthetic, intermediate-longevity substitute for cast-gold, gold-foil, porcelain jacket, or porcelain-fused-to-metal restorations in anterior teeth. It should be considered when a significant amount of anterior tooth structure and tooth strength remain but the patient's appearance demands new tooth-colored restorations. However, dentists should warn patients about the necessity to replace these restorations eventually, the requirement of avoiding excessively hard foods, and the availability of other stronger but more radical and expensive esthetic alternatives.

Tooth Preparations for Extracoronal Restorations

Designs for the preparation of teeth for crowns or onlays vary in details, depending on the individual operator and the individual tooth. The author's concepts of adequate tooth preparation are portrayed by shaded drawings and are described in the following sections.

MOD Gold Onlays

These restorations are used for rebuilding and strengthening single teeth, or they may be soldered together to provide splinting for several teeth. The MOD onlay covers the entire occlusal surface of the tooth and, therefore, provides the dentist with an opportunity to modify the occlusion. Research has shown that the onlay strengthens the buccal and lingual cusps instead of weakening them, as the intracoronal inlay does. The buccal and lingual gingival tissues are not irritated by margins inasmuch as these margins of the onlay are above the gingiva. They are also plainly visible and readily accessible for careful finishing. These restorations represent the most conservative treatment for badly involved carious teeth. They are excellent for teeth that have no carious involvement on the buccal or lingual surfaces and yet require a strong restoration. *The author does not recommend gold onlays for fixed partial denture retainers.*

Important cavity characteristics shown in Figure 9–37 are:

Outline Form. The buccal and lingual proximal extensions should be prepared to allow at least 0.5 to 1.0 mm clearance between the cavity preparation margin and the adjacent tooth. This provides space for adequate finishing and permits good cleansing of the margins by the patient.

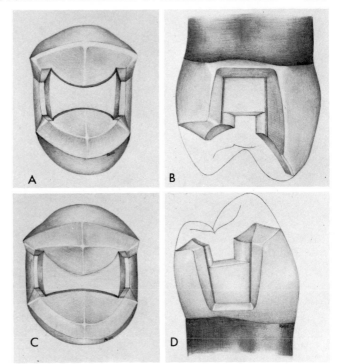

FIGURE 9–37 *A,* Occlusal view of MOD onlay preparation for a maxillary premolar. *B,* Proximal view. *C,* MOD onlay preparation for a mandibular premolar, occlusal view. *D,* Proximal view.

Resistance Form. One to 1.5 mm of gold should cover all the occlusal surfaces, except those at the bucco-occlusal line angle of maxillary teeth. This thickness of gold is sufficient for strength and provides adequate bulk for the reproduction of occlusal anatomy. For esthetic reasons the buccal coverage of maxillary teeth should be limited to 0.5 mm. Buccal cusps of mandibular teeth are usually the pestle or "chewing" cusps and should be covered with a sufficient amount of gold to provide optimal strength (1.0 to 1.5 mm).

Retention Form. Box forms should have very slightly divergent walls. Since the occlusogingival length of the tooth has been reduced, the restoration for the short crown needs maximal retention. Sharp internal angles made with hand instruments or carefully placed, pounded, parallel internal forms placed with No. 1170 or 1171 burs are advised.

Bevels. All cavosurface margins should be carefully beveled. Sharp angles should not be left at the external junctions of the occlusal bevels and at the proximal flares of the preparation. Bevels are best placed with No. 7901 or 7902 trimming and finishing burs.

Anterior Three-quarter Crown

This type of restoration is indicated (1) when the incisal angles of a single tooth have been weakened by proximal caries but the labial surface remains intact and (2) when an anterior tooth with an intact labial surface is needed as a fixed partial denture retainer.

Although used less than in past years, the anterior three-quarter crown may be a restoration that preserves the esthetic appearance and harmony of the tooth, or it may be unesthetic, with a large display of gold caused by poor treatment planning by the overextension of crown margins. A few years ago an esthetic appearance in fixed partial denture retainers for broken-down anterior teeth was difficult to achieve. The increased use of porcelain-fused-to-metal restorations has decreased the use of the three-quarter crown in the restoration of anterior teeth. Yet the anterior three-quarter crown, if properly prepared, remains an esthetic, strong, retentive, and long-lasting restoration. It should not be used in situations in which metal would be necessary on visible surfaces or in which the tooth has great translucence at the incisal edge. In such situations, a full-coverage esthetic restoration,

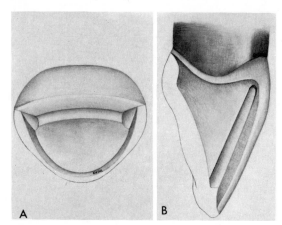

FIGURE 9–38 *A,* A three-quarter crown preparation for a maxillary central incisor, incisal view. *B,* Proximal view.

although more radical, is a better choice for the patient.

Important preparation characteristics illustrated in Figure 9–38 are:

Outline Form. The labial outline form should be parallel with the curvature of the adjacent tooth. This provides adequate extension for prevention of caries, and the outline of gold around the tooth blends into the shadows of the interdental embrasures. The proximal and gingival margins should extend adequately toward the gingiva for retention.

Resistance and Retention Form. A thickness of at least 1 mm of metal on the lingual surface of the tooth is advisable for resistance to the forces created by tooth-to-tooth contact. The incisal offset gives extra strength to the casting in the area that supports the maximal occlusal stress. The reduction of the incisal edge should be minimal (0.5 mm or less).

The casting is retained in place by the near-parallelism of all the walls of the preparation, the parallelism of the mesial and distal grooves, and the lingual surface of the preparation; additional retentive aids (pins, box forms, and so on) may be used when deemed necessary. The proximal grooves of the preparation should be parallel to the incisal two thirds of the labial surface. When the grooves are made parallel to the long axis of the tooth, there is a great tendency to overcut the angles of the tooth and create a square appearance.

Bevels. The proximal surfaces usually have a slight chamfer finish line. The lingual surface has a deep chamfer to facilitate parallelism between the proximal grooves and the lingual surface of the tooth. A slight bevel on the incisal edge provides adequate thickness of metal and supported enamel for finishing and does not detract appreciably from the esthetic result of the restoration.

Posterior Three-Quarter Crown

For years these restorations have been commonly used as retainers for posterior fixed partial dentures. Few restorations give the strength, retention, longevity, and esthetic result that a well-constructed posterior three-quarter crown provides (Fig. 9–39).

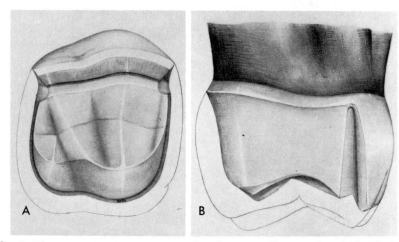

FIGURE 9–39 *A,* Three-quarter crown preparation for a maxillary molar, occlusal view. *B,* Proximal view.

However, these restorations are not used much by most dentists today.

A suggested variation in the usual tooth preparation technique is the use of pin and amalgam build-up in a broken-down tooth prior to the preparation for the three-quarter crown. The amalgam is treated as if it were dentin. The retention added by the stainless-steel pins and the decrease in sensitivity offered by the less conductive amalgam contribute to the success of the three-quarter crown.

Outline Form. Proximal clearance 0.5 to 1.0 mm from the adjacent tooth gingival extension slightly below the gingival margin provides optimal extension for caries prevention.

Resistance and Retention Form. Proximal grooves that are approximately parallel to the long axis of the tooth, and near-parallelism of all walls, retain the casting in place. One to 1.5 mm of metal over the occlusal surface should provide optimal strength. The occlusal offset gives additional resistance to masticatory forces.

Bevels. The same type of bevels and finish lines apply to this preparation as to the anterior three-quarter crown.

Seven-Eighths Crown

A situation often arises in which the mesiobuccal surface of a molar is the only surface that remains unaffected by dental caries or by an old restoration. The use of the seven-eighths crown gives maximal retention and a surprisingly good esthetic result in such cases. The preparation is basically the same as that for a conventional posterior three-quarter crown except that the distal extension is moved onto the buccal surface to approximately the center of the tooth. The parallel buccal and mesial grooves provide good retention (Fig. 9–40).

Porcelain Jacket Crown

Despite the advent of many new restorative materials and techniques, the porcelain jacket crown remains the most esthetic anterior restoration. Its most serious disadvantage is lack of strength. Over the past few years this objection has led to the expanded use of porcelain-fused-to-metal restorations in place of porcelain jacket crowns. A comparison of the tooth reduction necessary for both types of restorations shows that the porcelain jacket crown requires more lingual tooth reduction, but that the porcelain-fused-to-metal crown requires slightly more labial reduction (Figs. 9–41 and 9–42). This extra labial reduction is necessary to compensate for the additional thickness of the metal, opaque coating, and porcelain.

Porcelain jacket crowns or aluminous porcelain jacket crowns are indicated in patients who need a single, or possibly two or three, anterior crowns, and who have light occlusion on the anterior teeth and an absence of overt signs of adverse occlusal habit patterns. They may also be necessary, in spite of the occlusion, in those patients whose tooth color is extremely difficult to match or in patients with unusual esthetic demands. All patients should be warned of the fragility of these crowns and instructed in preventive maintenance.

The characteristics of the tooth preparation are illustrated in Figure 9–41.

Outline Form. Extension slightly below the gingiva on the facial aspect is essential for esthetics. However, the lingual margin may be placed supragingivally if adequate tooth length is present.

Resistance and Retention Form. At least 1 mm of porcelain over the entire surface of the preparation is necessary for strength. The gingival half of the labial surface should be nearly parallel with the lingual wall for retention.

Porcelain-Fused-to-Metal Crown

Adequate strength, good marginal fit, and acceptable esthetic appearance have made

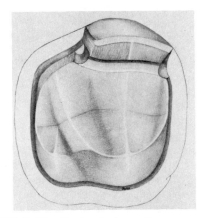

FIGURE 9–40 Occlusal view of a seven-eighths crown preparation for a maxillary molar.

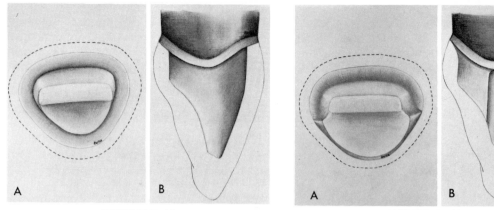

FIGURE 9–41   FIGURE 9–42

FIGURE 9–41   *A,* Porcelain jacket crown preparation for a maxillary central incisor, incisal view. *B,* Proximal view.
FIGURE 9–42   *A,* A porcelain-fused-to-metal crown preparation for a maxillary central incisor, incisal view. *B,* Proximal view.

this restoration very popular. Its esthetic limitations have been widely discussed. However, proper tooth preparation and the use of internal and external stains can produce acceptable esthetic restorations. At least 1.0 to 1.5 mm of tooth structure must be removed from the labial surface of the tooth to allow the ceramist to construct an esthetic and properly contoured restoration. Underpreparation is the most frequent error encountered in the construction of porcelain-fused-to-metal crowns and is a serious detriment to periodontal health.

Tooth preparation characteristics are shown in Figure 9–42.

Outline Form.   Extension slightly below the gingiva on the facial surface is essential for an esthetically pleasing result.

Resistance and Retention Form.   The casting is retained in place by near-parallel proximal walls and the near-parallelism of the labial half of the preparation with the lingual surface of the preparation.

The preparation of the lingual one half of the tooth is similar to that for an anterior three-quarter crown. Additional space for the porcelain must be provided at the contact areas.

Margins.   The lingual one half of the preparation has a chamfer margin; the labial one half of the tooth has a deep chamfer (near shoulder) to allow the placement of porcelain to the gingival margin. In posterior teeth or in areas where gingival appearance is not important, many dentists have used a bevel on the labial or buccal surface. In those situations, a collar of metal remains around the gingival area. Research has not supported the theory that such bevels produce more tightly adapted margins than butt-joint castings for porcelain-bearing metal surfaces.

Posterior Full Metal Crown

Full metal crowns are indicated primarily for the restoration of broken-down posterior teeth and as retainers for fixed partial dentures. Since the retention in a well-made three-quarter or seven-eighths crown may actually exceed that in a full crown, full crowns should not be used solely to gain additional retention. In many instances, pin and amalgam build-up are indicated prior to preparation for full-crown restorations.

A typical tooth preparation for the full gold crown is illustrated in Figure 9–43.

Outline Form.   Margins are located apically enough for adequate retention but need not be subgingival. A rubber dam and clamp may be used to retract the gingival tissue to facilitate the preparation and the seating of the crown. Gingival margins are better when placed on enamel than on dentin.

Resistance and Retention Form.   One to 1.5 mm of metal coverage is necessary for adequate strength and to provide thickness for the reproduction of occlusal anatomy.

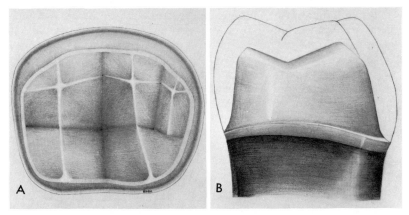

FIGURE 9–43 *A,* Full crown preparation for a mandibular molar, occlusal view. *B,* Proximal view.

Nearly parallel walls are necessary for retention. Grooves placed in the buccal and lingual surfaces may provide additional retention if necessary.

Dowel Crown

Treatment of an endodontically involved tooth is not complete until a strong restoration has been placed. The necessity for extracoronal coverage has already been emphasized. When there is little or no

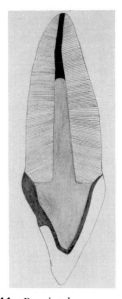

FIGURE 9–44 Proximal cross section of cast metal dowel crown, with a porcelain-fused-to-metal crown cemented over it.

supragingival tooth structure for retention of a crown, a dowel crown will provide an excellent restoration (Fig. 9–44).

The dowel should be prepared to approximately two thirds of the root length. A metal casting is made to fit into the root and to form a simulated crown preparation. The margins of the final restoration should cover the dowel and should terminate on solid tooth structure apical to the margins of the dowel. If, for some reason, the final restoration fails, it may be removed without endangering the root or the endodontic therapy.

One-Visit Post-and-Core Build-up. The technique of fitting a prefabricated stainless-steel post two thirds of the way down the root canal, placing two accessory pins mesial and distal to the post (TMS Minikin or similar product), and building up the coronal portion with composite or amalgam has nearly replaced the cast post-and-core procedure. Research and clinical use have supported such procedures, and the economy, efficiency, speed, and success of the technique assure its continuation.

Rehabilitation of One Side of the Mouth at a Time

Indications

Rehabilitation of one side of the mouth at a time provides an opportunity for the dentist to develop or to retain a functional occlusion for the patient who requires multiple restorations. It does not involve the problems that are often associated with restoration of all the teeth simultaneously, such as a change in vertical dimension and establishment of an entirely new occlusal pattern. The following characteristics make patients candidates for this treatment procedure: nonpainful, functioning occlusal relationship; no presence of serious occlusal interferences; adequate vertical dimension; no history of temporomandibular joint pain; and badly broken-down restorations that need replacing. These patients often have several posterior teeth that do not require occlusal coverage. Also, many times their anterior teeth are fundamentally sound and do not require full-coverage restorations. The restorations used in such dental reconstruction, therefore, may be either extracoronal or intracoronal.

Procedures

The following sequence of procedures is suggested for the restoration of the posterior teeth on one side of the mouth in a minimal amount of time.

Mounted Diagnostic Casts. It is desirable that accurate impressions of the patient's mouth be made and that casts be mounted correctly on the articulator. Occlusal interferences should be determined and provision made for their correction. A tentative treatment plan should be developed with the aid of these casts and full-mouth radiographs. The plan should be reviewed carefully and presented to the patient before final decisions are made and treatment is begun.

Initial Adjustment of Gross Occlusal Interferences. The technique described earlier should be used for correction of gross occlusal interferences determined by analysis of the diagnostic casts.

Rebuilding of Broken-down Teeth. The technique described previously for the use of amalgam or composite resin in rebuilding tooth structure may be used to provide a sound foundation before further tooth preparation. Tooth build-up for the entire mouth should be completed before final tooth preparation.

Occlusal Correction. Much of the occlusion is usually changed by the placement of the amalgam bases. Since all the teeth on one side of the mouth are to be rehabilitated, the occlusal interferences must be relieved before the teeth are prepared for ex-

tracoronal restorations and the working casts are mounted in the articulator.

Tooth Preparation. The author has recommended and illustrated several basic preparations for extracoronal restorations of broken-down teeth. The types of restorations used will depend on the problems presented by the patient. The most conservative preparations that can be used, in keeping with the specific functional and esthetic needs of the individual, should be chosen.

Depending on the ability of the patient to tolerate dental treatment and the speed of the operator, the preparation of teeth may be accomplished in one or two appointments. It is preferable to prepare all the posterior teeth on one side of the mouth in one appointment to eliminate the repetition of many procedures.

If all the preparations on one side of the mouth are to be made at one appointment, the maxillary and mandibular teeth to be treated should be anesthetized simultaneously. All the tooth structure removal to be done by one instrument is accomplished at one time. For example, if a flame-shaped diamond is used for proximal reduction, it should be used on the proximal surfaces of all teeth to be prepared before instruments are changed. Approximately 1.0 to 1.5 mm of occlusal clearance should be provided for placement of each occlusal coverage restoration. Therefore, following preparation, 2 to 3 mm of space will exist between the maxillary and mandibular teeth. (Figure 9–45 shows one quadrant of the preparation com-

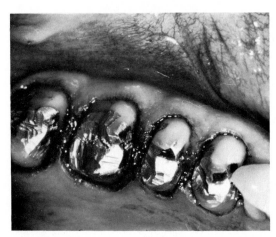

FIGURE 9–45 Crown preparations completed for the teeth shown in Figure 9–46. The amalgam cores were used as retentive structure.

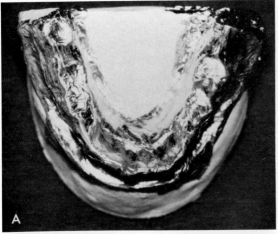

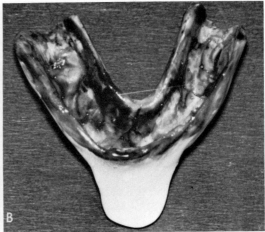

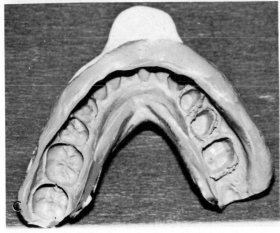

FIGURE 9–46 *A,* Mandibular cast ready for tray acrylic resin. Aluminum foil, which is used as a separating medium, can be applied rapidly; it is not necessary to remove wrinkles for this procedure. *B,* Acrylic resin tray with adhesive material applied, ready for impression. *C,* Completed rubber base impression.

pleted. The teeth used for illustration here are the same as those used for illustration of the amalgam build-up technique.)

Impressions. Polysulfide, addition or condensation reaction silicone, polyether, or hydrocolloid impression materials are excellent for making full-arch impressions. If rubber types of materials are used, custom acrylic resin trays provide the most accurate technique. A suggested technique is illustrated in Figure 9–46. Aluminum foil is adapted to a layer of wax over the occlusal surfaces of the teeth on the diagnostic cast (Fig. 9–46A). At least three "stops" should be provided for proper seating. The cast is then ready to receive the tray acrylic resin. Household aluminum foil provides an excellent separating medium and need not be free from wrinkles for this procedure. Figure 9–46B demonstrates the completed tray with adhesive applied, and Figure 9–46C illustrates the completed impression.

Interocclusal Records. The technique for accurate cast mounting has been described on page 418. A semiadjustable articulator (such as Whip-Mix) is recommended in reconstruction of one side of the mouth, since it is easy to use and sufficiently accurate for the necessary restorative treatment. The ear face-bow, developed for use with the Whip-Mix articulator, can be assembled easily on the patient (Figs. 9–47 and 9–48) and allows accurate maxillary cast mounting. Registrations in material of the operator's choice should be made in centric relation, protrusive, and right and left lateral excursions before the mandibular cast is mounted in the articulator. This articulator permits adjustment of the condylar inclination, incisal guidance, Bennett movement, and intercondylar distance. It is usually desirable to trim the dies after the casts have been mounted on the articulator. Figure 9–49 demonstrates the working casts with the dies

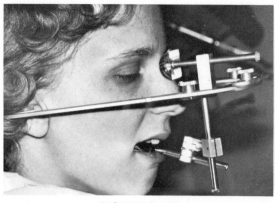
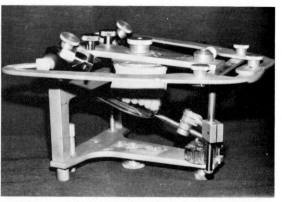

FIGURE 9–47   FIGURE 9–48

FIGURE 9–47   The ear face-bow applied to the patient. Note that the external auditory meatus and nasion are used as anatomic landmarks.

FIGURE 9–48   The face-bow applied to the articulator, relating the maxillary cast to the upper articulator member.

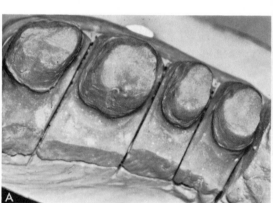
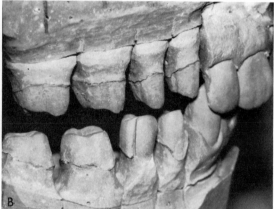

FIGURE 9–49   *A,* Dies trimmed and ready for waxing. *B,* Mounted maxillary and mandibular casts with the dies trimmed. Note adequate interocclusal space for development of functional occlusion.

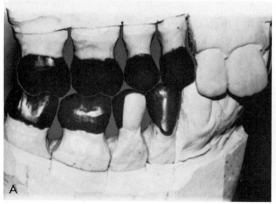
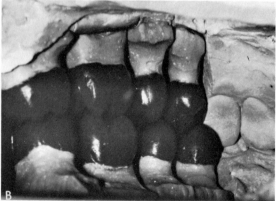

FIGURE 9–50   *A,* Completed wax patterns, buccal view. *B,* Lingual view. Note the centric contacts of the wax patterns.

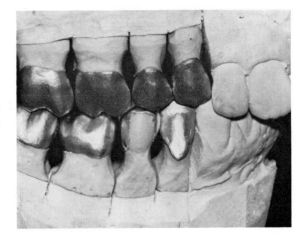

FIGURE 9–51 Raw castings ready to be tried in the mouth. Occlusion can be adjusted at this point when fit of castings is evaluated.

trimmed, ready for the construction of the restorations by the technician or dentist.

Construction of Restorations. The laboratory technician can develop an occlusion for the patient that is nearly ideal and is compatible with the previously adjusted occlusion on the other side of the mouth. Figure 9–50 shows the buccal and lingual aspects of the wax patterns. The importance of adjustment of the natural teeth on the uncut side of the mouth is obvious. If these teeth have interferences, the development of proper occlusion for the new restorations will be seriously hampered.

Try-in and Correction of Castings. It is often desirable to try in castings for porcelain-fused-to-metal restorations at the cast-

ing stage, before placement of any porcelain (Fig. 9–51). If a casting does not fit, this is the most opportune time to make a new impression. If occlusion is not adequate, remount is desirable at this time.

It is also suggested that, after the porcelain has been placed (Fig. 9–52), the dentist try in the restorations again. Margin fit, color match, and occlusion of the restorations may be checked at this time before the final glaze has been placed on the porcelain (Fig. 9–53). If the technician is close by, the restorations can be glazed, polished, and seated at this appointment. If the restorations must be sent out of the office, the final seating must be completed at another appointment.

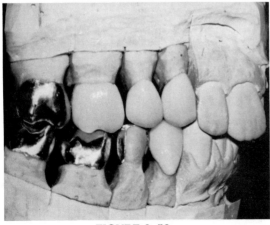

FIGURE 9–52

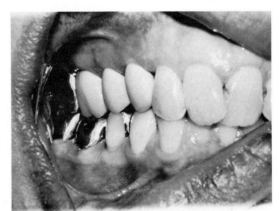

FIGURE 9–53

FIGURE 9–52 Ceramic restorations at high biscuit-firing stage, ready for try-in for color and occlusion.

FIGURE 9–53 Try-in of restorations at high biscuit-firing stage. Color and occlusion were adjusted.

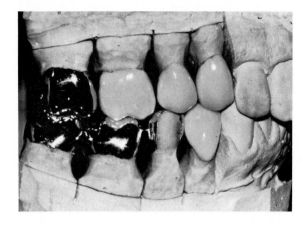

FIGURE 9–54 Completed restorations returned from the laboratory, ready for finishing of margins and cementation.

To facilitate occlusal adjustment during try-in stages, it is suggested that the restorations be tried without anesthesia. First, each restoration should be tried in the mouth individually. Second, all the restorations should be tried in simultaneously, and contact areas should be adjusted. Third, occlusal interferences, if any, should be determined and corrected. All teeth should contact with even pressure in centric occlusion and function as the restorations were planned on the articulator. Remounting the casts is usually not necessary.

Cementation of Final Restorations. Figure 9–54 demonstrates the final restorations as returned from the laboratory. After a brief try-in of the restorations without anesthesia for final checking of the occlusion, the patient is anesthetized, the margins are finished, and the restorations are cemented. Use of a rubber dam in seating inlays and onlays is an excellent procedure. However, a high-velocity evacuation device such as the Vac-Ejector* is extremely helpful during cementation of full crowns, when the routine use of the rubber dam is difficult (Fig. 9–55). This device retracts the tongue and simultaneously dries the maxillary and mandibular teeth on one side. Figure 9–56 shows the restorations for one side of the mouth cemented into place.

The dental rehabilitation process is then repeated for the alternate side of the mouth, beginning with tooth preparation. Occlusion of the alternate side of the mouth is adjusted

---

*The Erickson Vac-Ejector, Erickson Manufacturing Co., 72 Sea Way, San Rafael, CA 94901.

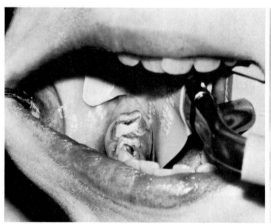

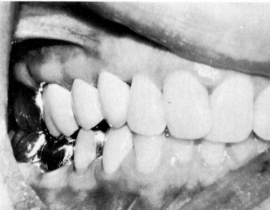

FIGURE 9–55

FIGURE 9–56

FIGURE 9–55 A high-velocity evacuation device is helpful during full crown cementation (Vac-Ejector).
FIGURE 9–56 Cemented restorations, maxillary and mandibular, right side.

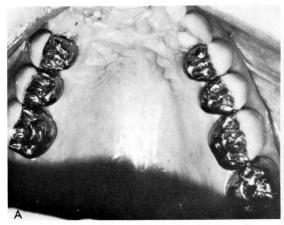

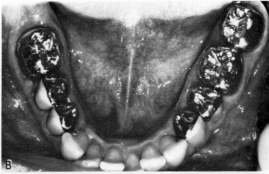

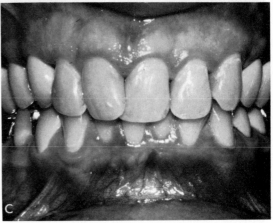

FIGURE 9–57 *A,* Occlusal view of completed maxillary restorations for entire mouth. *B,* Occlusal view of completed mandibular restorations for entire mouth. *C,* Labial view of completed full mouth treatment. Compare with Figure 23*A.*

to the pattern established for the first side.

The completed restorations for the entire mouth appear in Figure 9–57.

Simultaneous Restoration of All Posterior Teeth

Indications

In some clinical situations, the occlusal function of the mouth needs so much changing that all the posterior teeth require gross occlusal alteration. Those patients who need alteration of the vertical dimension of occlusion also require this type of treatment. In such cases, restoration of all posterior teeth on both sides of the mouth at the same time provides the best opportunity for development of a new occlusal relationship.

The differences between this method of dental rehabilitation and the one just described were shown in Table 9–2.

Procedures

The diagnostic casts of the illustrated clinical situation show the mandibular first premolars in lingual version (Fig. 9–58). Before restorative procedures were started, these teeth were orthodontically repositioned under the maxillary premolars (Fig. 9–59). Retention during the treatment phases was accomplished by soldering together the contact areas of the temporary metal castings. The final castings were also soldered together between the first and second premolars (Fig. 9–60).

The Stuart mandibular recorder was used to obtain tracings of the patient's condyle movement (Fig. 9–61). The Stuart articulator was adjusted to follow the recordings (Fig. 9–62). Diagnostic casts were mounted on the articulator and treatment was planned.

Tooth preparation was accomplished one quadrant at a time, and a sectional cast was made at the time each individual quadrant was prepared. (The dies of the sectional casts should accurately reproduce the gingival finish lines. They are used for making the temporary metal castings and for completion of the gingival finish lines for the wax patterns of the permanent castings. Gingival retraction is not repeated when the full-arch impressions are made. The gingival

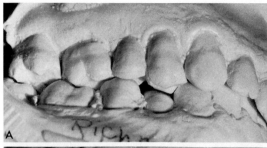

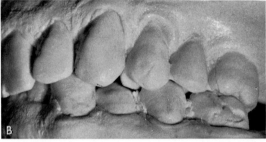

FIGURE 9–58

FIGURE 9–58 **A,** The mandibular first premolar was locked lingual to the maxillary first premolar on the right side. **B,** The left side was similar.

FIGURE 9–59 After space was created interproximally and the opposing occlusion was relieved, the teeth were repositioned buccally.

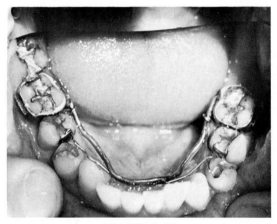

FIGURE 9–59

FIGURE 9–60 The finished casting of the mandibular premolar is made to occlude in the mesial fossa of the opposing maxillary premolar.

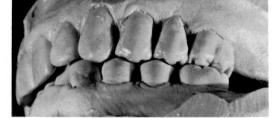

FIGURE 9–60

FIGURE 9–61 Tracings of mandibular movement are made by attaching the recording device rigidly to the maxillary and mandibular teeth.

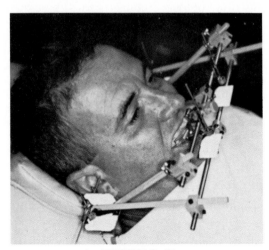

FIGURE 9–61

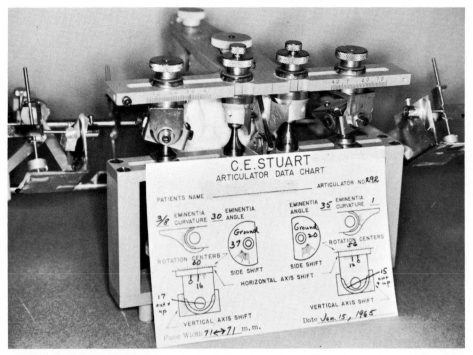

FIGURE 9–62 The controls of the articulator are adjusted to follow the tracings of the patient's mandibular movements.

areas of the full-arch casts are relieved with a round bur to prevent interference with gingival tissue areas.)

Metal temporary castings were made from sectional casts, for one quadrant at a time, and served the patient during the reconstruction. Full-arch casts were then made of all the tooth preparations and mounted in the articulator for the wax-up of the permanent castings (Fig. 9–63).

Formation of the wax patterns is started on the sectional die and transferred to the full-arch cast (Fig. 9–64). All the initial wax patterns are fully seated and joined together at the proximal contacts (Fig. 9–65A and B). They must be maintained as a rigid unit to avoid distortion of the undersurface of the wax during the occlusal waxing.

Reverse pin pontics were made from porcelain denture teeth and shaped to fit the

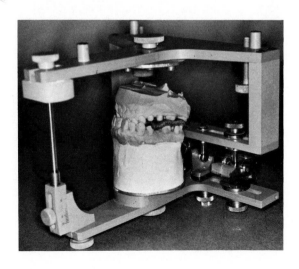

FIGURE 9–63 After the maxillary cast is mounted with the hinge-axis face-bow, the mandibular cast is related to the maxillary cast by means of an interocclusal centric relation wax record.

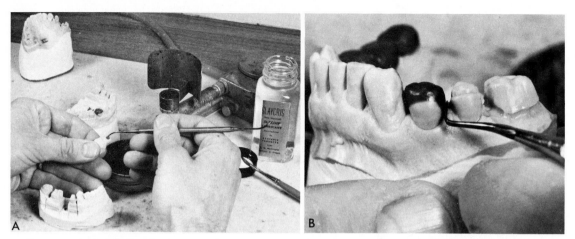

FIGURE 9–64 *A,* The quadrant sectional casts with removable dies are used to facilitate carving of external contours and finish lines in the wax patterns. *B,* The wax patterns, started on the sectional dies, are transferred to the articulated full-arch casts for development of the occlusal surfaces.

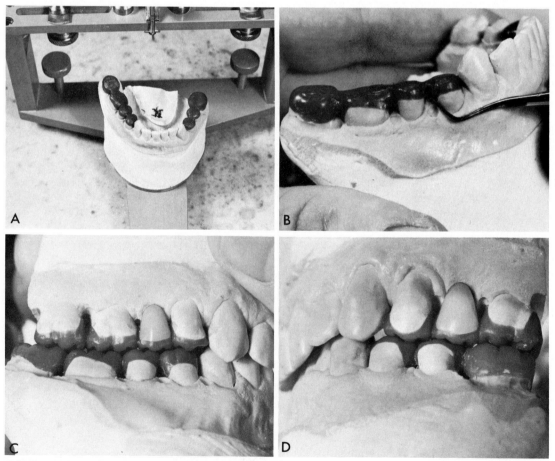

FIGURE 9–65 *A,* Before the occlusal anatomy is developed, the beginning wax patterns are luted together proximally on the full-arch casts (occlusal view). *B,* Proximal view. *C,* As soon as the lengths of the maxillary buccal cusps have been determined, the reverse pin pontics are placed in the edentulous spaces (right side). *D,* Left side.

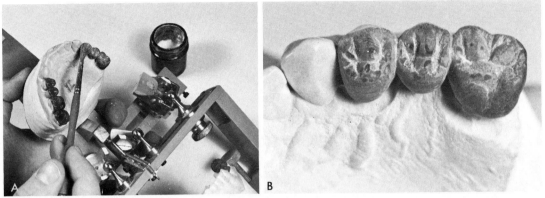

FIGURE 9–66 *A,* Zinc stearate powder provides a means of detecting opposing contacting surfaces in the wax, and it does not interfere with the burn-out or casting procedure. *B,* Occlusal contact with the opposing arch is shown by the darker areas.

edentulous spaces (Fig. 9–65*C* and *D*). Porcelain-fused-to-metal restorations may be used in place of these.

The occlusal surfaces are dusted with talcum powder or zinc stearate, and the articulator is gently closed (Fig. 9–66). Wax is reduced occlusally until the incisal pin contacts the table. Then the cones are located to start the occlusal waxing.

After the waxing of both arches has been completed (Fig. 9–67), the wax patterns are sawed apart with a very thin ribbon saw (Fig. 9–68). The individual sectional dies are again used to perfect the gingival finish line (Fig. 9–69).

After the restorations have been cast into metal, they are seated on the full-arch casts so that the proximal contacts may be adjusted. The castings then are tested in the mouth for final verification of proximal contact. The illustrations in Figure 9–70 show the small button projections that are placed on the buccal or lingual surfaces to aid in removal of the castings after they are tested on the patient's teeth. They are removed before final cementation.

No attempt is made to correct the occlusion on the stone working casts. Instead, separate remount casts are made and mounted in the articulator for the final perfection of the occlusion of the restoration.

Before the fabrication of the remount casts is begun, the soldering index for pontics is obtained in the mouth. When the fit of

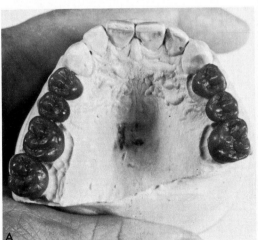
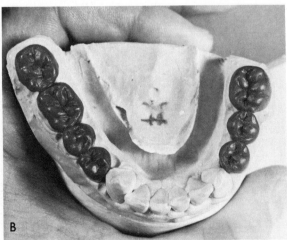

FIGURE 9–67 *A,* The finished wax-up with the wax patterns still joined proximally (maxillary arch). *B,* Mandibular arch.

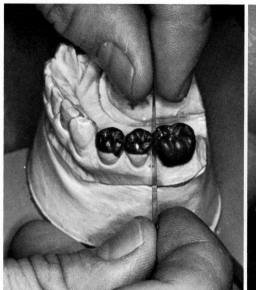
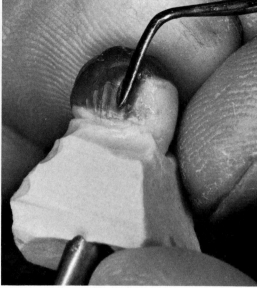

FIGURE 9–68   FIGURE 9–69

FIGURE 9–68   The wax patterns are separated proximally with a very thin ribbon saw.
FIGURE 9–69   The individual sectional dies are again employed to complete the waxing of the finish lines.

the margins of all the castings has been accepted and the soldering has been completed, the hinge-axis face-bow and centric relation records are made. Next, a reinforced acrylic matrix is made over the occlusal surfaces of the restorations (Fig. 9–71A). The matrix is adjusted and sized so that it will cover the occlusal surfaces of the restorations and will also allow an impression tray to pass over it without impingement (Fig. 9–71B). The matrix is used to make a zinc-oxide impression-paste index of the castings after they are fully seated on the patient's teeth (Fig. 9–72). An alginate impression is then made of each arch, with the matrix in place on the teeth. The castings are removed

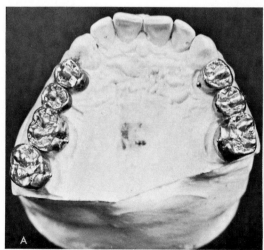
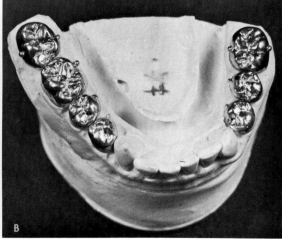

FIGURE 9–70   *A,* The castings are placed on the full-arch working casts so that the proximal contacts may be adjusted; no attempt is made to correct the occlusal surfaces at this time (maxillary view). *B,* Mandibular view.

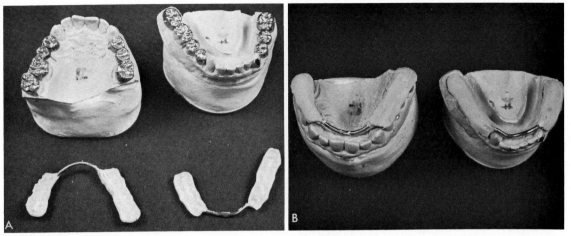

FIGURE 9–71 *A,* A rigid matrix made from acrylic and rigid coat hanger wire is constructed for each arch. *B,* The matrix is adjusted to size on the occlusal surfaces.

from the teeth and carefully seated in the matrix, which has become incorporated in the alginate impression (Fig. 9–73). Low-fusing metal is poured into the castings. Paper clip staples are heated and inserted into the metal for retention of the fast-setting stone, which is subsequently poured to complete the formation of the remount casts (Figs. 9–74 and 9–75).

The remount casts are mounted in the articulator for the final occlusal correction (Fig. 9–76). (The low-fusing metal provides a substantial support for the castings. The

stone working casts would break apart if they were used for occlusal corrections.) Cellophane ribbon, 0.001-inch thick, is used as a feeler gauge for the occlusal corrections. Adjustment is continued until each cusp holds the cellophane with equal tension in the centric position. As eccentric excursions are made, the cellophane pulls out (Fig. 9–77). The occlusal surfaces are finished with a wire brush and No. 1/4 round burs (Fig. 9–78). The corrections made on the remount casts compensate for any slight

Text continued on page 454

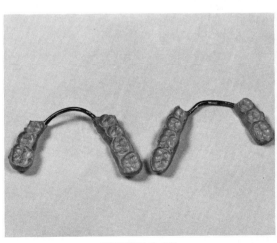

FIGURE 9–72

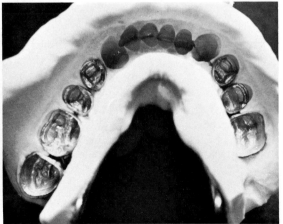

FIGURE 9–73

FIGURE 9–72 A zinc oxide–eugenol impression paste is used in the acrylic matrix to obtain an extremely accurate occlusal index of the castings in the patient's mouth.

FIGURE 9–73 The index is replaced in the mouth, and an alginate impression of the entire arch is made over it. Now the castings are seated in the firm occlusal index, held in the alginate impression.

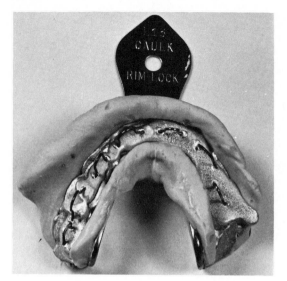

FIGURE 9–74 After the internal surfaces of the castings have been lubricated with silicone, a low-fusing metal is poured into the impression. Paper clip staples are then inserted in the metal.

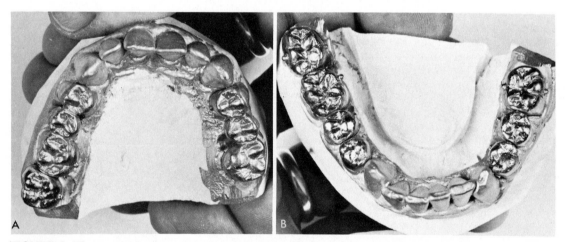

FIGURE 9–75 *A,* The remount casts are now ready to be mounted in the articulator for the final refinement of the occlusion in gold. The low-fusing metal is used instead of plaster or stone because it will not fracture when the casts are tapped together (maxillary cast). *B,* Mandibular cast.

FIGURE 9–76 The reference points previously tattooed on the patient (see page 418) are again employed during the hinge-axis transfer for mounting of the remount casts in the articulator.

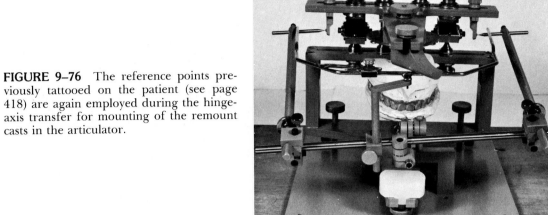

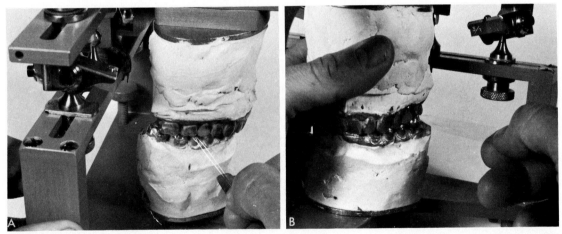

FIGURE 9–77 *A,* A cellophane strip, 0.001 inch thick, is used to judge the centric holding stops for all the castings. *B,* During the eccentric movements, the cellophane strip readily pulls out as the anterior teeth disocclude the posterior teeth.

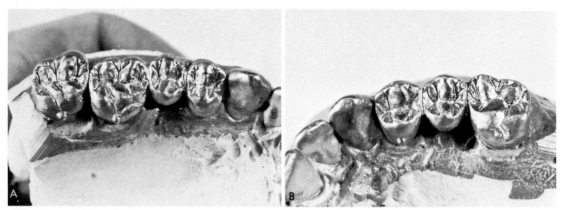

FIGURE 9–78 *A,* After the occlusal corrections have been completed, the developmental and supplemental ridges are refined with small inverted cone or round burs. The small round projections on the lingual surfaces, previously used to remove the castings from the patient's teeth, are now removed prior to final cementation (right side). *B,* Left side.

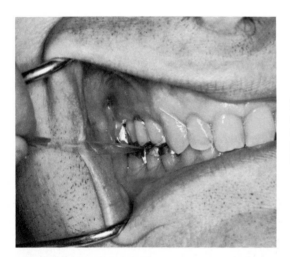

FIGURE 9–79 If the remount casts have been accurately fabricated and mounted, testing of the occlusion in the mouth with the cellophane feeler gauge will reveal the same occlusal relationships that were demonstrated on the articulator.

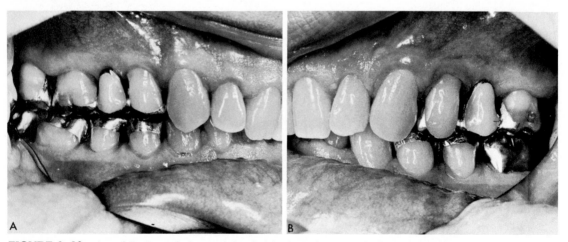

FIGURE 9–80 *A* and *B,* Buccal views of the finished castings, ready for cementation.

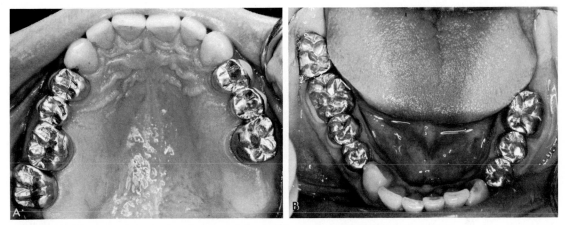

FIGURE 9–81   *A* and *B,* Occlusal views of the finished castings after cementation.

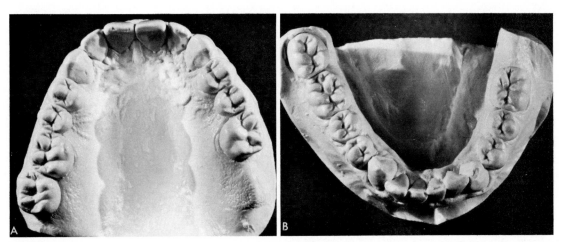

FIGURE 9–82   *A* and *B,* Stone casts of the finished castings show the extent to which the occlusal anatomy was reproduced in the gold.

changes in tooth position that may have occurred during the period when the final restorations were being made.

If all the mounting procedures have been accurately performed, the castings will have the same occlusal relationships in the mouth as were perfected on the articulator. No further occlusal correction is required in the mouth (Fig. 9–79). The finished castings are then ready for final cementation (Fig. 9–80).

Mirror views of the cemented castings are shown in Figure 9–81A and B, and Figure 9–82 shows the stone casts of the finished restorations.

COMPLICATIONS IN RESTORATIVE DENTISTRY

Occlusal Complications

Improper occlusion of restorations is a frequent complication that can cause mobility of the teeth and pain in the teeth, muscles, and temporomandibular joints.

Mobility of a tooth is one of the most important clinical signs of improper occlusion. It is often overlooked by the dentist because it can occur without pain. Slight movement of teeth can usually be seen by close visual inspection as the patient grinds his teeth. Also, palpation along the facial surface of the tooth with the finger will help to detect slight movement. Palpation is especially useful for detection of occlusal interferences of the anterior teeth.

Pain that occurs in a tooth after it has been restored may be the result of a pulpal trauma inflicted during tooth preparation or the result of occlusal trauma. It may be difficult to determine which factor is responsible for the pain; therefore, the occlusion should always be carefully evaluated and adjusted. Also, a periapical radiograph should be made for comparison of the apical area with that on previous films.

Occlusal interferences are difficult to locate on highly polished gold surfaces with any type of marking tapes. Sandblasting the occlusal surface of the gold prior to cementation is helpful, because interferences are clearly visible as burnished areas on the gold.

Pain in the muscles or the temporomandibular joints limits a patient's mandibular movements and interferes with the location of occlusal discrepancies. Except for the re-moval of obvious gross interferences, the occlusal adjustment should be delayed until the joint and muscle pain has been brought under control by other techniques, such as occlusal splinting.

Complications Involving the Pulp

Pulpal complications may occur despite the most careful operating technique and after all apparent necessary precautions have been taken. Methods for pulp protection have been suggested in the section, Biologic Considerations. Some common clinical problems associated with the dental pulp are described here.

Hypersensitivity of Teeth

Gold alloys conduct temperature changes much faster than does tooth structure. As a result, sensitivity in teeth after cementation of gold alloy castings is a common problem. Patients should be advised that some degree of sensitivity to hot and cold stimuli is to be expected for a few days following cementation.

Gold alloy restorations, if properly prepared, based, and seated, should not develop postoperative sensitivity in teeth. If sensitivity does not diminish rapidly after cementation, one or several procedures may have been performed incorrectly. The preparation of the teeth, the impression procedures, the temporary restorations, or the cementation may have injured the pulp. If the pulp has been damaged, replacement of the restoration probably will not decrease the sensitivity. If the base provided for the restoration is not thick enough, redoing the restoration may eliminate the sensitivity. It should be remembered that the pulp may have been irritated when previous restorations were placed and, therefore, may show sensitivity in spite of the most cautious technique.

If the sensitivity does not disappear after a period of a few days to several weeks, the dentist is obliged to remove the restoration or to perform endodontic therapy. A conservative decision, removal of the restoration, is usually indicated. A well-fitted temporary restoration, cemented with zinc oxide and eugenol, should be placed on the sensitive tooth. If the sensitivity diminishes within a few days, a new well-based cast restoration may be constructed. If the sensitivity is not relieved within a few days, however, vitality tests should be performed and a careful radiographic study made. Although often no adverse conditions will be found on the radiograph, the final decision will probably be in favor of endodontic therapy. The new restoration must then be designed to provide cuspal support for the tooth.

Pulpal Death

Patients for whom comprehensive restorative treatment is planned should be warned that endodontic therapy may be required for some teeth. Teeth with questionable pulps should be restored with onlays at least, rather than intracoronal restorations, to avoid the necessity of changing restorations in the event that endodontic therapy is needed. The endodontic therapy may then be accomplished through the existing restoration. An endodontically treated tooth has lost most of its internal support and may fracture unless adequate support is incorporated in the restorative design; therefore, for strength, the final restoration for the tooth should cover all the cusps.

Fractures Due to Improper Design of Restorations

Common examples of restoration failure are broken porcelain pontics or facings. There is no simple method for replacement of the porcelain. Fractures of porcelain-fused-to-metal restorations result from construction of improper metal frameworks or other inadequate laboratory procedures. Composite-resin porcelain repair kits have been shown to be useful in those situations in which trauma has caused the porcelain fracture. Porcelain breakage resulting from improper laboratory procedures is best repaired by redoing the crown or, if the restoration is a fixed prosthesis, by making a facio-lingual overcrown for the broken segment.

Fractures of teeth are usually created by failure to restore weakened cusps. Cusps, especially those of premolars, often break when inlays are used as retainers for fixed partial dentures. The broken tooth is treated by placement of a pin-retained amalgam foundation and repreparation of the tooth

for a partial-coverage or complete-coverage retainer.

Fixed partial dentures become loose when the abutment retainers lack sufficient retention. Retention for a gold casting is obtained by developing as much length as possible in opposing walls or grooves, by using parallel pins in the casting, or by placing mesial, distal, facial, and lingual grooves in the preparations. MOD onlays usually lack sufficient retention to be used as retainers for fixed partial dentures, because it is not possible to gain sufficient length in the parallel proximal boxes or grooves.

Complications Due to Poor Oral Hygiene

The importance of optimal oral hygiene measures cannot be overemphasized to patients receiving comprehensive restorative treatment. The patient's failure to maintain good oral hygiene can contribute to recurrent dental caries and periodontal disease; consequently, any dental treatment will fail, regardless of how well performed. It is discouraging to see a patient allow his oral health to degenerate after the effort has been exerted to rebuild his mouth. When this happens, several methods may be tried to restore and to maintain oral health.

Frequent Oral Hygiene Appointments

A patient who neglects oral hygiene procedures may need to have scaling and polishing procedures every 2 or 3 months, at which time carious lesions and incipient periodontal disease may be found and arrested. These appointments should include rigorous oral hygiene instructions. Eventually the patient may realize the importance of oral cleanliness and assume his responsibility in the maintenance phase of his treatment.

Topical Fluoride Applications

During the oral hygiene appointment, the patient should receive topical application of a fluoride solution. The additional protection that this provides is especially indicated for patients who have had extensive restorative treatment. Use of acidulated phosphate fluorides should be avoided where porcelain-fused-to-metal crowns have been placed, because the acid removes external stains.

Topical Fluoride Rinses

Routine fluoride rinses (0.2 per cent neutral sodium fluoride) provide additional protection against caries. The findings reported in recent studies on fluoride rinses appear very promising. The possibility is good that a daily rinse will remind the patient of his oral hygiene problem. Often a patient who neglects toothbrushing can be motivated to use mouthwash.

RELATIONSHIP OF RESTORATIVE DENTISTRY TO OTHER DENTAL SPECIALTIES

The more involved a general practitioner becomes in extensive restorative procedures (occlusal rehabilitation), the less time he has to maintain or to develop his clinical skills in other disciplines. The more he tries to satisfy the goal of preserving the natural dentition, the more he demands technical excellence in the performance of every procedure and therefore welcomes the assistance of recognized specialists.

The restorative dentist has greater opportunities to work with a periodontist than with any of the other dental specialists. In order to coordinate their efforts and to work together as a team, they must agree on methods of and a philosophy of treatment. The ideal arrangement is for the dentist and the periodontist to see the patient together initially to discuss the findings and to plan the overall treatment. At that time it should be possible to determine what restorative and periodontal procedures are necessary and how they will affect the prognosis. The patient can then be thoroughly informed about both. To avoid confusing the patient and to avoid confusion between the two offices, decisions should also be made as to who is going to be responsible for educating the patient in oral hygiene and for performing procedures common to both disciplines, such as occlusal adjustment, temporary splinting, and repositioning of teeth.

The working relationship of the restorative dentist with the endodontist consists primarily of referral of patients requiring endodontic treatment, but it should also include consultations. Many times, retention of the last remaining molar or root stump in a quadrant becomes a critical factor in the restorative treatment plan. The endodontist should be consulted about the possibility of successful endodontic treatment of this key tooth if it should be required at a later date. Some teeth cannot be treated endodontically. If the possibility of failure is known in advance of the treatment, the patient can be informed of the risk involved.

Extensive restorative treatment for adults is simplified by repositioning of malposed teeth prior to tooth preparation. Assistance of an orthodontist is often needed, but there are certain problems associated with adult orthodontics. Many adults object to wearing orthodontic devices on their teeth. They will accept removable appliances, but orthodontists, in many instances, are reluctant to use anything but fixed devices. Adult orthodontics is, however, becoming more common.

QUESTIONS

1. A complete diagnostic work-up for a complex restorative dentistry patient should include what items?

2. When should pin and amalgam build-ups be used before final tooth preparation?

3. When should pin and composite build-ups be used before final tooth preparation?

4. Should bases other than simple CaOH preparations be placed routinely beneath amalgam or composite cores?

5. Is occlusal adjustment indicated before all complex restorative dentistry therapy? Why?

6. Should intracoronal restorations be included in complex restorative dentistry treatment?

7. What are some of the methods used to lessen a patient's fears before extensive restorative therapy is begun?

8. Where should margins for crown preparations be placed in relation to the gingival tissue?

9. Should water spray be used all the time during tooth cutting for complex restorative procedures?

10. Are stainless-steel posts and composite or amalgam build-ups comparable in strength and acceptability to cast post-and-core restorations?

11. What are the advantages of onlay restorations over full crowns?

12. Why do porcelain-fused-to-metal crowns require more tooth reduction on the facial surfaces of teeth?

13. What advantages are offered by rehabilitation of the dentition on one side of the mouth at a time?

14. What disadvantages are offered by rehabilitation of the dentition on one side of the mouth at a time?

15. What disadvantages are seen in rehabilitation of one quadrant at a time?

16. What disadvantages does rehabilitation of all the posterior dentition at one time have?

17. What advantages does rehabilitation of all the posterior dentition at one time have?

18. What are the steps in rehabilitation of one side of the mouth at a time?

19. What are the steps in rehabilitation of all the posterior teeth at one time?

20. How should therapy interrelate between the other specialties and restorative dentistry?

See answers in Appendix.

REFERENCES

1. Baum, L.: Advanced Restorative Dentistry: Modern Materials and Techniques. Philadelphia, W. B. Saunders Company, 1973.
2. Brecker, S. C.: Crowns. Philadelphia, W. B. Saunders Company, 1961.
3. Charbeneau, G. T., et al. (eds.): Principles & Practice of Operative Dentistry. Philadelphia, Lea & Febiger, 1975.
4. Christensen, G. J.: Clinical application of research in tooth colored restorations. Northwest Dent., 50:343–346, 1971.
5. Christensen, G. J.: Current uses of cements in dentistry. J. Colo. Dent. Assoc., 50:29–32, 1972.
6. Christensen, G. J.: Making better fixed prosthodontic impressions. Oral Health, 69:37–39, 1979.
7. Christensen, R. P., and Christensen, G. J.: Comparison of instruments and commercial pastes used for finishing and polishing composite resin. Gen. Dent., 29:40–45, 1981.
8. Clark, J. W.: Clinical Dentistry. Hagerstown, Maryland, Harper & Row, 1976.
9. Dawson, P. E.: Evaluation, Diagnosis, and Treatment of Occlusal Problems. St. Louis, C. V. Mosby Company, 1967.
10. Kornfeld, M.: Mouth Rehabilitation: Clinical & Laboratory Procedures, Volume I, 2nd ed. St. Louis, C. V. Mosby Company, 1974.
11. Kornfeld, M.: Mouth Rehabilitation: Clinical & Laboratory Procedures, Volume II, 2nd ed. St. Louis, C. V. Mosby Company, 1974.
12. McLean, J. W.: The Science and Art of Dental Ceramics, Volume II. Chicago, Quintessence Publishing Company, Inc., 1980.
13. Ramfjord, S. P., and Ash, M. M., Jr.: Occlusion, 2nd ed. Philadelphia, W. B. Saunders Company, 1971.
14. Shillingburg, H. T., Jr., Hobo, S., and Fisher, D. W.: Preparations for Cast Gold Restorations. Chicago, Quintessence Publishing Company, Inc., 1974.
15. Smith, D. C., and Williams, D. F.: Biocompatibility of Dental Materials, Volume III. Boca Raton, CRC Press, 1982.
16. Tylman, S. D., and Malone, W. F. P.: Theory and Practice of Fixed Prosthodontics, 7th ed. St. Louis, C. V. Mosby Company, 1978.

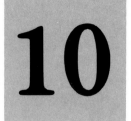

10

EMMETT R. COSTICH

ORAL SURGERY IN GENERAL PRACTICE

The principal objective of this chapter is to update the general practioner's knowledge of oral surgery so that he may provide better surgical care, particularly for patients in communities in which the services of an oral surgeon are not conveniently available.

The material included will be familiar to some practitioners; others will find new approaches to operations previously performed by different methods; and to still others, the procedures described will seem entirely new.

There is no uniform agreement among oral surgeons or general practitioners as to which procedures should be included in general practice and which should be reserved for the specialist. It would not be appropriate in this chapter, therefore, to attempt to establish sharp boundaries by preparing lists of operations for the generalist and for the specialist. A far more rational philosophy of treatment follows the principle that the general practitioner perform operations for which he feels he has the training, skill, and facilities to accomplish successfully without injuring the patient. The dentist who does not find satisfaction in performing surgery and who operates infrequently should not attempt advanced procedures. He should not, for example, attempt to remove an impacted third molar in order to save the patient the inconvenience of a visit to a specialist. People do well what they do often; the dentist who operates only occasionally does neither himself nor the patient a favor. If the practitioner plans to expand his interests in surgery, he should study, be equipped adequately, and operate regularly.

Consultation is an important aid to accurate diagnosis and treatment, and referral for consultation should be considered a regular part of the practitioner's service to his patients. Patients appreciate the general practitioner who has the foresight to refer difficult problems to a specialist. Whenever a patient shows concern about a procedure recommended by the practitioner, the dentist should suggest that the opinion of another dentist be obtained.

The general practitioner should also feel responsible for referring to oral surgeons those patients with lesions or injuries to the mouth or jaws that he does not choose to treat or does not feel qualified to treat. The letter to a consultant or specialist should be explicit in stating whether the patient is sent only for consultation or for consultation and treatment.

PREPARATION FOR ORAL SURGERY IN THE DENTAL OFFICE

The ordinary standard of cleanliness maintained in the dental office provides adequate health protection for patients during most dental procedures. However, patients are more susceptible to infection during surgery because of the exposure of deep tissues. The trauma of surgery alters the viability of tissues locally, and hematomas and necrotic tissue offer a culture medium for pathogenic organisms that may be introduced into deep tissues by surgical instruments. Proper care of instruments is therefore important to prevent the development

458

of infection in patients undergoing oral surgery. It is also important, in an office in which both surgical and other dental procedures are performed, to avoid cross-contamination of dental patients through instruments used in oral surgery.

Surgical Cleanliness

The cleansing of instruments after they have been used in patient care can be described as disinfection or as sterilization. Although the terms are sometimes improperly used synonymously, the two processes are distinctive and produce different results. *Disinfection* is the process by which many, but not all, microorganisms are killed. The important exceptions are most viruses and spore formers, such as the tetanus and the tuberculosis organisms. Examples of disinfecting techniques are boiling and the use of cold chemical solutions such as alcohol or benzalkonium chloride. *Sterilization* is the process by which all microorganisms, including spores and viruses, are killed. Examples of sterilizing techniques are autoclaving, dry heat, and gas sterilization.

Disinfection, if properly understood and accomplished, is adequate for some equipment in the dental office. Sterilization is mandatory for any instrument that penetrates tissue and becomes contaminated by blood or pus. Thus, instruments used for injection of local anesthetic solution and for endodontic treatment, periodontal therapy, and oral surgery must be sterilized. Once sterilized, they should be stored where they will remain sterile until used.

Methods of Disinfection

Scrubbing With Brush and Soap. Mechanical loosening of infected debris is accomplished by scrubbing. This procedure is a necessary prelude to sterilizing methods such as autoclaving, but when used alone, it cannot be relied upon to sterilize instruments, even when antiseptic soaps are employed.

Wiping With 70 Per Cent Isopropyl Alcohol. Mechanical cleansing with alcohol will remove superficial material. This procedure will reduce the number of organisms present but will not kill pathogens.

Boiling. Boiling is ineffective against spores and viruses.

Chemical Disinfection. Chemical agents rarely produce sterility, since they are ineffective against spores, viruses, and the tuberculosis bacillus. Also, cold solutions fail to penetrate adequately the crevices of instruments, lumens of needles, or oil films on instruments. In addition, they are inactivated by traces of soap that may remain on instruments after washing.

Under proper conditions, chemical solutions may be used safely for *disinfection* of instruments that do not contact blood or penetrate tissues. The instruments must be washed properly, adequate concentration of the solution must be maintained, and the instruments must be left in the solution for the proper length of time. The instruments should be thoroughly scrubbed with a brush and detergent soap and then rinsed and shaken free of most water before being placed in such a solution. Adherent debris could contain pathogens or could protect pathogens on the instrument from the disinfectant solution. Adherent water dilutes the solution and decreases its efficacy.

Cold solutions must be changed regularly because their effectiveness is lost with time. A solution should be replaced every 2 or 3 days, and a written record of the date of change should be kept. An automatic timer should be used to ensure that instruments are kept in contact with the solution for at least 30 minutes. During this time, additional instruments should not be added to the solution unless the time cycle is reset and lengthened to run 30 minutes from the time the last instrument is added. The manufacturer's instructions must be followed absolutely for chemical disinfection to be of any value.

Methods of Sterilization

Autoclaving. This is the most effective of all means of sterilization if the live steam reaches all portions of the materials being autoclaved. Instruments, therefore, must be free of debris and properly placed in the autoclave as directed by the manufacturer. The usual sterilization period is 15 minutes at 250° F, or 20 minutes if the instruments are wrapped in towels. Syringes and needles should be autoclaved at 250° for 30 minutes.

Dry Heat. Dry heat sterilization is effective if sufficient time is allowed for the heat to reach all parts of the material. Towels and gauze must be exposed to dry heat for 3 hours at 320° F. One hour is sufficient for unwrapped cutting instruments such as scissors and chisels.

Gas. Ethylene oxide gas is lethal to all bacteria, spores, viruses, and fungi. It is noncorrosive and will not injure fabrics, rubber, or plastics, provided it is used in accordance with the manufacturer's instructions. Instruments must be clean and free of all blood, mucus, and debris. More time is required for sterilization by gas than by steam, but less time is required for sterilization of metal or glass by gas (48 minutes at 140° F) than by dry heat. Heat-sensitive materials, which must be gas treated at room temperature, may require from 3 to 12 hours for sterilization, depending on the size and nature of the material.

Preparation of Office Equipment

The attainment of cleanliness sufficient for oral surgery procedures is limited by the design of dental equipment, but these shortcomings can be overcome.

Table and Light. In preparation for oral surgery, the unit table should be covered with a sterile towel. The operator should be careful not to touch the underside of the table as it is being moved.

The light handle should be wrapped with a clean towel or new aluminum foil before surgery is performed on any patient. The towel or foil becomes contaminated as the dentist readjusts the light during treatment, but when the towel or foil has just been changed, the dentist and his assistant need not wash their hands when the light is repositioned. A light with removable metal handles that can be autoclaved is preferable because a freshly sterilized light handle can be inserted before each patient is treated; a cover for the handle is then unnecessary.

Chair. Before a patient is seated, the headrest cover should be changed, and the arms of the chair and all adjustment levers or buttons should be wiped with 70 per cent isopropyl alcohol. The operator and the assistant should then wash their hands before the headrest and chair are adjusted for the patient; they should not make readjustments unless they again wash before and after touching the chair.

Water Syringe. A large autoclavable or disposable syringe should be used when irrigation is necessary. The unit syringe is difficult, if not impossible, to keep surgically clean.

Handpiece. Autoclavable handpieces are now available and are the only type that should be used in oral surgery.

Burs and Stones. All burs and stones must be autoclaved. Used burs must be carefully cleaned with a wire brush before the burs are autoclaved, so that debris is cleared from the flutings.

Suction Tips. Autoclavable metal tips are recommended. They should be carefully cleaned inside and outside before autoclaving. During surgical procedures, they should be flushed periodically to prevent the accumulation of clotted blood.

Gauze. Gauze squares (2″ × 2″ *without* cotton fill) should be wrapped in paper in groups of ten, sterilized by autoclaving, and stored in a sterile canister. Individual packs can then be removed with transfer forceps. This method conserves sponges and prevents contamination.

Surgical Instruments. Instruments should be scrubbed after use, autoclaved, placed on a sterile towel, and covered by another sterile towel in a closed cabinet. Individual instruments may be removed from the cabinet with surgically clean pick-up or transfer forceps.

Local Anesthetic Equipment. Disposable needles are ideal; their use assures the operator a new, sharp, sterile needle for each patient. Syringes should be autoclaved and stored in the same way that surgical instruments are stored. Cartridges of local anesthetic solutions, if unpacked without contamination, may be placed in sterile containers and removed with sterile pick-up forceps as needed. Anesthetic cartridges should never be stored or immersed in disinfectant solutions because the cartridge contents may become contaminated with the disinfectant through capillary leakage around the stoppers or through corrosion of the metal band.

The use of the aforementioned precautions in preparation for oral surgery will reduce the possibility of cross-contamination and provide a safe environment for the patient.

Minimum Equipment for Oral Surgery

Table 10–1 lists the basic instruments that should be properly sterilized, stored, and kept ready for use in oral surgery. The

TABLE 10–1 Minimum Instrument List

1.	Scalpel	Bard-Parker handle No. 3
2.	Scalpel blades	Bard-Parker type No. 15 (Nos. 11 and 12 optional)
3.	Periosteal elevator	Molt No. 9
4.	Forceps	Upper universal No. 150 Lower universal No. 151 Lower cowhorn No. 23
5.	Scissors	Dean type, straight or angled
6.	Bone file	Doubled ended (Hu-Friedy No. 21)
7.	Curets	Double ended, Miller standard surgical Nos. 10, 12, and 13 (Hu-Friedy)
8.	Rongeur forceps	Standard pattern or Blumenthal type
9.	Mosquito hemostats	Curved or straight
10.	Needle holder	Gardner, 5 or 6 inch
11.	Irrigating syringe	10 ml Luer type
12.	Trochar needle	Silver, for attachment to Luer syringe (Sklar No. 15) or 1½-inch blunt 18-gauge needle
13.	Rubber mouth prop	Small and medium (McKesson Nos. 872 and 874)
14.	Root-tip picks	Heidbrink No. 2 and 3 (Hu-Friedy)
15.	Elevators	Straight Nos. 1 and 80 (Hu-Friedy) Cryer Nos. 44 and 45 (Hu-Friedy) Root Nos. 190, and 191 (Hu-Friedy) Potts Nos. 6, and 7 (Hu-Friedy)
16.	Tissue retractor	Austin (Hu-Friedy)

high-speed handpiece is ideal for cutting teeth and bone. Supplemental irrigation from a 10-cc syringe is necessary, however, to prevent thermal damage to bone. Adequate suction is mandatory for efficient surgical procedures. Sharp instruments, such as rongeurs and files, will make surgical treatment more rapid and less traumatic. Hemostats should not be used as needle holders because they do not hold the needle rigidly and such use damages the beaks for their intended use.

MANAGEMENT OF THE PATIENT IN ORAL SURGERY

Assessment of the Patient's Condition

The importance of the medical history in planning treatment for the dental patient has been discussed in Chapter 3 (Oral Medicine in General Practice). The general health of the patient is of special significance when oral surgery is considered. Bleeding tendencies, diabetes, cardiovascular disease, and hepatitis, as well as the drugs used in the treatment of these conditions, or radiation therapy to the jaws may influence decisions as to the desirability of oral surgery. The choice of anesthetics, premedication, or antibiotics to be administered in conjunction with oral surgery is also dependent upon the health of the patient.

In addition to obtaining a medical history, the dentist can assess the general health status of the patient by noting his or her physical appearance, even before an oral examination is begun. An awkward gait or slurred speech suggests that the patient has had a stroke and thus could be taking anticoagulant drugs. Blueness of the lips and clubbing of the fingertips may indicate pulmonary or cardiac disease.

The oral examination may also reveal signs of systemic disease. Scars on the lips and tongue and fractured tooth cusps could indicate epilepsy. Paleness of the mucous membranes, multiple petechiae, and ulcerations or bleeding from the oral tissues may suggest anemia or blood dyscrasia. Clinical examination of each patient should include observation of the entire oral cavity, with special attention to the soft tissue. The soft tissue examination is not complicated, requires little time, and may be lifesaving if malignant disease is detected in an early stage.

Any abnormal physical finding during clinical examination requires an explanation by the health history or by medical consultation if the patient is to be served properly. Before treatment is begun, the medical and dental history, clinical examination, radiographs, and results of laboratory or clinical tests are correlated in order to make possible a differential diagnosis and a treatment plan in the best interest of the patient.

Accurate diagnosis and proper planning of treatment depend to a great extent on well-positioned, properly processed radiographs that show all borders of a lesion or the roots of teeth to be removed. Panoramic films frequently distort root images and fail to provide good detail for adequate differential diagnosis of opacities and radiolucencies. They are excellent screening tools but are not suitable substitutes for periapical and occlusal films. Time employed in producing good films may save time that might have to be spent later doing unplanned work. The evaluation of the film, including an estimation of bone density, will aid in planning the surgical approach.

In analyzing the patient's oral condition, it is important to know when not to treat a problem surgically. For example, an asymptomatic root tip or an impacted third molar in a 70-year-old patient with cardiovascular disease generally requires observation only. On the other hand, in a healthy 20-year-old patient, a third molar that will probably not erupt further should be removed. There are numerous patients who require removal of third molars in later life when the potential for bone regeneration is reduced and when a deep periodontal pocket exists distal to the second molar. The periodontal condition probably could have been avoided by early removal of the third molar.

The complete evaluation of the patient will inform the dentist not only of the patient's health problems but also of the patient's attitude regarding dental care. A health problem can be a contributing factor to the patient's fear of dental operations; for example, the patient may fear the effect of surgery on his cardiac condition or his diabetes. Since fear itself may affect the physical reaction to treatment, it is important that the dentist assess the patient's mental attitude in planning premedication and pain control prior to surgery.

Instructions to the Patient

In order to be properly prepared, the patient should be told at an appointment prior to the visit for surgery what to expect from surgical treatment and should be given an estimate of length of time he may be away from work and of the amount of swelling he may experience. If there is danger of complications such as perforation of the maxillary sinus or postoperative paresthesia, the patient should be informed in a way that will not alarm him.

Specific instructions should be given regarding diet, since the patient may be concerned about the necessity for fasting before and after the operation. The patient should not fast before an operation to be performed under local anesthesia. If the dentist plans to use intravenous sedation, the patient should fast in accordance with the directions of the particular dentist. The need for ice bags, special foods, drugs, and mouthwashes may be discussed before the visit for surgery. The requirements of the individual patient may be modified by his reaction to the operation, but for most procedures the dentist will be able to judge the patient's needs ahead of time. The patient will be grateful for the suggestions that he use juices, baby foods, commercial high-protein diet supplements, instant breakfast preparations, and soft drinks during the first postoperative days. He should be made to understand that his fluid and caloric needs must be met and that to go without fluid and nourishment postoperatively may jeopardize his speedy recovery.

Scheduling the Appointment for Surgery

Sufficient time should be allowed in the day's schedule for unhurried completion of planned procedures. Careful and realistic preoperative evaluation of the extent of the surgical problem will permit an accurate estimate of the time required.

Surgery in general practice should be scheduled for early in the day. Complications are less likely to develop if the dentist and patient are rested. If complications should develop, consultants are more readily available, since they will have the remainder of the day in which to rearrange appointments. Also, if the patient experiences immediate postoperative problems of pain or bleeding, he will be able to contact the dentist or his assistants while they are still in the office.

Use of Drugs in Oral Surgery

Pain Control

One of the keys to successful dental practice is painless treatment. The successful relationship between dentist and patient is frequently determined by the skill and finesse with which pain is controlled.

Premedication. Some form of premedication should be offered to any patient requiring extensive oral surgery under local anesthesia. However, while premedication administered in tablets or capsules is helpful, it is not always reliable. The action depends on the time interval since the last meal, the patient's state of nervousness, the absorption rate, and individual variations in drug response. The intravenous route of administration of hypnotics is easy, convenient, and more certain to give the desired results. Diazepam (Valium), 10 to 20 mg, or sodium pentobarbital, 75 to 125 mg, given slowly intravenously before the local anesthetic is administered, makes the surgical experience less upsetting to the apprehensive patient. The state of sedation can be determined easily by keeping the patient engaged in conversation. As the patient's speech becomes slowed and slurred, the dentist knows that the patient is appropriately sedated. In this way the dentist can be certain that the patient has not been over- or undersedated.

Prior to the administration of any medication, the patient's drug history should be reviewed. Sensitivity to sedatives and hypnotics need not prevent the patient from receiving good sedation. Other drugs such as diphenhydramine (Benadryl) or promethazine (Phenergan) are also effective hypnotics. If the patient is being treated medically with an antihypertensive drug, it is probably safer to give him hypnotics intravenously than in tablet form, since the dose required may be smaller than that for the average patient. Intravenous administration can prevent a hypotensive episode, because it permits the dentist to titrate the amount of drug given through observation of its effect on the patient while it is being administered.

Intravenous Infusion. The intravenous (IV) route permits administration of drugs directly into the circulation, where they can become effective rapidly, and their effectiveness can be determined during the course of the administration. The advantages are many: Gastrointestinal problems that may be present will not be a factor in drug absorption; the irritating properties of the drug are not a factor because it is rapidly diluted in the infusion media and the blood; doubt about how much active agent reaches the circulation is eliminated; a small portion of the drug can be administered as a test dose to determine whether the patient will have an allergic response to the drug—if an allergic or other untoward response is detected, the administration of the drug can be stopped immediately; the patient need not come to the office groggy from heavy sedation; the patient receives only sufficient medication to achieve the desired effect.

Lifesaving procedures frequently depend on having the ability to administer drugs by the intravenous route. The successful completion of an intravenous injection in a patient who is experiencing a severe reaction is extremely difficult if the dentist has not maintained skill in administering drugs intravenously. Thus, the intravenous route is not only an extremely desirable method of administering drugs but is one that should be used often to keep the dentist "in practice."

Intravenous infusion has not been a regular part of general dental practice. However, the increased frequency of patients receiving medications for health problems of a nature that could precipitate a crisis in the dental office mandates the need for knowing how to administer an intravenous infusion during the process of dental treatment. A patient who may have had a cardiovascular collapse of a precipitous nature will understand the need for an intravenous infusion and feel comforted during the procedure to know that the dentist is well prepared to treat an incipient emergency. Disposable intravenous infusion sets are available and make it very easy for the dentist to maintain the proper equipment in his office.

Fluids commonly given as intravenous infusions are normal saline solution, 5 per cent glucose in 0.2 per cent saline, 5 per cent glucose in water, and lactated Ringer's solution (Hartman's solution) with or without 5 per cent glucose. The patient with healthy, functioning kidneys generally will tolerate whatever type of solution is administered. However, if questions arise regarding intravenous infusion, the patient's physician should be consulted for his recommendation. The objective in giving these solutions to patients with potential problems is simply to have ready a route by which emergency drugs can be administered intravenously.

Occasionally, patients returning to the dental office following surgical procedures will be weak and dehydrated because of their fear of eating and possibly injuring the site of surgery. For these patients, intravenous infusion of 5 per cent dextrose in 0.2 per cent saline will bring about a remarkable recovery of the feeling of well-being.

A 50-ml vial of 50 per cent glucose solution should be kept in the office for intravenous administration to a patient in insulin shock. Attempting to give an unconscious or semiconscious patient solutions by mouth courts disaster because of the possibility of

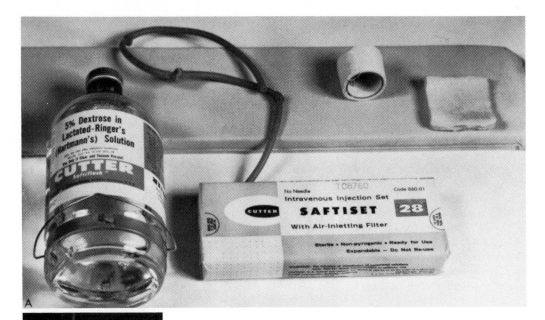

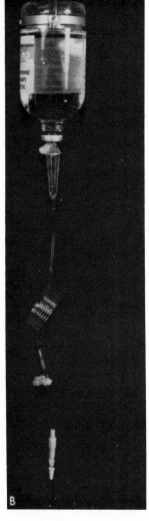

FIGURE 10–1 *A,* The materials needed for an intravenous infusion. The infusion solution, a rubber tourniquet, adhesive tape, and 2×2 inch sterile sponges are on the arm board. The prepackaged sterile tubing, drip chamber, stopcock, and injection bulb are in the box. *B,* The assembled infusion set. From the top are shown the bottle of solution, drip chamber, tubing partially uncoiled, stopcock, rubber injection bulb, and 1½-inch 20-gauge needle. (From Costich, E. R., and White, R. P.: Fundamentals of Oral Surgery. Philadelphia, W. B. Saunders Company, 1972.)

aspiration of the solutions into the lungs or from a laryngeal spasm. The intravenous administration of 50 per cent glucose will correct hypoglycemia rapidly. This concentration of glucose is extremely irritating and therefore must be given intravenously; it must not be given intramuscularly.

The technique for intravenous administration of drugs is quite simple and can be mastered easily by every dentist.

Equipment. A tourniquet is necessary for distending the veins to be injected. Generally a short length of rubber tubing is used, since it can be released easily with one hand. The syringe should be sterile, of 3 or 5 ml capacity, and disposable. Disposable sterile needles, 20 to 25 gauge, 1½ inches in length, are recommended. Alcohol sponges are needed to clean the top of the drug vial and the injection bulb of the intravenous set that will be penetrated by the needle. Adhesive bandages or gauze sponges are used to cover the puncture site in the skin after the injection or infusion is completed. An arm board, an intravenous injection set, and the intravenous solution complete the needed equipment (Fig. 10–1).

Technique. The rubber diaphragm of the drug vial is wiped with an alcohol sponge before the needle is inserted. The plunger of the syringe is placed at the appropriate volume mark, depending on the quantity of drug to be withdrawn. When 10 to 20 mg of diazepam is to be used, the volume will be 2 to 4 ml (5 mg/ml). The needle is pushed through the diaphragm, air is injected into the vial, and the plunger is then slowly withdrawn to remove a quantity of solution equal to the volume of air injected (Fig. 10–2). The plastic cover is replaced to protect the needle from contamination while the injection site is prepared.

The intravenous infusion requires the placement of the needle in an area in which it will not penetrate the wall of the vein during motion of the patient's hand or arm. The antecubital fossa is an undesirable place for infusion. The back of the hand is the preferred location because it remains flat when the wrist is flexed.

The tourniquet is placed on the midforearm and the patient is instructed to make a fist. This will usually distend the veins, but if they cannot be palpated easily, gently slapping the area, applying warm compresses, or allowing the arm to hang to-

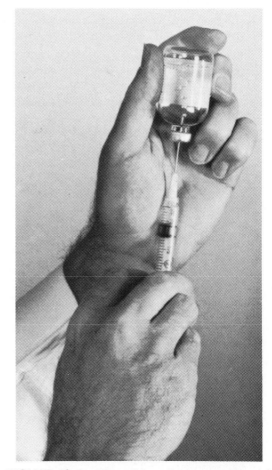

FIGURE 10–2 The rubber diaphragm of a vial is perforated by the needle; a volume of air equal to the volume of solution to be withdrawn is injected into the vial, and the solution is then withdrawn. (From Costich, E. R., and White, R. P.: Fundamentals of Oral Surgery. Philadelphia, W. B. Saunders Company, 1972.)

ward the floor may help to engorge the veins. Rapidly repeated clenching of the fist together with these maneuvers will also help.

A likely vein is selected, and the area is wiped with alcohol. The operator grasps the patient's hand, tensing the skin in the area over the vein. The needle is grasped in the operator's other hand with needle bevel away from the patient's skin; the needle is pushed quickly through the skin and then passed into the vein. The sensation of a needle entering the vein is similar to that of a needle pushing through a sheet of rubber dam or passing through the buccinator muscle when a zygomatic block is performed. There is initial resistance, but after the

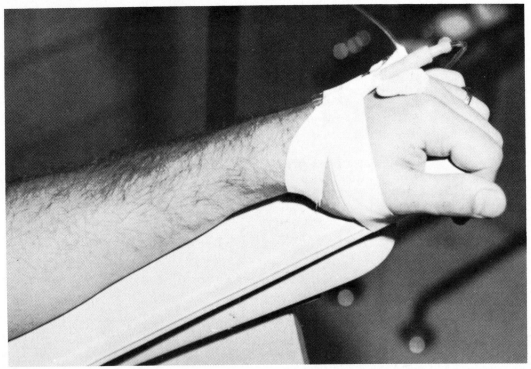

FIGURE 10–3 An intravenous infusion is being given into a vein in the back of the hand. The needle is held in place by adhesive tape; the hand is taped to an arm board to stabilize it in a comfortable position. The injection bulb is supported by a gauze sponge. (From Costich, E. R., and White, R. P.: Fundamentals of Oral Surgery. Philadelphia, W. B. Saunders Company, 1972.)

needle has penetrated the outer wall into the vein, there is little or no resistance to forward motion.

The needle can be maneuvered gently in such a way that it usually can be observed as it is threaded 5 to 10 mm into the vein. Gentle pinching of the injection bulb on the infusion set will serve to aspirate blood, demonstrating that the needle is in the vein. If a "butterfly" (a needle with flat plastic wings and a short length of tubing attached before the hub) is used, the blood will flow back into the tubing and should reach the hub before the latter is connected to the tubing from the infusion set. At this point, the tourniquet is released, the drip started, the needle taped into position, and the hand and arm taped to the armrest or a board (Fig. 10–3).

Occasionally, the needle may perforate but not enter a vein, resulting in a hematoma or subcutaneous collection of intravenous fluid. In such an event, the fluid flow should be stopped and the needle immediately withdrawn. Gentle pressure and milking will express blood and/or fluid through the skin perforation. A new attempt should then be made using the patient's other hand or another vein on the same hand. Such events happen to the best phlebotomists and should not be any more distressing than occasionally fracturing a root.

The flow control on the IV tubing is opened wide to assure rapid washing of the sedative drug from the smaller peripheral veins. The rubber injection bulb is wiped with an alcohol sponge, and the injection of the drug is made at the rate of 1 ml per 30 seconds. The tubing is pinched as each advancement of the syringe piston is made to prevent backflow of the drug toward the IV solution reservoir. The tubing is released as soon as the piston stops so that the drug is washed on into the vein. Diazepam causes a slight stinging or burning sensation as it enters the vein. It may cause some irritation and occasionally a mild phlebitis that is treated by applying warm compresses. The fast flow of the intravenous solution minimizes such events. The flow is slowed to a "keep open" rate (20 drops per minute) after the medications are administered. The patient is asked to inform the operator when he feels any altered sensation. Most patients will soon report a pleasant sensation of drowsiness, and the operator will note ptosis of the eyelids. When the desired level of sedation is achieved, the needle is withdrawn.

The patient will be cooperative and perhaps talkative. Hypnotics do not relieve pain, but some, such as pentobarbital, may relieve inhibitions. The reaction is similar to that produced by several alcoholic drinks. For this reason some dentists prefer to give meperidine first to raise pain thresholds. Following this type of sedation, the patient should not leave the office unescorted and for about 24 hours should not drive a car or do anything requiring good judgment and good reflexes. The hypnotic drug depresses reflexes, and even when it does so very effectively, its effects may not be perceptible to the patient. Since the dentist is legally and morally responsible for any drug that he prescribes or administers, be it local anesthetic, antibiotic, or hypnotic, he must have a thorough understanding of its actions and side effects and must know how to manage any adverse reactions.

Topical Anesthesia. In most instances, patients appreciate topical anesthesia prior to injections because it eliminates the discomfort associated with the insertion of the needle. The use of a disposable needle for each surgical procedure eliminates most of the pain; however, topical anesthetic ensures absence of pain from penetration of the needle. Topical anesthetics have an added psychologic value in that their use demonstrates that the dentist is concerned about the patient's comfort.

Topical anesthetics are available in liquid form for painting or spraying, and in ointment form. Application of the liquids to a limited area is difficult to control, and when applied as a spray, they may be used to excess. The easiest forms to apply are the ointment and viscous forms.

The mucosal surface to be anesthetized should be gently wiped dry and the ointment then applied with a cotton swab or cotton roll. The cotton roll technique is very convenient: A small amount of ointment is "buttered" on the roll, and the treated surface of the roll is then placed against the dried mucosa over the proposed injection site. After a minute, the cotton roll is moistened with water to prevent it from sticking to the mucosa and it is removed. The area is again wiped dry and the injection carried out.

Local Anesthesia. As soon as the patient is comfortably adjusted to a relaxed state, the dentist may proceed to administer the local anesthetic. The waiting period is generally not more than a minute. The dentist rarely has difficulty with the technique of administering local anesthesia. If he does experience a series of anesthetic failures occasionally, he can overcome the difficulty by simply reviewing the steps in injection procedures and then following them slowly and deliberately. Anesthetic failures by experienced dentists usually represent laxity in technique.

Local Anesthetic Agents. The drugs commonly used as local anesthetic agents are listed in Table 10–2. The volume of local anesthetics administered throughout the world each day is staggering. The solutions used in any city during the course of a year would probably fill a small lake. Yet, in spite of the widespread use of the drugs, reactions are exceedingly rare. In cases in which toxicity has been reported, the reactions are usually in response to large volumes of solutions used in general surgery. The toxic dose for lidocaine is about 400 to 500 mg. The dentist rarely administers a dose of more than 288 mg (eight cartridges containing 1.8 ml of a 2 per cent solution of anesthetic) and probably averages about 37 to 72 mg for each patient at a single visit.

It is apparent, therefore, that few of the "reactions" to local anesthetics administered in dentistry are toxic. Most reactions are probably psychogenic. Patients who have fainted and convulsed slightly are misdiagnosed as having a toxic or allergic reaction

TABLE 10–2 Local Anesthetic Agents

Generic Name	Proprietary Name
I. Ester	
Procaine*	Novocain†
Propoxycaine	Ravocaine
II. Amide	
Lidocaine*	Alphacaine
	Octocaine
	Xylocaine
Mepivacaine*	Arestocaine
	Carbocaine
	Isocaine
Prilocaine	Citanest

*Marketed under the generic name as well as under the proprietary name.

†"Novocain" is a term used by some patients as a synonym for any local anesthetic.

to the anesthetic agent. The dentist may forget that simple syncope (fainting) is occasionally accompanied by a brief convulsive episode.

Management of Reactions to Local Anesthesia. Untoward reactions to local anesthesia may be psychogenic, toxic, or hypersensitive. Management of the patient depends on the type of reaction.

Syncope, the most common reaction, is not related to the drug itself but to a complex of factors associated with the injection episode: the sum of the patient's previous medical and dental experiences; the amount of pain suffered preceding the appointment; the sights, sounds, and smells of the office, and the sight of the syringe and needle. All may contribute to the reaction elicited. Fainting can be prevented by placing the patient in an almost horizontal position when injecting the solution. Kind words, gentle handling of the tissues, and the use of topical anesthetics and hypnotics will minimize, if not eliminate, the problem.

Toxicity reactions are next in frequency of occurrence and usually result from fast intravascular injection or the use of a large volume of the drug. Symptoms of toxicity include initial excitement with talkativeness and signs of apprehension. This state progresses to central nervous system depression (reactions to aniline anesthetics such as lidocaine and mepivacaine may begin with CNS depression) manifested by slurring of speech, drowsiness, depressed respiration, and convulsion. Treatment involves the use of oxygen, administered by a mask and bag, if the respiration is slow, shallow, or absent. Diazepam (5 mg/ml) is given intravenously in the least amount needed to control persistent convulsions. Medical assistance should also be obtained. Epinephrine, 0.3 to 0.5 mg (0.3 to 0.5 ml of 1:1000 solution), may be given intravenously or intramuscularly if there is a severe drop in blood pressure.

Allergic reactions to local anesthetics are extremely rare. They may be mild or severe in nature and immediate or delayed in onset. The major types of allergic reactions are contact dermatitis, delayed serum sickness, and anaphylactic or accelerated reaction.

Contact dermatitis is characterized by localized rash and eruption where the drug has touched the tissues. It is usually associated with ester (procaine) type anesthetics. Management of such a reaction involves the

oral administration of an antihistamine such as diphenhydramine (Benadryl), 50 mg, and avoidance of subsequent use of the anesthetic.

Delayed serum sickness reaction is characterized by onset 4 to 10 days after the drug has been given. There may be fever, skin eruption, urticaria, arthralgia, and lymphadenopathy. Occasionally the joints swell and the patient may have diarrhea. Treatment is symptomatic, with aspirin and antihistamines. Epinephrine and steroid therapy are rarely necessary. Usually the course of this reaction is benign. The patient should be told the nature of the reaction and the exact name of the drug involved and should be instructed to inform subsequent doctors of the problem before treatment.

Anaphylactic reaction is extremely rare in association with local anesthetics. It is an accelerated, severe, life-threatening reaction characterized by sudden severe loss of vasomotor tone resulting in deep shock, absent pulse, loss of blood pressure and poor and inadequate respiration. Treatment involves immediate support of respiration and circulation. Artificial respiration is induced by means of oxygen applied with bag and mask or by mouth-to-mouth resuscitation. Closed chest cardiac massage and possibly epinephrine, 0.3 to 0.5 mg (0.3 to 0.5 ml of 1:000 solution), injected intravenously or intramuscularly, are used to support the circulation. Immediate medical consultation is also indicated.

It is imperative that syncope and toxicity reactions be distinguished from true allergic responses so that the patient is not misinformed following a reaction. If a patient has one of these reactions, he should be told its exact nature. If a true allergic reaction occurs, the drug involved and the nature of the reaction should be recorded. A written report should be given to the patient to be presented to the treating doctor whenever subsequent treatment is necessary.

Management of the Patient With a History of Allergic Reactions. In spite of the rarity of true allergy to local anesthetics, a history of reactions must be taken seriously and investigated before any injection is given. Should the patient give a history of previous reactions, the following steps are recommended.

1. If possible, determine the exact nature of the previous reaction by calling the doctor

in attendance during the reaction. If the patient can give a detailed history, he may describe a reaction that was not allergic, and a local anesthetic may be given safely.

2. If the patient knows the exact drug that produced the reaction, use a drug from another chemical grouping. (The major classifications are shown in Table 10–2.) For example, if a reaction was associated with a para-amino-benzoic acid ester, then an aniline derivative may be used.

3. Do not test for drug sensitivity in the dental office. A person who is truly allergic may have a serious reaction to the dilute solution used in sensitivity testing. Furthermore, sensitivity tests for local anesthetics are difficult to interpret. A detailed, accurate history is the most valuable procedure in determining allergy. If the dentist is unable, by means of history, to rule out a true sensitivity, the patient should be referred to an allergist to determine what local anesthetic may be used safely.

4. In the unlikely event of allergy to all local anesthetic drugs, dental treatment can be performed under general anesthesia if an anesthetic is required.

Use of Epinephrine in Local Anesthetic Solutions. Because it is a superior vasoconstrictor, epinephrine continues to be used widely in anesthetic solutions. Epinephrine is present in physiologic amounts in the body at all times, and under stressful circumstances, such as emotional upset caused by fear or pain, the adrenal glands liberate large amounts that have a definite effect on the heart. Local anesthetics containing epinephrine give deeper and longer-acting anesthesia than local anesthetics without this agent, thus greatly reducing the chance for pain-induced release of the body's epinephrine. Furthermore, the extremely small amounts of epinephrine given for dental purposes, even when injected intravascularly, seldom produce a systemic effect.

It is currently recommended that not more than 0.2 mg of epinephrine be used for healthy patients at any one dental appointment. Eight ml of local anesthetic solution containing 1:100,000 ephinephrine has only 0.08 mg of epinephrine, which is less than one-half the maximal allowable dose. Patients with cardiac problems should not receive more than .04 mg of epinephrine or two cartridges of local anesthetic containing 1:100,000 epinephrine. Tricyclic antidepressant drugs are the only drugs that necessitate the use of a local anesthetic without a vasoconstrictor. In such instances mepivacaine 3% or prilocaine 4% may be used.

Control of Infection

For the acutely sick patient, one must carefully consider the administration of antibiotics. This decision is made by weighing the possible benefits of antibiotic therapy against its disadvantages.

If antibiotics were completely innocuous, they could be prescribed in every case of infection in the hope that they might be of some benefit. However, a number of dangers are associated with their indiscriminate use, and these must be understood and appreciated.

Preliminary Considerations
Dangers of Antibiotic Therapy. Antibiotics may give the dentist a false sense of security and cause him to depend on the drug rather than on sound surgical principles. For instance, abscesses that are fluctuant should be drained; to fail to do so will only prolong the course of therapy.

Resistant strains of bacteria may be produced by improper use of antibiotics, so that in the long run they become ineffective as therapeutic agents. Also, use of antibiotics may result in moniliasis, enterocolitis, pneumonia, and wound infection through suppression of normal bacterial flora with overgrowth of resistant pathogens.

Like all drugs, antibiotics may produce untoward reactions. Toxic reactions may occur, especially with misuse of streptomycin and chloramphenicol. Sensitization of the patient, especially by the use of topical antibiotics, may result in serious allergic reactions. Tetracyclines, if given to children during the first 4 years of life, may cause unsightly discoloration of the anterior teeth.

Indications for Antibiotics. Antibiotics usually are not necessary in treatment of normal patients requiring multiple extractions, alveolectomy, extraction of chronically abscessed teeth, drainage of localized abscesses, removal of small cysts (less than 1.5 cm), or simple impaction surgery, nor are they necessary for most patients with pericoronal infections or localized osteitis. In these situations, however, antibiotics may be required as a prophylactic measure for patients with uncontrolled diabetes or congenital or acquired heart disease, with prosthetic

TABLE 10–3 Suggested Oral Antibiotic Dosage

Drug	Adult Dose	Child's Dose
Penicillin		
Tablets and capsules, 125 and 250 mg	250 mg 4 times/day	125 mg 4 times/day
Suspension	5 ml (1 tablespoon) 4 times/day	2½ ml (½ teaspoon) 4 times/day
Erythromycin		
Tablets and capsules, 100 and 250 mg	250 mg 4 times/day	100 mg 4 times/day
Suspension		
40 mg/ml	6 ml (1 tablespoon) 4 times/day	—
20 mg/ml	—	5 ml (1 teaspoon) 4 times/day
Tetracyclines		
Tablets and capsules, 50, 100, and 250 mg	250 mg 4 times/day	15 mg/kg/day in three or four divided doses. Tablets, suspension, or syrup may be used (should be avoided in children under 7 years of age)
Suspension, 250 mg/15 ml		
Syrup, 125 mg/ml	—	

heart valves and hip replacement, or with a history of radiation therapy to the jaws as well as those on corticosteroid therapy.

Antibiotics are usually indicated in the following circumstances even if the patient has no other health problem:

1. acute dentoalveolar abscess with systemic signs and symptoms, such as an oral temperature of 101° F (102° F rectally), difficulty in swallowing or managing saliva, trismus, swelling causing noticeable distention of tissues, severe pain when the area is palpated, or indications of obvious toxicity and illness,
2. compound facial fractures and osteomyelitis, and
3. acute periocoronitis with marked systemic signs and symptoms.

Choice of Drug

Administration of Antibiotics. Most oral infections, both in adults and in children, are best treated with penicillin. If the patient is allergic to penicillin, erythromycin should be substituted. The third choice of drug when sensitivity tests have ruled out penicillin and erythromycin is a tetracycline. This last group should be avoided in treatment of young children during the years when the crowns of the anterior teeth are forming. Fortunately, few children are troubled by acute dental infections before 5 years of age.

Whenever pus is present, it must be drained, and a specimen should be sent to the laboratory for culture and antibiotic sensitivity testing. If the patient has not responded to penicillin by the time the test results are received, he should be placed on the antibiotic suggested by the results of the laboratory tests.

The antibiotic drug should be given systemically in the recommended dosages (see Table 10–3 and 10–4). It should be prescribed for 5 days, and the patient should be instructed not to discontinue it before the

TABLE 10–4 Suggested Oral Antibiotic Dosage for Prophylaxis Patients With Congenital Heart Disease, Prosthetic Heart Valves, or Prosthetic Joint Replacements

Drug	Adult Dose	Child's Dose
Penicillin V	2.0 gm 30 to 60 minutes before surgery, 500 mg every 6 hours for 8 doses after surgery	For children over 27 kg*—same as adult. For children under 27 kg— 1.0 gm 30 to 60 minutes before surgery; 250 mg every 6 hours for 8 doses after surgery
Erythromycin (if patient is allergic to penicillin)	1.0 gm 1½ to 2 hours before surgery, 500 mg every 6 hours for 8 doses after surgery	20 mg/kg 1½ to 2 hours before surgery. 10 mg/kg every 6 hours for 8 doses after surgery

*1 kilogram = 2.205 lb, ∴ about 10 mg per lb.

end of that period, even if his condition improves before that time. A full 5-day course prevents development of mutant, resistant bacterial strains and is more likely to eliminate the infection completely.

Topical use of antibiotics should be avoided, since sensitization occurs most often by this route. Even if the drug is given systemically, however, the patient should be forewarned of the possibility of a hypersensitivity (allergic) reaction. He should be told to discontinue the drug in the event of a rash, hives, itching, or difficulty in breathing.

The cause of the infection should be treated as early as possible by endodontic methods, periodontal therapy, or removal of the tooth, and the patient's progress should be observed closely. The condition of the patient with an infection requiring antibiotic therapy should be monitored daily, if possible.

Antibiotic Effectiveness. The effectiveness of the treatment is evaluated first by observation of changes in the patient's general condition. If the infection is subsiding, the patient should have less pain, a temperature approaching normal, and improved ability to open the mouth, move the jaws, and swallow. The effects of the drug should also be evidenced by improvement at the site of the infection, as manifested by reduced swelling, modified pain, and less trismus.

If there is no improvement within 48 hours, the diagnosis and the choice of the antibiotic should be reviewed. The results of the antibiotic sensitivity test, at times available in 48 hours, may aid in determining whether therapy should be altered. Sometimes the dosage of the drug initially administered may be increased, or the route of the administration may be changed. Therapy with a different antibiotic may begin while the original one is continued to complete its 5-day course. One should also consider the need for consultation and possible hospitalization of the patient.

ORAL SURGICAL PROCEDURES

Surgical Removal of Teeth and Root Tips

Adherence to good surgical principles in the removal of teeth and root tips should result in more efficient treatment procedures, less tissue loss, less postoperative discomfort, more rapid recovery, and fewer residual defects following healing.

Flap Reflection

The dissection of tissue to expose the underlying structures is referred to as flap reflection. This procedure is necessary in removing retained roots, residual cysts, or periapical pathologic tissue in some endodontic therapy and to expose exostoses and impacted teeth.

Although flap reflection if frequently neglected in removal of many teeth and fractured roots, it is desirable because it speeds the operation by permitting controlled removal of bone and roots under direct vision. The careful reflection of a well-designed flap also reduces the trauma to the tissue and thus helps to prevent postoperative discomfort, edema, and delayed healing.

The keys to success in the reflection and replacement of soft tissue flaps are:

1. careful planning to ensure a wide base to the flap and a good blood supply;
2. clean, sharp incisions perpendicular to the surface;
3. incisions over bone that will not be removed during the surgical procedure;
4. incisions completely through periosteum and not less than 5 mm from the margin of any bony defect if the flap is being reflected over bone;
5. careful dissection of the flap along a surgical plane, such as fascia, muscle, or bone;
6. reflection of a sufficiently large and adequate flap;
7. extreme gentleness in handling and retracting the flap; and
8. careful and accurate repositioning, with adequate sutures to hold the flap in position.

Every flap should be large enough to expose an area adequate for performing surgery without injuring the flap and surrounding tissues. The instruments used in retracting the flap should rest on bone whenever possible and not on soft tissue.

The most desirable type of flap is the envelope, made by a gingival crevice incision and flap reflection (Fig. 10–4). If adequate exposure without tension on the flap is not possible by this method, an oblique incision should be made anterior to the field of sur-

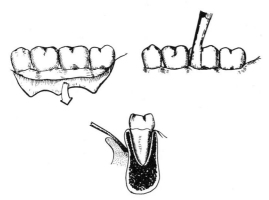

FIGURE 10–4 The envelope flap is reflected after an incision is made in the gingival crevice. The mucoperiosteum is reflected and includes the interdental papillae. (From Costich, E. R.: The role of oral surgery in preventive dentistry. Dent. Clin. North Am., July 1965, pp. 429–34.)

gery (Fig. 10–5). The trap-door flap, created by two oblique incisions, one on either side of the surgical field, has a compromised blood supply and is difficult to return to place.

The base of the flap should be broader than the free end in order to preserve a good supply to the margin. Any oblique incision should be placed at least one tooth beyond the region of anticipated bone removal so that when the flap is returned to place, the oblique cut will rest on a bony surface and not fall into the bony defect.

The oblique or vertical incision should terminate in the interproximal area and not on the midlabial or midbuccal aspect of the root. The tissue is thin over the root prominence, and after healing, any resulting irregularity due to scar contracture or poor technique may trap debris and thus affect the underlying structures. Also, the incision should not split the interdental papilla, since this area tends to collect debris. The papilla should remain intact in the embrasure (Fig. 10–6).

It is important that the periosteal elevator pass beneath the periosteum, which will then be reflected with the mucosa. The larger capillaries are located between the mucosa and the periosteum. Splitting the mucosa

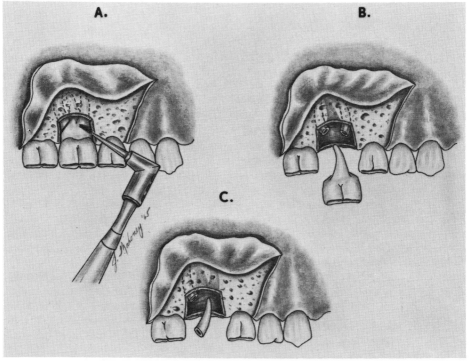

FIGURE 10–5 *A,* A gingival crevice incision and a vertical incision at the anterior end of the gingival incision have been made to permit a higher reflection of the mucoperiosteal flap. Sufficient buccal bone is then removed to permit access for sectioning the buccal roots. *B,* After the two buccal roots have been sectioned, the crown and palatal root are removed in one segment. *C,* The buccal roots are then removed. (From McCarthy, F. M.: Emergencies in Dental Practice. Philadelphia, W. B. Saunders Company, 1967.)

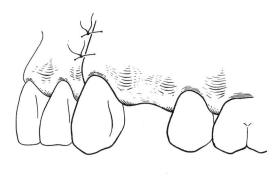

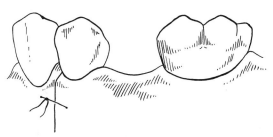

FIGURE 10–6 The interdental papilla was not split when the vertical incision was made for the flap reflection. The tissues have been approximated and are held in position by sutures that have been slightly angled and tied without tension to prevent irregularities at the gingival margin of the incision. (From Schram, W. R.: A Manual of Oral Surgery Techniques. Philadelphia, W. B. Saunders Company, 1962.)

from the periosteum produces much bleeding, causes distortion of the mucosal flap, and thus makes bone surgery messy. The flap should be designed in such a way that damage from the incision to vital anatomic structures such as the mental nerve or greater palatine vessels and nerve is avoided.

When surgery is performed to reach the periapical areas of teeth, the flaps should be reflected by incisions in the gingival crevice, and the interdental papillae should be included with the flap; the papillae should not be amputated. Since periosteum is not elastic, the mucoperiosteal flap is not distorted by shrinkage and can easily be repositioned and sutured. Healing is more rapid with this type of incision than with the apical mucosal incision, and scarring is minimal. Incision in the attached gingiva also results in no distortion of the tissues in the vestibular folds, as sometimes occurs with the mucosal semilunar incision beyond the margins of the attached gingiva.

Bone Removal

Once the flap has been reflected, sufficient bone should be removed to allow free passage of the root of the tooth from the socket (Figs. 10–5 and 10–7). If burs are used to remove bone, water irrigation from a syringe should be employed to prevent overheating or burnishing of the bone. After the teeth or roots are removed, the bony margins should be filed smooth, the defect irrigated to remove loose debris, the flap returned to position, and an appropriate number of sutures placed.

Tooth Sectioning

Molar teeth with widely divergent roots present problems in removal. These problems can be simplified by reflection of an envelope flap and removal of the crest of bone buccal to the tooth being removed. The bifurcation of the roots is thus exposed, and one or more roots may be cut from the crown to simplify removal (Figs. 10–5 and

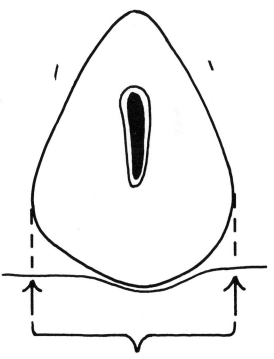

FIGURE 10–7 Sufficient bone must be removed from the labial aspect of a maxillary canine in order to remove the tooth easily. (From Costich, E. R., and White, R. P.: Fundamentals of Oral Surgery. Philadelphia, W. B. Saunders Company, 1972.)

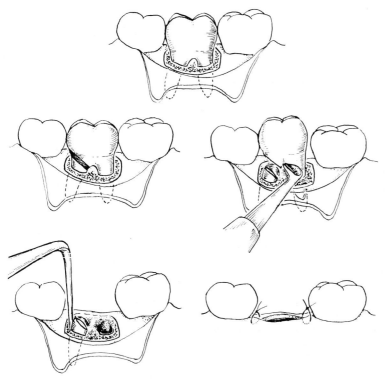

FIGURE 10–8 An envelope flap and the removal of the buccal alveolar crest can provide adequate exposure of the roots of a lower molar. If the roots are divergent, one may be sectioned and removed after the crown and attached root have been removed. (From Hayward, J. R., and Costich, E. R.: The use of elevators. Pract. Dent. Monogr., March 1957.)

10–8). The tooth should be manipulated with the forceps before the roots are cut. This loosens the roots and makes their removal easier.

Recovery of Fractured Root Tips

Blind picking for a root tip is courting the problem of loss into deeper structures; it also wastes time and causes needless discomfort for the patient. Root tips must be seen to be removed. The simple act of reflecting a flap will often make the tip visible. If flap reflection does not reveal the tip, the removal of the buccal crest of bone will complete the exposure. By use of good suction, irrigation, and a root-tip pick, the root end may be dislodged. If this method does not bring satisfactory results within a minute, a small, round bur should be used to cut root and bone around the circumference of the root. This creates space for the insertion of the pick and provides space into which the root can be rocked and from which it can subsequently be dislodged (Fig. 10–9).

If the root tip is close to the maxillary sinus, inferior alveolar canal, or a lower second or third molar, it is wise to reflect a flap and immediately relieve the buccal wall and remove bone adjacent to the root tip. This will assure a space into which the tip can be dislodged and from which it can be removed easily with suction or apical root picks. Occasionally, a tiny (3 mm) maxillary third molar tip can be ignored if the tooth has been asymptomatic and the radiographs show no periapical pathology.

Removal of Retained Roots

The incidental findings of previously undiagnosed root tips on radiographs introduce some problems. If they have been present for years, are symptomless, and show no radiographic evidence of pathologic changes and if there is no medical or dental indication for removal, they may be left undisturbed. However, if fixed or removable prostheses are to be placed over the area, these retained roots should be removed. It is easier to remove retained roots or teeth prophylactically than to treat infections associated with their exposure by bone resorption.

Multiple x-rays will localize the tip relative to the remaining teeth and anatomic landmarks such as the maxillary sinus. If the position of a root tip is to be determined in an edentulous jaw (either maxillary or mandib-

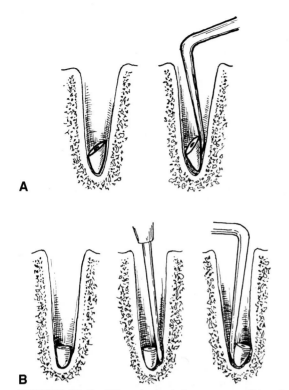

A

B

FIGURE 10–9 The gingival tissues are reflected as an envelope flap to permit direct view of the tooth socket so that the root-tip pick will not be used blindly. These diagrams of a cut-away view of the socket show *(A)* how the pick is used after flap reflection and *(B)* how the pick is used after the bur has created space for the pick. (From Hayward, J. R., and Costich, E. R.: The use of elevators. Pract. Dent. Monogr., March 1957.)

ular), the mucosa can be anesthetized and a suture needle placed in the alveolar mucosa to serve as a landmark on the radiograph taken just before the surgery. After the position of the tip has been determined, a long, curved incision is made, bypassing the area of bone through which the root will be removed. Maxillary root tips will generally be residual portions of the buccal roots. The buccal bone is thin so that generally the root tips may be easily removed with an elevator after the reflection of a mucoperiosteal flap. If it is necessary to remove bone, then only buccal bone should be removed. The crest of the alveolar ridge should not be altered. In the rarer instance, when a retained palatal root tip is encountered, a palatal mucoperiosteal envelope flap is reflected. The overlying palatal bone is removed by the use

of a bur, and the root tip is removed with an elevator.

Closure with braided silk is best for intraoral surgery because it causes minimal tissue reaction and the least discomfort for the patient. Resorbable gut sutures are occasionally used, especially if the patient lives some distance away and cannot return for a postoperative visit. However, gut is stiff, and since the cut ends are sharp, they may cause some discomfort.

Impacted Teeth

The term "impaction" implies that the tooth is prevented from erupting because it is blocked by another tooth or teeth or by overlying bone. During the course of development the tooth may have formed in an unusual position, which prevents it from following the normal pathway of eruption. Thus, it assumes an abnormal position within the alveolar process. The teeth that are impacted most frequently are the mandibular third molars, followed by the maxillary canines and the mandibular premolars. Maxillary third molars frequently fail to erupt and are regarded as impacted teeth.

Any teeth that have failed to assume a normal, functional position within the alveolar arch and are completely unerupted or only partially erupted and serving no useful function should be removed to prevent further complications, such as the development of dentigerous cysts, periodontal lesions, dental caries, and chronic irritation to adjacent tissues.

Third Molars. In this day of excellent dental care, the young person who is receiving good dental therapy should have all third molars removed before the age of 17 years. For this patient, it is usually not a matter of the teeth being impacted or unerupted but simply is good preventive dentistry. It is unusual for lower third molars to erupt into adequate occlusion, with good exposure of the distal surfaces for oral hygiene; thus, these teeth frequently become a focus of periodontal disease and may be the cause of other complications (Figs. 10–10 to 10–12). It is easier to remove these teeth in the young individual because the patient tolerates the procedure better. Young people also recover more quickly and the potential for periodontal complications following surgery is less.

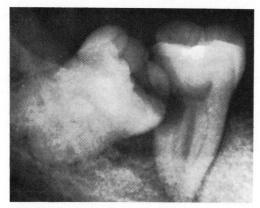

FIGURE 10–10   Failure to remove the impacted third molar resulted in distal caries, pulp necrosis, and periapical abscess of the second molar. (From Costich, E. R., and White, R. P.: Fundamentals of Oral Surgery. Philadelphia, W. B. Saunders Company, 1972.)

Even though a tooth fails to erupt, its root development continues, and the growing roots will be deflected by anatomic structures already present. For example, careful inspection of the roots of mandibular third molars will often reveal that they have been deflected by the mandibular canal during their development. This indicates that the canal may be disrupted during the extraction procedure, or that the curved root may fracture, with great potential for its displacement into the mandibular canal. This same type of deflection is also seen in the maxillae, where the roots of impacted canines and premolars deviate and pass along the walls of the maxillary sinus. Thus, when planning surgery for any impaction, the dental radiographs should be studied carefully to determine the tooth's relationship to anatomic structures as well as its form and position in the arch.

At some time most dentists will feel obliged to remove an impacted tooth. The principles for removing impacted teeth are the same as for fully erupted teeth but, because of their abnormal locations, impacted teeth present problems of access and visibility. A plan must be developed carefully before these teeth are approached, so that they can be removed with a minimum of trauma to the adjacent soft tissue and supporting bone and in as short a time as possible.

The anatomy of the area should be viewed before the operation. The lingual nerve is close to the alveolar crest in the mandibular third molar region, and the inferior alveolar nerve and vessels may be exposed as this tooth is removed. Also, the mandible is very thin beneath the third molar and roots can be easily pushed into the floor of the mouth. Exposure is gained by the reflection of an adequate soft tissue flap and removal of sufficient bone to enable the tooth to be seen and, if necessary, divided into segments for removal. The division of the tooth must be planned so that whatever segment of the tooth is to be removed next in the sequence will be visible and can be manipulated easily (Fig. 10–12).

The usual path of rotation of the maxillary third molar is to the buccal and distal aspects. This tooth may be displaced into the maxillary sinus, the pterygomaxillary fissure, or the buccal fat pad. Maxillary molar impactions are rarely divided.

The most common type of impaction is the mesial angular impaction, and as a general rule, this is the easiest of the impactions to remove. The distal angular and vertical impactions are probably the most deceptive of all impactions. In these instances, the tooth appears to be in a normal vertical relationship when viewed on the radiograph and therefore appears to be simple to remove. However, such is not the case, for these impactions actually are most difficult to remove. The natural path of delivery of a third molar usually is in the distal direction, but if the roots of the impacted third molar are in such close proximity to the roots of the second molar that very little interdental alveolar process can be seen, it will generally be extremely difficult to remove the impacted tooth (Fig. 10–13). A frequent error

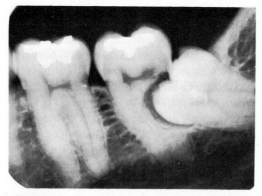

FIGURE 10–11   An impacted third molar causing root resorption of a second molar. (From Costich, E. R., and White, R. P.: Fundamentals of Oral Surgery. Philadelphia, W. B. Saunders Company, 1972.)

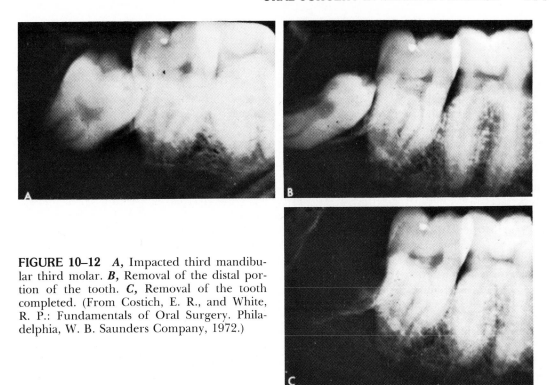

FIGURE 10–12 *A,* Impacted third mandibular third molar. *B,* Removal of the distal portion of the tooth. *C,* Removal of the tooth completed. (From Costich, E. R., and White, R. P.: Fundamentals of Oral Surgery. Philadelphia, W. B. Saunders Company, 1972.)

is to section the entire crown from the roots and to deliver it occlusally. When this is done, it is impossible to remove the remainder of the tooth without doing extensive bone surgery. The tooth can be removed by sectioning only the distal portion of the crown and then, if necessary, more of the crown and the distal root. These cuts must

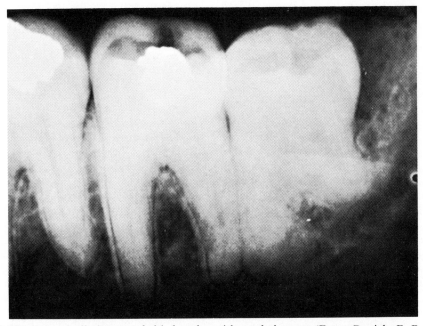

FIGURE 10–13 A vertically impacted third molar with angled roots. (From Costich, E. R., and White, R. P.: Fundamentals of Oral Surgery. Philadelphia, W. B. Saunders Company, 1972.)

be planned and executed carefully to be certain that adequate tooth structure is retained for visualization and manipulation.

The following steps are suggested in removing third molars:

1. Reflect a generous envelope flap. For mandibular teeth, the incision distal to the second molar must stay over the anterior border of the ramus to avoid cutting the lingual nerve. For the maxillary teeth, there should be a vertical relaxing incision at the distobuccal line angle of the first molar. Elevate the flaps using the periosteal elevator and then use the broad end of the Austin retractor to maintain exposure.

2. Use a round bur (No. 6) to cut a trench adjacent to the buccal and distal surfaces of the third molar. The trench should penetrate the cortical bone to medullary bone so that the tooth can be luxated easily. This is generally not possible for the maxillary molar. Instead, the bone on the buccal surface is removed to the level of the third molar's cementoenamel junction.

3. A. For mandibular teeth there are several approaches. A traction hole can be cut in the mesiobuccal surface of the third molar and a No. 190 or 191 elevator inserted in the hole and the tooth elevated, using the buccal alveolar rim as the fulcrum. The tooth may be cut vertically with the bur to split it in half or to remove a segment of the distal part of the crown. The tooth may be cut to permit elevation of the distal crown and root followed by the mesial crown and root.

B. For maxillary teeth a straight No. 1 or No. 80 elevator is worked between the crown and the alveolus at the mesiobuccal line angle. The tooth is elevated bucally and distally. If removal is not accomplished easily, the appropriate Potts' elevator (No. 6 for the left and No. 7 for the right) is worked into the third molar crypt on the mesial surface and rotated so that it slides around the mesiolingual line angle and forces the tooth bucally.

Regardless of the elevator used, the process is facilitated by having the patient close his mouth slightly and move the mandible to the side being operated. This provides better access and visibility and lessens the possibility of losing the tooth in the buccal fat pad or the pterygopalatine fissure.

4. The bone margins are smoothed using a bone file or the No. 6 bur. Remnants

of the follicle are removed by grasping them with the rongeurs or hemostat and pulling them away from the bone. Sharp dissection may be necessary if they are attached to soft tissue. Retract the flaps, flush generously, and aspirate to be certain that all specks of bone that may be trapped at the junction of bone and periosteum are removed.

5. In the mandible, a suture between the first and second molar and a suture distal to the second molar should be placed to re-establish the gingiva. The incision should not be sutured further distally. This technique provides a vent for decompression of any submucosal oozing and minimizes ecchymosis. In the maxilla, place one suture to reposition the interdental papilla between the first and second molar; no distal sutures are required.

6. Place one or two damp 2×2 inch gauze sponges over the gingiva and in the buccal vestibule and have the patient close to provide gentle pressure over the extraction sites. Try to avoid getting the sponges between the teeth, since the object is to keep pressure on the extraction sites. These packs can be left in place for several hours and then replaced as needed.

Maxillary Canines. The second most frequently impacted member of the dentition is the maxillary canine. Such an impaction should be detected early and the tooth exposed so that it is given every opportunity to erupt into normal position. The location of impacted canines must be established carefully and the appropriate labial or palatal exposure created with care to avoid injury to adjacent erupted teeth. Exposure must provide a pathway large enough for the crown of the tooth to pass freely through bone. If the tooth is so deep that it will likely be covered rapidly by soft tissue during healing, a surgical pack or periodontal dressing should be placed to prevent this and should be maintained for a period of 3 to 4 weeks. If the tooth cannot be brought into function, it should be removed.

Mandibular Premolars. The mandibular premolars are the third most frequently impacted teeth. The crowns of the premolar teeth usually lie close to the lingual cortical plate and occasionally may perforate the plate but not the overlying mucosa. On many occasions, the lower premolar tooth erupts from its impacted location and is malposed lingually.

Periapical dental x-rays taken at several

angles, including an occlusal view, will help establish the precise position of the crown and root of the impacted premolar tooth. A lingual approach for the removal of this tooth is the one most frequently used. Adequate exposure will be provided by a gingival crevice incision along with reflection of an envelope flap on the lingual surface. The flap should extend from the midline of the mandible to the molar area. The mucoperiosteum strips easily from the lingual bone. It is important that the incision be made in the gingival crevice because it facilitates repositioning of the flap and permits more rapid healing. Incisions made in the mucoperiosteum of the lingual surface midway between the gingival crest and the floor of the mouth are difficult to reposition and suture and will heal very slowly, with much discomfort to the patient.

With the flap reflected, the overlying bone is removed carefully to expose the crown of the impacted tooth, without involving the roots of the adjacent teeth. At times, simply exposing the crown and drilling a hole into it is all that is necessary to provide a traction point for an elevator to permit the tooth to be lifted from its position. If it is necessary to remove a portion of the crown to gain a pathway, sectioning must be planned carefully so that the remaining tooth segment will be visible and large enough for placement of traction points and for grasping with a hemostat or forceps.

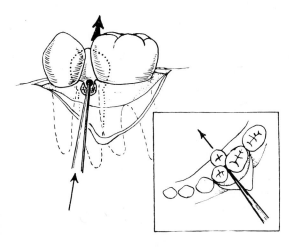

FIGURE 10–14 Elevator application in zones of limited access. (From Hayward, J. R., and Costich, E. R.: The use of elevators. Pract. Dent. Monogr., March 1957.)

Malposed Mandibular Premolar. The mandibular premolar that is lingually malposed and prevented from assuming its normal relationship in the dental arch may be a challenge when it is difficult to grasp the crown because of the danger of displacing the adjacent teeth during manipulation. In this instance, a buccal envelope flap may be reflected and a hole drilled into the impacted premolar tooth through the available space between the normally aligned teeth. A straight elevator (or a straight root-tip pick) that has been blunted then can be inserted in the hole and the handle gently tapped with a mallet, forcing the tooth upward and lingually from its position in the alveolar socket without disturbing the adjacent teeth (Fig. 10–14).

Soft Tissue Procedures

Lacerations

All intraoral wounds over 4 mm in length or depth should be sutured. The first step in management is to inspect the wound carefully to be sure that there are no foreign materials present. If teeth have been chipped and the remaining stump of a tooth is in the area of a laceration, soft tissue radiographs should be made to be certain there are no tooth fragments in the wound.

Deep lacerations are closed in layers. Muscle is sutured with size 3-0 gut, plain or chromic. The mucosal layers are closed with 3-0 black silk. Skin is closed with 5-0 silk or nylon. Skin closure, because of cosmetic implications, should be done by a person who has been properly trained.

It is best if definitive treatment of fractures requiring open reduction is completed before lacerations are closed. If that is not possible, the wounds should be closed to reduce blood and fluid loss, to minimize the chances for infection, to make the patient more comfortable, and to facilitate nursing care.

Biopsy

If the dentist has any reason to suspect the presence of malignant disease, he should do a biopsy rather than a cytologic smear. A negative smear from an unusual lesion does not eliminate the need for a biopsy, since oral cytology yields 25 per cent false negative reports. In addition, a positive cytologic

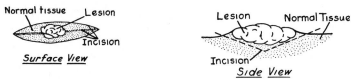

FIGURE 10–15 Excisional biopsy. Illustrated is the complete removal of a small lesion by elliptical surface incisions that include an area of normal tissue encircling the entire lesion. The elliptical surface incisions are demonstrated in the surface view by the solid lines around the normal tissue. The convergence of the incisions in the underlying tissue is shown by the dotted lines in the surface view and by the broken lines in the side view. (From Rovin, S.: The role of biopsy and cytology in oral diagnosis. Dent. Clin. North Am., July 1965, pp. 429–34.)

report must be confirmed by biopsy. Therefore, the point cannot be stated too strongly. If a lesion is suspicious, a biopsy must be done.

The following rules for biopsy are simple, as is the technique itself:

1. Anesthetize the area by block anesthesia, if possible. Avoid infiltration directly into the area in which the biopsy is to be done. If conduction anesthesia is not possible, a field block or infiltration around the biopsy site will prevent distortion of the lesion.

2. Tiny lesions must be removed completely to obtain sufficient material for the pathologist. A rule of thumb is: "If it is small, take it all." A superficial lesion about 5 mm in diameter or less can be considered small (Fig. 10–15).

3. If the lesion is too large to be removed in its entirety, excise a wedge of tissue that is approximately 4 mm wide and generally not less than 4 mm deep. Do not "skin" the surface of a lesion, but penetrate into it so that

a representative specimen is taken (Fig. 10–16). If the lesion is very superficial, however, deep cuts are not necessary.

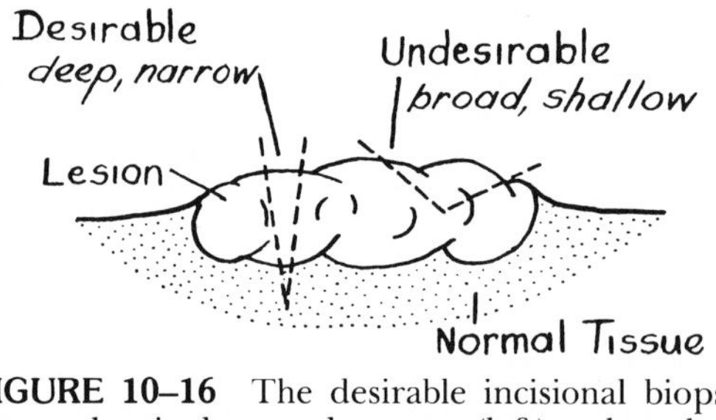

4. If a large tumor or an area of hyperkeratosis varies in appearance in different regions, perform multiple biopsies (Fig. 10–17) and place each specimen in a separate bottle. Draw an outline diagram indicating the areas from which each of the biopsies is taken; each bottle should be labeled with a number or letter corresponding to the area on the diagram from which the specimen is taken. Record this information and drawing on the patient's chart as well as on the biopsy form.

5. The specimen bottles should contain 10 per cent neutral formalin. Since a thin section of tissue may curl in the fixative, the tissue should be placed on a piece of paper towel and then immersed in the fixative with the paper to minimize distortion.

Knowledge of the orientation of the specimen in the mouth is often helpful to the pathologist in interpreting tissue changes. A large lesion with a wide base may require marking to indicate its orientation. This can be done by attaching a suture to the anterior pole and noting the suture location on an accompanying diagram.

A negative biopsy, when malignant disease was the clinical impression, requires another biopsy. In some cases as many as four repeat biopsies have been done to finally confirm a suspected malignancy. A biopsy that is positive for malignant disease imposes a serious obligation on the dentist; he must make every effort to see that the patient receives immediate attention.

Care of Fractured Jaws

If a fracture is suspected on the basis of history of an accident, altered occlusion, or

FIGURE 10–16 The desirable incisional biopsy is one that is deep and narrow (left) rather than broad and shallow (right). The deeper biopsy reveals the deeper changes that may be more significant than those revealed by the shallower biopsy. (From Rovin, S.: The role of biopsy and cytology in oral diagnosis. Dent. Clin. North Am., July 1965, pp. 429–34.)

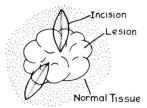

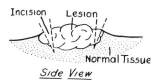

FIGURE 10–17 Incisional biopsy. In large lesions, it may be necessary to excise more than one section of the lesion in order to obtain areas representative of the disease process. In the illustration at the left, the solid lines show the elliptical surface incisions, including both normal and diseased tissue. The side view in the illustration at the right shows the surface incisions converging to form a V in the underlying tissues. (From Rovin, S.: The role of biopsy and cytology in oral diagnosis. Dent. Clin. North Am., July 1965, pp. 429–34.)

pain or deformity, a careful clinical and radiographic examination is required. Bimanual palpation and manipulation of the jaws by grasping different quadrants and attempting to move the segments will help to locate fractures. Maxillary fractures that run through the infraorbital canal may produce numbness of the cheek and upper lip. Fractures of the body of the mandible may cause numbness in the mental nerve area. The skin over the face should be checked with a pin to locate any areas of numbness that would help to localize a fracture. If the clinical examination suggests a fracture, radiographs should be taken to confirm the diagnosis. If a suspected fracture cannot be

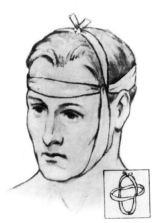

FIGURE 10–18 The modified Barton bandage (barrel bandage) supports the mandible without creating pressure over the chin that might displace the parts posteriorly. Thus it prevents displacement of the tongue and airway obstruction. (From Massler, M., and Schour, I.: Atlas of the Mouth in Health and Disease, 2nd ed. American Dental Association, 1958.)

confirmed radiographically, the patient should be treated as if a fracture exists and consultation should be requested.

Emergency Care

Emergency treatment for fractured jaws can be administered at the scene of an accident, in the dental office, or in the hospital and is intended to be lifesaving and pain reducing. The essentials of emergency care are: (1) Be sure the patient has a good airway and can breathe adequately, (2) control the bleeding, and (3) make the patient as comfortable as possible. One procedure may sometimes accomplish all three objectives.

The mandible should be brought forward to keep the tongue from blocking the airway. Bleeding can be controlled by pressure packs to intraoral and extraoral wounds. Immobilization of the jaws with a bandage will maintain the mandible in a forward position and apply pressure to the bleeding points. By keeping the parts motionless, the bandage also reduces pain and helps to control the bleeding by preventing clot disruption due to movement. A modified Barton's bandage that passes under the mandible to hold it up and forward is suitable for this purpose (Fig. 10–18). Pressure on the anterior part of the mandible that displaces the jaw posteriorly should be avoided because it may compromise the airway.

Definitive Care

Following the emergency care, the severely injured patient should be referred immediately to an oral surgeon, if possible. If other injuries require immediate attention, treatment of fractured jaws can be delayed as long as 10 days. However, every day of delay makes definitive care more difficult.

The three steps necessary for definitive care of fractured jaws are: (1) reduction of the fractures, (2) fixation of the parts in place, and (3) immobilization of the jaw. Less than this may result in nonunion or malunion of the bone.

Simple fractures in patients with an adequate dentition can be managed by wiring the teeth in occlusion. The key to success in immobilization is to be sure that the wires between the jaws maintain occlusion and prevent motion of the parts.

Edentulous patients require special care. They should be referred to an oral surgeon. If the patient has dentures, he should take them to the oral surgeon even if they are broken and parts are missing. The dentures can be used as splints and wired or pinned to the jaws to provide immobilization and maintenance of proper intermaxillary distances.

Transplantation of Teeth

Allogenic tooth grafting has been practiced at least since the earliest days of recorded history. The surgical procedures and postoperative care for autografting and allografting are similar. It is difficult to offer any well-supported opinions of these procedures because there have been no large, longitudinal studies done on them. Many factors, such as age of the patient, development of the graft, status of the natural dentition, utilization of abutment teeth, and general health, play a definite role in the success of tooth grafts. Survival of allografts is unpredictable. The impression from the literature is that in most cases the roots have resorbed completely within 2 years.

Autograft success depends on a few known factors and some still unknown factors. Mandibular third molars with one half to two thirds of the roots developed and of appropriate mesiodistal measurement can be repositioned in mandibular first and second molar sockets immediately after removal of the latter teeth and may be retained for many years (Fig. 10–19 and 10–20). The average survival time ranges from 8 to 10 years, with many reports of survival for more than 20 years.

The most frequently transplanted or surgically moved tooth is the maxillary canine. It is the second most frequently impacted tooth and is a key tooth in regard to occlusal stability and esthetic appearance. It is unfortunate that its failure to erupt is not treated earlier in more instances by orthodontic therapy. Once the tooth is fully formed and impacted, orthodontic treatment is difficult and sometimes not acceptable to the older patient. Orthodontic therapy is, however, the method of choice, since the results are more predictable. Exposure of the canine crown and placement of a threaded pin in the crown, a bonded plastic bracket, or a wire lasso around the neck of the tooth provide a traction point for the orthodontist. The lasso procedure is difficult and requires experience.

When orthodontic treatment has been ruled out, surgical repositioning is the second method of choice (Fig. 10–21). Age, however, is a factor, and success is best assured if the procedure is done in individuals under 20 years of age, since bone regeneration seems to be more complete for younger patients. The apex of the fully formed, palatally impacted canine is usually sharply angled superiorly where it lies along the anterior wall of the sinus. This relationship makes it difficult to remove the tooth intact, resulting in more extensive bone loss than for the simple removal of the canine by sectioning the crown from the root. If the angled apex of this tooth fractures during removal for transplantation, it will not affect the transplant. The tip should be recovered if it does not require the removal of additional bone. If the tip is not removed, the patient should be so informed and the fact noted in the record. While the process of tip recovery takes place, if it is necessary, the canine is stored in the floor of the mouth, under the patient's tongue. The socket is prepared and the tooth tried in place. Because the tooth is slippery and difficult to handle without touching the root, a Williams mesenteric clamp with rubber tubing over the ends (Fig. 10–22) is used to grasp the tooth at the crown. If the angled apex causes problems in positioning, it can be cut off with a fissure bur cooled by a copious flow of normal saline. The tooth is held with the Williams clamp during this procedure.

The basic steps in transplantation are

fairly simple and can be modified as the situation and good judgment dictate. The steps are as follows:

1. Check to be sure that there is room for the transplant in the new position, as estimated by measurements on radiographs and by oral examination. Be sure that the impacted tooth can be extracted without damage and without removing bone to the extent that other teeth are endangered.

2. Explain to the patient the possibilities of failure. The discomfort will be no worse than in the removal of an impaction without transplantation.

3. Obtain written permission from the patient or a parent for the procedure.

4. Reflect a buccal envelope flap to expose the tooth to be transplanted.

5. Loosen and move the transplant to make sure that it can be removed intact. If it cannot be retained in its socket while the

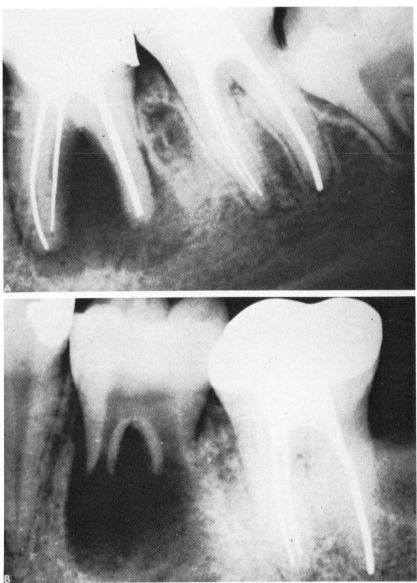

FIGURE 10–19 *A,* The mandibular first molar was endodontically treated without success and the patient refused further treatment. For that reason it was removed, and the third molar was transplanted into its place. *B,* The immediate posttransplant radiograph, before splinting. (From Costich, E. R., and White, R. P.: Fundamentals of Oral Surgery. Philadelphia, W. B. Saunders Company, 1972.)

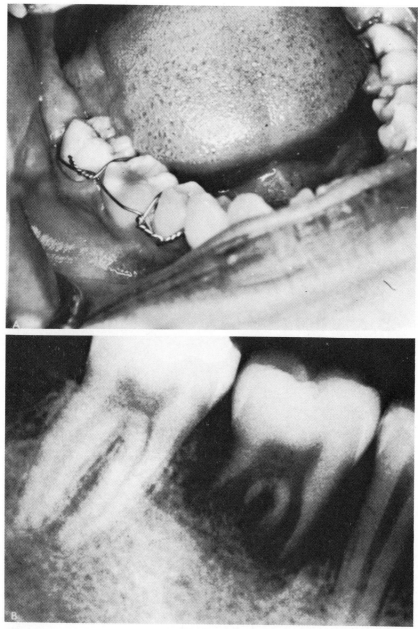

FIGURE 10–20 *A,* Six weeks prior to this photograph, the lower right third molar had been transplanted to the first molar site. The wires for splinting were removed at this time. *B,* Radiograph of the tooth immediately after removal of wires. Healing of the alveolar socket is progressing. (From Costich, E. R., and White, R. P., Fundamentals of Oral Surgery. Philadelphia, W. B. Saunders Company, 1972.)

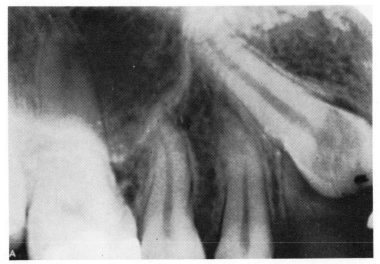

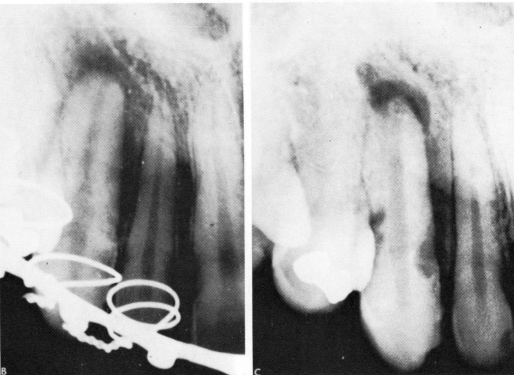

FIGURE 10–21 *A,* An impacted canine in an 18-year-old girl with a retained primary canine. Note the deviation of the canine root tip along the maxillary sinus wall as well as the deviation of the first premolar root ends to accommodate the impacted canine. The roots of the second premolar conform to the sinus wall. *B,* The canine has been placed in a new socket created after the primary canine was removed. The apex of the canine was cut off to facilitate placing it in the new socket. Because the patient had spaces between all teeth, a segment of the annealed arch bar was used in splinting the repositioned tooth. *C,* Three months after surgery, root resorption on the mesial and distal root surfaces is very noticeable. There is an obvious periapical radiolucency.

Illustration continued on following page

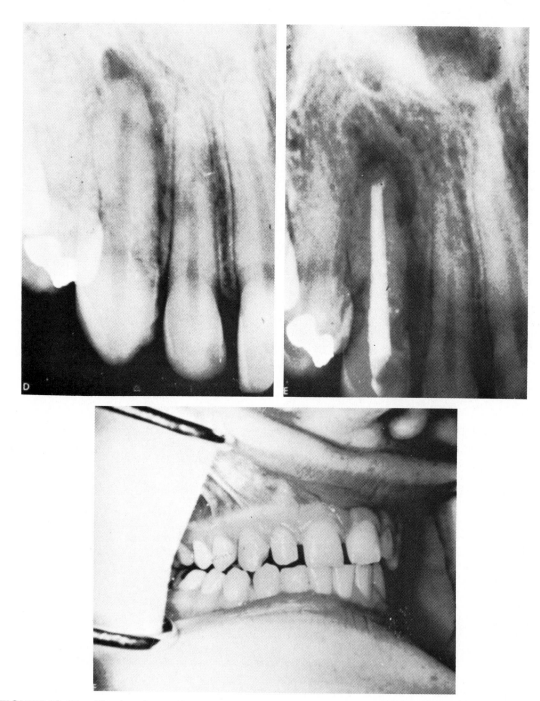

FIGURE 10–21   *(Continued)*   *D,* Six months after surgery, the two prominent areas of root resorption have undergone repair or remineralization. The apical area of radiolucency is smaller but still present. *E,* One year after surgical repositioning and immediately after the completion of endodontic treatment. The root shows evidence of continuing fluctuation of resorption and repair. *F,* Photograph of the right canine taken at the same time as radiograph *E.* The gingival condition is good. Five years after surgery, the tooth is still in position. (From Costich, E. R., and White, R. P.: Fundamentals of Oral Surgery. Philadelphia, W. B. Saunders Company, 1972.)

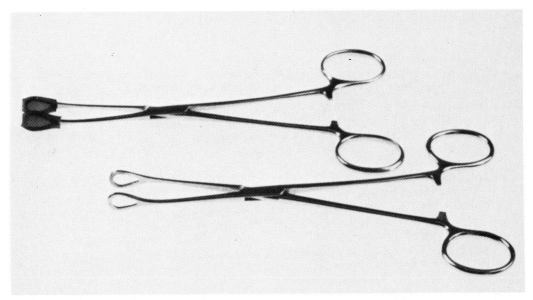

FIGURE 10–22 The Williams mesenteric clamp can be modified to handle teeth in transplantation procedures by putting rubber tubing over the ends of the beaks. (From Costich, E. R., and White, R. P.: Fundamentals of Oral Surgery. Philadelphia, W. B. Saunders Company, 1972.)

new site is prepared, place it under the patient's tongue. Any remnants of periodontal membrane or follicle should be left attached to the tooth.

6. Prepare the new site by removing all bony septa with a bur. Do not injure the adjacent teeth.

7. If the root or the crown of the transplant must be shaved so that the tooth will fit, use a diamond stone while holding the tooth with the Williams clamp and cooling with saline.

8. Immerse the tooth in 2 per cent sodium fluoride in a sterile dish for 2 minutes.

9. Rinse the tooth with sterile normal saline, and then insert it in its new position.

10. Suture the flap into position.

11. Splint the tooth using 27- or 30-gauge stainless-steel wire, and cover the wire on the labial surface with the clear acrylic used for restorations or temporary crowns. An alternative technique is to acid etch the transplant and two teeth on both sides and then to cement a wire to the teeth using composite as the bonding material. This gives added stability.

12. Postoperative care should be similar to that for any tooth removal. Antibiotics are not needed.

13. The patient should be seen weekly for 6 to 8 weeks, after which time the splints can be removed.

14. If the dentist feels that endodontic treatment should be given, because perhaps the pulp was extirpated when the root tip was cut from the canine or because radiographs indicate that such treatment would be advantageous, it can be begun at any time after gingival attachment is established.

Implantation

Various materials can serve as replacements for teeth or be made into devices for the attachment of crowns or bridges. Bone, ivory, acrylic resin, lead, iron, gold, platinum, stainless steel, carbon, and ceramics such as simple crystal sapphire are the materials most frequently described. The shape of the implants varies from conforming to the shape of the tooth root to hollow tubes, meshwork, screws, or thin, flat plates (blades). The implant is either subperiosteal or intraosteal.

Implants are intriguing because the body tolerates many completely buried foreign materials acquired either by accident or by intention. Plates used to hold bones apart or together are tolerated and generally remain in place without causing trouble.

"Dental Implants: Benefits and Risks," An NIH-Harvard Consensus Development Conference, held in 1978, reviewed the status of alloplastic implants. Four categories for use were identified: *Unrestricted*—adequate data available for a favorable 5-year prognosis; *Use With Guidelines*—reason for a specific restricted application, even though there may be adequate data available for a favorable 5-year prognosis; *Clinical Trials*—insufficient data to provide the basis for prognosis; and *Human Application Contraindicated.*

It was the consensus of the conference that no implants had achieved the "Unrestricted" category. Three applications of implants were placed in the "Use With Guidelines" category, based on the recommendation of more than 75 per cent of the voting participants. They were: (1) the full-arch subperiosteal mandibular implant placed on basilar bone opposing a complete tissue-borne denture; (2) the metallic blade implant in the free-end application; and (3) the blade in the interdental application when contributing to the support of a fixed bridge where there is adequate available bone, adequate intermaxillary space, and a treatment plan that favors a fixed prosthesis. All shapes, styles, and materials that are described in the literature were not reviewed at the conference because of the difficulty of accumulating sufficient data to make judgments. Controlled long-term studies by more than one investigator are not yet available to justify the designation of "Unrestricted" for any of the alloplastic implants. Practitioners who choose to use implants should review "Dental Implants: Benefits and Risks." The fact that a specific type of implant was not included in that publication, however, does not mean it is unacceptable. Selection should be made based on critical evaluation of published articles in refereed journals.

One planning to use implants should take advantage of a continuing education course, preferably one that includes manikin experience and the opportunity for supervised clinical participation.

SURGICAL PREPARATION OF THE MOUTH FOR PROSTHODONTICS

The surgical preparation of the mouth for dentures may involve soft tissue, bone, or both. The need for such surgery is determined by clinical and radiographic examination.

Clinical Examination

The importance of examining all the oral tissues as well as the denture-bearing surfaces cannot be overemphasized. Abnormalities of any area of the oral mucosa must be diagnosed. Biopsy usually will provide the diagnosis of an abnormality and may also eliminate the condition.

All clinically visible or palpable lumps and bumps that could be traumatized by the denture, including papillomas or polyps of the buccal mucosa, lips, and tongue, should be removed. Such lesions are generally traumatized by new prostheses, either fixed or removable.

The common bony abnormalities requiring preprosthodontic surgery include tori, mandibular third molar lingual crests, internal oblique ridges (mylohyoid ridges), buccal bulge of the maxillary tuberosities, and postextraction irregularities of the alveolar ridges. Occasionally the genial tubercles are enlarged and close to the crest of atrophic ridges; these too may have to be removed.

Abnormal frenum attachments or bands of scar tissue sometimes require correction. The maxillary labial frenum is the most common problem of this type and the lingual frenum the least common.

Roentgenographic Examination

Radiographs are an absolute necessity when oral surgery on or adjacent to a bony surface is indicated. Although some dentists use occlusal films to screen the jaws, these films have very limited value for surgical planning. Periapical or panoramic films will reveal unerupted or impacted teeth, retained roots, enostoses (localized sclerotic bone), odontomas, residual cysts, and other pathologic bone conditions. In addition, periapical or panoramic films show the thickness of the soft tissue over the crest of the alveolar ridge. If a panoramic film reveals a questionable shadow, the area should be evaluated further with a periapical or lateral oblique film. Panoramic radiographs give information about the size of the maxillary sinus, the location of the mental foramen, and the position of the inferior alveolar canal but do not provide good, "in focus" details.

Conditions Requiring Preprosthetic Surgery

Fibrous Tuberosity

Chapter 11 (Prosthodontics in General Practice) emphasizes the need for solid tissue support to provide stability for removable dentures. Fibrous tuberosities and flabby alveolar ridges are the most common conditions requiring preprosthetic surgery.

The tuberosity is easily reduced by removal of multiple wedges of tissue. An elliptical incision is made along the crest of the ridge, and a V-shaped wedge of tissue is removed, with the apex of the wedge at the surface of the alveolar crest. The palatal and buccal mucosa are then undermined to re-move wedges of tissue that have their apex toward the alveolar crest incision and their base on the bone. The buccal and palatal wedges are freed from the bone with a periosteal elevator; the periosteum is taken with the fibrous tissue. The remaining two flaps of tissue, about 2 mm thick at the margins, are easily pressed into place on the alveolar crest. If the flaps overlap, the excess tissue is removed to allow the edges to abut and the sutures to bring them together for a primary closure (Figs. 10–23 and 10–24).

If the buccal alveolar bone is bulbous or if there is limited space between the ramus and the maxilla, the excess buccal bone can be removed after the wedges of fibrous tissue have been removed and the buccal flap is elevated. Rarely is it necessary to reduce the height of the bony alveolar crest (Figs. 10–23D and 10–24C and D).

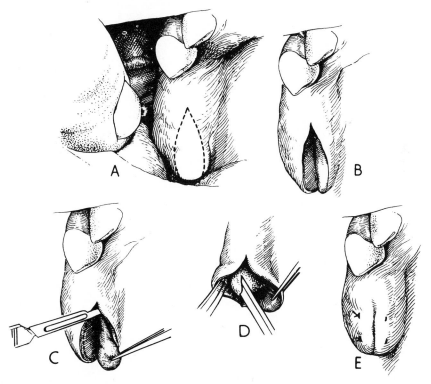

FIGURE 10–23 The technique for excision of soft tissue and bone from tuberosities, as viewed from the surface of the alveolar crest. **A,** The dotted line shows the shape of the incisions along the surface of the crest. **B,** The first wedge of tissue has been removed. **C,** The dotted line to the left shows where the cut will be made to undermine the buccal mucosa. At the right, this wedge of palatal tissue is shown being removed. **D,** The position of a chisel in removing a buccal bulge of bone is shown. The rongeurs, a file, or a bur may be equally effective. **E,** The remaining tissue flaps have been brought into place on the alveolar crest and sutured. (From Howe, G. L.: Minor Oral Surgery, 2nd ed. Baltimore, Williams & Wilkins, 1971.)

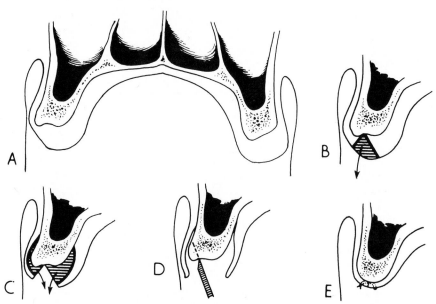

FIGURE 10–24 *A,* The soft tissue and bone to be removed from fibrous bulbous tuberosities is shown in frontal section. The striped segments in *B* and *C* represent the wedges of tissue excised. The bulbous bone is cut in *D*. *E* shows the closed, reduced tuberosity. (From Howe, G. L.: Minor Oral Surgery, 2nd ed. Baltimore, Williams & Wilkins, 1971.)

Flabby Ridges

This condition of the alveolar ridge, which usually occurs in the area between the premolars, may exist in either jaw but is seen more frequently in the maxilla. In these sec-

tions, the alveolar processes are narrower than in the tuberosity areas, so that generally only a single V-shaped wedge along the surface of the crest needs to be removed to firm the tissue (Fig. 10–25). In the maxillary

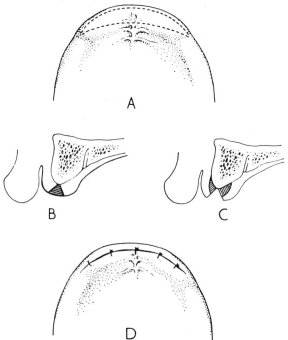

FIGURE 10–25 The surface incisions are indicated by the dotted lines in *A*. The flabby anterior ridge generally requires the excision of only a single V-shaped wedge of tissue along the crest, as shown in *B*. Occasionally the tissue may be undermined and extra tissue excised, as shown in *C*. *D*, The remaining tissue is sutured. (From Howe, G. L.: Minor Oral Surgery, 2nd ed. Baltimore, Williams & Wilkins, 1971.)

anterior region, the operator must be careful to keep the wedge over the crest. If the incisions are made too far to the labial aspect, all the attached gingiva may be removed; consequently, when the margins are sutured, the labial mucosa will be pulled onto the crest, thus distorting the gingival sulcus in the area. The incisive papilla presents no deterrent to surgery in the maxillary anterior segment. The papilla can be removed, and there is no contraindication to cutting the structures emerging from the incisive canal. The patient's denture, if available, may be lined with tissue conditioner and seated immediately after surgery to serve as a splint. The patient must be instructed to carefully clean the denture after eating and not to wear the denture at night. New denture fabrication can be initiated in 4 to 6 weeks.

Shallow Mandibular Vestibule

Increased depth of the mandibular labial vestibule can be gained using Gamble's modification of a vestibuloplasty described by

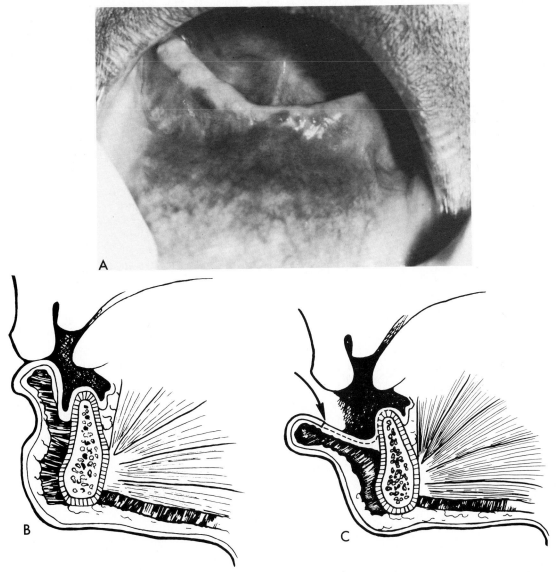

FIGURE 10–26 Patient with high mentalis attachments, and the mucosal incision and dissection. (From Kethley, J. L., and Gamble, J. W.: The lipswitch: a modification of Kazanjian's labial vestibuloplasty. J. Oral Surg., *36*(8):701–705, 1978.)

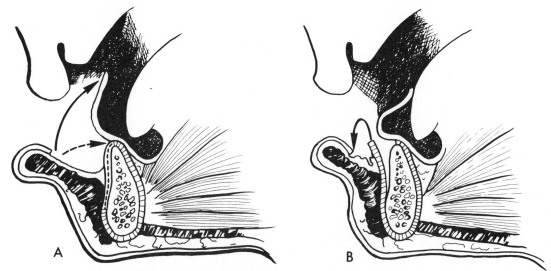

FIGURE 10–27 Retraction of the mucosal flap, incision of the periosteum, and reflection of the periosteal flap. (From Kethley, J. L., and Gamble, J. W.: The lipswitch: a modification of Kazanjian's labial vestibuloplasty. J. Oral Surg., *36*(8):701–705, 1978.)

Kazanjian and by Clark. An incision is made in the labial mucosa, and the mucosa is reflected to the depth of the sulcus. The reflection is then extended from the mandible supraperiosteally in a crestal direction, with the periosteum retained on the mandible and alveolar bone (Fig. 10–26). The reflection of mucosa usually is terminated at the mucogingival junction. The periosteum is then incised at that level and reflected from the mandible to the depth of the desired sulcus (Fig. 10–27). The periosteum is sutured to the lip, covering the areas denuded of mucosa, and the mucosal flap is sutured so that the incised margin is at the depth of the sulcus (Fig. 10–28).

The transposition of the flaps of mucosa and periosteum greatly reduces the relapse and loss of vestibular depth associated with the single-flap procedures of Kazanjian and of Clark. The modified procedure is an excellent operation that can be performed on an outpatient basis, using local anesthesia without the need for grafts or splints.

Frena

At times the maxillary labial or the lingual frenum must be eliminated. Only occasionally do other frena present surgical problems.

Before the incision is made, the frenum is stabilized with two small hemostats; for the maxillary frenum, one is clamped perpen-

dicular to the lip and the other perpendicular to the alveolus; for the lingual frenum, one is clamped along the tongue and the other along the floor of the mouth. The tissue immediately adjacent to the hemostats is cut from underneath them, and the instruments are thus freed with the frenum. This procedure leaves a surprisingly large mucosal defect. The mucosa is brought together with the first suture placed in the center of the incision (Fig. 10–29). For the labial frenum, this is at the level of the height of the vestibule. The labial side of the incison is sutured next, and the tissues usually approximate without difficulty. If tension is required to close this section, the margins should be undermined to facilitate the closure. The alveolar portion is closed last. If this portion cannot be adapted tightly, there is little cause for concern, since the area will granulate and heal. Problems in closing are usually due to excision of too much tissue.

In the case of the lingual frenum, the tongue side is closed first. The excision procedure and suturing are made easier if a suture is placed through the tip of the tongue so that the assistant can put traction on the tongue to stabilize it and facilitate excision and suturing (Fig. 10–30). The suturing is started at the junction of the floor of the mouth and the ventral surface of the tongue. As in all instances of cutting and suturing in

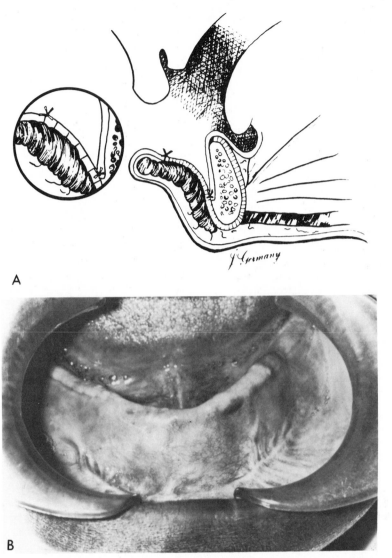

A

B

FIGURE 10–28   The mucosal flap sutured to the depth of the new vestibule and the periosteum sutured to the original mucosal incision and the vestibule 8 months postoperatively. (From Kethley, J. L., and Gamble, J. W.: The lipswitch: a modification of Kazanjian's labial vestibuloplasty. J. Oral Surg., *36*(8):701–705, 1978.)

the floor of the mouth, the operator must be careful not to damage the sublingual salivary ducts or their orifices.

Papillomatosis

Papillomatosis is a condition seen on the palate, usually in the relief area under complete denture bases. It is occasionally seen in dentulous patients with mouths characterized by high palatal vaults and poor oral hygiene. In areas where the palatal bone has resorbed beneath a denture, hyperplastic papillomatous tissue forms to fill the space.

If the patient does not wear the denture for 7 to 10 days, the redness will subside, and the multiple small papillomas will shrink but not disappear. The tissue must be removed, or it will proliferate under a new denture, because debris accumulates and bacteria thrive in the grooves and crevices of the pebbly papillomatous surface.

The entire area of involvement should be removed by scraping with a sharp Molt curette or by supraperiosteal dissection with a No. 15 blade. After the tissue has been removed and the surface has been wiped with gauze sponges to remove the loose fragments, a moist gauze pack is placed over the raw surface to apply pressure and to stop the oozing. The old denture is lined with a tissue conditioner and seated immediately after the sponges have been removed. This controls bleeding, provides a protective covering for the tissue, and acts as a temporary denture until a new one can be prepared after healing takes place. Sutures from alveolar crest to alveolar crest may be used to retain gauze packs if a denture is not avail-able or cannot be retained. Specimens of the tissue removed, regardless of the surgical technique, should be sent to the pathologist for examination.

Tori

All maxillary tori that have undercuts, all sessile maxillary tori with an elevation of more than 5 mm, and all mandibular tori should be removed. The time and inconven-

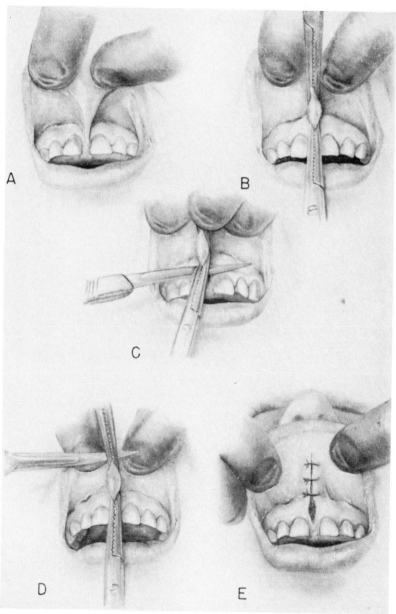

FIGURE 10–29   The technique for removal of an undesirable labial frenum. (See text for description.) (From Archer, W. H.: Oral Surgery, 4th ed. Philadelphia, W. B. Saunders Company, 1966.)

ience involved in removing these structures are insignificant compared with the difficulty they impose in fabricating dentures and the subsequent discomfort, worry, and irritation they cause the patient.

Palatal Tori. Maxillary tori are covered by a very thin and easily traumatized mucosa. The torus is dense, hard bone and does not resorb as do the alveolar ridges. For this reason, the torus becomes a pivotal area on which the denture rocks. Palatal ulceration is commonly associated with this condition.

In the removal of palatal tori, the area involved is anesthetized by bilateral greater palatine blocks and infiltration between the anterior pole of the torus and the incisor teeth. If the torus extends to the posterior border of the hard palate, it may be necessary to infiltrate a few drops of anesthetic solution distal to the torus.

An incision is made in the midline of the palate so that when the mucoperiosteum is elevated, two large flaps with wide bases parallel to the posterior teeth are present. The exposed torus is cut vertically and crosswise

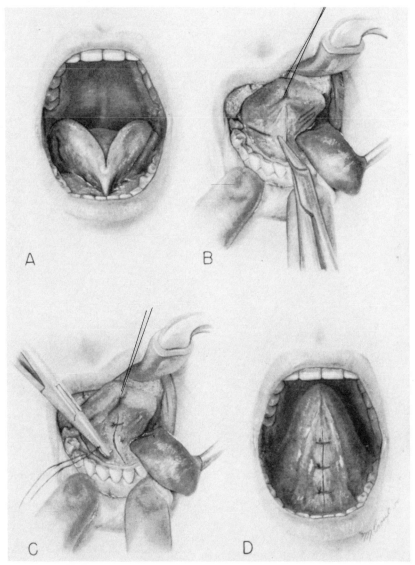

FIGURE 10–30 The technique for removal of an undesirable lingual frenum. Note that in *B* a suture has been placed through the tip of the tongue so that the assistant can use gentle traction to keep the tongue elevated, extended, and motionless during the operation. (From Archer, W. H.: Oral Surgery, 4th ed. Philadelphia, W. B. Saunders Company, 1966.)

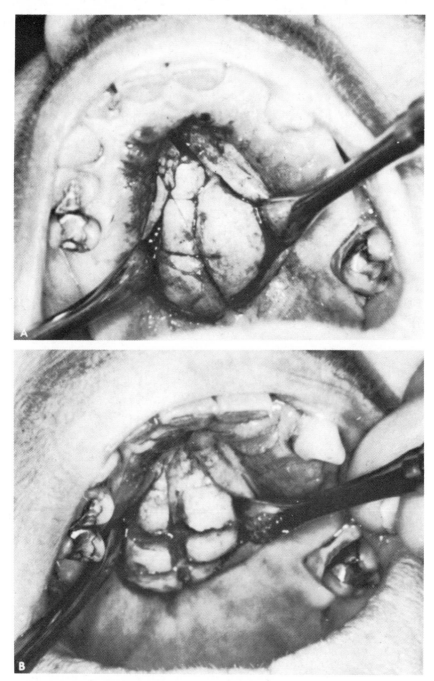

FIGURE 10–31 Removal of maxillary torus. *A,* Exposure of the torus. *B,* Crosshatching made with a bur.

Illustration continued on opposite page

with a fissure or round bur, creating a checkered pattern of grooves (Fig. 10–31). A broad gouge elevator or bone chisel is placed in the grooves, and the segments of bone are pried out. The small rim of torus remaining, and small spicules left projecting, can be trimmed with a No. 6 to 8 round bur and fi- nally smoothed with a bone file. The area should be irrigated and the flaps sutured into place. A previously prepared acrylic splint or an old denture lined with tissue conditioner is then placed to keep the tissue in close contact with the palate during heal- ing and to prevent a hematoma from form-

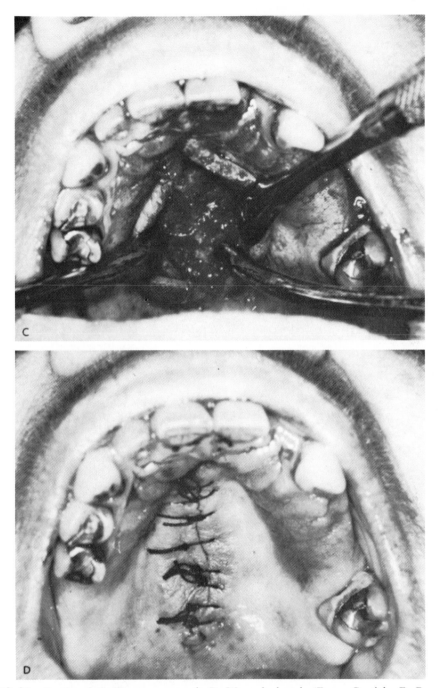

FIGURE 10–31 *Continued* **C,** Torus removed. **D,** Wound closed. (From Costich, E. R., and White, R. P.: Fundamentals of Oral Surgery. Philadelphia, W. B. Saunders Company, 1972.)

ing. Sponges can be placed and retained by sutures spanning the palate if no other support can be retained.

Mandibular Tori. Mandibular tori in dentulous patients are more difficult to remove than those in the edentulous patient. Nonetheless, their removal is indicated if

they will interfere with a lower removable prosthesis.

The incision is made in the gingival crevice, where teeth are present, and along the alveolar crest in edentulous areas (Fig. 10–32). The interdental papillae are reflected with the flap to facilitate closure. If the tori

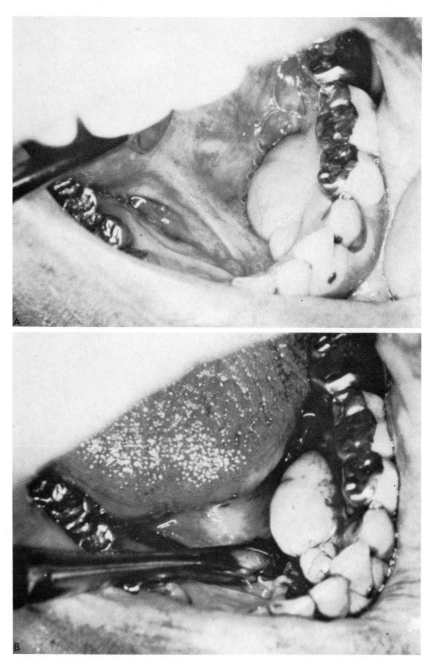

FIGURE 10–32 *A,* Mandibular torus. *B,* Torus exposed.

Illustration continued on opposite page

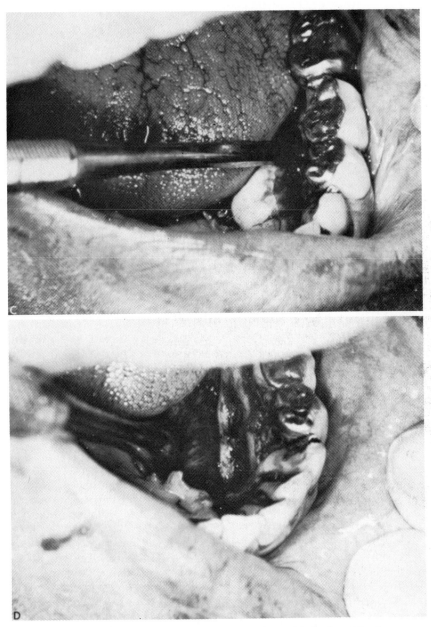

FIGURE 10–32 *Continued* **C,** The torus being broken away by a chisel placed in the cut made by a No. 702 bur. **D,** Torus removed and the margins of the defect smoothed.

Illustration continued on following page

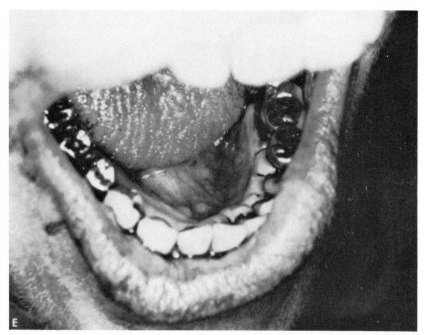

FIGURE 10–32 *Continued E,* Wound closed. (From Costich, E. R., and White R. P.: Fundamentals of Oral Surgery. Philadelphia, W. B. Saunders Company, 1972.)

are large, the operator must be careful to avoid perforating the flap when elevating it for reflection around the inferior surface, since the lingual mucosa is very thin and easily damaged. A large torus can be cut with a bur (see the procedure described for palatal tori) or amputated flush with the lingual surface by use of a No. 704 fissure bur or a No. 6 round bur in a high-speed handpiece, accompanied by a copious flow of water. The area is then carefully irrigated to remove all bone debris, the flap is repositioned, and sutures are placed.

Retained Roots, Teeth, and Cysts

In preparation for complete dentures, retained teeth are removed. The same is true of all retained root tips. All radiolucent bone lesions should be investigated; they are frequently residual cysts that also should be removed.

The surgical approach to removal of a cyst is the same as for a tooth or root, with one exception: never cut into a radiolucent area in bone without first aspirating the defect to determine whether the lesion is solid, cystic, or vascular. An 18- to 20-gauge needle is recommended for this procedure. If the overlying bone is thin, these needles are strong enough to pass through the bony plate. If the bone resists the needle, reflect a flap and, using a No. 4 round bur, carefully remove a small amount of bone; again attempt to push the needle through. After repeated removal of small amounts of bone, followed by attempts to insert the needle, entry will be gained to the radiolucent area. If the area is found to be vascular, it may be fatal to operate without hospitalization and available blood replacement; if it is solid, only an incisional biopsy is indicated; if it is cystic, as determined by the characteristic straw-colored fluid, then the operation may proceed.

Surgical technique for the operation in the edentulous mouth is slightly different from that for a dentulous jaw. The incision should be kept over bone and in mucoperiosteum insofar as possible. It is important to remember that the mandible flares laterally in the molar area. An incision made straight posteriorly, passing off the alveolar ridge, will be unsupported by bone and may cut the lingual nerve.

The incision should be long and slightly curved so that the suture line will not be directly over a surgically created defect (Fig. 10–33). It is important to remember the location of the mental foramen and greater

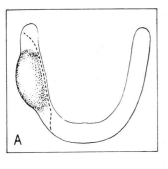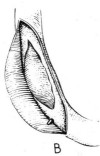

FIGURE 10–33 **A,** The incision for enucleation of a cyst has been placed so that the suture line will rest on bone when the wound is closed. **B,** Note that the mental nerve has been located and identified to prevent injury. The bone has been removed lateral to the crest of the ridge to preserve the ridge. (From Howe, G. L.: Minor Oral Surgery, 2nd ed. Baltimore, Williams & Wilkins, 1971.)

palatine vessels so that the nerves and vessels in these areas will not be cut. If the operation is being performed near a large vessel or nerve, they should be dissected out first so they can be seen and easily avoided during the remainder of the procedure. In order not to reduce the height of the alveolar crest, the operator should work from the buccal, lingual, or palatal aspect, if possible. Enough bone should be removed so that roots can be located easily, and a path should be created for their removal either whole or in sections. The same is true for teeth. Generally, it is best to section retained teeth. High-speed handpieces make sectioning simple. The operator should feel no pride in removing large unsectioned roots of retained teeth at a great sacrifice of bone.

Holes should be drilled into the roots of sectioned teeth to provide traction points for elevators. Wedging maneuvers with elevators sometimes block removal of tooth sections. A traction hole for a direct lift is a simple but quick way to remove tooth fragments (Fig. 10–34). Bone that has been used as a fulcrum should be freshened with a large bur or bone file. This prevents separation and sloughing of a piece of devitalized bone at a later time.

The operative field should always be irrigated and carefully suctioned before it is sutured. The operator should carefully inspect the periosteal side of the flaps at their attachment to bone to be sure that no debris or chips are retained in these areas. The flap should be returned to position and sutured, leaving no gaps. If most of the incision has been in mucoperiosteum, the flap will close easily and neatly.

If the patient has a denture, it should be lined with tissue conditioner and seated. The sutures should be removed no sooner than 4 days and no later than 8 days postoperatively. Impressions for new dentures may be made as early as 3 weeks after surgery. If old dentures or splints have been lined with tissue conditioner, they should be examined at least weekly and the tissue conditioner replaced frequently until the new dentures are placed.

Postoperative Care

Instructions should be given to the patient regarding possible problems with pain, swelling, or bleeding. Following elective removal of noninfected teeth, root tips, or ex-

FIGURE 10–34 The buccal bone at the alveolar crest is removed to facilitate placement of the traction hole. An elevator is then placed in the traction hole to pry or lift the root. (From Hayward, J. R., and Costich, E. R.: The Use of Elevators. Pract. Dent. Monogr., March 1957.)

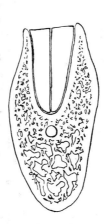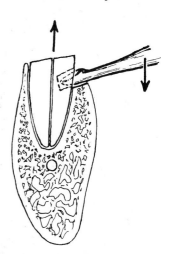

ostoses, it is well to suggest application of an ice pack to the external facial region (a schedule of 20 minutes on and 10 minutes off for the first 6 hours postoperatively). *Heat is not recommended* in the postoperative period, since it may encourage edema. Oral hygiene must be maintained by brushing and gentle rinsing. Normal caloric intake must also be maintained; soft foods, juices, soft drinks, and diet supplements such as Ensure should be suggested to the patient.

MANAGEMENT OF INFECTIONS

In this era of fluoridation and antibiotics, extensive infections of odontogenic origin are not seen so frequently as in earlier times. Infections still constitute, however, the most common nonelective surgical problem encountered in dental practice.

Factors Influencing the Course of Infection

Oral infections undergo resolution, fluctuation, or extension. Resolution is healing without pus formation, whereas fluctuation is the occurrence of central necrosis in the infected area with the formation of pus. Extension is the spread of the infection to adjacent tissues along fascial or anatomic spaces or by the blood stream. The course that an infection takes is dependent upon the nature of the infection, the anatomic location, the extent of involvement, and the resistance of the host.

Nature of Infection

Odontogenic infections are usually mixed bacterial infections, but one should consider the possibility of a resistant bacterial infection or a fungus infection, especially if the condition does not improve rapidly under treatment.

Extent of Involvement

Patients with an acute infection have an elevated temperature, an increased pulse rate, and an increased rate of respiration. Many common analgesics are also antipyretics; thus, the patient on such medication may be very sick yet still not have an elevated temperature. Swelling may be firm and diffuse (cellulitis) or fluctuant (abscess), and the skin may be warm to the touch and discolored. Enlargement and tenderness of the regional lymph nodes are also present. A complete white blood cell count will reveal an increase in total white cells with a high proportion of polymorphonuclear leukocytes.

Anatomic Location

The location of the apices of teeth in relation to muscle attachments and the lines of least resistance determine the direction of spread of dental infections. Periapical abscesses of mandibular first molars in children frequently drain extraorally because the apices of the roots are below the attachment of the buccinator muscle. Pericoronal infections of the lower third molars extend to the lateral pharyngeal area. Regardless of the surgical spaces involved, basic principles of management apply to all infections.

Resistance of the Host

The localization and resolution of the infection are to a large extent dependent on the general state of health of the patient. Patients who are debilitated or who have some systemic disease such as blood dyscrasia or uncontrolled diabetes present special problems.

Aims of Therapy: Altering the Course of Infection

Intervention by surgical means or by antibiotic therapy is an attempt to alter the course of the infection by inhibiting fluctuation and extension and encouraging resolution.

Localized infections in the oral cavity are usually relieved by the release of pus and the removal of the cause of infection. Advanced caries and periodontal disease are the predominant causes of oral infections. Endodontic or periodontic therapy may preserve the teeth. However, if it is determined that the tooth or teeth cannot be salvaged, then the removal of the teeth involved is generally the immediate first step in treatment. If the teeth are to be saved, then pus must be released by incision and drainage. Opening the pulp canal will provide only minimal drainage and should not be the only method used to drain fluctuant areas. The release of pus removes bacteria and toxins and reduces the distention of tissues caused by the presence of pus. This decompression improves circulation to the area and so aids natural defenses by increasing the blood supply.

The host resistance can be improved by supportive measures that help in overcoming the infection. The patient should be required to rest in bed, should be ordered to force fluid intake in the form of juices, soft drinks, water, and soups, and should have a diet high in protein. Dietary supplements are available at pharmacies and are fine for augmenting diets. The instant breakfast foods may be helpful as supplements, since they contain vitamins and minerals as well as carbohydrates and some protein.

If antibiotics are used, they should be used wisely. Pus specimens should be sent to a hospital or commercial pathology laboratory for culture and sensitivity tests that will identify the organisms responsible for the infection and also determine the susceptibility of the predominant organism to various antibiotics.

Treatment of Common Infections

Apical Pathology Without Cellulitis

Diagnosis of apical pathology is made by history, percussion, pulp testing, and radiographic findings as described in Chapter 6 (Endodontics in General Practice). Suitability of the tooth for endodontic therapy should be considered.

If the decision is made to remove the tooth, adequate anesthesia is often a problem. Ineffective or marginally effective infiltration anesthesia may be supplemented by block anesthesia. In a maxilla, a zygomatic, greater palantine, or infraorbital block may produce more effective anesthesia than will infiltration. If pain still persists, administration of a hypnotic or narcotic may prove helpful. If the tooth remains sensitive to manipulation, intraseptal or periodontal ligament injection or injection directly into the pulp may be effective, or the pulp chamber may be opened and a sedative dressing placed. Referral to an oral surgeon for general anesthesia is occasionally necessary for complete elimination of pain during the extraction.

Antibiotics are not required for the treatment of apical infections unaccompanied by cellulitis unless there is some specific medical indication for their use. Patients with uncontrolled diabetes or rheumatic or congenital heart disease, patients with heart valve or hip prostheses, and patients on steroid therapy do require antibiotics.

Facial Cellulitis

For patients with facial cellulitis, the following steps are advocated:

1. Determine the etiology of the cellulitis. Cellulitis may be a sequel to pulpitis, but it may also be due to infection of a salivary gland or trauma, or it may be a manifestation of allergy (angioneurotic edema). The history and radiographs are important in ruling out odontogenic infection.

2. If the cellulitis is of other than odontogenic origin, or if it is extensive and the practitioner does not feel comfortable with the responsibility of management, the patient should be referred immediately to an oral surgeon.

3. If the infection is of odontogenic origin, the primary aim of treatment is to control and to eliminate it. Antibiotic therapy and *intraoral* heat in the form of warm mouthwashes should be part of the treatment. With antibiotics and intraoral heat, resolution may take place without pus formation. In the event that pus does form but an attempt is to be made to preserve the tooth, the canal should be opened and drainage established by incision. If the tooth is to be extracted, it should be removed immediately. If the less desirable decision has been made to wait for the cellulitis to subside before extraction, it is imperative that the patient understand that the source of infection must be eliminated when the swelling is gone, or the condition can be expected to return.

Pericoronitis

Pericoronitis is an inflammatory process in the tissue adjacent to an erupting tooth or in the tissue covering a tooth that has erupted but is partially covered by gingiva. The term is generally used to refer to the inflammation surrounding partially erupted lower third molars. It may be initiated by bacterial action, decomposing debris in the crevice, or trauma from an overerupted upper third molar.

Emergency Treatment. If trismus is present, antibiotics and warm irrigation in the retromolar area are recommended; frequently, extraction of the opposing tooth is recommended if the opposing tooth is a source of trauma.

Definitive Treatment. If sufficient room for proper eruption of the third molar does not exist, immediate extraction or extraction as early as possible is required. The opposing tooth should also be extracted, because passive eruption results in the loss of normal contact with the adjacent tooth, which in turn results in food impaction, caries, and periodontal disease. If the opposing tooth has strategic importance, however, such as for a posterior retainer for a fixed or removable partial denture, then it should not be removed.

Postsurgical Infections

When a patient returns with an infection following extraction or other surgical procedure, a re-evaluation of the medical history is important. A postoperative infection may be a clue to systemic diseases such as diabetes or a blood dyscrasia.

A radiograph should be taken in order to determine whether there are any local foci of infection or infectionlike local reactions to pieces of amalgam, chips of enamel or root, bone spicules, or tips of instruments. If severe systemic signs and trismus are present, the patient should receive antibiotics and the infected area should be treated with warm irrigations. Incision and drainage should be performed if an abscess has developed. If a specific cause for the infection is found, it should be eliminated as quickly as possible.

Infections in Children

Odontogenic infections in children differ in some respects from infections in adults. Dental infections in children are more likely to spread because of large marrow spaces. Systemic effects are often more pronounced, e.g., sudden high-temperature elevation. Infections may involve buds of permanent teeth and may cause enamel hypoplasia. Because of the relation of the apices of partially erupted teeth to muscle attachments, cellulitis and cutaneous abscesses may occur in locations where they would not in an adult.

Removal of the involved primary tooth results in early relief of pain, prevents the further spread of infection, allows for drainage through the socket, and removes the source of possible injury to the developing permanent tooth. In such cases, consideration of space maintenance is important. Pulp therapy, combined with incision and drainage and with antibiotic therapy, should be considered for infected permanent teeth.

As with the adult, a good history and examination, good radiographs, and the observance of basic surgical principles will lead to proper treatment for the child.

COMPLICATIONS IN SURGERY

Routine oral surgery occasionally produces complications. It is necessary to recognize the nature of a complication when it occurs and then to deal with it in an effective manner.

Prevention of Complications

Some complications result from overlooking the basic steps in the management of the patient. Good management is based on good history, radiographs of good quality, a well-formulated plan of treatment, and referral of the patient when the contemplated surgery requires the help of a specialist.

Postoperative infection may be minimized or avoided by attention to the principles of surgical cleanliness discussed earlier in this chapter. The use of an autoclave and of disposable needles and an awareness of how the dentist and his assistants may transfer infection will help to prevent postoperative infections.

Complications During Surgery
Sinus Involvement in Maxillary Surgery

The maxillary sinus probably is opened frequently without the dentist's being aware of it and with no untoward sequelae. When the operator is aware that the sinus has been opened but that no roots have been forced into it, the flaps should be sutured as usual, a piece of gauze should be placed over the socket, and precise instructions should be given to the patient. The patient should be told to avoid coughing, sneezing, blowing the nose, and smoking for 8 hours to prevent displacement of the clot. The gauze should be left in place for 1 to 2 hours, and no rinsing should be allowed for the remainder of the day. Neo-Synephrine nose drops (0.25 per cent) should be prescribed to help drainage from the sinus into the nose. Antibiotics are indicated if the opening exceeds 5 mm in diameter or if pus has drained from the socket.

If a maxillary molar root tip disappears during attempted removal, perforation of the sinus should be suspected. The patient is instructed to pinch the nostrils shut and gently blow the nose. If the sinus is perforated, air will pass through the socket into the oral cavity, causing bubbling in the socket. If the sinus wall is intact, the tip may be lying between the membrane and the bony floor of the sinus, may be beneath the buccal mucoperiosteum, or may have been removed from the mouth by suction or on a gauze sponge.

As the first step in management of the problem radiographs should be made. The radiographs should include the floor of the sinus not only in the immediate area of surgery but also in the adjacent areas. If no root tip can be seen on radiographic examination, it can be assumed that it is not in the sinus area of surgery. The dentist should examine the sponges and the contents of the suction bottle; it is very comforting to have the assurance that the tip has been removed. If the tip is not found but is not visualized on radiographs, it may be presumed that it has been removed.

If the fragment is visible in the radiographs but the sinus is not perforated, the buccal alveolar mucosa over the socket should be palpated. The fragment may be beneath the mucoperiosteum on the buccal surface, from which it can readily be removed. It may also be between the bony floor and the intact sinus membrane. In this situation an envelope flap is reflected, the buccal wall of the socket is removed to permit access to the area, and a curet is used to gently lift the sinus membrane and pull the root fragment into the socket. In some instances, an assistant will recover the tip with the suction while the surgeon has the membrane elevated.

If the root tip has penetrated the sinus, it may be recovered by flushing the sinus. This is done by flowing saline gently into the sinus from a 10-ml syringe via a blunt 18-gauge needle. The needle is placed in the opening and the gentle flow of saline frequently brings the root tip to the opening, where it is recovered by the suction or by a curet. If these steps do not result in recovery of the fragment, the patient should be referred to an oral surgeon.

Although this situation is not an emergency requiring an immediate visit, the consultant should be called and an appointment made for the patient. Certainly no attempt should be made to enlarge the opening, and gauze should not be packed into the defect. The patient should be informed of the problem, the wound closed with sutures, and the patient given any instructions that may have been suggested by the oral surgeon who will complete the operation.

Occasionally, an entire root is accidentally forced into the sinus. This is a problem best treated by the specialist, who will usually perform a Caldwell-Luc procedure to recover the root. The dentist has fulfilled his duty to the patient if he has exercised care, skill, and good judgment in management of the patient and if he has taken adequate radiographs, informed the patient of the problem, and arranged referral.

Fracture of the Labial or Buccal Bone and the Tuberosity

Fracture of supporting bone during tooth extraction usually can be prevented by proper preoperative assessment of the surgical problem. If the tooth does not move easily, it should be removed only after reflection of a flap and removal of marginal bone; if the tooth is found to be multirooted, sectioning of the roots from the crown may be required. If, unexpectedly, bone is found to be attached to the tooth being removed and the bone already has been largely detached from the periosteum, it is best to remove the bone fragment with the tooth. The bony margins of the defect should be smoothed, the wound irrigated, and sutures placed, if necessary.

When the tuberosity has been fractured and the tooth cannot be separated from the bone without disrupting its periosteal attachment, the tooth and tuberosity are removed; the margins are smoothed, the wound is irrigated, and the mucosa is sutured. If, however, the tuberosity can be separated from the tooth, it should not be removed with the tooth; the mucosa should be sutured over the bone to help to stabilize it. If at least half the periosteum has remained attached to the bone, reattachment can be expected.

Excessive Bleeding During Surgery

Hemorrhage may be a complication during, as well as following, surgical procedures. The most frequent causes of hemorrhage during surgery are poor planning and lack of care in handling tissues. The patient with loose, periodontally involved teeth and the patient with large periapical granulomas should be expected to bleed profusely.

Radiographs showing large periodontal spaces in a patient with swollen, red gingivae may signify that the patient might lose as much as 500 ml of blood in the routine removal of ten mobile teeth. Such problems can be avoided by careful preoperative planning of the sequence of extraction and the removal of granulation tissue.

Patients with a history of high blood pressure may also have bleeding problems. The blood pressure of hypertensive patients should be checked before any surgery is started; these individuals may experience increased blood pressure as a result of the worry or excitement of the operation. Premedication with hypnotics usually helps in reducing the blood pressure, making the operation easier. Medical consultations should be arranged before surgery for patients with persistent diastolic pressure over 100 mm Hg (see Chapter 3, Oral Medicine in General Practice).

Fewer than 1 per cent of the population have inherent blood dyscrasias that cause prolonged bleeding. Such patients can usually be identified if a good history is taken and a careful examination is performed. They should be managed by referral to a center where a hematologist and an oral surgeon can cooperate in treatment.

Granulation Tissue. If clinical and radiographic examination suggest large quantities of granulation tissue, bleeding can be minimized if the following procedures are observed: (1) Begin the surgery in the posterior part of the mouth. Remove only a few teeth at a time; then, using curets or scissors, remove all granulation tissue from the sockets and gingival tissues. Granulation tissue is extremely vascular, and any tear or cut in this tissue ruptures many small vessels. Total removal of the granulation tissue eliminates the major sources of bleeding. (2) If hemorrhage is excessive during removal of granulation tissue, have the patient close on gauze sponges that have been packed into the wound. Ordinarily the bleeding will cease after 2 minutes. Remove the sponges and proceed with the removal of the granulation tissue. As soon as the operation is resumed, bleeding may once again occur and may be brisk enough to require a second packing and waiting period. When all the granulation is finally removed, the bleeding will be minimal. Any fragments of granulation tissue that are inadvertently left may result in a delayed hemorrhage and a night call to stop the bleeding. Since patients with large quantities of granulation tissue usually have very irregular and sharp alveolar processes, the alveolar process should be gently smoothed and any spurs of bone rounded before the sutures are placed. The dentist who removes teeth and leaves granulation tissue because he thinks it is "part of the healing process" has been misled and is doing the patient a disservice. Such granulation, in addition to being a source of postoperative bleeding, may contain sequestering bone and beginning cysts.

Bleeding from Nutrient Canals. Occasionally, large nutrient channels in the alveolar septa, especially in the lower anterior region, will bleed vigorously. In some patients, blood may even be seen spurting from these openings. Bleeding from nutrient canals is controlled by burnishing or crushing the adjacent bone into the opening.

In elderly people with thin septa between sockets, it may be difficult to burnish bone without fracturing a septum. It is easier to place a hemostat or needle holder in the sockets so that the separated beaks straddle the septum with the bleeding foramen. The beaks are then gently squeezed several times so that the crestal bone is pinched and the bleeding canal is collapsed. This procedure requires care to avoid fracturing the septum (Fig. 10–35). After the bone is burnished or crushed to occlude the bleeding points, the assistant must be warned not to run the suction over the site. Such suctioning will remove the plug, and bleeding will recur.

Patients Receiving Anticoagulant Therapy. Patients who have had coronary artery occlusion or a cerebrovascular accident, or who have peripheral vascular disease, may be taking anticoagulant drugs. Al-

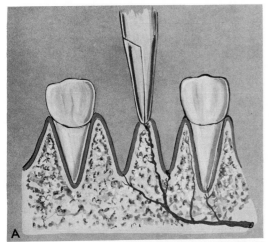

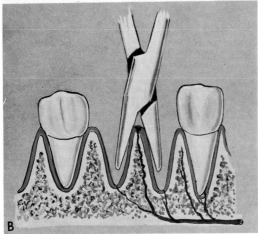

FIGURE 10–35 *A,* The needle holder or hemostat is used to crush bone into the canal to control excessive bleeding. *B,* If the septum is unsupported and too thin to permit pressure at the crest without the danger of fracture, the separated beaks are placed straddling the septum and then gently squeezed to compress the crestal margins without crushing them.

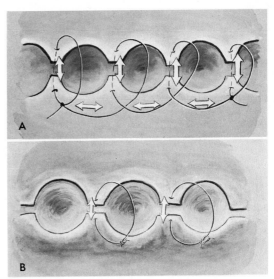

FIGURE 10–36 *A,* The continuous suture produces tension in two directions (as shown by the arrows), thus providing more chance for movement of the flap. If a suture cuts through the tissue at any point, the whole flap is loosened. *B,* Interrupted sutures produce tension in only one direction; if a single suture pulls through the tissue, it does not loosen the other sutures.

though it is not necessary to stop the anticoagulant therapy for oral surgery, the following precautionary procedures are recommended:

1. In cooperation with the patient's physician, the drug dosage should be adjusted to bring the patient's prothrombin time to 1½ times the normal level of the laboratory control blood sample.

2. The surgery should be performed in the usual manner, with the same care that is always exercised in the incision and reflection of tissues. Any bleeding foramina should be controlled and all granulation tissue removed.

3. Flaps should be sutured so that few raw, cut edges are exposed. Interrupted rather than continuous sutures should be used, so that the entire flap will not be loosened if a suture cuts through the flap (Fig. 10–36).

4. The patient should be instructed to use gauze packs postoperatively to exert moderate pressure on the wound. Fresh gauze sponges should be wet with warm water and then squeezed until damp before being placed. The moisture reduces the gagging and irritation sometimes caused by dry sponges. The packs should be maintained for 6 hours and replaced thereafter as needed to control oozing (Fig. 10–37).

It is rarely necessary for the dentist to use drugs or hemostatic agents to control hemorrhage in oral surgery. Vitamin K is of no value unless there is a demonstrated vitamin K deficiency. Gelatin sponges and oxidized cellulose are rarely needed to control bleeding in normal patients. However, these agents are occasionally useful for a patient with a

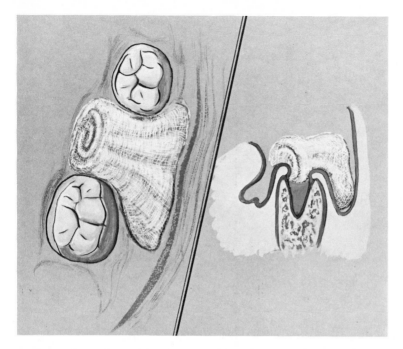

FIGURE 10–37 *Left,* The gauze pack is placed to occlude the socket opening and support the buccal tissue flap if it has been reflected. *Right,* The patient should understand that the gauze must rest over the socket; it should not be held between the remaining teeth, thus leaving the socket open.

prolonged prothrombin time resulting from anticoagulant therapy.

Postoperative Complications

Pain that increases in intensity after the anesthetic is no longer effective and that does not respond to ordinary analgesics warrants investigation. Such pain may be due to a fractured or displaced interseptal, buccal, or lingual plate of bone or to the presence of a foreign body. A local anesthetic should be given, a radiograph taken, and the socket explored. If a cause can be found for the pain, it should be corrected. If no cause is evident, a narcotic such as codeine (60 mg) or meperidine (50 mg) should be prescribed. The medication may be taken every 4 to 6 hours when needed to relieve the pain. Six to 8 tablets should control the acute phase of pain due to trauma. If infection is suspected, as indicated by a temperature over 101° F, possibly chills, and increased swelling, then antibiotics should be prescribed as discussed earlier.

Dry Socket

Pain that has it onset 2 to 10 days after an extraction, in the absence of signs of generalized inflammation, usually indicates delayed healing and local infection. The pain frequently radiates to the area of the ear, the temporomandibular joint, or the neck. The onset of pain, foul taste, bad oral odor, and radiation of the pain is characteristic of localized alveolar osteitis, or "dry socket." One frequently sees no inflammation of the gingiva, and the wound may appear closed. By gently inserting the closed beaks of cotton pliers into the cleft of the healing wound and allowing the beaks to spread and open the socket, one can see the socket. It may contain food debris, a degenerating clot, or only bare bony walls. Such a socket is treated by irrigation with sterile normal saline or water or mouthwash and by the application of a sedative dressing. The dressing is prepared by incorporating a mixture of Vaseline, zinc oxide powder, and eugenol to make a white, semisolid grease, with ¼-inch selvage-edge gauze ribbons. One to 1½-inch lengths of dressing can be cut as needed and a drop or two of eugenol placed on the ribbon before it is placed in the socket. The dressing serves three purposes: (1) It is slightly antiseptic and anesthetic because of the eugenol, (2) it reduces space for food accumulation, and (3) it acts as a drain, keeping the gingival margins open.

Occasionally, there are instances in which the eugenol effect is lost so rapidly that symptoms return within a day. The effectiveness can be extended by incorporating a soft doughy mix of zinc oxide and eugenol with the dressing. This provides more eugenol that can leach out over a longer time. This latter type of dressing hardens. Therefore, it must be placed carefully so that it can be withdrawn painlessly after several days.

Dressings should be changed every 2 days. Zinc oxide and eugenol dressings that harden may remain 3 or 4 days. Dressings are usually not continued for longer than 5 to 7 days. If the problem persists, it would be wise to seek consultation with an oral surgeon.

Postoperative Hemorrhage

The best remedy for postoperative bleeding is good preventive care at the time of the operation, e.g., removal of granulation tissue, crushing of nutrient canals, and careful suturing.

If the patient calls on the telephone and complains of bleeding following the operation, he should be instructed to place gauze over the bleeding point and to close his jaws to exert pressure. The patient without opposing teeth will require a large amount of gauze to produce pressure on the bleeding point. If the bleeding resumes after half an hour of pressure, the patient should be seen at the office.

Some patients may be very disturbed and nervous because of bleeding. They can be calmed with intravenous injection of a sedative or hypnotic drug. Then, before the area of bleeding is anesthetized, the bleeding point should be sought. The vasoconstrictor in the anesthetic will frequently stop the bleeding; if this occurs before the bleeding point is located, it will be difficult to provide treatment, and bleeding may resume when the anesthesia wears off. Once the bleeding point has been located by the use of suction and sponges, the area can be anesthetized. This procedure must be done with care because of postoperative pain and tenderness in the area of the surgery.

Postoperative bleeding in the first 24 hours generally may be controlled by resuturing. Occasionally the bleeding will come from large nutrient canals in the alveolar bone, and the bone around the bleeding point will need to be crushed. Delayed bleeding after a week or more may be due to traumatized granulation tissue. Exuberant granulation tissue bulging from the socket should be removed and the wound sutured.

If the patient appears to be in poor physical condition, with a fast, thready pulse, low blood pressure, ashen skin color, and cold, clammy hands, the blood loss may have been substantial. After emergency packing, this patient should be seen by an oral surgeon. The consultant should be called immediately. He may advise that the patient go directly to a hospital for treatment.

There are occasions when the dentist may be requested to treat postoperative bleeding in a patient for whom he did not perform surgery. As a protection for himself and the patient, he should x-ray the area of bleeding before giving definitive treatment. Root tips, bone fragments, pieces of calculus, and broken instruments may cause formation of exuberant granulation tissue and so stimulate spontaneous bleeding. Foreign bodies in the tooth socket must be removed, but their presence may not be evident without an x-ray. A posttreatment film should be made to record the corrected condition for the completion of the record of treatment.

RELATIONSHIP OF GENERAL PRACTICE AND ORAL SURGERY

Oral surgery is closely associated with the practice of general dentistry. As a specialist, the oral surgeon depends on his colleagues for referred patients. In turn, the oral surgeon refers to the general dentist many patients who come to him seeking surgery for problems better treated by nonsurgical techniques. In addition, the general dentist restores teeth needed for splinting when corrective jaw surgery is contemplated. He also constructs restorations for edentulous areas following definitive care for trauma or correction of jaw deformities.

A congenial relationship helps to bring the best possible care to patients with congenital, acquired, or traumatic deformities of the face and jaws. The oral surgeon's careful evaluation of the mouth and jaws to detect potential hazards to dental health, as well as the surgical procedure he performs to effect early prophylactic elimination, can be a valuable service to the general practitioner. Early removal of impacted third molars, ankylosed primary teeth, odontomas, cysts, and all abnormal tissue will save time and money and suffering for the patient.

The oral surgeon can do his part in preventive dentistry only if patients are referred to him. The general practitioner may wish to treat these problems early, before complications develop; such procedures are well within his province if he feels comfortable performing them. Regardless of who renders the treatment, the patient must be cared for and potential dangers cannot be ignored.

QUESTIONS

1. How can the operatory be prepared for oral surgery so that an aseptic technique can be maintained?

2. What are the disadvantages of the panoramic x-ray film in diagnosing and planning oral surgery procedures?

3. List the advantages of intravenous sedation over the use of oral sedation.

4. What is the dose of epinephrine used to treat an anaphylactic or a cardiovascular collapse drug reaction?

5. How do you manage a patient who gives a history of "allergic reaction" to a local anesthetic?

6. What are some of the health problems associated with the administration of antibiotics when one considers the risk versus the benefit of prescribing such a drug?

7. What factors are important in carrying out soft tissue flap reflection?

8. What are the advantages of early removal of third molars (before 17 years of age)?

9. What anatomic features must be kept in mind when doing third molar surgery?

10. When doing multiple biopsies in various parts of the mouth or from a single large lesion, how do you fix the specimens, and how do you inform the pathologist about the multiple biopsies?

11. What are the three essentials of emergency care in caring for patients with fractured jaws?

12. Describe and diagram the procedure for reduction of fibrous tuberosities.

13. What are the advantages of the correction of a shallow mandibular vestibule using the transposition of mucosal and periosteal flaps?

14. When operating on the lingual surface of the mandibular alveoli, why is a lingual gingival crevice or alveolar crest incision used?

15. Prior to biopsy or definitive surgery involving a lytic lesion within bone, describe what diagnostic test must be carried out and why.

16. Describe how one differentiates between an abscess and cellulitis.

17. A patient in good health comes to your office with a temperature of 101° F, in pain, with a swelling of the mandibular buccal vestibule adjacent to the left first molar. The tooth is beyond periodontal and endodontic therapy and the patient will accept only extraction. When do you extract? What is your postoperative medication? What factors enter into your decisions?

18. What is accomplished by placing a dressing in a "dry socket"?

19. How do you determine whether an unerupted third molar could be transplanted to a first molar position following removal of the first molar?

20. List the similarities and dissimilarities of infections of dental origin in adults and children. Why the difference?

See answers in Appendix.

REFERENCES

1. Andreasen, J. O.: Effect of extra-alveolar period and storage media upon periodontal and pulpal healing after replantation of mature permanent incisors in monkeys. Int. J. Oral Surg., *10*:45–53, 1981.
2. Archer, H. W.: Oral and Maxillofacial Surgery, 5th ed. Philadelphia, W. B. Saunders Company, 1975.
3. Ash, M. M., Costich, E. R., and Hayward, J. R.: A study of periodontal hazards of third molars. J. Periodont. Res., *33*:209–219, 1962.
4. Brown, R. D.: The failure of local anesthesia in acute inflammation—some recent concepts. Br. Dent. J., *151*:47–51, 1981.
5. Bruce, R. A., Frederickson, G. C., and Small, G. S.: Age of patients and morbidity associated with third molar surgery. J. Am. Dent. Assoc., *101*:240–245, 1980.
6. Bysledt, H.: Antibiotics in Oral Surgery. Stockholm, Karolenska Institute, 1979.
7. Catellani, J. E., Harvey, S., Erickson, S. H., and Cherkin, D.: Effects of oral contraceptive cycle on dry socket (localized alveolar osteitis). J. Am. Dent. Assoc., *101*:777–780, 1980.
8. Costich, E. R., and White, R. P., Jr.: Essentials of Oral Surgery. Philadelphia, W. B. Saunders Company, 1971.
9. Gonty, A. A., and Costich, E. R.: Severe facial and cervical infections associated with gas-producing bacteria: Report of two cases. J. Oral Surg., *39*:702–707, 1981.
10. Hayward, J. R., and Costich, E. R.: The use of elevators. Prac. Dent. Monogr., March 1957.
11. Hayward, J. R. (ed.): Oral Surgery. Springfield, Ill., Charles C Thomas, 1976.
12. Hinds, E. C., and Freg, K. F.: Hazards of retained third molars in older persons. Report of 15 cases. J. Am. Dent. Assoc., *101*:240–250, 1980.
13. Howe, G. L.: Minor Oral Surgery, 2nd ed. Baltimore, Williams & Wilkins, 1971.
14. James, R. A.: Treatment planning for the implant patient. J. Oral Implant., *9*:352–356, 1981.
15. Jastak, J. T., and Yagiela, J. A.: Regional Anesthesia of the Oral Cavity. St. Louis, C. V. Mosby, 1981.
16. Kethley, J. L., and Gamble, J. W.: The lipswitch: A modification of Kazanjian's labial vestibuloplasty. J. Oral Surg., *36*:701–705, 1978.
17. Killey, H. C.: Fracture of the Middle Third of the Facial Skeleton. Bristol, John Wright and Sons, 1965.
18. Killey, H. C., and Kay, L. W.: Impacted Wisdom Tooth, 2nd ed. New York, Churchill Livingston, 1975.
19. Malamed, S. F.: Handbook of Medical Emergencies in the Dental Office. St. Louis, C. V. Mosby Company, 1978.
20. Mahajan, S. K., and Sidhu, S. S.: Effect of fluoride on root resorption of autogeneous dental replants. Clinical study. Aust. Dent. J. *26*:42–45, 1981.
21. Richards, A. G.: The buccal object rule. Dent. Radiogr. Photogr. *53*:37–56, 1981.
22. Schnitman, P. A., and Shulman, L. B. (eds.): Dental Implants: Benefits and Risks. Bethesda, Md., U. S. Dept. Health and Human Services, Public Health Service, National Institutes of Health, 1980.
23. Sims, W.: The problem of cross-infection in dental surgery with particular reference to serum hepatitis. J. Dent. *8*:20–26, 1980.
24. Syrgänen, S. M., and Syrgänen, K. I.: A new combination of drugs intended to be used as a preventive measure for the postextraction complications. A preliminary report. Int. J. Oral Surg., *10*:17–22, 1981.
25. Von Wowern, N., and Winther, S.: Submergence of roots for alveolar ridge preservation: a failure (4-year follow-up study). Int. J. Oral Surg. *10*:247–250, 1981.

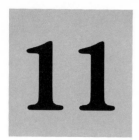

GERALD N. GRASER

PROSTHODONTICS

This chapter deals with four components of prosthodontics: removable partial dentures, overdentures, complete dentures, and maxillofacial prosthetics. The first section presents general principles of prosthodontics applicable to all four components. Subsequent sections relate the practical application of techniques in each specific area, based on present scientific and clinical knowledge. Methods are presented for treating anatomically, medically, and emotionally compromised prosthodontic patients. Patients with identifiable problems in using a prosthesis or patients for whom problems are anticipated through careful evaluation and diagnosis require special management techniques and advanced treatment procedures. These management techniques and treatment procedures, which also may be used for the more routine patient, are emphasized throughout the chapter.

It is assumed that the reader has a basic understanding of and clinical experience with routine prosthetics as it relates to removable partial dentures and complete dentures. Therefore, the chapter will not present basic techniques considered fundamental to routine removable prosthodontic practice. It is also assumed that the majority of laboratory procedures will be carried out by skilled, knowledgeable dental laboratory technicians. For this reason, the chapter will not present detailed laboratory procedures except when necessary to clarify and reinforce clinical concepts and procedures.

OBJECTIVES

Upon completing this chapter, the dentist should be able to do the following:

1. Differentiate between the accepting patient and the demanding patient and use appropriate methods to treat them.

2. Determine the prognosis for a complete denture based on the anatomic structures of the mouth.

3. Describe conservative methods by which the tissues of the mouth can be prepared for prostheses in order to minimize the need for surgery.

4. Make a preliminary and final impression for the edentulous patient at the same appointment without making an acrylic resin custom tray.

5. Establish and verify maxillomandibular jaw relations so that the remount procedure can be eliminated at the time of delivery of the prosthesis.

6. Develop a more natural appearance for the patient based on several guides that can be used to set teeth even when the patient is not present.

7. List the critical components of a removable partial denture and be able to incorporate them into the designs for the most commonly used removable partial dentures.

8. Provide treatment with an overdenture for the patient in whom a removable partial denture is contraindicated.

9. Have a better understanding of, and provide treatment for, maxillofacial prosthetic patients with certain types of congenital defects such as cleft palate and amelogenesis imperfecta, patients with an acquired defect such as a fractured jaw, or cancer patients during or after radiation or surgical treatment.

10. Treat many complications that may result from the use of a removable prosthesis.

GENERAL PRINCIPLES OF PROSTHODONTICS

Philosophy of Patient Management

Getting to know the patient is an especially important consideration in prosthodontics. The success of the prosthesis may depend on it. Before obtaining complete mouth radiographs or making impressions, the dentist should sit down and talk with the patient to know him as a person as well as a patient. An office, if available, rather than a dental chair can be much less threatening to the "problem" prosthodontic patient.

In addition to the patient's past medical and dental history, the dentist should find something out about the patient's social history. Questions concerning what he does in his free time, such as hobbies and special interests, not only allow the patient to relax and talk about himself but also give the dentist a better insight into the type of patient.

Generally, people can be classified broadly into "accepting" patients and "demanding" patients. The accepting denture patient might be considered easy-going, philosophic, or indifferent, whereas the demanding denture patient may be exacting, difficult, unreasonable, or overbearing. There are degrees to which individual patients fit into these two classifications. Some will be very demanding, whereas others will be only moderately so. Clues about which of the two groups the patient represents can be gained from his or her bearing, handshake, and manner of grooming and dress (Fig. 11–1). A previous dental history in adjusting to any other prosthesis can be another clue. The patient with the bag of dentures or even one denture that appears to be well made, who complains of continual soreness, the inability to eat, or that the dentures are not tight enough, may well represent the demanding category. Patients with a "burning" mouth or temporomandibular pain are others who may be in this demanding group.

Of course, there will always be some people who are difficult to categorize, even after several appointments. It is with these patients as well as with the demanding denture patient that extreme care and thoughtfulness in approach may mean the difference between success and failure. One should remember that as the dentist evaluates the patient the patient evaluates the dentist for an "accepting" or a "demanding" attitude. Frequently, little things help in the development of a good relationship between the patient and the dentist and can spell the difference between success and failure. Giv-

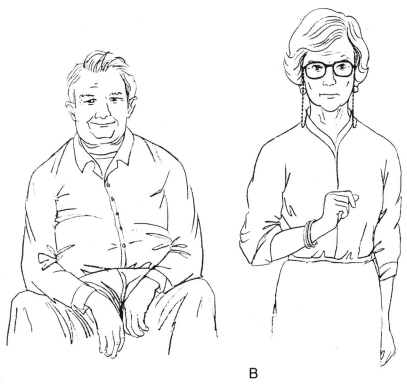

A   B

FIGURE 11–1 **A,** The accepting patient is often characterized by an easy-going, congenial manner. **B,** The demanding patient may be recognized by a meticulous, regimented manner.

ing a warm handshake and a gentle smile, helping the patient with his coat, asking about his family, or offering a magazine or a cup of coffee may contribute as much to the success of the prosthesis, as far as the patient is concerned, as all the time spent on exacting technical aspects of treatment.

The dentist must remember also that there are some things dentists cannot change regardless of their ability, interest, or knowledge. A few patients are simply unable to become accustomed to wearing a removable prosthesis because the slightest amount of movement disturbs them or because of some emotional factor connected with having something "removable" in their mouth. The dentist must learn to identify these patients and to modify his management and treatment techniques accordingly.

Patient History

The denture patient's primary concern can be discussed even before his medical history is reviewed. If he has a dental prosthesis and does not like it, he should be encouraged to present his feelings in detail. His past dental history should be reviewed carefully. Who was his last dentist? Why did he leave him? How long has he had the prosthesis? How many has he had? What problems has he encountered? What does he like about the prosthesis? The answers to these questions should be written down and reviewed periodically during treatment so that the dentist does not forget problems of importance to the patient. The patient should be told some possible limitations of a removable prosthesis should his expectations be too high but not in such a manner that it would seem impossible for him to adapt (Table 11–1). When the limitations are discussed before treatment, they are explanations; when discussed after treatment, they become excuses.

The medical history for the prosthodontic patient is of utmost importance and should

TABLE 11–1   Limitations of Removable Prostheses

Short-term	Long-term
Feels strange in the mouth	Some movement
	Some food beneath
Difficulty with speech	Less biting force than nat-
Difficulty with eating	ural dentition

be thoroughly reviewed with particular attention to medications, endocrine disorders, and the cardiovascular system. Certain drugs, such as anti-inflammatory agents for arthritic patients, and endocrine disorders, such as diabetes, may make the tissues more susceptible to irritation and delayed healing. Diuretics may cause fluid loss from the mucosa and contraction of tissues, thereby decreasing denture retention. The tooth-supported removable partial denture may be a better treatment than fixed partial dentures for some medically compromised patients. Less sophisticated prosthetic procedures may represent superior treatment for the cardiovascular patient. The appointments are shorter and involve less stress.

Patient diet should be reviewed, especially for the patient unable to wear a well-fitting prosthesis when no other medical problems are present. Elderly patients living alone frequently receive inadequate nutrition, a factor that affects their ability to wear a prosthesis comfortably.

Should questions arise about the medical suitability of the patient to receive prosthodontic care, his physician should be contacted (see Chapter 3, Oral Medicine in General Practice).

Examination

The examination should begin with a thorough evaluation of the head and neck. External tissues, including the temporomandibular joint regions, should be palpated bilaterally. Pain in the joint may be an indication that the occlusion or vertical dimension is inadequate. As the patient opens the mouth, abnormal or excessive jaw or tongue movements should be observed. Such movements may adversely affect the prognosis of a removable prosthesis. The amount and consistency of saliva should be noted; minimal saliva or a thick, ropy saliva can result in decreased retention of a prosthesis. The teeth and intraoral soft tissues are then examined thoroughly and abnormalities noted for subsequent correction as necessary.

Prognosis

Knowledge of the emotional make-up of the patient must be accompanied by an evaluation of the anatomy of the mouth as it relates to the prognosis for wearing a remova-

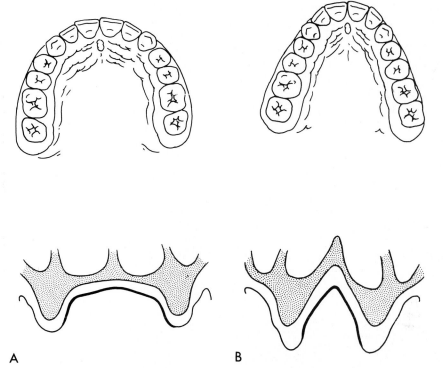

A   B

FIGURE 11–2 *A,* The broad, flat hard palate provides a favorable prognosis for the stability and retention of a denture. *B,* The small, narrow palate with a high vault provides a poor prognosis for denture stability and retention.

ble prosthesis. The anatomy of the maxilla, mandible, and contiguous soft tissue is an important factor in the determination of the prognosis for both partial and complete dentures. A poor prognosis may mean that an extra effort should be made to save some "hopeless" teeth. If they are extracted, the patient may become a dental cripple when a retentive complete denture cannot be made. Two factors that significantly affect the stability and retention of a complete denture are the size and the shape of the mouth.

Maxilla

Hard Palate. The large, firm, flat palate presents the best prognosis for a complete denture, whereas the small V-shaped palate presents the worst prognosis (Fig. 11–2). The ovoid palate is between these two extremes.

Soft Palate. The mobility and angle of descent of the soft palate is another consideration. The soft palate with little movement and a slight drop from the hard palate has the best prognosis, and the soft palate with

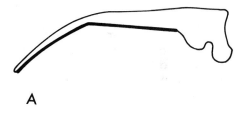

A

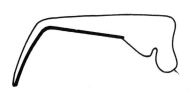

B

FIGURE 11–3 *A,* The soft palate that gradually slopes from the hard palate and has limited mobility has a good prognosis for denture retention. *B,* The soft palate that drops abruptly from the hard palate has great mobility, and a more exacting placement of the posterior palatal seal is necessary.

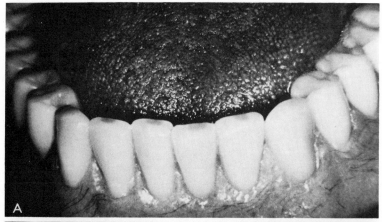

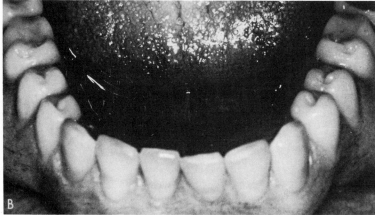

FIGURE 11–4 *A,* The anterior tongue position provides the best prognosis for mandibular denture retention. *B,* The retruded tongue position provides the poorest prognosis for mandibular denture retention.

the most mobility and an abrupt drop has the poorest prognosis (Fig. 11–3).

Mandible

Tongue. A good tongue position is observed when the mouth is opened and the tongue remains forward, surrounding the lingual of the lower anterior ridge or teeth; a poor prognosis is associated with a tongue that drops back as the mouth opens. (Fig. 11–4). This allows a denture to be unseated, rather than maintaining the peripheral seal.

Floor of the Mouth. The sublingual fold space is one of the most critical areas for achieving good retention of a mandibular denture. A flat floor of the mouth with a well-defined fold of tissue formed by the sublingual gland and ducts from premolar to premolar provides the best prognosis. The floor of the mouth that drops abruptly behind the ridge with no sublingual fold space has the poorest prognosis (Figs. 11–5C and *D*).

Buccal Fold. A very flexible, prominent buccal fold of tissue, from the pterygoman-

dibular ligament to the external oblique ridge, provides a favorable condition. Conversely, taut buccal tissue, which makes the fold almost nonexistent, presents an unfavorable condition (Fig. 11–6B).

BIOLOGICAL CONSIDERATIONS

Without regular recall and maintenance programs, the effects of removable prostheses of any kind can be detrimental to the hard and soft tissues of the mouth. On the other hand, properly motivated patients who exercise effective plaque control and participate in regularly scheduled recall appointments can contribute much to the success of the prosthesis. The importance of a daily plaque control program and regular recall appointments in reducing the incidence of new carious lesions and in the control of gingival inflammation cannot be overemphasized.

It has been documented that overdentures and removable partial dentures increase masticatory effectiveness compared with complete dentures. This is an important consideration, especially for the elderly. In addition, removable partial dentures, when properly designed and maintained, do not have to lead to increasing mobility of the abutment teeth. With overdentures, tooth mobility may decrease after the abutment teeth have been reduced in height.

Residual ridge resorption is another important biologic consideration. The presence of two mandibular cuspids beneath an overdenture can reduce anterior bone loss as much as eight times more than that experienced by an edentulous patient. If for no other reason, this is justification enough to maintain what few teeth remain and to fabricate a removable partial denture or overdenture.

With proper patient selection, tissue preparation, and design and maintenance of the prosthesis, removable prosthodontics can be a very important component of the total health of an individual.

Planning the Treatment

Using recent complete mouth radiographs, diagnostic casts, and information from the patient interview and examination, the most appropriate type of prosthesis to be fabricated is determined. When only one or two teeth remain, an overdenture or complete denture are not the only choices available. A removable partial denture may function adequately. The decision should be

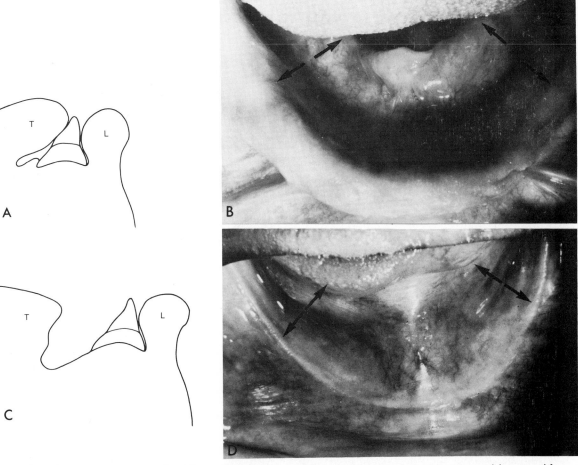

FIGURE 11–5 *A,* The good sublingual fold space combined with an anterior tongue position provides the best prognosis for a mandibular denture (T=tongue, L=lips). *B,* Intraorally, the good sublingual fold can be seen as a valley between the fold of tissue and the residual ridge (between the left and right sets of arrows). *C,* The floor of the mouth that drops abruptly with no sublingual fold space and has a retruded tongue position has the poorest mandibular denture prognosis. (T=tongue, L=lips). *D,* Intraorally, the poor sublingual fold space is seen when the floor of the mouth drops abruptly between the tongue and the residual ridge (between the left and right sets of arrows).

Illustration continued on following page

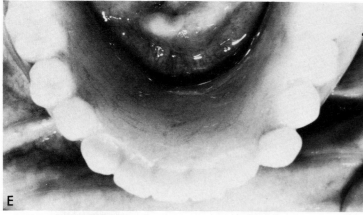

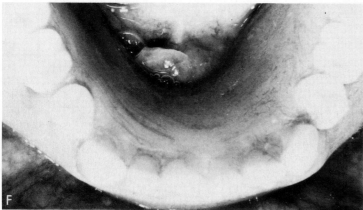

FIGURE 11–5 *Continued* *E,* Poor mandibular denture retention is seen when the lingual flange does not completely fill the sublingual fold space. *F,* The same patient with a new denture that fills the sublingual fold space and greatly enhances retention.

predicated upon the patient's previous prosthesis and whether it is functioning satisfactorily. Second, the amount of periodontal support and tooth mobility of potential abutments play a role. The removable partial denture may be a better choice if the prognosis for a complete denture or overdenture is not good.

All efforts should be made to save teeth. This is especially true for terminal abutments whose retention will avoid distal extension denture base partial dentures and for cuspids that are in a critical position to provide support for removable prostheses. Teeth with advanced furcation involvement should generally be resected in order to provide abutments that can be maintained plaque-free.

Instead of simply saying clinical judgment should be used in the selection of abutment teeth, specific guides can be cited. It must be remembered that these guides do not constitute hard and fast rules but are a place to begin abutment evaluation. When 50 per cent or more of the vertical bone height remains for support, a removable or fixed par-

tial denture should be considered. When 25 to 50 per cent (3 to 8 mm) of bone is present, an overdenture or fixed partial denture should be considered. If less than 25 per cent (less than 3 mm) of bone remains, extraction is probably indicated (Fig. 11–7C). This is a very simplistic approach to abutment selection. Many other factors, such as plaque control, periodontal health, tooth mobility, and abutment number and position, should be considered before a final treatment plan is devised.

It may be advantageous to develop more than one treatment plan. Variations may reflect anatomic conditions, financial considerations, the patient's desires, and appropriateness of specific types of treatment. These alternative treatments, their prognoses, and possible complications should be discussed with the patient. The final decision should involve both dentist and patient.

Mouth Preparation

The oral tissues must be in good health before impressions are made for any pros-

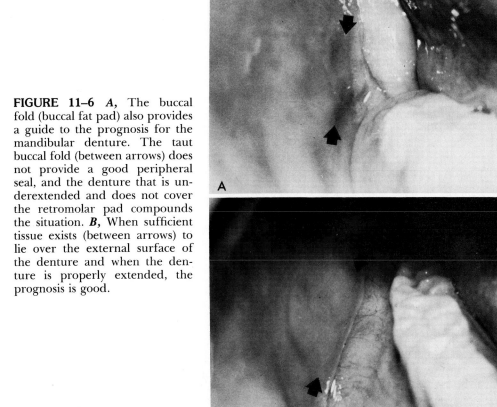

FIGURE 11–6 *A,* The buccal fold (buccal fat pad) also provides a guide to the prognosis for the mandibular denture. The taut buccal fold (between arrows) does not provide a good peripheral seal, and the denture that is underextended and does not cover the retromolar pad compounds the situation. *B,* When sufficient tissue exists (between arrows) to lie over the external surface of the denture and when the denture is properly extended, the prognosis is good.

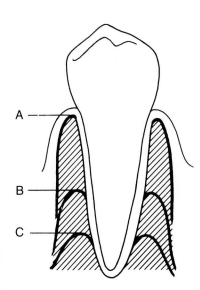

FIGURE 11–7 One consideration in the evaluation of abutments for removable prosthodontics is the amount of bone support available. Abutments with 50 to 100 percent bone height (*A* to *B*) may be used as removable partial denture abutments; 25 to 50 percent bone height (*B* to *C*) can be considered for overdenture abutments; teeth with less than 25 percent bone support (below *C*) should probably be extracted. (Note: owing to root tapering, 50 percent bone height has less than 50 percent bone support remaining.)

thesis. Anatomic and pathologic conditions that do not allow proper tissue coverage and functional jaw movement must be corrected. Periodontal treatment and restorative dentistry must be completed before *definitive* prosthetic care is provided. *Interim* immediate prostheses can be made following the extraction of teeth, before periodontal and restorative treatment.

There are several conditions directly related to prosthodontic therapy that can often be corrected without surgery. Conservatism should be the rule with preprosthetic surgery. Nothing should be removed unnecessarily. Upon healing, alveolar bone resorbs beyond that which is removed during surgery. The patient should be informed that an attempt will be made to fabricate the prosthesis and that surgery will be avoided unless absolutely necessary.

Soft Tissue

Epulis Fissuratum. Epulis fissuratum refers to the folds of redundant oral mucosa caused by overextended or sharp denture flanges. When the condition has not been present for more than a few months, simply cutting away the offending flange and lining the denture with tissue-conditioning material can bring about resolution of the epulis in several weeks (Fig. 11–8). Lesions present for a longer duration may necessitate surgery.

Papillary Hyperplasia. The inflammation and size of the papillary lesions will decrease with the use of tissue-conditioning material. In conjunction with a candida infection, topical application of an antifungal agent* to the denture and removal of the denture at night should be stressed. Once the inflammation is resolved, a new denture may be constructed over the existing papilla (Fig. 11–9B). Only in severe, widespread conditions does papillary hyperplasia necessitate surgery.

Denture Stomatitis. A generalized soreness and inflammation of the denture-bearing tissues are usually indicative of denture

*Nystatin Ointment, Squibb & Sons, Inc., Princeton, N.J.

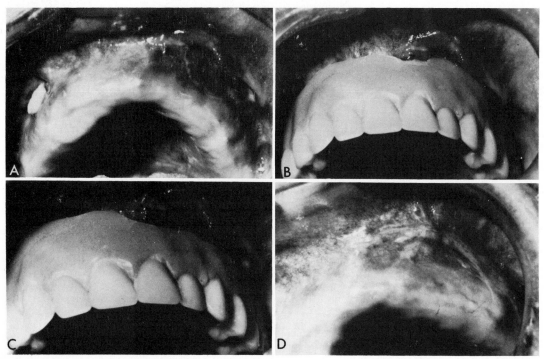

FIGURE 11–8 *A,* An epulis fissuratum that has been present for several months. *B,* The offending denture, with its sharp labial flange. *C,* Relief is provided by cutting away a portion of the denture flange. *D,* Resolution of the epulis approximately 6 weeks following denture adjustment, with no surgery required.

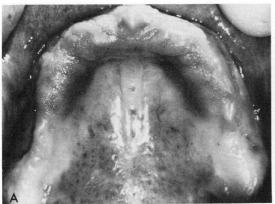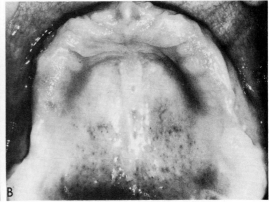

FIGURE 11–9 *A,* Papillary hyperplasia is often associated with poor oral hygiene habits and with a poorly fitting denture that has been worn night and day. *B,* Following several changes of tissue-conditioning material and the improvement of oral hygiene habits, the inflammation begins subsiding. The papillae become reduced in size but generally will not disappear completely.

stomatitis. Trauma and microbiotic infection are two contributing factors. When a fungal infection is present, soaking the denture in an antifungal agent (1 part Clorox,* 2 parts Calgon,† 8 parts water), applying a topical antifungal medication‡ to the affected area, and placing tissue-conditioning material in the denture will often alleviate the problem. Subsequently, the denture must be relined or remade.

Shallow Vestibule. The result of trying to provide more ridge through vestibuloplasty is not always good. Patients who have a great deal of residual ridge resorption have the poorest prognosis. Therefore the patient with the "flat" ridge benefits least from this procedure.

Fibroepithelial Hyperplasia. Unless the hyperplasia involves the majority of the residual ridge, one can put less pressure on this flabby tissue and more on the firm bearing areas by using a selected pressure impression technique (Fig. 11–10). When more than half of the residual ridge has flabby tissue and denture stability is compromised, surgical procedures can help produce a better foundation.

Frena. Most frena do not present a problem with denture retention. It is when they attach very close to the crest of the ridge, as in the case of the high lingual frenum, that surgical elimination can be beneficial.

*Clorox Co., Oakland, Calif.

†Beacham Products, Pittsburgh, Pa.

‡Nystatin Ointment, Squibb & Sons, Inc., Princeton, N.J.

Hard Tissue

Sharp Spiny Ridge. Surgery on the sharp spiny ridge generally will result in another sharp edge until very little ridge remains, unless it has a broad base. Again, if less pressure is placed on the ridge and more on the other denture-bearing areas, a satisfactory denture can be made without surgery. Similarly, relief of the denture for a sharp mylohyoid ridge, except when very large and undercut, may be all that is necessary.

Tori. Most maxillary tori can be accommodated by providing adequate relief in the denture base with pressure disclosing paste at the time of insertion. Only if tori are very large, are undercut, or approach the soft palate do they present a problem necessitating surgery (Fig. 11–11*A*). Mandibular tori are more of a problem for complete dentures than for removable partial dentures. If the tori are so large that adequate peripheral seal cannot be obtained, they should be removed.

Tuberosity Reduction. Tuberosity reduction is one of the important surgical procedures that allows proper basal seat coverage with the prosthesis. It may involve both hard and soft tissue. Sufficient room must be present for coverage of the tuberosity and the retromolar pad (Fig. 11–12). If the space present is questionable, it may be better to wait until the denture teeth are arranged at the correct vertical dimension of occlusion to make the final determination about the need for surgery. Reduction of buccal undercuts, unilaterally or bilaterally, may be necessary, depending on the depth

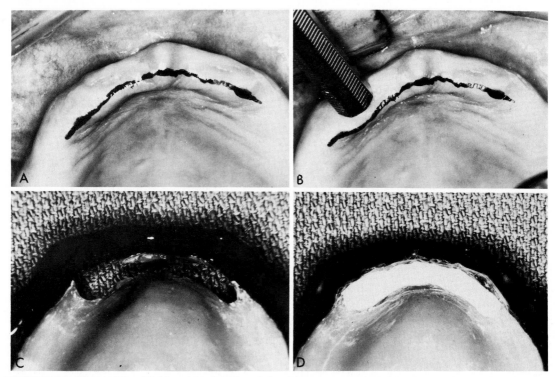

FIGURE 11–10 *A,* The "flabby ridge" with minimal bone support as it exists in the resting state. *B,* Displacement of the same ridge illustrates the lack of residual ridge support. *C,* In this impression technique, cutting a hole in the tray minimizes displacement of the movable tissue. *D,* The hypermobile mucosa is recorded by painting quick-setting stone on the tissue after the impression tray is placed in the mouth.

of the undercut and the path of insertion. Small undercuts may be negotiated by relieving the inside of the denture flange, without sacrificing retention. When surgery is necessary, the use of diagnostic casts that outline exactly what should be removed is helpful in obtaining adequate reduction and in avoiding excessive reduction.

Extruded Teeth. Extruded teeth may be altered so that they have a better occlusal

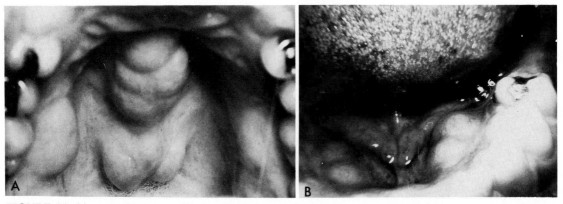

FIGURE 11–11 *A,* A large maxillary torus that should not have a complete denture constructed without surgery. *B,* Mandibular tori that could be maintained for removable partial dentures but should generally be removed if making a complete denture. (Courtesy of Dr. Bejan Iranpour, Rochester, N.Y.)

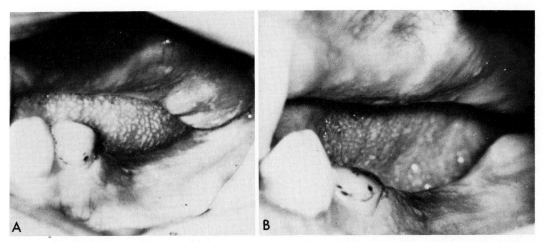

FIGURE 11–12 *A,* A tuberosity reduction is needed to obtain adequate tissue coverage for both the maxillary and the mandibular prosthesis at the existing vertical dimension of occlusion. *B,* Surgical reduction of the tuberosity provides the space necessary for proper denture coverage. (Courtesy of Dr. Aaron Fenton, Toronto, Ont.)

plane. They may be reduced in height, with or without crowning them. Endodontic therapy along with posts and crowns may be necessary if more reduction is needed. Orthodontic intrusion and surgical repositioning are two other methods of treatment that should be considered before extraction.

ILLUSTRATIVE TECHNIQUES

Once the mouth has been properly prepared, there are some general principles that apply to clinical techniques for all aspects of removable prosthodontics. The characteristics of a good impression, an accurate record base, and a correct centric jaw relation record will be discussed. Methods are offered that are especially useful when treating the difficult patient. Tooth selection and arrangement along with delivery and care of the prosthesis will conclude this section.

Impressions

In order to have a stable and retentive denture, there must be a stable and retentive impression. There are many techniques for developing a stable impression. The important point is to know when the impression is completed, providing the best possible opportunity for a well-fitting denture.

Although the laboratory usually makes an acrylic resin custom tray for the secondary impression to be made at a subsequent appointment, any of a variety of conditions may make it advantageous to complete the preliminary and secondary impressions at the same appointment. One method that does not involve having the laboratory fabricate a custom tray is as follows.

The preliminary impression is made using block compound* in a stock tray (Black)† (Fig. 11–13A). The stock tray can be shaped through bending or cutting in order to provide a good initial impression. The material is then removed from the metal tray after chilling. A heavy-gauge metal coat hanger is bent to provide a reusable handle.

After the handle is attached to the preliminary impression with compound, the various sections are border-molded in order to allow normal functional movements, such as opening, closing, swallowing, and movements of the lip and tongue. *Exaggerated movements should not be made,* or the compound will be overshortened. Low fusing stick compound* (132° F) can be traced along the posterior aspect of the maxillary impression and any other peripheral areas that are underextended. The impression must extend to the hamular notches and completely fill the buccal and labial vestibules of the maxilla. The mandibular impression must cover the retromolar pads,

---

*Sybron/Kerr, Romulus, Mich.
†I-Den Dental Mfg., Dayton, Ohio.

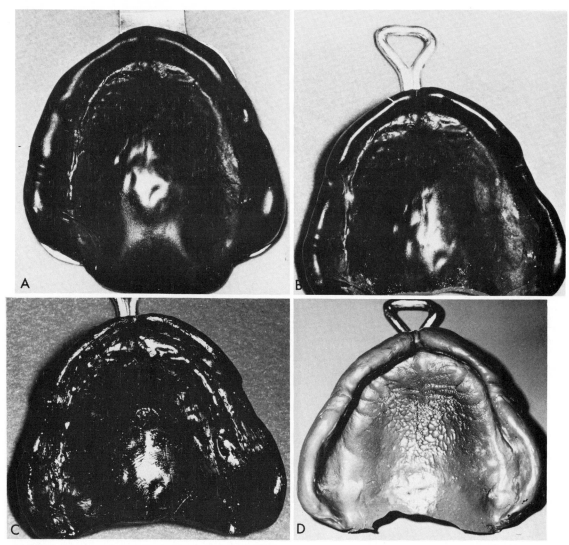

FIGURE 11–13 *A,* A block-compound impression formed in a stock tray. *B,* The compound is removed from the tray, a metal handle is attached with stick compound to the undersurface of the impression, and the tray is border-molded, section by section. *C,* The compound impression is relieved of undercuts and vented, and suitable adhesive is applied. *D,* The final impression is made using the material of choice.

run parallel to the external oblique ridge, and fill the buccal and labial vestibules. The distal extent of the lingual flange should drop straight down from the end of the retromolar pad and curve into the retromylohyoid space. The S-shaped curve of the mylohyoid muscle then proceeds to the sublingual fold space area. The sublingual fold space is the most critical area and must be completely filled. Additional compound can be added and manually molded into the area to develop good retention. The preliminary impression now should be retentive and stable.

Undercuts and soft displaceable tissues are relieved in the compound. A vent is placed in the height of the palate. A suitable adhesive is applied and the secondary wash impression is made with the material of choice such as polysulfide, polyether or silicone (Fig. 11–13D). The material used for the secondary impression is not nearly as critical as developing a good preliminary impression and using similar functional movements while the secondary impression is made.

When the mouth opening is limited, the use of a custom-made acrylic resin tray for the mandible may be helpful. The tray is made from the cast of the initial compound impression.

The completed maxillary and mandibular impressions should exhibit stability and retention. Stability can be evaluated by alternating pressure from front to back and from side to side. There should be minimal move-

ment, usually less for the mandibular impression than for the maxillary impression. Retention is evaluated by the force necessary to displace the impression when lifting or pulling on the handle as well as if the impression stays in position during the functional movements of the lips, tongue, and mandible.

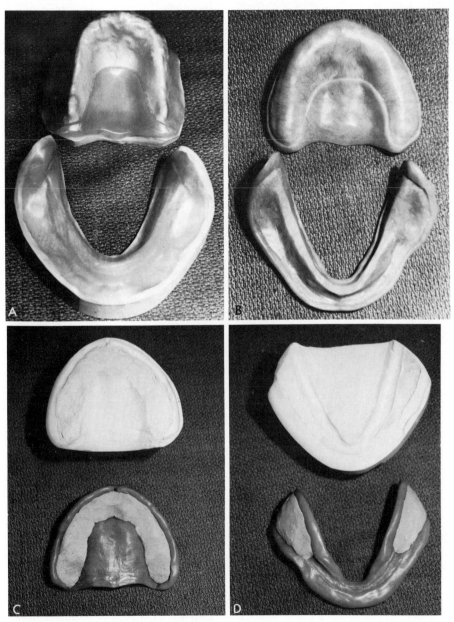

FIGURE 11–14 *A,* The casts are waxed for processed denture bases after filling the peripheral sulcus with beading wax. *B,* The casts have been flasked and processed with heat-cured acrylic resin, resulting in completed denture bases. *C* and *D,* The undercuts of the heat-processed denture bases are blocked out, and stone mounting casts are made. A mounting cast must be made, since the original cast from the final impression is destroyed when the processed base is retrieved.

Record Bases

Once the impressions are completed, the next step usually involves making some kind of temporary record base, using wax or self-curing acrylic resin. Temporary bases have inherent weaknesses caused by blocking out undercuts and by not completely utilizing the periphery of the cast so that the base can be removed. The temporary base does not fit the mouth the same as the completed denture. For these reasons, the use of *heat-processed completed bases* can make all of the subsequent steps much easier to accomplish and is strongly advocated for the problem patient (Fig. 11–14).

The heat-processed acrylic resin base is the same material used for the final denture and becomes a part of the final denture. The teeth are attached by a second processing for a longer time at a lower temperature. The processed bases offer several advantages. They allow for an evaluation of the fit of the final denture before a centric jaw relation record is made. A more accurate maxillomandibular relation can be made because the bases are stable and retentive, and the greatest deformation in the acrylic resin is released before the centric jaw registration is made, not after. During the try-in appointment, both the dentist and the patient are more comfortable, since the processed bases are more retentive. Finally, the need to remount at the delivery appointment can be eliminated, since the artificial stone is removed from the denture after the second processing, *before* the occlusion is adjusted on the articulator. If the split-cast method is used, the occlusion is adjusted and then the cast is removed, releasing the strain in the acrylic and resulting in an occlusal error and the need for a remount record at the time of insertion of the dentures.

The heat-processed completed base can be used with removable partial dentures and overdentures as well. The step-by-step technique can be done by the dental laboratory. The details of this technique have been published by the author.

Maxillomandibular Relations

Establishing the correct vertical dimension of occlusion remains one of the more difficult procedures in removable prosthodontics. For the partially edentulous patient with some natural teeth in occlusion, this vertical dimension should be the one used. Removable partial dentures should not be used to increase the vertical dimension of occlusion. The natural teeth *must* contact. When no teeth are present, esthetic appearance and phonetic ability are important guides. However, as a place to start, a total vertical dimension of 37 mm from flange to flange in the region of the cuspid can give an average value for a tentative vertical dimension of occlusion (Fig. 11–15). In the posterior area, the bases are placed so the ridges are parallel, and the occlusal plane of the mandibular wax rim extends from the height of the cuspid to halfway up the retromolar pad. If the laboratory sets the rims on the record bases at the 37 mm vertical to start, the bases then can be evaluated more carefully intraorally by using the *ssss* sound. The lower occlusal rim should come to within 1 mm of the upper occlusal rim in the anterior region. This is the "closest speaking space." For Class II occlusions, the 1mm approximation occurs in the premolar region. Starting with the average value vertical, it usually is necessary to adjust the vertical dimension only about 3 mm in either direction to arrive at a correct vertical. There will be a few patients with a greater variation, but they are exceptions to the rule. The final determination of the correct vertical dimension should occur when the anterior and posterior teeth are arranged.

Once the tentative vertical dimension has been selected, the centric jaw relation record is made. Any number of methods for recording this position have been advocated.

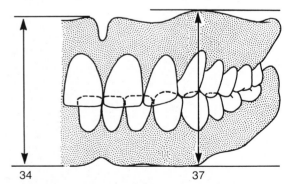

34   37

FIGURE 11–15 An average value for the tentative vertical dimension of occlusion from the edge of the flanges is 37 mm in the region of the cuspids and 34 mm in the region of the central incisors.

There is probably no one best method; just how far posterior the mandible should be positioned is another unresolved question. What has been agreed upon, however, is that an *accurate* centric jaw relation is one of the most important records. No matter how it is recorded or with what type of material, the important thing is that it be verified. Even if the centric jaw relation is recorded correctly with the patient, an error can be made when the casts are mounted on the articulator.

One method that can produce an accurate centric jaw relation record is to use three metal points* on the maxillary base against three wax blocks on the mandibular base (Fig. 11–16A). Since minimal contact will be

made between points and wax, the chance for error from distortion of the material is reduced. The upper and lower bases are carefully supported with quick-setting stone and then mounted on the articulator (Fig. 11–16D).

The jaw relation is then verified through the use of Centric Check Points* (Fig. 11–17). These consist of sets of points that allow for verification in three dimensions, since an error can be present in the horizontal plane either anteroposteriorly or mediolaterally or can be present in the vertical plane. The latter type of error is probably the most critical, since the teeth will not contact on both sides simultaneously.

The technique for setting up the check

*Teledyne Hanau, Buffalo, N.Y.

*Teledyne Hanau, Buffalo, N.Y.

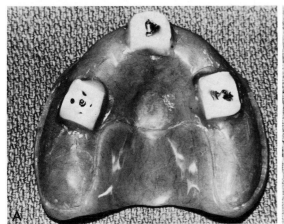
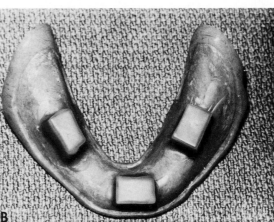
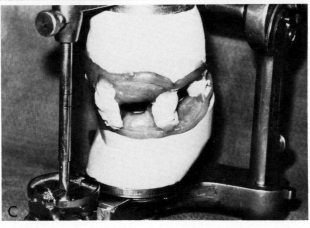

FIGURE 11–16 *A* and *B,* Three metal points on the maxillary denture base are arranged to oppose three wax blocks on the mandibular denture base. *C,* Once the record has been made, the bases are carefully positioned into the indentations and are secured with quick-setting stone to prevent movement. The mandibular mounting cast is then placed on the articulator. The maxillary mounting cast had previously been attached to the articulator following a face-bow recording.

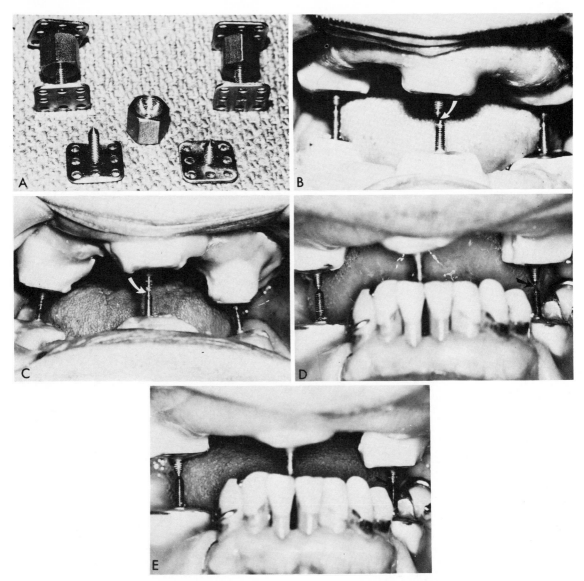

FIGURE 11–17 *A,* Centric Check Points and cups are used in the verification of centric jaw relation. *B,* An error (arrow) in centric jaw relation as demonstrated intraorally with Centric Check Points. *C,* Following a new maxillomandibular record and the resetting of the check points on the articulator, this second jaw registration is verified as being correct (arrow). *D,* Centric Check Points can be used to verify maxillomandibular records for the partially edentulous by aligning one or more points to a cusp tip or incisal edge as necessary. An error is apparent (arrow) in the patient's left molar region. *E,* The error has been corrected (arrow) by making a new maxillomandibular record and by remounting and reverifying.

points can be readily accomplished by the laboratory technician or dental assistant. Once set point to point on the articulator, this same relationship should occur when the record bases are taken to the mouth. If an error exists, it can be seen easily, without excess recording material or denture teeth blocking the view (Fig. 11–17*D*). The correction can be accomplished with the metal

cups provided. The bases are then secured with stone in this new position, and one of the casts is remounted. The technician or assistant can reset the points, and the position can be checked intraorally. It is checked until found to be correct by having all three points contact simultaneously (Fig. 11–17*E*).

Although the procedure requires a little more time at this stage, once the correct centric jaw relation has been verified, the posterior teeth can be positioned accurately. When this procedure is used in combination with processed bases, the remount procedures can be eliminated at the delivery appointment, saving time in the end.

The check points can be used for the complete denture opposing the removable partial denture as well as for overdentures or two removable partial dentures. This is the time to know that what the laboratory has mounted on the articulator is correct! Once the teeth are placed on the bases, it becomes very difficult to detect small errors.

Tooth Selection and Arrangement

Anterior Teeth

Various guides for tooth selection, including old photographs, diagnostic casts, or old partial dentures with anterior teeth, may play a role in determining the proper tooth. Using the size and shape of the face or the nose has not been shown to be totally reliable for predicting the size and shape of the natural anteriors. Nonetheless, from an esthetic viewpoint, teeth that blend into the frame of the mouth and face are more pleasing than those that do not.

The shade of the teeth should also blend with the patient's complexion and hair color. At times the dentist may be able to improve upon what nature originally provided.

The teeth can be set in position while the patient is present, but if time does not permit, or if teeth must be ordered, they can be arranged before the patient is seen at the next appointment, using average values as a guide (Fig. 11–18). The teeth and shade should be selected by the dentist, taking into

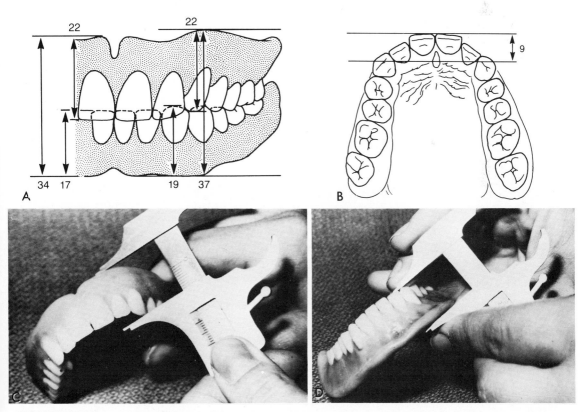

FIGURE 11–18 **A,** The vertical position of the anterior teeth can be tentatively arranged by using average values. The maxillary central incisal edge is 22 mm from the denture flange, while the mandibular central incisal edge is 17 mm; the maxillary cuspid is 22 mm from the denture flange, while the mandibular cuspid is 19 mm. **B,** The horizontal position of the anterior teeth can be approximated by placing the labial aspect of the central incisors 9 mm anterior to the center of the incisive papilla. The center of the incisal edge of the cuspids is in line with the center of the incisive papilla. **C** and **D,** A Boley gauge may be used to position the anterior teeth in relation to the denture flange.

consideration what the patient liked or did not like about his natural teeth or old denture. Block posterior teeth* may be used during the initial try-in, since they can be set up in minutes, and the vertical dimension of occlusion can be changed quickly if necessary. The same guides for the occlusal plane are used. Parallel ridges and the tip of the mandibular cuspid to halfway up the retromolar pad provide a place to start.

This average value set-up is tried-in, and necessary adjustments are made to provide satisfactory phonetic ability and esthetic appearance. The sibilant sounds are used to determine the closest speaking space; the anterior teeth are approximately 1 mm out of contact during the *ssss* sound.

For a pleasing appearance, following the

---

*Dentsply International, Inc., York, Pa.

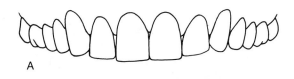

A

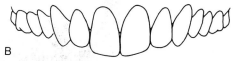

B

FIGURE 11–20 *A,* A masculine-appearing tooth is provided by flattening the incisal and interproximal surfaces and using a tooth with a flat labial surface. *B,* A more feminine-appearing tooth is created with anterior teeth by rounding the incisal and interproximal surfaces as well as using a tooth with a curved labial surface.

smile line of the lower lip and allowing some mandibular anterior teeth to show while speaking are very important considerations (Fig. 11–19). The buccal corridor should not have all teeth filling the lateral aspects. Females tend to show more of the maxillary incisal edge, whereas males show more of the mandibular incisal edge. The amount of maxillary incisal edge that shows decreases with age. Adjusting the shape of tooth surfaces can provide a more feminine or a more masculine appearance (Fig. 11–20). A more feminine appearance is provided by teeth with curved incisal and labial surfaces; a more masculine appearance has flatter incisal and labial surfaces.

Posterior Teeth

The most frequent question dentists ask regarding posterior tooth selection is whether to use an anatomic or nonanatomic tooth. They both have a place, with specific indications for each type.

Nonanatomic teeth are very useful when the dentist is confronted with a patient with a great deal of abnormal movement of the

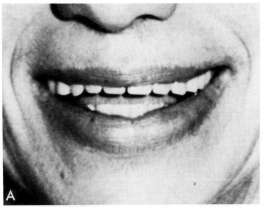

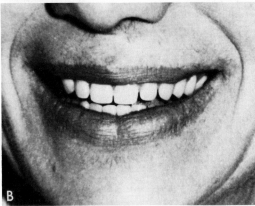

FIGURE 11–19 *A,* The "denture look" is emphasized when the maxillary anterior teeth follow the upper lip when smiling. *B,* The "natural look" is created by arranging the maxillary anterior teeth so that they follow the curvature of the lower lip when smiling.

FIGURE 11–21 Anatomic posterior teeth allow for vertical overlap of the anterior teeth while still providing for a balanced occlusion in the protrusive position, as seen on the left side of the illustration. Nonanatomic teeth set with a flat occlusal plane cannot provide for balance in the protrusive position when a vertical overlap of the anterior teeth is required for appearance or speech, as seen on the right side.

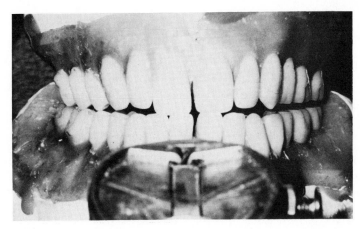

mandible. If a large discrepancy exists between centric jaw relation and the neuromuscular (habitual) position, properly balanced zero-degree teeth allow for a range of closure. This is especially useful for Class II occlusions. For elderly patients and patients with minimal residual ridges, nonanatomic teeth can minimize lateral stresses and should be considered. Nonanatomic teeth may be recontoured in the maxillary premolar buccal region to provide a more natural appearance.

Anatomic posterior teeth may provide a better esthetic appearance. They allow more anterior vertical overlap, a point that may be important for both proper esthetics and phonetics. This greater vertical overlap shows

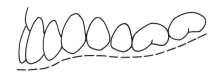

A

B

FIGURE 11–22 *A,* A masculine appearance is created by arranging the posterior teeth with a flat occlusal plane. *B,* A feminine appearance is created by arranging anatomic posterior teeth with a curved occlusal plane, rising in the cuspid and first premolar region and again in the second molar area.

more anterior tooth, given the same vertical dimension of occlusion for nonanatomic teeth (Fig. 11–21). Minimal or no anterior vertical overlap should be present with zero-degree teeth unless an equal amount of horizontal overlap is present. The posterior teeth can also be set to provide a more feminine or masculine appearance (Fig. 11–22). Complete bilateral balanced occlusion to the height of the cusp can be an important asset for the problem patient with anatomic posterior teeth. As the patient closes in various positions, the pressure seats, rather than dislodges, the denture. Cusped posterior teeth also allow for more lateral movement and proper tissue coverage when potential interference from the tuberosity exists, by increasing the vertical dimension while moving up the cusp inclines.

The question of whether acrylic resin or porcelain teeth should be used is a common one. Generally, porcelain teeth are used when sufficient space exists. Because of their lack of wear, their good surface detail, and a luster that remains after repeated brushings, they can provide a natural appearance for many years. Acrylic resin teeth should be used when space is minimal and neuromuscular control is not good, and, with some elderly patients, to minimize the "clicking" sound. Acrylic resin teeth should also be used over the abutment teeth of an overdenture and next to the clasp of a removable partial denture to provide a more natural appearance by placing the tooth as close as possible to where the natural tooth was. A harder acrylic resin tooth* now available

---

*Trubyte IPN, Dentsply International, Inc., York, Pa.

may reduce some of the wear of conventional acrylic resin teeth.

The Try-in
Office Try-in

When the dentist is satisfied with the appearance of the teeth, the patient is allowed to see the dentures. A large wall mirror should be used rather than a hand-held mirror so the patient can get an overall picture and not just concentrate on the teeth. If substantial changes have been made from the old dentures, the reasons for and the effects of these changes should be explained to the patient. A notebook with magazine clippings of people smiling and talking with natural dentition allays the patient's fear that too much tooth is showing. Proper examples of a natural smile line can be emphasized (Fig. 11–23).

When the patient is reluctant to accept changes that avoid the denture look, he should have the opportunity to spend more time getting used to the different appearance. The "home try-in" is such an opportunity. Most people want to look better, even when they say they do not care. In some sit-uations, a compromise must be reached between what the patient and dentist feel is esthetically pleasing.

Home Try-In

The patient is offered the opportunity to take the dentures home in the waxed try-in stage. The dentures are sealed in a bag of water. Processed bases allow the patient to be comfortable during this home try-in, since they fit like the completed dentures. Family members or friends can comment on the appearance of the dentures at this time.

If speaking is a problem, the patient can read aloud to see if he can adapt to the changes. The patient is cautioned not to eat or drink with the dentures at this wax-up stage. He should wear them for only 15 to 20 minutes at a time; otherwise, body temperature might soften the wax. When not in the mouth, the dentures should be kept in room-temperature water. The home try-in gives the dentist one more opportunity to evaluate the vertical dimension of occlusion. If it is excessive, the posterior teeth will be pushed into the wax and the vertical dimension of occlusion must be decreased. Any changes that the patient or others would like

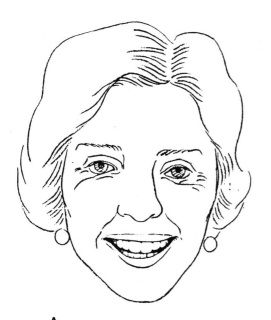
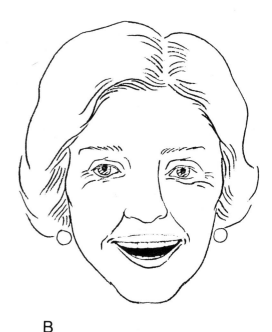

A

B

FIGURE 11–23 *A* and *B,* Photographs, magazine clippings, or other illustrations can be used to show the patient the "natural look" (*A*) as opposed to the "denture look" (*B*).

to see made should be written down so they can be incorporated at the next appointment.

For the demanding patient very concerned about appearance, this stage can often involve the greatest amount of time in the fabrication of the dentures. It may consist of several home try-in appointments until final approval is received. It is better to spend the time while the teeth are in wax, than to have the patient dissatisfied after they are processed in acrylic resin. The home try-in can be used for removable partial dentures, overdentures, or complete dentures.

Once final approval has been received, the dentures may be processed. The shade of the soft tissue and gingival acrylic resin should be matched. This is especially important for removable partial dentures in which the flange must blend with the gingival tissues in order to have as natural an appearance as possible.

When processed bases are used, the second processing is done at a lower temperature (138° F) for a longer time (12 hours minimum). The laboratory can refine the occlusion after remounting, and the dentist can check the occlusion after the dentures have been *deflasked* and polished, since they still fit the articulated mounting casts. This is an advantage over conventional, one-stage processing of dentures using the split cast, since once the stone is removed from the denture, the occlusion cannot be checked again, and an error is produced when the stone is removed. This necessitates a remount procedure with the patient. When centric check points and processed bases are used properly, the remount procedure need not be done. If the occlusion or vertical dimension is wrong, this will be readily apparent on the articulator, and the dentures should be returned to the laboratory to be corrected.

Delivery Appointment

Delivery of the denture should represent the shortest appointment in the series, if each of the previous steps has been done carefully. The need for remounting has been eliminated. The dentures have been completed before insertion, not after insertion. The impression was checked using processed bases to evaluate retention and stability. The centric jaw relation was verified using centric check points. The vertical dimension of occlusion, esthetic appearance, and phonetic ability were carefully evaluated by dentist and patient during the office and home try-in. The dentures are now inserted and the responsibility is shifted from the dentist to the patient. The dentist has done everything as carefully as possible to provide a good prosthesis. It now becomes the patient's responsibility to learn to function with the new denture.

The first-time denture wearer may require more guidance than previous denture wearers. Many booklets are available with advice about dentures. Some are so involved they might shake the confidence of the new denture wearer. They describe all the problems that can occur, when the patient usually encounters only a few of these. It is better to have the patient start slowly, giving him only a few key suggestions, such as telling him to place several small pieces of food on the fork so they can be placed on both the right and the left side of the denture when chewing, in order to balance the prosthesis during mastication. When biting into objects such as sandwiches, the sandwich should be pushed in and up, rather than pulled down and forward, in order to keep the maxillary denture in place. The patient should be cautioned that sticky foods can prove difficult and should be eaten only after simpler foods are tried. The importance of tongue position for retention of the lower denture can be re-emphasized. Further difficulties can be discussed at the adjustment appointments as necessary.

COMPLICATIONS

Adjustments

The patient should be seen within 24 hours after the insertion of any prosthesis. If the patient has difficulty with the prosthesis and must wait 2 or 3 days following the delivery of the denture, he may build up hostility against the dentist. Depending upon the severity of the problem, he can then be given another appointment within 24 to 48 hours. Specific appointments should be made until the patient is comfortable. He should not be squeezed in between other patients once the dentures are delivered. The dentist must be truly concerned about any problems the patient presents.

Special Problems

It is extremely difficult at times to make the true xerostomia patient completely comfortable. The use of artificial saliva* may be of some benefit. A heat-processed soft liner is not necessarily the most comfortable base for this kind of patient, and sometimes a highly polished acrylic resin undersurface may be better.

The "burning" mouth patient is another prosthodontic concern. This patient's problem often has a strong emotional component and should be handled jointly by the physician and dentist when no deficiencies are seen in the prosthesis. Other possible causes may include nutritional deficiencies and pernicious anemia.

Another problem that might be present with the denture patient is gagging. Gagging may be a problem at the impression stage and at the time of delivery of the dentures. At the impression stage, it is usually when the dentist is attempting to make the maxillary impression that the patient starts to gag. The use of block compound in a stock tray can prevent this. The compound tray can be removed quickly and then reinserted until a good preliminary impression is developed. The completed preliminary impression can then be followed by the use of a functional impression material† inside the compound tray, which again will allow placement and replacement several times if gagging occurs. Any excess impression material that may flow over the posterior border can be trimmed, and the impression can be reseated. Often, it is the excess material that potentiates the gag reflex.

Gagging at the time of insertion may be caused by the posterior border of the maxillary denture or by overextension of the distal lingual flange of the mandibular denture. It is just as likely that the posterior border of the maxillary denture is too thick and should be *thinned* before *shortening* the denture eliminates the posterior palatal seal section of the denture.

Should the posterior palatal seal or another small area such as a flange or a frenum area, need to be extended, this can be done by placing compound on the area and border-molding it. The patient should then make sure that the problem is corrected by wearing the denture for several hours. He should, of course, be cautioned not to drink anything hot. The denture can then be removed and a localized, self-curing acrylic resin addition completed.

Another cause for gagging is an excessive vertical dimension of occlusion. If there is no other indication for gagging, the vertical dimension should be re-evaluated and decreased if it appears excessive.

One other problem that may occur with any denture technique is that of improper speech. Sometimes this is just a question of the patient's lips, cheeks, and tongue adapting to different contours. If, however, after 4 to 6 weeks a problem is still present, the following possibilities should be considered: (1) When the patient has a lisping sound, too little air is being allowed through the anterior portion of the palate and tongue. Using pressure-indicating paste,* the tongue contact can be delineated and the acrylic thinned in the offending region. (2) If a whistling sound is present, then too much air is escaping between the tongue and palate. The use of soft wax placed behind the maxillary anterior teeth will show if this is the problem. When the correct palatal contour is determined, processing self-curing acrylic resin in that area can correct the problem. If the speech problems are not corrected in this manner, it may be necessary to reset the anterior teeth.

Maintenance

Once the patient is comfortable, a 6-month recall for dentulous patients and a 1-year recall for edentulous patients should be established. Instructions on the care of the prosthesis should be given to the patient upon delivery and at the 24-hour appointment. The instructions are repeated at 24 hours, since the patient may not always give his undivided attention on the day the new prosthesis is inserted. Written instructions can be very helpful for the new denture patient. In addition to stressing the importance of removing the prosthesis for 6 to 8 hours each day to promote tissue health, the dentist should remind the patient of the importance of massaging the tissue. In order to prevent dimensional change, it should be empha-

---

*Orex, King's Dental Specialty Co., Fort Wayne, Ind.
†Coe-Comfort, Coe Laboratories, Inc., Chicago, Ill.

---

*Spot-chek, SAEES, P.O. Box 92566, Rochester, N.Y.

sized that the denture must be kept in water when not in the mouth.

The use of a *soft* bristled brush (denture brushes usually are too stiff) and a partial denture clasp brush* should be demonstrated to the patient. If the inside of the clasp is not properly cleaned, the plaque will be placed right back on the tooth, with the possibility for decay.

Although soap and water can keep a prosthesis clean, many patients like to use a solution to soak their denture. An effective and inexpensive solution can be prepared by the patient using 1 part Clorox, 2 parts Calgon, and 8 parts water. This solution can be used for 15 to 30 minutes each day or for

overnight soaking twice a week. It should *not* be used with metal frameworks.

A commercial denture cleaning product* has been shown to be very effective in removing plaque if the patient does not want to prepare his own solution. This may be used with all types of prostheses for 15 to 30 minutes of cleaning, but not with metal frameworks for regular overnight cleaning. If a long-term soft liner has been used, then cleaners containing sodium hypochlorite (Clorox, Mersene) should not be used. Instead a cleaner such as Prolastic Denture Cleaner† or Kleenite‡ is recommended.

*John O. Butler Co., Chicago, Ill.

*Mersene, Colgate-Palmolive, New York, N.Y.
†Young Dental Mfg. Co., Maryland Heights, Mo.
‡Kleenite, Richardson-Vicks Inc., Wilton, Conn.

Removable Partial Dentures

Removable partial dentures are frequently reported to be harmful to the remaining dentition or are not worn after being fabricated. Some reasons cited by patients for not using removable prostheses include soreness, interference with speech, gagging, food catching under the denture base, or unsatisfactory esthetic appearance. When evaluated by dentists, removable partial dentures have been implicated in increasing caries and periodontal disease as well as in not allowing patients to get their natural teeth into occlusion.

This portion of the chapter will discuss when and why a removable partial denture should be fabricated; it will also show when not to use such a prosthesis. Factors critical to the success of the prosthesis will be emphasized. Some specific designs for distal extension partial dentures will be presented based upon the concern to preserve what remains and still satisfy the patient.

Principles of Removable Partial Denture Therapy

Indications

One frequently cited rule is to use a fixed partial denture whenever possible. In many situations this rule is simply impractical. For example, if all the molars and a first premolar are missing, but the second premolar

remains, the replacement of the first premolar with a fixed partial denture while the molars are replaced with a removable partial denture is an impractical solution. The expense of the three-unit fixed partial denture may be twice the expense of the removable partial denture, and the single missing premolar can be incorporated easily into the design and fabrication of the removable partial denture at no appreciable increase in cost to the patient. Removable partial dentures are generally indicated for the following situations and reasons.

Distal Extensions. When posterior teeth are missing and masticatory function is compromised or when opposing teeth could extrude and there is no distal abutment, the removable partial denture may be the treatment of choice.

Long Spans. When there are four posterior teeth or five or more anterior and posterior teeth missing on the same side of the arch, the span is generally too long for a fixed partial denture.

Financial Considerations. Because a removable partial denture can be fabricated for considerably less than a fixed partial denture, the removable prosthesis may be the patient's choice.

Esthetic Appearance. Appearance becomes a factor owing to the loss of a large segment of the maxillary alveolus, to a high smile line, or to the need for lip support. Improved appearance can best be provided by the flange of a removable partial denture.

Congenital Anomalies. Anomalies such as a cleft palate may be treated with a removable partial denture, especially in early childhood.

Maxillofacial Prosthetics. Prosthetic reconstruction of the maxilla or mandible following surgical resection because of cancer can often be done only by using a removable partial denture.

Occlusal Stabilization. In order to stabilize mobile teeth, the removable partial denture directs forces to be distributed over the entire arch. Generally, the tooth mobility is

decreased only while the prosthesis is in place.

Contraindications

The following factors contraindicate the use of a removable partial denture.

Emotional Factors. Some patients feel that they can never wear something removable in their mouth.

Poor Plaque Control. Following adequate oral hygiene instructions, if poor plaque control continues, the longevity of a removable partial denture is compromised.

Advanced Periodontal Disease. Extremely mobile teeth with 50 to 75 per cent bone loss may not be good abutments for a

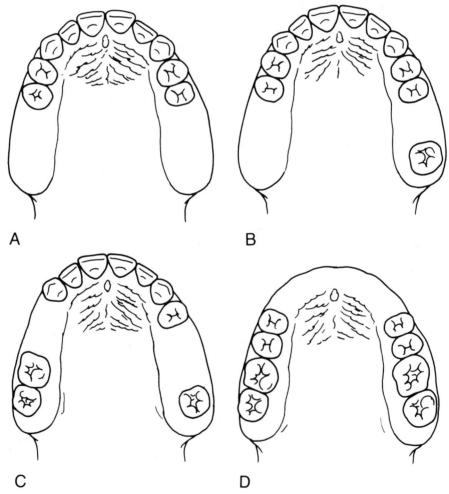

FIGURE 11–24   Four of Kennedy's classifications for the partially edentulous mouth include **A,** Kennedy Class I—bilateral edentulous areas posterior to remaining teeth, **B,** Kennedy Class II—a unilateral edentulous area posterior to remaining teeth, **C,** Kennedy Class III—a unilateral edentulous area with teeth anterior and posterior, and **D,** Kennedy Class IV—a single edentulous area located anterior to the remaining teeth and crossing the midline.

removable partial denture. An overdenture may be the treatment of choice.

Age of the Patient. Advanced age combined with poor health results in a poor prognosis for wearing any new prosthesis.

Premolar Occlusion. Although all molar teeth are missing, sufficient teeth remain for proper masticatory function. A full complement of 28 to 32 teeth is not always necessary.

Advantages

The removable partial denture has the following advantages: (1) It is more economical than a fixed partial denture. (2) Usually shorter and fewer appointments are required than for a fixed partial denture. (3) Less tooth preparation is necessary than for a fixed partial denture. (4) Good oral hygiene is possible when the prosthesis is removed.

Disadvantages

The following disadvantages may be attributed to removable partial dentures: (1) The risk of caries or gingival disease is increased if plaque control is not adequate. (2) Improper design and maintenance can result in mechanical trauma. (3) An esthetic appearance is compromised if clasps are visible. (4) There may be some movement of the prosthesis.

Design

The dentist is the only one who can make the proper decisions involved in the treatment plan and design of a removable partial denture. The technician cannot decide what is biologically acceptable for a patient. The dentist has both a moral and a professional responsibility to design the removable partial denture.

Classification. The Kennedy classification will be used throughout this chapter. This classification simplifies communication and provides a method for grouping similar situations when thinking about the design of the prosthesis (Fig. 11–24). Although designs cannot be provided for the infinite variety of situations that occur, examples are provided for the most common. The dentist can use these to extrapolate other configurations and conditions. The components that are most important to the long-term

success of the prosthesis are emphasized here.

Critical Components. Since so many different designs succeed, it would appear that there is no one best type of clasp for each classification of partial denture. There are, however, some *critical* factors in the design of a removable partial denture that, when not taken into consideration, can lead to the destruction of the oral structures or to the patient's refusal to wear the prosthesis.

Rigid Connectors. The first *critical component* is that there must be *rigid major and minor connectors.* The palatal or lingual connector joining the components of the removable partial denture between each side of the arch should have sufficient thickness and bulk so that it does not flex when the patient closes on the distal extension base. It could also flex each time the patient swallows. Only with a rigid connector can the forces be distributed throughout the arch, avoiding undue stress in any one area (Fig. 11–25).

The greater the length of the distal extension, the more bulk will be needed to provide rigidity. It is also better to have the palatal connector wide and thin rather than narrow and thick. Full palatal coverage should be considered when the remaining maxillary teeth have less than ideal support, when the residual ridges are severely resorbed, or when the opposing occlusion is composed entirely of natural dentition. The minor connectors joining the major connector and clasps must also be rigid. This is necessary, again, to distribute the forces throughout the arch.

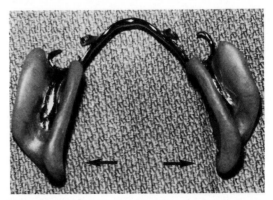

FIGURE 11–25 A rigid major connector is necessary to minimize lateral forces distributed to the teeth and edentulous ridge. Normally, the lingual bar should be approximately 2 mm thick and 5 mm high.

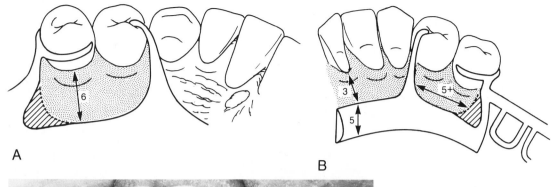

A

B

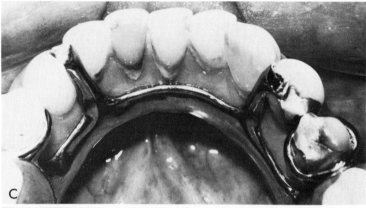

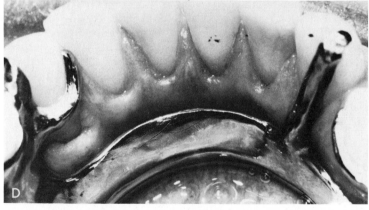

C

D

FIGURE 11–26 *A,* The maxillary major connector should be at least 6 mm from the free gingival margin and should follow the contour of the distally most prominent rugae. Designing the junction between the major and minor connector, as shown in the striped area, allows freedom from tissue encroachment. *B,* In order to avoid irritation to the soft tissue of the mandible, the major connector should be at least 3 mm from the free gingival margin. There should also be at least 5 mm between vertical components of the prosthesis. The lingual bar should be approximately 5 mm in height in order to be rigid. *C,* Clinically, this photograph shows the incorrect position of the lingual bar. *D,* The lingual bar is correctly placed when at least 3 mm from the free gingival margin.

Location of Connectors. The *location* of the major connector is another *critical component.* The superior edge of the lingual bar should be kept a minimum of 3 mm away from the free gingival margin. In the maxillary arch, the palatal connector can usually be even farther (a minimum of 6 mm) from the gingival margin. The anterior border of a palatal strap should be placed just behind the distally most prominent rugae when posterior teeth are replaced (Fig. 11–26). The anterior palatal U-shaped connector (horseshoe) should be avoided if possible, since it interferes most with speech. For a rigid mandibular major connector, a minimum of 7 to 8 mm is needed from the gingival margin to the floor of the mouth in normal function. With this need in mind, the major connector is referred to as the *sublingual* bar when it is placed into the sublingual-fold space, much as would be done for the lingual flange of a complete denture (Fig. 11–27). If 7 to 8 mm is not available, alternatives exist, such as rotating the bar horizontally (Fig. 11–28*B*).

When the floor of the mouth is very high and the dentist wants to avoid covering the free gingival margin, a cingulum bar may be

FIGURE 11–27 *A* and *B,* There should be approximately 8 mm between the free gingival margin and the floor of the mouth when using the lingual bar (*A*) or the sublingual bar (*B*).

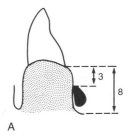

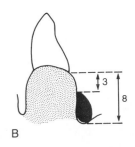

used as the major connector (Fig. 11–28*C* and *D*). The cingulum bar can provide rigidity with normal function and will not lead to potential gingival problems.

Guide Planes and Surfaces. Guide planes are two or more vertically parallel surfaces of abutment teeth. Guide planes should be used only on interproximal surfaces of tooth-bounded spaces and kept to the occlusal half of the tooth. This prevents impingement on the gingival tissues (Fig. 11–29). A flat surface should not be placed on the distal as-

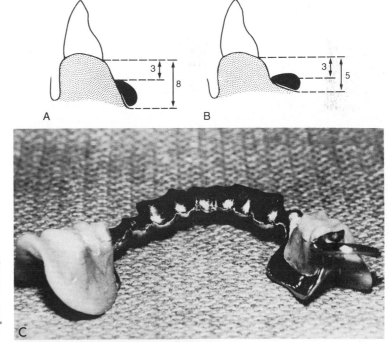

FIGURE 11–28 *A* and *B,* Should less than 8 mm of space be available, the lingual bar can be rotated so that the top edge of the bar remains 3 mm from the free gingival margin. *C* and *D,* The cingulum bar may provide an alternative method of achieving a rigid mandibular major connector and avoiding encroachment on the free gingival margin, especially when the floor of the mouth is high.

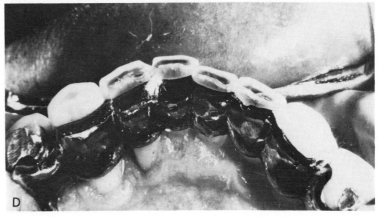

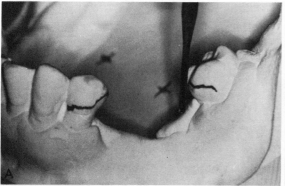
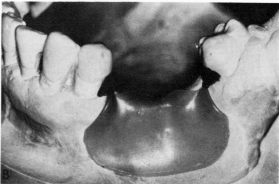

FIGURE 11–29 **A,** Guide planes are created on the proximal surfaces of a tooth-bounded edentulous space to approximately halfway down the tooth, lowering the height of contour and increasing the retention and stability of the prosthesis. **B,** The gingival half of the cast's interproximal tooth surface is then blocked out with wax to keep the partial denture framework away from the free gingival margin.

pect of the last tooth of a Kennedy Class I or II removable partial denture, with the clasp in intimate contact. This flat surface will only create torque on the distal abutment if the two flat surfaces (clasp and tooth) are in contact during movement of the prosthesis, since during function the prosthesis does not move straight up and down.

Guide surfaces are broad axial surfaces of the teeth that are parallel to the path of insertion. They should be used to allow the reciprocal clasp arm to be placed on the tooth at the same level as the retentive arm when in an active position. Having the reciprocat-

ing arm at the same level as the retentive arm is a *critical component.* As the clasp passes over the tooth, the retentive tip does not move the tooth each time the prosthesis is inserted and withdrawn. Placing the reciprocating arm at the same level as the retentive arm may be accomplished by recontouring the tooth or by providing a vertical or horizontal lingual reciprocating surface. Since a vertical reciprocating arm crosses the free gingiva, a situation to avoid, a compromise is to have a *wide* lingual reciprocating arm, which prevents having to recontour the lingual aspect of the tooth, especially when a

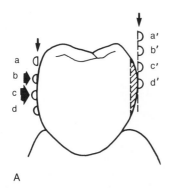
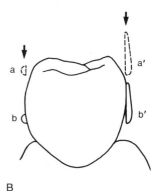

A   B

FIGURE 11–30 **A,** Clasp reciprocation is a very important component in the design of a removable partial denture. If the retentive arm (a) and the reciprocating arm (a') are not at the same level as the clasp goes over the tooth, force will be directed against the tooth (c), causing it to move. This can be prevented by reshaping the tooth (shaded area) so the height of contour is lowered on the lingual surface. **B,** An alternative method for clasp reciprocation is to provide a wide lingual clasp arm (a') so that as the retentive clasp tip (a) goes over the height of contour, the lower border of the reciprocating arm is at the same level as the tip of the retentive clasp when seated (b, b').

large undercut is present (Fig. 11–30).

Rests. Rests are another *critical component.* Unless proper rest preparations are made to provide support, the tooth can move or the prosthesis can settle into the tissue. The occlusal rest preparation should have sufficient depth so that the rest can have adequate thickness for strength and yet not interfere with occlusion. The incisal and cingulum rests must be designed in such a manner that they prevent tooth movement when forces are applied to the tooth. The cingulum rest has a lower fulcrum point than the incisal rest and is not visible (Fig. 11–31*A*). However, it is sometimes more difficult to achieve the necessary depth in en-

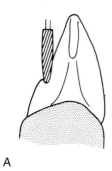

A

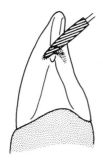

B

FIGURE 11–31 *A,* The cingulum rest lowers the fulcrum point on the tooth and can be used when the tooth has a prominent cingulum, since a groove is placed into the tooth to prevent the tooth from moving away from the partial denture rest. *B,* The incisal rest is formed by making a groove on the incisal edge of the tooth, primarily on the lingual but also onto the labial surface, in order to prevent tooth movement. Both the incisal and the cingulum rest are important to prevent gingival movement of the partial denture.

amel to maintain tooth position unless a restoration is placed in the tooth. If the dentin is penetrated, a restoration can be placed. The incisal rest on mandibular cuspids may be the choice if appearance is not a critical factor. The incisal rest can be made more esthetic if placed on the distal incisal edge of the tooth. Finishing burs* with twelve flutes are very useful for tooth alteration because they produce a smooth enamel surface.

Denture Base. Another *critical component* is the denture base. The denture base has two important aspects. The first is that sufficient area be covered to best support the forces applied in order to decrease forces distributed to the abutment teeth. For example, both the external oblique ridge and the retromolar pad should be covered. The second point is that the distal extension area should be formed functionally through the use of a secondary impression. This is accomplished by placing the soft tissue of the distal extension ridge under slight pressure, by making a functional impression of the edentulous area after the framework has been made. A completed base and altered cast is then formed as shown in the Illustrative Techniques section on p. 548.

Clasps. The actual clasp design used does not seem to be as important as its relation to the gingiva, the amount of undercut it is placed into, and the proper function of the reciprocating arm. Various clasps have been tested in laboratory experiments on distal extension removable partial dentures. No one best clasp or partial denture design for tooth-tissue–supported removable partial dentures has been demonstrated, in vitro or in vivo. The circumferential and bar clasp (T clasp and I clasp) designs seem to be able to function without undue stress to distal abutments when designed properly. Whether the clasp is cast or wrought wire does not seem to be a significant factor either. All of the aforementioned clasps can be designed to be esthetic and still encircle the tooth at least halfway to prevent tooth movement. The other elements previously designated as critical components along with a knowledge of the forces acting on the prosthesis appear to be more important. These factors, coupled with proper oral hygiene, will allow the removable partial denture to be a good prosthesis for replacing missing teeth.

---

*Midwest American, Des Plaines, Ill.

Concepts of Design. When the dentist understands the various ways a removable partial denture moves as forces are applied during function and knows how to use a surveyor, he can then employ the basic design concepts to fabricate a prosthesis that has minimal movement and is esthetically pleasing.

Forces. When considering design, one must visualize three possible movements of the prosthesis. They occur around vertical, horizontal, and perpendicular axes (Fig. 11–32). When vertical forces are applied to the distal extension base while chewing food or when sticky food lifts the base away from the tissue, rotation occurs around the horizontal axis. Indirect rests help to counteract this force. Horizontal forces occur primarily when the patient swallows and the tongue puts lateral forces on the distal extension bases, allowing for possible rotation around the vertical axis. A rigid major connector helps to counteract this force. Food masticated on one side may result in a tilting action around the perpendicular axis along the ridge crest. Bilateral chewing and bilaterally balanced occlusion help to minimize this third movement. The removable partial denture should be designed to counteract the rotational movements of the denture related to these three axes.

Use of Surveyor. The surveyor is useful in determining if sufficient undercut exists on a tooth to provide adequate retention, produce a better cosmetic result, eliminate interferences, and develop guide planes. The best placement of the cast on the surveyor is in a horizontal plane similar to the way the removable partial denture might function intraorally (Fig. 11–33A). The cast may be tilted in order to equalize the depth of undercuts, improve appearance, or minimize interferences. The teeth to be clasped should be analyzed for the location and amount of undercut. If undercut areas are not present, the abutment teeth must be recontoured or restored. Tilting will not necessarily provide retention. When anterior teeth are missing, the cast is usually tilted posteriorly to minimize the interference of the anterior ridge and improve esthetic appearance, by allowing the labial flange to approximate the labial portion of the ridge (Fig. 11–33B). When posterior teeth are missing, the cast may be tilted to the posterior, right or left, primarily to improve the appearance of clasp position and the amount of retention (Fig. 11–33E and F). Soft tissue interferences may sometimes be reduced by tilting the cast. Guiding surfaces (e.g., proximal or lingual surfaces parallel to the path of insertion) are the last considerations (Fig. 11–33G and H). The most intelligent compromise is made for the four components—esthetic considerations, retention, interferences, and guiding surfaces—as they best suit each situation. The path of insertion is then marked with three widely distributed points, or three lines scribed on the side of the cast, in order to relay the desired path of insertion to the laboratory.

Abutments. Teeth that have approximately 50 per cent or more bone support or at least 6 mm, whichever is greater, should

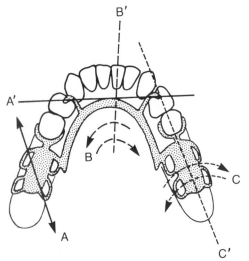

FIGURE 11–32 Three of the forces acting on a removable partial denture are illustrated. Representation of forces to and away from the gingival tissues in a vertical direction is shown in A. It occurs around the fulcrum A′. These forces are resisted by rests and good denture base coverage when applied in a gingival direction and by the retentive clasps when acting in an occlusal direction. B represents horizontal forces acting on the distal extension bases, such as occur from lateral pressures from the tongue during swallowing. The fulcrum is at B′. These forces are resisted by a rigid major connector. C represents a tilting force acting on one distal extension base, such as might occur when chewing unilaterally. The fulcrum is represented by C′, and the force is best resisted by chewing bilaterally.

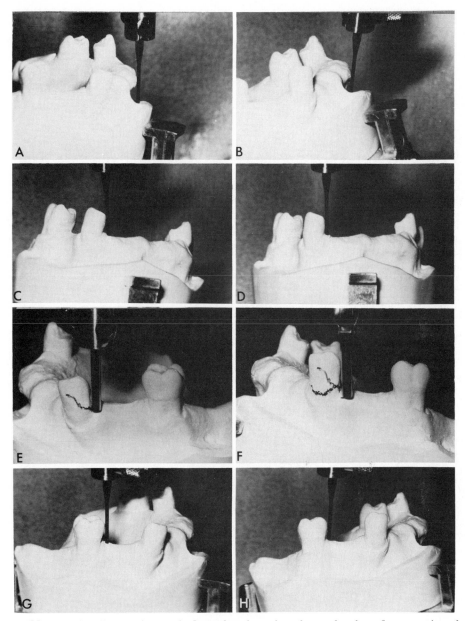

FIGURE 11–33 *A,* The diagnostic cast is first placed so that the occlusal surfaces are in a horizontal plane when analyzed with the surveyor, similar to the way the prosthesis would be positioned intra-orally. *B,* When anterior teeth are missing, the cast usually is tilted to the posterior in order to minimize undercuts of the anterior residual ridge. *C* and *D,* The cast may also be tilted from left to right in order to equalize the proximal undercuts on either side of the most anterior abutments. *E* and *F,* Tilting the cast to the posterior also lowers the height of contour on the mesial of the tooth. This can be particularly important if it is an anterior tooth—the visibility of the clasp will be minimized. *G* and *H,* The correct position of guide planes and surfaces is then determined based on the path of insertion that best meets all of the aforementioned criteria.

be considered for removable partial denture abutments. Tooth mobility generally should not exceed 1 millimeter. When a prosthesis is properly designed and maintained, teeth with limited mobility can function satisfactorily. Splinting of abutments for distal base extension partial dentures should not be done on a routine basis. A slight amount of

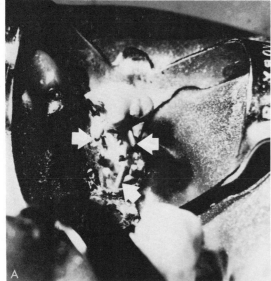

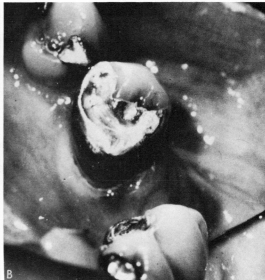

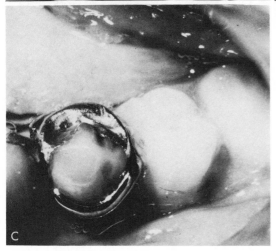

FIGURE 11–34 *A* and *B,* The use of pins (arrows) can allow many teeth that might otherwise have been extracted to be restored. *C,* The pin amalgam may be used as a potential abutment for removable partial dentures. (Courtesy of Dr. Ross Tallents, Rochester, N.Y.)

mobility can be acceptable in the absence of inflammation, as long as the mobility is not gradually increasing. Third molars should be maintained whenever possible, as they can be the difference between the more stable tooth-supported prosthesis and the less stable tooth-tissue–supported prosthesis.

Badly broken-down abutments with adequate periodontal support can be restored. Although the complete cast crown would normally be the restoration of choice, there may be occasions when a pin amalgam can function adequately as a clasped abutment (Fig. 11–34C). A potential abutment tooth should not be extracted just because the patient cannot afford a cast crown.

Illustrative Techniques

Mouth Preparation

Mouth preparations should be done in a specific order. Guide planes and surfaces precede rest preparations. These are followed by retentive dimples if indicated. The occlusal rest will be partially obliterated if the guide planes are prepared after the rest. The axial surfaces are recontoured where necessary in order to lower the position of the clasp on the tooth (Fig. 11–35D). Following the necessary rest preparations (Fig. 11–36), additional retention may be achieved through the use of retentive dimples when necessary.

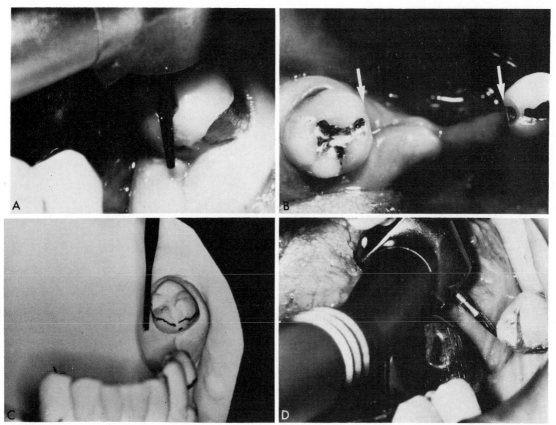

FIGURE 11–35 *A,* The use of a Midwest 7205 bur can provide smooth, flat, parallel guide planes. *B,* Guide planes (arrows) can be beneficial when placed on the proximal surfaces of tooth-bounded edentulous spaces. *C,* Frequently, owing to normal tooth form, the height of contour is higher on the lingual than on the buccal aspect. *D,* The recontouring of the tooth allows this height of contour to be lowered.

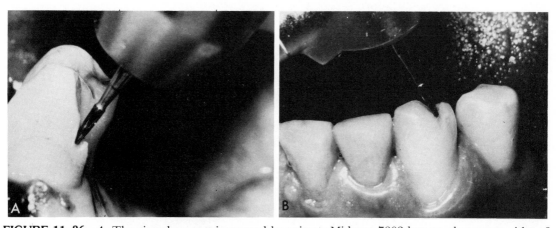

FIGURE 11–36 *A,* The cingulum rest is created by using a Midwest 7802 bur on abutments with sufficient enamel. *B,* The incisal rest also is created with the Midwest 7802 bur and can be made quite inconspicuous when placed on the distal aspect of the cuspid.

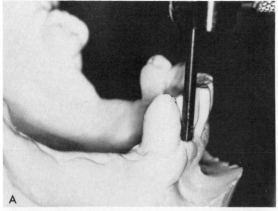

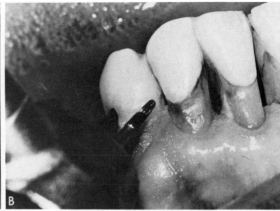

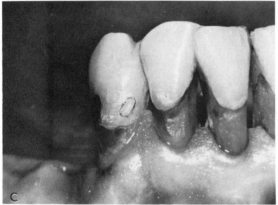

FIGURE 11–37 **A,** When an abutment lacks sufficient undercut only at the desired path of insertion, the use of the dimple preparation may provide it. **B,** The Midwest 7802 bur may be used to provide an oval indentation for retention. **C,** The dimple preparation should follow the contour of the gingiva, just above the free gingival margin, and be approximately 1 mm × 2 mm and 0.5 mm deep.

Retentive dimples are a very useful and simple method to create undercuts for clasp retention. They are used when the desired path of insertion is selected and the tooth lacks sufficient undercut. Rather than crowning the tooth, a small oval dimple is cut into the enamel (Fig. 11–37). The patient should be informed before proceeding with any preparations that only very small amounts of enamel will be recontoured in order to provide a proper prosthesis.

Following mouth preparations, a preliminary impression is made and poured in quick-setting stone to assure that the preparations are correct for the desired path of insertion (Fig. 11–38); if they are not correct, alterations are made. Once correct, the final impression is made in irreversible hy-

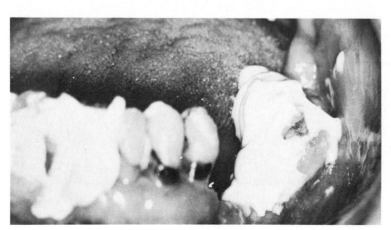

FIGURE 11–38 Irreversible hydrocolloid is first painted around the abutment teeth and then around the remaining teeth to prevent the entrapment of air in critical areas such as rests, guide planes, and surfaces that will be contacted by the clasps.

FIGURE 11–39 Three casts are usually made of the arch. The first is the diagnostic cast, used to determine the design of the prosthesis (*A*). The second, a preliminary cast made in quick-setting stone, is used to determine if the mouth preparations are adequate and may also be used to draw the design of the prosthesis (*B*). The third is the master cast that will be used for the construction of the partial denture framework (*C*). The cast with the design of the prosthesis and the master cast are sent to the dental laboratory.

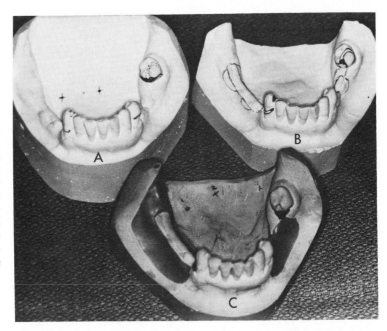

drocolloid. The master cast is made in die stone to provide a hard, accurate cast. The path of insertion should be marked on the master cast with three widely distributed points, for reproduction in the refractory cast by the laboratory.

The design is then drawn in detail on the diagnostic cast, not on the master cast. Areas of tooth reduction are marked in red, and the partial denture framework is outlined in blue. The diagnostic and master casts along with a complete laboratory prescription are forwarded to the dental laboratory technician (Fig. 11–39). The three-dimensional drawing on the cast is much more useful

than a drawing on the prescription, since the exact position of each component of the prosthesis can be illustrated. Having the laboratory *return the wax-up for inspection* permits errors to be corrected before the casting is made, thus preventing costly remakes (Fig. 11–40).

Specific Designs

A few examples for possible designs in Kennedy Class I, II, III, and IV removable partial dentures incorporating some of the general principles already discussed are presented. These examples are not to be mis-

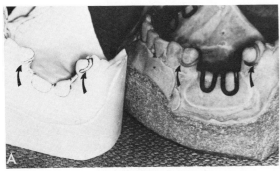
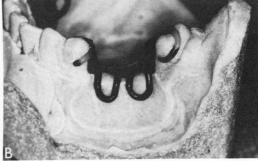

FIGURE 11–40 *A,* The wax-up is returned for inspection. Should the exact design drawn on the diagnostic cast not be followed as shown here (arrows), it can easily be corrected at this stage. *B,* The corrections can be made in the dentist's office, or a note listing the necessary changes may be sent to the laboratory.

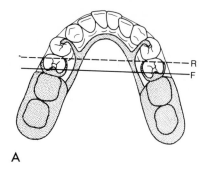

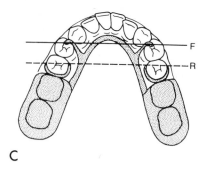

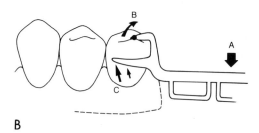

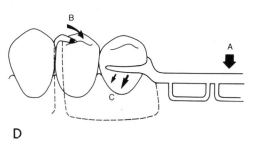

FIGURE 11-41 *A,* When the rests are placed between the distal extension base and the retentive clasp tips, a Class I lever system is created. R, Retentive clasp tips. F, Fulcrum line. *B,* The potential for creating greater forces on the abutment teeth exists with a Class I lever system. A, Force on denture base. B, Center of rotation. C, Force on tooth. *C,* When the retentive clasp tips are placed between the rests and the distal extension base, a Class II lever system is formed. *D,* Smaller potential forces are created on the abutment teeth with a Class II lever system.

construed as the only correct designs, for there are many designs that can function for each classification. Thoughtful consideration of the forces acting on the prosthesis results in appropriate designs for a Kennedy Class I removable partial denture, with rest placement and retentive clasp tips providing Class II instead of Class I lever systems, decreasing the forces on abutment teeth (Fig. 11-41). Many feel that one of the best ways to accomplish the Class II lever design is not to place the rest on the distal of the terminal abutment. This improved lever design coupled with the incorporation of the critical *components* just reviewed will result in removable partial dentures that function effectively (Fig. 11-42).

Other Procedures

Altered Cast. The use of a functional impression and altered cast technique for Kennedy Class I, Class II, and some Class IV designs is very important. Before the impression is made the framework should be tried-in. Any discrepancies can be corrected following the use of disclosing wax* (Fig. 11-43). The functional impression provides for a decrease in mobility of the edentulous area, which is important in counteracting the forces applied to the prosthesis (Fig. 11-44). A completed base (Fig. 11-45) can be made that has numerous advantages as discussed in General Principles, p. 541. A second processing attaches the teeth.

Attachments. Although numerous attachments are available, it must be remembered that they increase the cost and complexity of treatment. Most removable partial dentures can be designed to be esthetic without the use of special attachments. Precision attachments may be used when a tooth-supported situation exists. When distal extension bases and six maxillary anteriors re-

---

*Sybron/Kerr, Romulus, Mich.

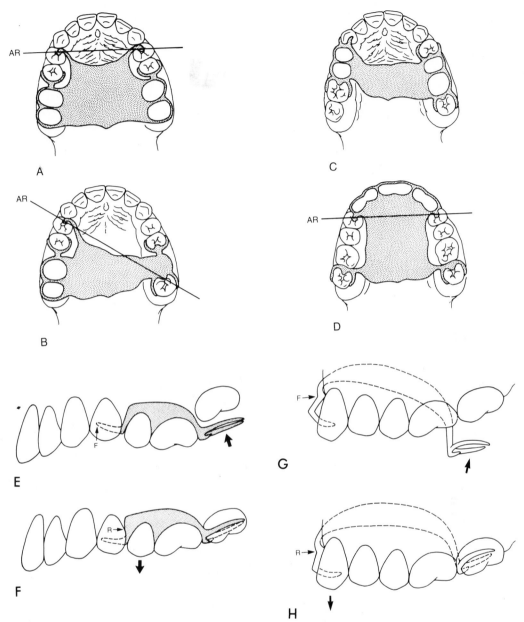

FIGURE 11–42 *A, Kennedy Class I.* The most posterior teeth on each side of the arch are clasped, with the rests placed as far anterior as is practical. AR, axis of rotation. *B, Kennedy Class II.* For the distal extension area, the same rules apply as for the Class I. For the dentulous side with only one or two missing teeth, the teeth adjacent to the missing tooth are retained with the simplest clasp (circumferential) and the retentive tip is placed into a distobuccal undercut for the anterior abutment and a distobuccal undercut for the posterior abutment. If no teeth are missing on the dentulous side, the clasps are placed as far anterior and posterior as is practical. *C, Kennedy Class III.* When edentulous spaces exist on both sides of the arch, all four abutments adjacent to the edentulous areas should have the simplest clasp possible. *D, Kennedy Class IV.* This is the reverse situation of the Kennedy Class I. Should a number of anterior teeth be missing, the prosthesis could rotate around the axis of rotation (AR). *E,* A dual path of insertion may sometimes be used to eliminate the clasps on two of the four abutments for the Kennedy Class III arch. The prosthesis rotates into place at the fulcrum (F). *F,* Once seated, retention is gained at R, resisting displacement along the path illustrated with an arrow. *G* and *H,* A dual path of insertion can be used to provide an esthetically pleasing prosthesis for the Kennedy Class IV arch. Definite rests are placed on the abutments adjacent to the edentulous space, whereas clasps are placed on the most posterior abutments, engaging distobuccal undercuts.

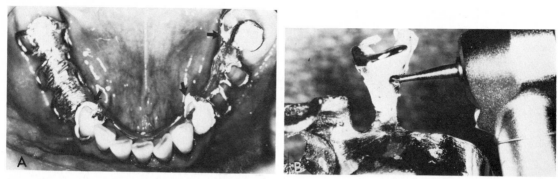

FIGURE 11–43 *A,* The framework is carefully fit to the abutments using disclosing wax (arrows). *B,* Adjustments can be made using a small, round bur in a high-speed handpiece.

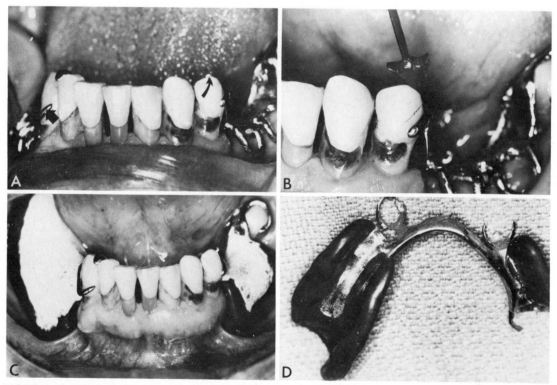

FIGURE 11–44 *A,* Following complete seating of the framework, the casting is also adjusted to allow some movement of the clasp around the distal abutment when pressure is placed on the distal extension base (large arrow). Note elevation of the rest on patient's left side (curved arrow). *B,* The difference between the line and the top of the clasp represents the amount of movement of the framework before a functional impression is made of the distal extension area. *C,* A functional impression of the edentulous distal extension area is formed using modeling compound to provide maximal stability and coverage and minimal movement when force is placed on the distal extension base. *D,* The completed functional impression has increased the stability of the distal extension partial denture by displacing unattached mucosa.

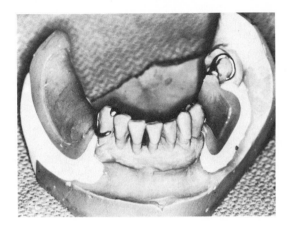

FIGURE 11–45 A heat-processed acrylic resin completed base is used with the distal extension partial denture to provide maximal stability and accuracy during the establishment of maxillomandibular relations, and the base becomes part of the completed denture. The master cast is altered to accept the processed base.

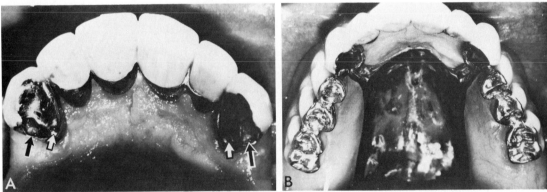

FIGURE 11–46 *A,* The Thompson dowel attachment is a semiprecision attachment consisting of a well (black arrows) and a lingual dimple (white arrows), requiring no prefabricated attachments. *B,* The distal extension prosthesis incorporating the Thompson dowel attachment allows for some movement of the distal extension base without putting undue pressure on the abutments and avoids a clasp on the labial of the cuspid.

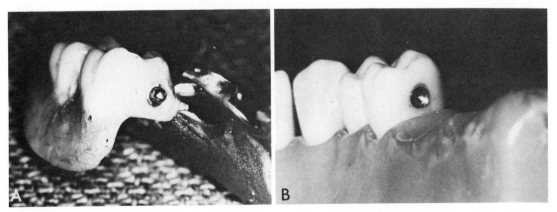

FIGURE 11–47 *A,* Another semiprecision attachment that allows for some movement of the distal extension base is the IC attachment. *B,* The preformed dimple may not always be necessary, but when used can be cemented in place on the distal aspect of the abutment tooth.

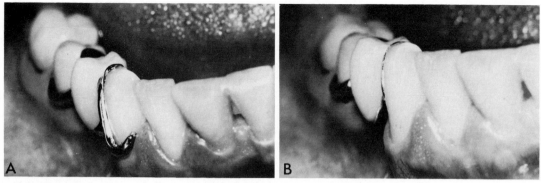

FIGURE 11–48 *A,* The conventional cast clasp provided from the laboratory may be more than is necessary for retention. *B,* Recontouring to minimize the display of metal can improve appearance without sacrificing retention as seen in this Kennedy Class IV removable partial denture.

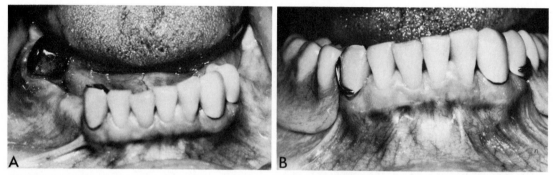

FIGURE 11–49 *A,* The use of a distal abutment for a patient with a poor periodontal prognosis adds excellent stability to a distal extension partial denture. *B,* The partial denture is seated intraorally.

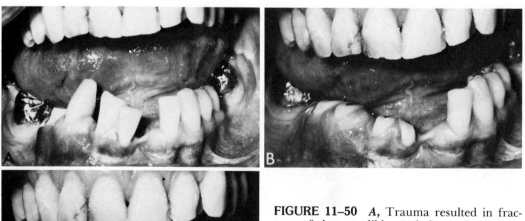

FIGURE 11–50 *A,* Trauma resulted in fracture of the mandible, and the patient's right anterior teeth occluded with the palate after the fracture had been treated. *B,* The teeth were reduced following endodontic therapy to provide support. *C,* The removable partial overdenture as seen intraorally.

main, a semiprecision attachment might be used to avoid the display of clasps. The design may involve a recess incorporated in a complete crown and a retentive lingual arm on the denture as first described by Thompson (Fig. 11–46). An IC* attachment represents another type that is prefabricated and requires minimal tooth preparation (Fig. 11–47). Remember, the more complicated the attachment, the more complicated the adjustments and repairs. Often, cast clasps can be recontoured or positioned to be made more esthetic (Fig. 11–48B).

Partial Overdentures. There are many applications for a removable partial denture as an overdenture. One of the simplest is to use a posterior tooth that is not strong enough to be a clasped abutment but when reduced in height can serve as a posterior stop to increase the stability of a distal extension base removable partial denture as well as to maintain the alveolar process (Fig. 11–49). Other situations such as trauma, wear, and congenital defects may also be aided by partial overdentures (Fig. 11–50).

*APM-Sterngold, San Mateo, Ca.

Complications in Removable Partial Denture Treatment

Biologic Complications

The importance of a good level of oral hygiene cannot be overemphasized. This may be the most critical component leading to a successful removable partial prosthesis. When a high level of plaque control is not maintained, the best removable partial denture can fail, and a poor one will fail sooner. Increasing tooth mobility combined with plaque can be detrimental to the periodontal attachment level. When clasps are not cleaned properly, they can harbor bacteria, leading to demineralization of enamel (Fig. 11–51).

When a removable partial denture is inserted and the natural dentition is not in occlusion, it is very important that the partial denture be adjusted. All too often the partial denture opens the vertical beyond the patient's correct vertical dimension of occlusion. This should be checked visually and by using occlusal registration strips,* so that the

*The Artus Corp., Englewood, N.J.

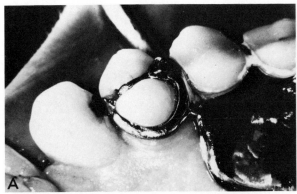
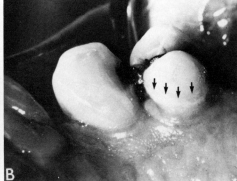
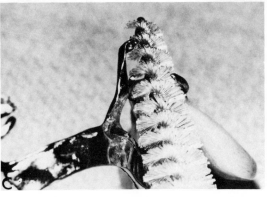

FIGURE 11–51 *A* and *B,* Although the natural dentition may be carefully cleaned, unless the prosthesis is also cleaned internally as well as externally, the tooth may decay under the clasp (*B* arrows). (Courtesy of Dr. Sean Meitner, Rochester, N.Y.) *C,* The partial denture clasp brush can prevent build-up of plaque on the internal surface of the prosthesis.

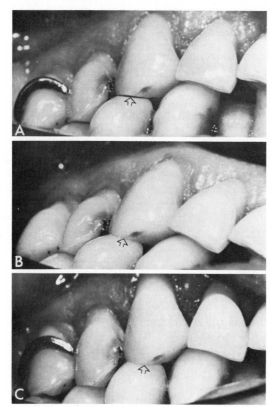

FIGURE 11–52 *A,* A frequent problem with removable partial dentures is an excessive vertical dimension of occlusion caused by the prosthesis. Note the space in the cuspid region when the prosthesis is inserted (arrow). *B,* The vertical dimension must be closely evaluated by observing the occlusion of the natural dentition without the prosthesis. *C,* The occlusion of the natural dentition must look and feel the same when the prosthesis is in place as when it is not present; the occlusion with the prosthesis in place is seen here following adjustment of the denture occlusion.

natural teeth and the artificial teeth have similar resistance to removal of the strips (Fig. 11–52).

With time, a change in the residual ridge will occur. This can be monitored on recall, by the position of the rests for the distal extension denture base (Fig. 11–53). It can be corrected by a relining procedure that uses modeling compound to reposition the rests in their proper position, which adjusts the occlusion, and that then uses a functional impression material* to register the tissue of the edentulous areas (Fig. 11–54).

Technical Complications

When insufficient thickness has been provided or when a void is present in the casting, the framework of a removable partial denture may be stressed beyond its limit, resulting in fracture. Fractured frameworks can often be soldered or welded back together by the laboratory. A clasp may sometimes have to be replaced, using wrought wire secured to the base with acrylic resin.

The clinical procedure for these repairs involves making an impression with the prosthesis in place in the mouth. The impression is then poured with the prosthesis in the impression after the undercuts of the removable partial denture have been blocked out (Fig. 11–55). If a major portion

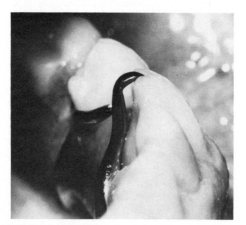

FIGURE 11–53 The need for relining a partial denture may be evident by observing the position of the rests when force is placed on the distal extension base.

*Coe-Comfort, Coe Laboratories Inc., Chicago, Ill.

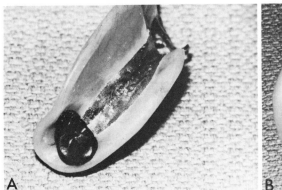

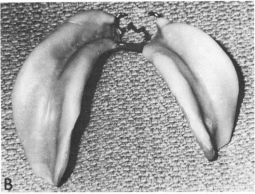

FIGURE 11–54 *A,* The removable partial denture may be repositioned with compound so that the framework is fitting properly, and then the occlusion can be modified. *B,* The use of a functional impression material can provide a good impression for relining the removable prosthesis.

of the framework is broken, the prosthesis may have to be held in position with compound or self-curing resin intraorally in order to keep the proper alignment before the impression is made.

Fracture of the flange can best be avoided

by bringing the retentive loops well over the ridge crest (Fig. 11–56*B*). Fracture of individual teeth or groups of teeth can be avoided by using tube teeth or Steele's facings when replacing anterior or single posterior teeth (Fig. 11–57).

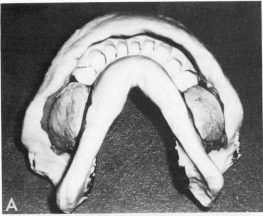

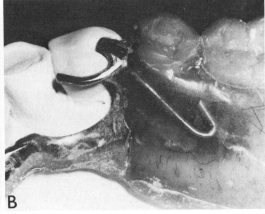

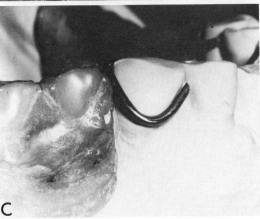

FIGURE 11–55 *A,* When a removable partial denture framework needs to be repaired, making an impression with the prosthesis in place and then blocking out undercuts on the distal extension base will allow the prosthesis to be removed from the cast after it has been poured. *B* and *C,* Wrought wire clasps can be used to repair fractured clasps after the cast has been poured.

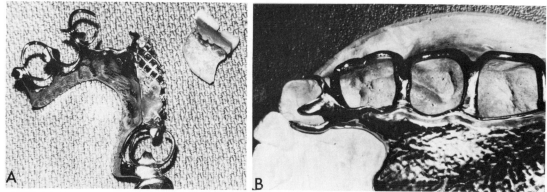

FIGURE 11–56 *A,* Fracture of a flange is often a result of using retentive mesh with small openings that end at the crest of the ridge. *B,* The potential for fractured flanges can be reduced by bringing retentive loops over the crest of the ridge with large spaces for placement of the denture teeth.

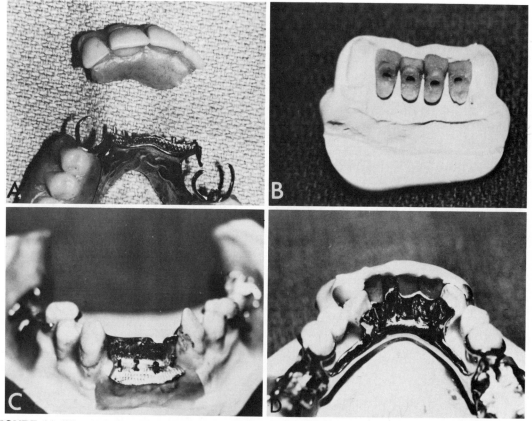

FIGURE 11–57 *A,* A frequent problem is the fracture of individual teeth or small segments of teeth. *B,* The use of tube teeth can prevent this problem. Acrylic denture teeth are selected for proper size and shade and tried in before the final cast is sent to the laboratory. An index is made of the correct position of the teeth, and holes are placed into the lingual aspect. *C,* The framework is waxed to the teeth and is cast so that the teeth are supported by metal. *D,* The index allows the teeth to be placed in the same position on the cast as when they were tried in previously. A large bulk of acrylic resin is avoided on the lingual aspect.

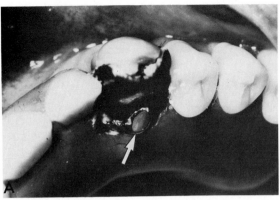
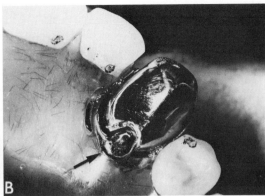

FIGURE 11–58 *A,* Placing or replacing crowns on abutments that have an existing clasp can be done in a direct manner when the patient cannot be without the prosthesis. Self-curing resin followed by marginal waxing will allow the restoration to be made to the existing clasp and rest (arrow) if the margins are not subgingival. The incisal edge has not been completely waxed. *B,* The casting is tried in and occlusion is checked before cementing the crown. The crown should be cemented with the prosthesis being seated at the same time as the crown. Check the rest (arrow) to be sure it is positioned properly.

Should clasp retention diminish with time, it can be improved by bending the clasp *down* and *in,* not just *in,* so it is placed into a greater undercut. If the clasp is just bent *in,* the increased retention will last only a short time.

When abutment teeth for an existing partial denture must be restored with complete cast crowns, the restoration can be done directly or indirectly. Contouring a pattern directly can allow the patient to function normally, without relinquishing the prosthesis (Fig. 11–58). An alternative method would be to make a temporary removable partial treatment denture of acrylic resin, and then restore the tooth using the indirect technique (Fig. 11–59).

When the removable partial denture is properly designed and maintained, it can be a very effective prosthesis. The *critical components* must be incorporated into the prosthesis to preserve the teeth that remain.

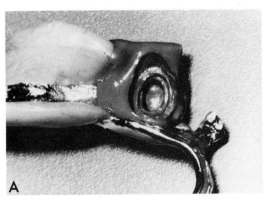
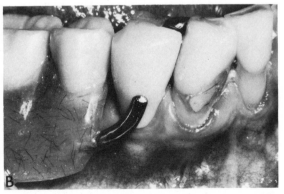

FIGURE 11–59 *A,* The indirect method of making crowns for an existing prosthesis involves making an acrylic tray over the clasp and an impression of the prepared abutment. The prosthesis is used in the laboratory while the crown is fabricated to the clasp. *B,* The crown is then cemented while the removable partial denture is seated.

Overdentures

An overdenture provides an alternative to a complete denture when the remaining teeth are periodontally compromised and unable to provide support for a removable partial denture. Reducing the crown-root ratio reduces the lever arm, so that with time, tooth mobility may decrease, allowing mobile teeth to function satisfactorily as abutments for an overdenture. Maintaining the abutments allows for the preservation of anatomy and the restoration of function to a higher level than if the few remaining teeth were extracted and complete dentures were fabricated.

Principles of Overdenture Therapy

Indications

Few Remaining Teeth. Generally, a few remaining teeth that are compromised in alveolar support (25 to 50 per cent bone support) are used as abutments for a conventional overdenture (Fig. 11–60). Even one tooth can be of value. Patients who have a poor prognosis for plaque control may also be considered for overdentures by submerg-

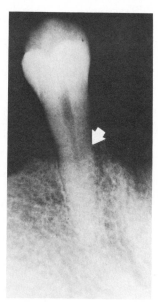

FIGURE 11–60 The typical overdenture abutment will have approximately 25 to 50 percent of its alveolar support remaining, as seen in this radiograph. Other criteria must also be used in selection of overdenture abutments.

ing the roots. Vital and nonvital root submergences have been performed successfully. When a poor prognosis for complete dentures is made, it is even more important to try to save some teeth, so that the stability and retention of the denture can be improved.

Long Edentulous Spans. A single tooth can be helpful in stabilizing a distal extension removable partial denture, although several teeth may be indicated in other situations. The Kennedy Classes I, II, and IV would be three examples in which questionable abutments for clasping can be used as abutments beneath a partial overdenture (Fig. 11–61).

Congenital or Acquired Defects. There are several conditions with complete or almost complete complements of natural teeth that can be covered with the unconventional overdenture. It is a reversible technique, since no tooth reduction is required.

Congenital defects for which overdentures are appropriate therapy are cleft palate, oligodontia, microdontia, amelogenesis imperfecta, cleidocranial dysostosis, and Class III patients with a prognathic mandible.

Acquired defects requiring overdenture therapy are caused by trauma, erosion, and abrasion.

All of these situations usually provide a sufficient number of teeth to serve as abutments for a fixed prosthesis. However, these teeth are often not considered good abutments because they are too short, are too few, or have inadequate periodontal support (Fig. 11–62). For patients such as those with a cleft palate or prognathic mandible, there is also a need for increased maxillary lip support that can be provided by an overdenture.

Contraindications

Emotional Contraindications. The patient has difficulty accepting something that is removable. The possibility exists that the few remaining teeth can be splinted with a fixed prosthesis, or implants may be considered (Fig. 11–63).

Poor Plaque Control. The remaining teeth will be very likely to fail in a short pe-

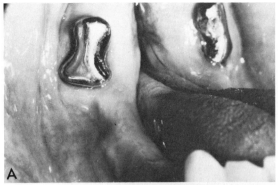

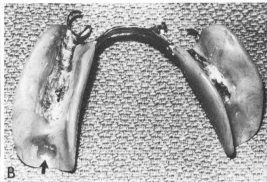

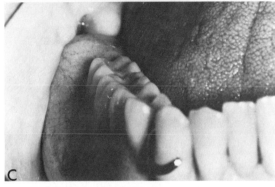

FIGURE 11–61 *A,* The partial overdenture using only one abutment to support the distal extension base can greatly increase the stability of the denture base. *B,* The internal view of the removable partial overdenture with one distal abutment (arrow). *C,* The partial overdenture intraorally, with less need for coverage of the entire retromolar pad owing to support from the abutment.

riod of time if the patient does not take responsibility for plaque control. When the patient is not interested in the surgical procedure of root submergence, the teeth may have to be extracted.

Limited Financial Resources. The patient is unable to meet the added expense of possible endodontic and periodontal therapy along with restoration of the teeth. It must be remembered that endodontic therapy is

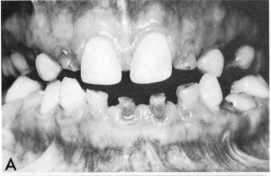

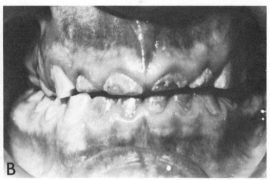

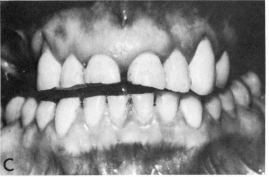

FIGURE 11–62 *A,* Congenital defects such as oligodontia may be corrected with the complete overdenture. *B,* Amelogenesis imperfecta is another congenital condition that can be treated with an overdenture. *C,* Acquired defects such as wear of the natural dentition can also be treated with overdentures.

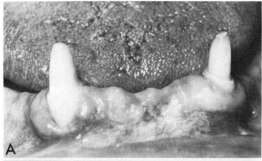

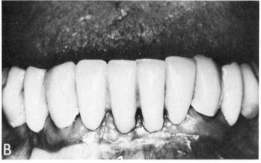

FIGURE 11–63 *A,* Two abutments may serve as retainers for a 10-unit fixed partial denture. *B,* When opposed by a removable denture with a carefully balanced occlusion, the forces are much less than when opposing all natural teeth, so that cantilevered pontics may be used with the fixed partial denture.

not always necessary, especially in older individuals with pulpal recession.

Advantages

The advantages of the overdenture far outweigh the disadvantages. Stability and retention are two advantages directly related to the number and position of overdenture abutments. The improved appearance, better masticatory function, and greater acceptance by the patient are other advantages. Once the selected teeth have been reduced in height, the procedures involved are basically the same as those for a complete denture patient. Should an abutment tooth be lost, the area can be filled with self-curing acrylic resin, without having to remake or reline the entire prosthesis.

Disadvantages

The disadvantages include the fact that if poor oral hygiene continues after treatment, caries and periodontal disease will occur. The prosthesis is somewhat bulkier than a fixed or removable partial denture, but the increased bulk is generally minimal and compensated by a better esthetic result.

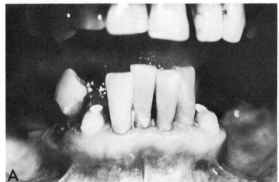

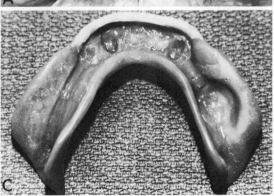

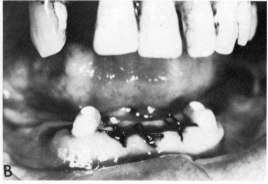

FIGURE 11–64 *A,* The overdenture abutments are prepared for the mandibular interim overdenture before any extractions. *B,* The remaining mandibular teeth are extracted. *C,* The interim overdenture, made of self-curing acrylic resin, is ready for insertion. (From Brewer, A. A., and Morrow, R. M.: Transitional Overdentures. *In* Brewer, A. A., and Morrow, R. M.: Overdentures, 2nd ed. St. Louis, The C.V. Mosby Company, 1980.)

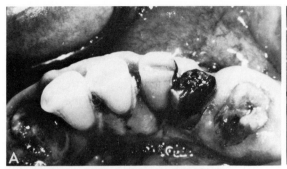
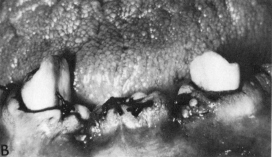
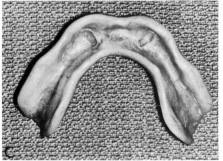

FIGURE 11–65 *A,* The immediate overdenture is fabricated following similar steps for the conventional immediate denture, except that at the time of insertion, the abutments are prepared before the extractions. *B,* The other teeth indicated for extraction are removed. *C,* The heat-processed immediate overdenture is inserted. It can be relined locally after final tooth preparation.

Types of Overdentures

Conventional Overdentures

Interim Overdenture. The interim overdenture is a temporary denture to be used for a short time, generally 3 to 12 months. It often involves converting an existing partial denture to a complete overdenture with self-curing resin (Fig. 11–64). Its advantage over an immediate denture is that it allows for a try-in of all teeth during the making of the definitive overdenture and eliminates the need for relining during the first year. The ability of the patient to maintain good oral hygiene can be evaluated to determine if a definitive overdenture or conventional complete denture should be made.

Immediate Overdenture. An alternative to the use of the interim overdenture is to use the immediate overdenture. It should be used when the teeth to be reduced and extracted are in the correct position. The prosthetic replacements can then be put in the same position, since a try-in is not possible for the teeth that are to be extracted (Fig. 11–65). As with other immediate dentures,

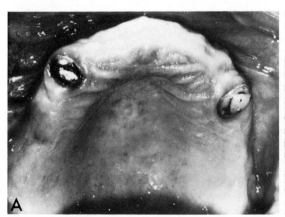
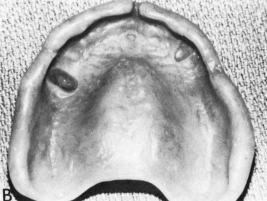

FIGURE 11–66 *A,* The definitive overdenture is fabricated similarly to the conventional complete denture after the abutments have had final preparation and after restoration following the interim denture. *B,* The definitive heat-processed overdenture is inserted after evaluating tissue contact around the abutments.

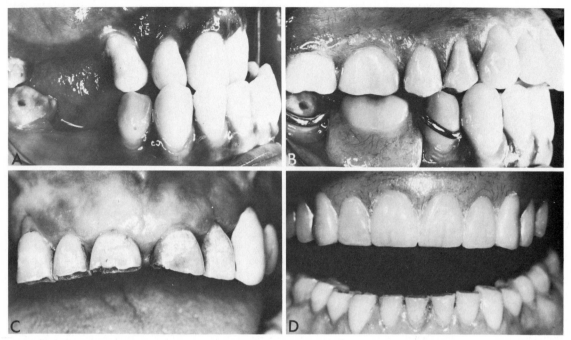

FIGURE 11–67 *A,* The unconventional overdenture is used to correct malocclusions that cannot be treated orthodontically or surgically. *B,* The prognathic mandible is one condition that can be treated with the overdenture. *C* and *D,* Acquired defects such as severe abrasion can also be corrected with unconventional overdentures.

the patient should be told of the need for relining during the first year.

Definitive Overdenture. The definitive overdenture is made after the interim overdenture. Following the proper contouring and restoration of the abutments, the steps in the fabrication of the definitive overdenture are very similar to a conventional complete denture (Fig. 11–66).

Unconventional Overdentures. Unconventional overdentures are used for congenital and acquired defects (Fig. 11–67). The procedure generally does not involve altering the natural teeth; therefore, it is a reversible procedure. If the patient does not like the prosthesis, he can return to his original condition or try an alternative method of treatment.

Abutment Selection

As a general rule, teeth are selected for conventional overdentures that have a minimum of 25 per cent and maximum of 50 per cent of bone remaining (3 to 8 mm). Teeth with less than 25 per cent bone (3 mm) generally should be extracted. Teeth with more than 50 per cent bone can usually serve as abutments for removable partial dentures

(Fig. 11–68*A*). Although oversimplified, this rule provides a guide to the use of abutments for conventional overdentures. The type of prosthesis must also be based upon other factors, such as plaque control and the prognosis for periodontal therapy and the opposing dentition. Acceptable overdenture abutments often exhibit greater than 1 mm of mobility and consequently are not considered good abutments for removable partial dentures. However, when the potential abutment has periodontal pockets within 3 mm of the apex, or has less than 3 mm of the bone support, it is contraindicated as an abutment even for overdentures.

The second consideration is the number of teeth and their position in the arch. It is better to have teeth on both sides of the arch, providing cross-arch stability. Ideally, the best situation is to have four abutments, such as two cuspids and two first molars. This does not mean that five or more teeth cannot be used, but as the number of abutments increases, fixed or removable partial dentures are more likely to be indicated.

The third consideration is the relation to the opposing dentition. When mandibular anterior teeth are functioning with a removable partial denture and when there are po-

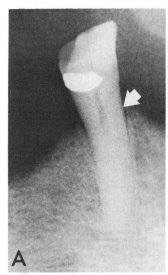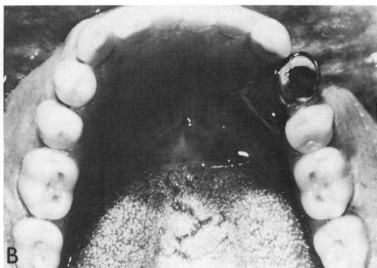

FIGURE 11–68 *A,* The tooth with 50 percent or more bone support and no mobility may be considered as an abutment for a conventional removable partial denture. *B,* Even one tooth may function with a removable partial denture, as this one has for over 20 years.

tential overdenture abutments in the maxillary arch, such as the cuspids or central incisors, the maxillary teeth should be used for an overdenture. This prevents resorption of the maxillary anterior residual ridge from pressures created by the mandibular anterior teeth.

Another consideration is whether there are labial or buccal bony undercuts. If large undercuts exist, they may compromise the retention obtainable with the prosthesis. At times this can be circumvented by surgical correction, such as grafting tissues to fill in the undercuts. Using a soft liner in the prosthesis to snap over the undercut and maintain peripheral seal is another alternative.

When three adjacent teeth are possible abutments for an overdenture, eliminating the one in the middle keeps the load distributed over a large area and may provide a better environment for periodontal health. If only two approximating teeth remain, it is better to keep both of them if one abutment is questionable and there are no financial restrictions.

Sequence of Treatment

The usual sequence of treatment, once the diagnosis has been made as to which abutments will be maintained, is as follows:

1. *Endodontic therapy* on selected abutments. There will be a few situations (e.g., in some elderly patients) in which pulpal recession has occurred to such a level that the teeth can be reduced and are not sensitive without endodontics. There may also be some teeth in which endodontic therapy is contraindicated owing to extreme curvature of the apex or calcifications. The majority, however, should receive root canal therapy.

2. Preparation of an *interim denture.* Following endodontic therapy, impressions are made with proper peripheral extensions. The casts are mounted on an articulator. Instructions to the laboratory must indicate those teeth to be removed from the cast and those to be reduced as abutments. The proper mold and shade of denture teeth must also be included. If a partial denture does not involve anterior teeth and if the patient can be without it for a few days, the partial denture can be used as part of the interim denture. If not, all the teeth can be set up and an interim denture made with self-curing acrylic resin.

If an *immediate overdenture* is used, then similar procedures used for a conventional immediate denture are followed, except for the overdenture abutments.

3. *Reduction* of the endodontically treated teeth. When the transitional prosthesis is completed by the laboratory, the clinical procedure resumes. The abutment teeth are reduced to approximately 2 to 3 mm above the gingiva.

4. *Extraction* of unsalvageable teeth. Once

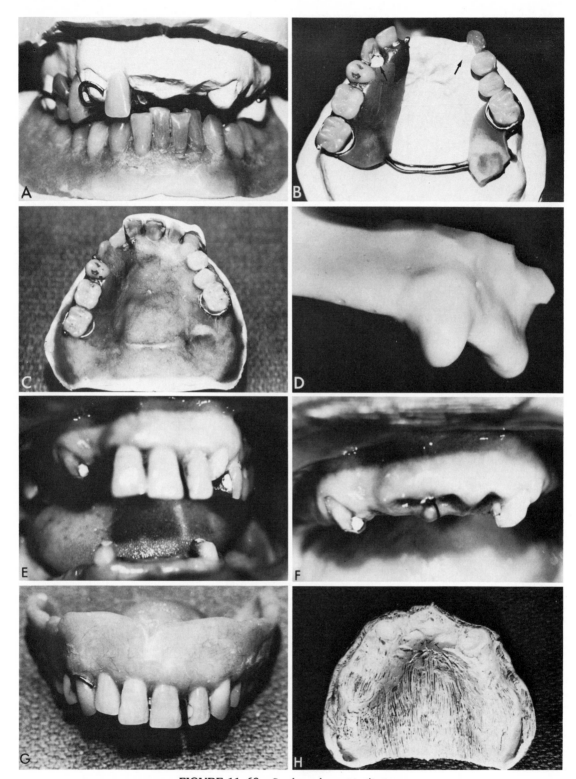

FIGURE 11–69 *See legend on opposite page*

the abutment teeth are reduced, the other teeth are extracted. Reducing the abutments *before* extractions prevents contamination of the surgical site.

5. *Insertion* of the interim or immediate overdenture. The interim or immediate overdenture is inserted, and the peripheral extensions and occlusion are checked. The prosthesis may be lined locally with a temporary soft liner if necessary, especially in the region of the overdenture abutments.

6. *Periodontal therapy.* Following adequate healing in the area of recent extractions (6 to 8 weeks), any necessary periodontal therapy can be accomplished. When the periodontal procedures are completed and the areas have healed (6 to 8 weeks), the definitive prosthesis can be constructed. If an immediate overdenture was made, then it is relined locally around the abutments following periodontal treatment and abutment restoration.

7. *Definitive overdenture.* A definitive overdenture is fabricated after the interim overdenture. Following healing of the tissues (3 to 4 months), final contouring and restoration of the abutments are accomplished. After the abutments have been restored, the steps in the fabrication of the definitive overdenture are similar to those for the conventional complete denture.

Illustrative Techniques

Interim Overdenture

If the patient has a removable partial denture that can be relinquished for a short time, an impression is made with the prosthesis in the mouth. While the prosthesis is still in the impression, undercuts are blocked out and a cast is made. The prosthesis and cast are sent to the laboratory. The casts are mounted on an articulator, using a centric jaw relation record at the proper vertical dimension of occlusion (Fig. 11–69). The overdenture abutments are reduced *slightly less* than they will be following intraoral preparation. The denture teeth that have been selected are carefully ground into position to replace the reduced abutment teeth and any other missing teeth (Fig. 11–69B). The interim overdenture is completed using self-curing acrylic resin (Fig. 11–69C). If no prosthesis exists, all the teeth can be set up and an interim denture made with self-curing acrylic resin.

When the abutment teeth are reduced intraorally, the coronal aspect of the tooth being cut is held, to prevent any chance of its being swallowed or aspirated. The height and contour are reduced a little more than prepared on the cast, to allow for easier insertion of the interim denture (Fig. 11–69E). The abutment contour of the interim overdenture can be checked by placing alginate into the abutment indentations of the denture just prior to reducing the teeth (Fig. 11–69F). Teeth indicated for extraction are removed, and the interim overdenture is inserted (Fig. 11–69G and H).

Immediate Overdenture

If an immediate overdenture is used, procedures similar to those used for a conventional immediate denture can be followed. A good impression is made, usually using a custom tray. After mounting of the cast from the final impression on the articulator, the teeth to be extracted are removed by cutting every other one from the cast. Denture teeth are substituted as they are cut (Fig. 11–70). The abutments are then reduced in height *slightly less* than they will be intraorally.

Once the denture is processed, the abutment teeth are reduced in the mouth, and the other teeth are extracted (Fig. 11–71). Contact

FIGURE 11–69 *A,* The interim overdenture may be fabricated by converting an existing removable partial denture. An impression is made with the prosthesis in the mouth, and a cast is poured and then articulated. *B,* The teeth are reduced on the cast to the level of the gingival margin if they are to be extracted or are reduced to a dome shape if they are to be used as abutments (arrows). *C,* Cold-cure acrylic resin is used to convert the partial denture to an overdenture after denture teeth have been placed with a stone index. *D,* An alginate impression of the internal surface of the interim overdenture will provide a guide to the size and shape of the abutment. *E,* The abutments are then reduced intraorally until they are slightly smaller than they were on the cast. *F,* The extractions follow the abutment preparation. *G,* The interim overdenture is finished. *H,* Pressure-indicating paste is placed at the delivery of the overdenture. (From Brewer, A. A., and Morrow, R. M.: Transitional Overdentures. *In* Brewer, A. A., and Morrow, R. M.: Overdentures, 2nd ed. St. Louis, The C. V. Mosby Company, 1980.)

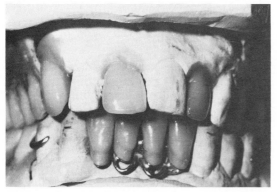

FIGURE 11–70 The immediate overdenture is fabricated similarly to the conventional immediate denture by replacing every other tooth so that the natural teeth may be used as guides. Acrylic resin teeth are usually placed in the area of the overdenture abutment, but porcelain teeth may be used elsewhere.

is checked with disclosing wax, and if no contact is made with the abutments, they can be lined locally with a tissue-conditioning material. After the extraction sites heal, necessary

periodontal therapy and abutment restoration are completed. (The final tooth preparation and restorations are described in the definitive overdenture section.) The abutment recesses in the overdenture are relined with an autopolymerizing resin to provide intimate contact with tooth and tissue.

Definitive Overdenture

The definitive overdenture is usually made 3 to 12 months following the interim overdenture. This allows adequate time for the tissues to heal following extractions and periodontal therapy. It also allows time to determine whether the patient's level of oral hygiene is adequate to maintain the abutments.

Tooth Preparation. The first step is to prepare the final height and contour of the abutments and to provide the necessary restoration. The height depends upon the mobility and periodontal support. A firm tooth with fair to good periodontal support may be kept 2 to 3 mm above the gingiva, but a tooth with more mobility and minimal per-

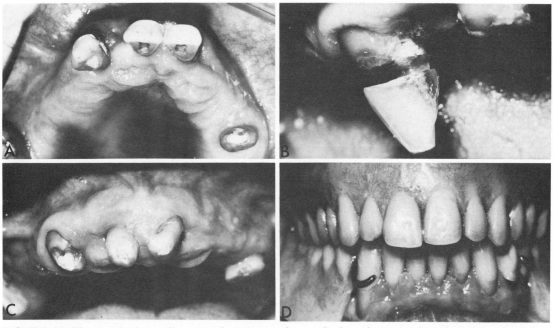

FIGURE 11–71 *A,* The immediate overdenture can be used when the natural teeth to be extracted or reduced for abutments are in a position approximately where the replacement teeth should be, since no try-in is available to determine what changes in tooth position will do to speech and appearance. *B,* When reducing a tooth for overdentures, the bulk of the tooth can be removed by cutting through the tooth and holding onto the remaining coronal section. This will prevent the tooth from being swallowed or aspirated. *C,* All the teeth are reduced slightly smaller than they were on the cast. *D,* Any necessary extractions are performed, and the complete overdenture is inserted.

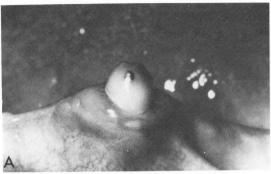
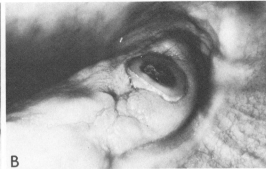

FIGURE 11–72 *A,* The overdenture abutment is normally reduced 2 to 3 mm in height and formed with a dome-shaped contour to allow placement of the denture tooth in the same position as the natural tooth. *B,* To what degree the abutment is reduced depends on the periodontal support and mobility of the tooth. When the prognosis is poor, the abutment should be reduced to the gingival margin to minimize lateral forces on the abutment. Even then, plaque accumulation may remain a problem.

iodontal support should be reduced to the level of the gingiva or only slightly above (Fig. 11–72).

Reducing the tooth so that it has a flat surface on top and 2 to 3 mm of natural root contour above the level of the gingiva has not been shown to be a significant factor in good periodontal health. Therefore, reducing the tooth to a dome-shaped contour allows for more natural placement of the artificial tooth and a greater bulk of acrylic in the region of the abutment (Fig. 11–73*B*). This reduction will prevent fracture of the denture in this region.

Tooth Restoration. The tooth may be restored simply by placing amalgam into the endodontic access or by covering the tooth with a composite resin (Fig. 11–74). Originally, gold copings were used almost rou-

tinely, but it has been found that they wear with time and that they have the potential to create periodontal problems if the margin is located at or below the gingiva. Therefore, amalgam is now used when abutment teeth are not badly decayed or broken-down. This decreases the expense to the patient and reduces potential periodontal problems. However, for some patients, a significant amount of wear on the abutment teeth may occur. Therefore, if copings are needed owing to wear of the abutments, they should be fabricated with a nonprecious alloy.

Attachments. Attachments are used only if indicated. If a poor prognosis exists for retention, and stability of the denture and the periodontal health of the abutments are good, then attachments may be used. Usually, the abutments do not have good perio-

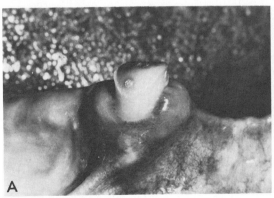
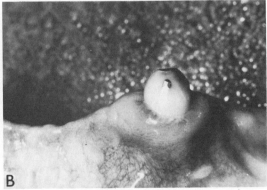

FIGURE 11–73 *A,* Maintaining the natural root contour does not appear to be advantageous to the health of the periodontium. *B,* The dome-shaped contour is used primarily because it may minimize lateral stresses to the abutment and allow a natural-looking denture tooth replacement.

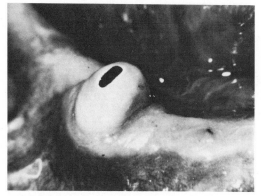

FIGURE 11–74 Sealing the canal with amalgam is one of the simplest and most cost-effective means of restoring the overdenture abutment.

dontal support, and the attachments would cause more stress to the abutments than if no attachments were used. Most frequently, adequate retention can be achieved using good prosthodontic principles and no attachments.

If attachments are indicated, generally something such as the Micro-Ring* or Ceka

---

*Howmedica, Inc., Chicago, Ill.

attachments* can be used (Fig. 11–75). More recently, magnets have been introduced as a possible attachment.† These can provide additional retention and allow for some functional movement. Stress to the abutment that produces torque should be kept to a minimum.

Following abutment reduction and restoration, the definitive overdenture is made. The technique is the same as for a conventional complete denture except that acrylic teeth are usually placed in the region of the abutment as described for the interim and immediate overdentures. The base must be inspected so that it properly fits the gingival tissues around the abutment (Fig. 11–76). With overdenture patients, the denture contact around and over the abutments should be checked with pressure disclosing paste at the time of insertion and at subsequent appointments as necessary. Intimate contact with no undue pressure to the soft tissue is desirable.

---

*J. F. Jelenko & Co., Armonk, N.Y.
†University of Sydney, Department of Prosthetic Dentistry, N.S.W. 2010, Australia.

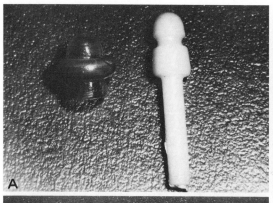

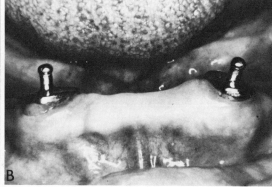

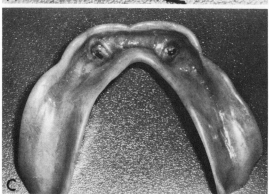

FIGURE 11–75 *A*, The Micro-Ring is one of several types of attachments that use a small O ring that fits over the post. *B*, The posts may be custom made and then cemented in place on the abutment teeth. *C*, The internal surface of the overdenture using O rings.

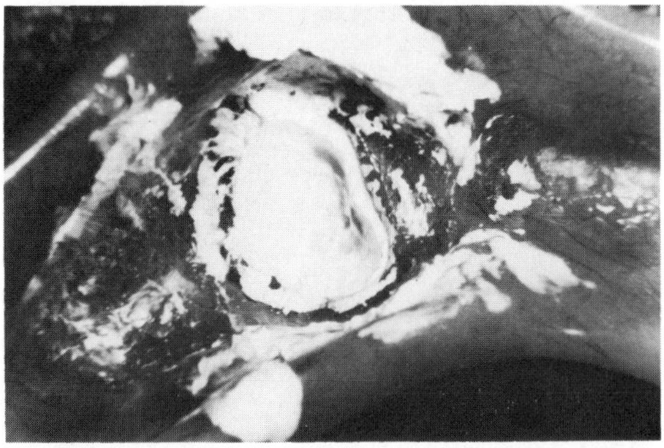

FIGURE 11–76 Pressure-indicating paste should be used to carefully fit the overdenture so that it intimately contacts the tooth and gingival margin around the abutment in function.

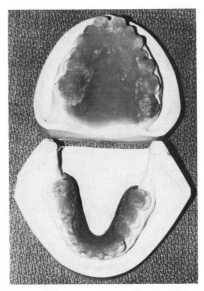

Unconventional Overdentures

The technique for fabricating unconventional overdentures varies slightly from that of the conventional overdenture. An accurate impression is made of both arches using irreversible hydrocolloid. The impression is poured in stone. The cast is then surveyed, and particular attention is given to the anterior teeth to determine the path of insertion of the prosthesis that will provide the greatest tissue-denture contact (Fig. 11–77). The cast is then sent to the laboratory to have the teeth and soft tissue undercuts blocked out. It is then duplicated, and a base is made on one of these duplicated casts (Fig. 11–78). The vertical dimension of occlusion may be varied by increasing the thickness of the occlusal surface of the base with self-curing resin intraorally. The patient wears the base for several weeks; if it is comfortable while functioning, then the interocclusal distance is adequate.

If adequate interocclusal distance exists (approximately 2 to 3 mm for each overdenture), then the casts are placed on a semiadjustable articulator at this selected vertical dimension of occlusion. The maxillomandibular relation is verified using the shortest centric check points on one base and is aligned so that the check points contact three cusps on the opposing natural dentition (Fig. 11–79).

In areas where the acrylic resin denture base may be thin, the laboratory can make chrome-cobalt castings to provide strength and minimize wear (Fig. 11–80). The proper mold and shade of tooth is then ground very

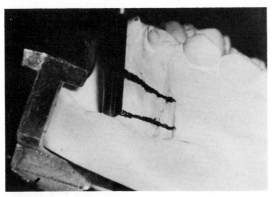

FIGURE 11–77 The technique for making the unconventional overdenture involves surveying an accurate cast of the dentulous arch so that undercuts around the teeth and soft tissue (between the two lines) may be blocked out and the cast duplicated.

FIGURE 11–78 An acrylic resin stent can then be fabricated at an increased vertical dimension that will allow for an assessment of the patient's ability to function at a new vertical dimension of occlusion. It can also be used to form a base for verifying centric jaw relation and to set up teeth for a try-in.

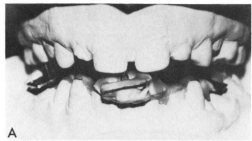

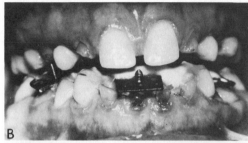

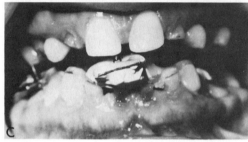

FIGURE 11–79 *A,* The casts are mounted on a semiadjustable articulator, and the maxillomandibular relation is verified with Centric Check Points to determine if an error is present. Three places on the opposing cast are selected to set the check points. *B,* The relationship is examined until proven correct with the check points. An error is seen with the initial record. *C,* Following the recording of a new centric jaw relation and resetting of the Centric Check Points, the relationship is verified.

thin and abutted to the teeth on the cast (Fig. 11–81). At this stage the dentures are tried-in. Following acceptance by the patient the dentures are flasked and processed (Fig. 11–82).

At the delivery appointment, disclosing wax is used to determine any areas that are preventing complete seating of the prosthesis. When completely seated, the length and thickness of the flange may be reduced so that it does not make the lip appear too full. If both the maxillary and the mandibular teeth are to receive an overdenture, then this procedure is used for both arches simultaneously.

Complications in Overdenture Treatment

The complications involved with overdentures can be divided into five areas: (1) periodontal problems, (2) caries, (3) fracture, (4) wear, and (5) relining or rebasing.

Periodontal Problems

Overdentures do not, by themselves, lead to a significantly higher incidence of periodontal problems. As with other prostheses, if the patient is motivated to maintain proper levels of plaque control through personal oral hygiene procedures and periodic recall visits to the dentist, then periodontal disease is not a problem. However, if the patient's oral hygiene practices have been poor in the past, they should be closely monitored (Fig. 11–83). The overdenture patient must pay particular attention to care of the abut-

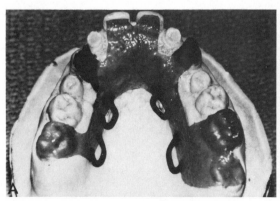

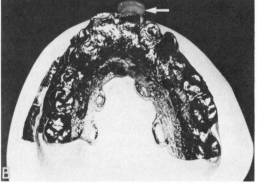

FIGURE 11–80 *A,* A wax-up is prepared to provide a chrome-cobalt casting. *B,* The casting minimizes wear and helps reduce fracture of the overdenture. An acrylic resin tooth (arrow) is carefully ground so that it is closely abutted to the natural tooth and is attached over a layer of tinfoil.

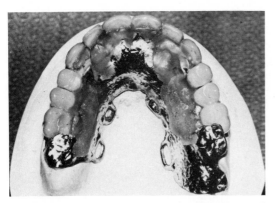

FIGURE 11–81 The remaining denture teeth are fitted in a similar manner and the prosthesis is waxed and tried in.

ments. The abutments should be cleaned with a very soft bristled brush. In addition, the gingival tissues should be massaged. A rubber polishing cup can be placed on the handle of the toothbrush for cleaning of the rounded abutment.

Caries

Fluoridated toothpaste should be recommended for all partially edentulous patients. A water-free 0.4 per cent SnF_2 gel* applied into the indentation of the wet overdenture once a day is useful as a decay-preventive

*Dunhall Pharmaceuticals, Inc., Gravette, Ark.

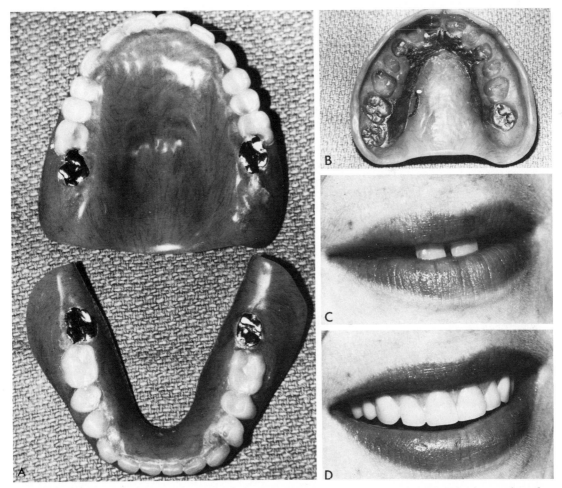

FIGURE 11–82 *A,* The overdentures are completed and ready for insertion. *B,* The internal surface of the overdenture shows the metal framework used to strengthen the overdenture. *C,* The smile of the patient as she appears before the overdenture. *D,* An improved appearance with the overdenture.

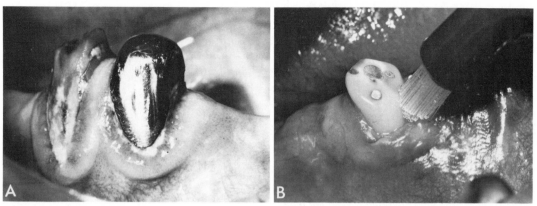

FIGURE 11–83   *A,* One of the potential problems of overdenture abutments is the periodontium. *B,* The need for a very high level of plaque control cannot be overemphasized to the patient.

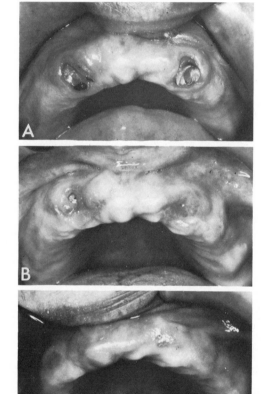

FIGURE 11–84   *A,* Abutments that the patient is not able to maintain might be considered for root submergence. Copings fell off these abutments owing to caries. *B,* The abutment is reduced to the level of the bone. The area is allowed to heal by secondary intention, or it can be closed surgically. (Courtesy of Dr. Gary S. Rogoff, Boston, Mass.) *C,* Two months following the root submergence procedure, the area has filled in nicely.

measure. For those with a greater caries potential, such as patients undergoing radiation therapy or patients whose own teeth have not been reduced but are covered with an overdenture, added protection should be provided. After using a fluoride dentifrice at bedtime, the patient can carry the 0.4 per cent SnF_2 to all tooth surfaces with a toothbrush. The gel should be swished for 10 seconds and held for 1 minute before expectorating. No further rinsing is done.

Professional applications of fluoride should

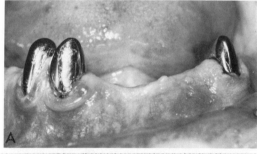

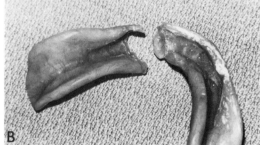

FIGURE 11–85   *A,* Abutments that were not reduced sufficiently in height. *B,* Fracture of the overdenture is usually the result.

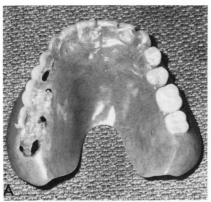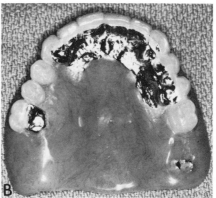

FIGURE 11–86 *A* and *B,* Fracture of an all acrylic resin unconventional overdenture can be a problem. The use of a metal casting within the overdenture that has natural teeth that have not been reduced can help to prevent fracture.

be given on a 6-month basis, using APF (acidulated phosphate-fluoride) (0.31 per cent F, pH 4.0) followed by 0.4 per cent SnF_2 solution.* Two 1-minute rinses with APF should be followed by two 1-minute rinses with SnF_2.

Vital or nonvital root submergence is a

---

*Dunhall Pharmaceuticals, Inc., Gravette, Ark.

potential alternative, if oral hygiene is poor (Fig. 11–84). Root submergence eliminates the need for periodontal therapy, and vital root submergence avoids the additional expense of endodontic therapy. However, some reports have shown a high incidence of dehiscences. Some of these exposed roots formed a secondary layer of dentin over the pulp, eliminating the need for endodontics. If the root is exposed to the oral environment, good oral hygiene becomes necessary.

Fracture

Fracture of the prosthesis can be minimized in three ways. First, the abutments under the conventional overdenture must have sufficient reduction with no sharp edges. If left too high, the acrylic resin is so

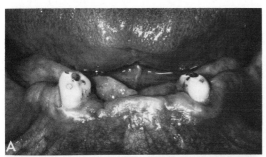

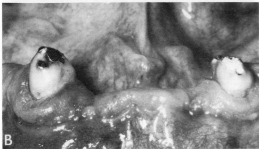

FIGURE 11–87 *A* and *B,* Another problem with overdentures is the wear of the abutment. This is more evident in some individuals than others and is possibly due to vigorous brushing. These are the same abutments following 2 years of wearing an overdenture.

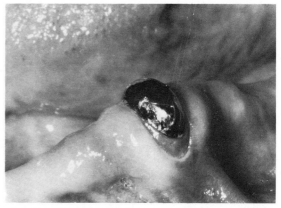

FIGURE 11–88 Should wear of the abutment be a problem, a nonprecious metal casting can reduce the amount of wear.

thin that it fractures (Fig. 11–85). The tooth should be reduced so that it is not more than 2 to 3 mm above the gingiva. The acrylic resin denture base should be at least 2 mm thick.

The second method of reducing fractures is to use a high-strength acrylic resin.* This is indicated especially when fabricating overdentures for the natural dentition that has not been reduced, as discussed under the unconventional overdentures.

The third method is to use metal castings to reinforce thin sections and reduce wear of the areas that may eventually fracture. Metal castings are also indicated when making overdentures for the unaltered natural dentition (Fig. 11–86).

Wear

Wear of the abutments is currently documented as evidenced by the lack of fit of the overdenture with the abutment, or by the

*Lucitone 199, L. D. Caulk Co., Milford, Del.

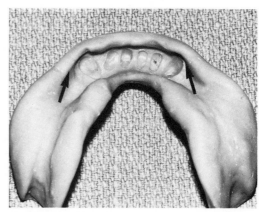

FIGURE 11–89   Heat-processed silicone liners can be useful to allow the overdenture to take advantage of undercuts sometimes present around the labial aspect of the abutments (arrows).

amalgam restoration being reduced or falling out of the endodontic access where it was sealing the canal (Fig. 11–87). Daily topical application of fluoride hardens the tooth

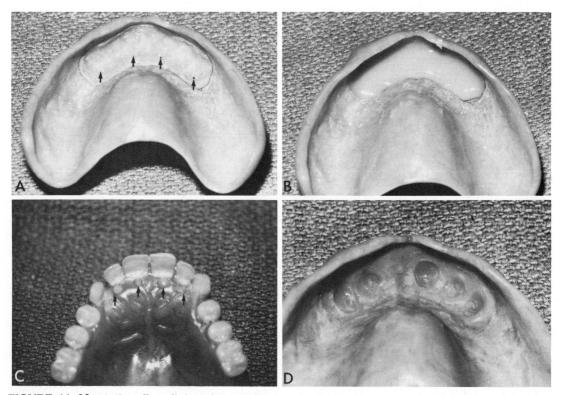

FIGURE 11–90   *A,* Locally relining the overdenture in the region of the abutments may be accomplished by relieving the denture around the abutments, placing holes on the lingual aspect (arrows), and putting a butt joint around the periphery. *B,* Self-curing acrylic resin is then placed in the overdenture, and it is seated intraorally. *C,* The holes permit complete seating of the prosthesis by providing an escapeway for the excess material (arrows). *D,* Excess material is removed and the local relining is complete.

surface and may reduce the wear. Another method is to use a metal coping that can be fabricated with a nonprecious alloy and locally relining the denture (Fig. 11–88). This technique can also be used if the abutment becomes seriously decayed and needs a coping after the overdenture is completed.

Relining or Rebasing

Another complication is the fit of the overdenture. Small undercuts around abutments can be negotiated without using a soft liner and still have adequate retention. The use of soft liners* may be indicated for some overdenture patients with larger undercuts.

*Molloplast-b, Mollosil, Buffalo Dental Manufacturing Co., Inc., Brooklyn, N. Y.

The soft liner is an acceptable alternative to extraction of the tooth with large bony undercuts that cannot be corrected surgically. It can be processed locally in the area of the undercut or may be used for the entire denture undersurface (Fig. 11–89).

The fit of an overdenture is also changed when an abutment is extracted. If this occurs, it is a simple matter of placing a small vent on the lingual aspect of the abutment indentation and placing a butt joint around the periphery of the abutment and locally relining it with self-curing acrylic resin. If the labial facing is thin, then the same shade as the tooth should be used, but if adequate thickness is present, then denture base resin may be used. The same procedure may be used locally to reline the overdenture in the region of the abutments if the contact is not proper (Fig. 11–90).

Complete Dentures

Methods for treating the routine denture patient or the patient with a poor anatomic prognosis were presented in the section on general principles. Therefore, this section will concentrate on management of the difficult, emotional patient with special needs or demands. A different denture concept that can be used for this most "demanding" denture patient will be presented. It is called the *diagnostic denture technique* and involves a method in which the dentures are not completed until the patient has had a chance to use them. If the patient's expectations cannot be met, the dentures are not finished and the dentist does not become involved with an unhappy patient who has made unrealistic demands. Only when the patient is satisfied does the dentist complete the dentures.

Principles of Diagnostic Denture Therapy

The *diagnostic denture technique* has a number of unique characteristics. At the beginning of treatment, a preliminary impression is all that is made. The final impression is not made until the insertion of the dentures.

The final impression material consists of functional or tissue-conditioning material. Three of the most critical factors in complete denture technique are impressions, vertical dimension of occlusion, and centric jaw relation. With the use of the diagnostic denture technique, these critical factors are determined by the patient through the use of the final impression material during function. The patient determines if and when the denture is comfortable and should be completed.

Neither dentist nor patient is committed to an impossible goal. Some patients cannot be satisfied, however skillful the dentist's diagnostic and technical abilities may be. The diagnostic denture technique will ensure many satisfied patients for whom dentists might previously have been reluctant to make dentures because of expressed discontent. The patient is also happier, since he knows that he is not obtaining another denture to add to an unused collection.

Indications

The technique is most useful for the patient who has several sets of dentures, the patient who is unable to eat with a set that appears to be well made, the patient who continues to have soreness after numerous adjustments, or the patient who wants a guarantee for the dentures.

Contraindication

The diagnostic denture technique is usually not needed when working with the accepting patient. This does not mean that it cannot be used for the accepting patient, but, as will be seen in the advantages and disadvantages of the technique, it is usually more expedient to use the conventional denture technique for the *accepting* patient and the diagnostic denture technique for the *demanding* patient.

Advantages

An advantage to this technique is that the dentist does not have to say that the new dentures will be any better than the ones the patient has. Even if a technically better set of dentures can be made, there is no assurance that they will meet the expectations of the patient. In the diagnostic denture technique it is the patient, not the dentist, who decides whether or not the new dentures are better than the old dentures before they are completed. Any necessary adjustments are made during the trial functioning period, and if the patient is satisfied that improvements have been made over his old dentures and the new dentures meet his expectations, then the new dentures are completed. The patient then pays the entire fee. Should the new dentures not be a significant improvement over the old or not meet patient expectations, then the dentures are returned and the patient pays only a predetermined portion of the fee. If it appears that the expectations of the patient cannot be met, the dentist can also stop the treatment. In either case, the patient will pay only for materials used and laboratory costs, usually one quarter to one third of the fee. This initial fee is agreed to and collected at the beginning of treatment. Although the dentist will spend time in fabricating the dentures to the point of termination of treatment, it is often the hours spent after insertion, when the patient is dissatisfied with the dentures, that involve a greater expense and mental duress, to which a price cannot be fixed.

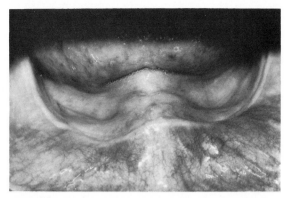

FIGURE 11–91 The *diagnostic denture technique* (as illustrated with this mandibular residual ridge) can be used with the demanding patient who has either a poor emotional attitude or a poor anatomic prognosis.

Disadvantages

One disadvantage is that more time may be involved initially with the technique, but the ability to treat more patients satisfactorily outweighs this drawback. The procedure includes some slightly new techniques, but most are variations of those the dentist may already be using, and the laboratory procedures are easily followed by a dental laboratory technician.

Illustrative Techniques

Once it has been determined that the patient will be treated with the diagnostic denture technique, the dentist must decide if it will be used for both dentures or only one. Most often, it is the mandibular denture that is the problem, so the maxillary denture can be made with a conventional technique if desired.

The problem mandibular denture will be used as an example (Fig. 11–91). The preliminary impression of the mandibular arch is made using irreversible hydrocolloid (Fig. 11–92), while a preliminary and final impression is made of the maxilla. No custom or "final" impression is necessary for the mandible. The approximate coverage of the denture base is outlined on the cast, undercuts are blocked out, and a self-curing acrylic resin record base is fabricated to the outline (Fig. 11–93). An accurate centric jaw relation record is made at a tentative vertical dimension of occlusion (Fig. 11–94*B*). This record is not verified with centric check

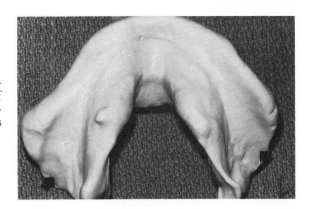

FIGURE 11–92 The diagnostic denture technique involves making an alginate impression of the edentulous arch covering all the denture-bearing areas, including the retromolar pads (arrows) and a little beyond.

points as is done with the conventional technique, since the final impression and maxillomandibular relation are not made until the end of the treatment.

The same care is taken in the selection and arrangement of teeth, as discussed under General Principles, although the arrangement can be changed before the final processing if necessary (Fig. 11–95). Once approval is received regarding appearance and speech, the denture is processed with

heat-cured acrylic resin to the preliminary mandibular cast (Fig. 11–96).

At the time of insertion, after any undercuts are removed, a layer of functional impression material* is placed inside the lower denture base (Fig. 11–97), and the patient is allowed to make functional movements such as talking, drinking and moving the tongue, lips, and cheeks for 5 to 10 min-

*Coe-Comfort, Coe Laboratories, Inc., Chicago, Ill.

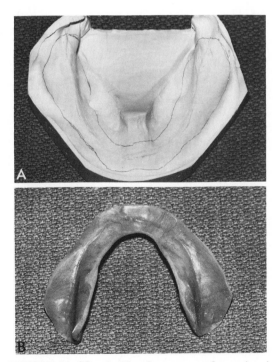

FIGURE 11–93 *A,* The denture configuration is outlined on the cast. *B,* A self-curing acrylic resin record base is made on the cast to approximate the denture base outline.

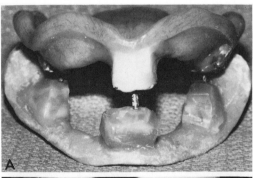

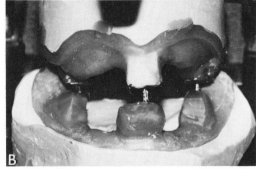

FIGURE 11–94 *A,* An accurate jaw relation is made using check points on the maxillary completed base and three wax blocks on the mandibular temporary base. *B,* The casts are mounted on the articulator.

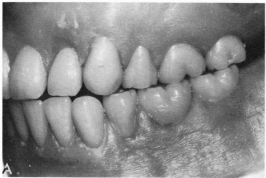
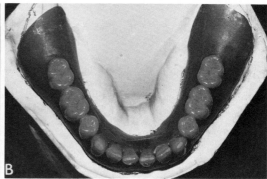

FIGURE 11–95 *A* and *B*, The teeth are set up and balanced (left working excursion shown here), and the wax-up is completed and tried in.

utes. It is important that the functional impression material be carefully measured and mixed for the same length of time before every insertion to ensure comparable consistency each time. The denture is then removed, and a diagnosis is made as to whether the material is underextended or overextended and the vertical dimension of occlusion is too little or too great (Fig. 11–98). Adjustments are then made to the denture base so that when a new layer of functional impression material is placed, no acrylic resin base shows through the impression material (Fig. 11–99). This may require two to three applications to accomplish. The

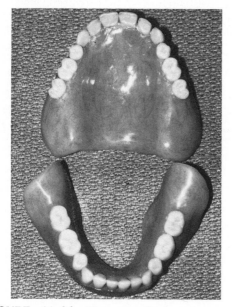

FIGURE 11–96 The mandibular denture is processed to the cast made from the preliminary impression.

occlusion must be correct, with good bilateral contact upon initial closure (Fig. 11–100).

The patient is then sent home and asked to return *the next day.* This is important, because if the patient is not seen for 2 or 3 days and is having a problem, he can become upset and lose confidence in the dentist. When the patient returns, he is asked how he accommodated to the denture. If there are numerous problems, the dentist should write them down as the patient is talking. This not only assures that none is forgotten but also shows the patient that the dentist has a sincere interest in his well-being. The mouth and denture base are now examined. Generally, oral areas that are sore will have corresponding areas on the base where the acrylic resin shows through the impression material. These areas are adjusted by marking the area of the denture base with a pencil and then relieving them with a carbide bur. If retention is not adequate, the dentist should check the borders of the base. When the base material shows through the impression material, the base is probably overextended. When the functional impression material has a thin sharp edge, it is usually underextended.

Another important area of the denture base requiring careful inspection is the crest of the alveolar ridge. When the entire denture base shows through the ridge crest, an excessive vertical dimension of occlusion is probably present. If a uniform thickness of material is present, then the vertical dimension of occlusion is correct or might need to be increased by adding another layer of material over the existing layer. This can be determined by evaluating appearance and

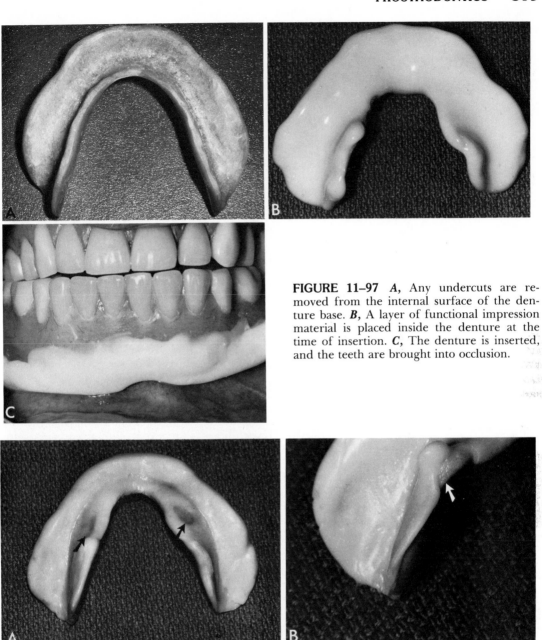

FIGURE 11–97 *A,* Any undercuts are removed from the internal surface of the denture base. *B,* A layer of functional impression material is placed inside the denture at the time of insertion. *C,* The denture is inserted, and the teeth are brought into occlusion.

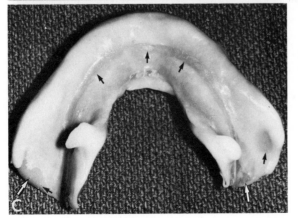

FIGURE 11–98 *A,* Areas of excess pressure or overextension can be located where the denture base is showing through the impression material (arrows). *B,* Areas where the material is thin around the flanges indicates insufficient impression material (arrow). *C,* When the material is thin over much of the denture base (arrows), it is an indication that the vertical dimension of occlusion is excessive.

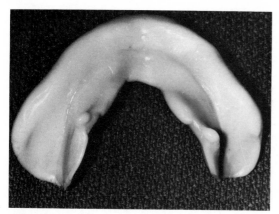

FIGURE 11–99 A good impression formed with the functional impression material.

speech. Usually, the *ssss* sound or closest speaking space, as described in the general principles section, is the best guide for determining the correct occlusal vertical dimension.

Once these corrections are made, and the old layer of material is removed, a new layer of material of the same consistency is placed in the denture. This procedure is repeated until the patient is comfortable and his expectations are met. The material is generally changed and adjustments made once or twice per week. If numerous adjustments are necessary over a 2- to 3-month period and the patient has seen no improvement with problems such as TMJ discomfort, burning, generalized soreness, inability to eat, or looseness, then one or both parties may decide that treatment should be discontinued. If so, the dentures are returned to

the dentist, and the patient pays no additional fee beyond the predetermined amount paid at the beginning of treatment.

If on the other hand, the dentures are an improvement as attested to by the patient, then the dentures are taken for completion, and the patient pays the balance of the fee at the final delivery appointment. The actual completion steps involve placing the new functional impression material of the same consistency into the relieved denture after removing the old material and allowing the patient to wear the denture overnight, so he has had at least one meal with the new material in place. He then returns early the next day, and as long as everything has remained satisfactory, the dentures are taken for completion. At this point, completion is basically a relining of the tissue surface, which must be done very carefully to preserve all that has been captured in the material. The correct vertical dimension of occlusion, centric jaw relation, and peripheral extension will have been recorded and must be maintained. The small amount of new acrylic that is processed to the tissue surface of the denture as compared with processing the entire bulk of acrylic in the conventional technique can add to the accuracy of the completed denture (Fig. 11–101).

The "functional basing" of the edentulous ridge allows for the true denture-bearing area to be recorded (Fig. 11–102). It usually results in a larger denture base (Fig. 11–103). The patient is able to adapt much more readily to this increased coverage, since it was formed while he was using it.

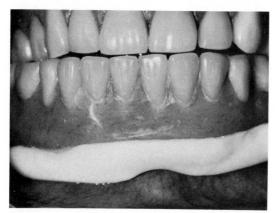

FIGURE 11–100 An error in the occlusion as evidenced by the mandibular denture being too far anterior.

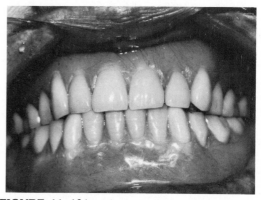

FIGURE 11–101 The completed prosthesis following the functional basing of the mandibular denture in the proper occlusion.

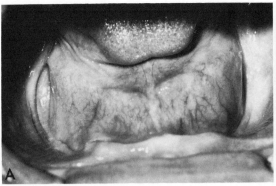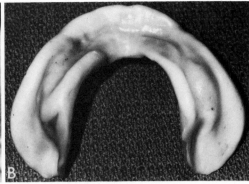

FIGURE 11–102 *A,* The severely resorbed residual ridge is a good indication for using this technique. *B,* An impression made with a functional impression material.

Complications in Diagnostic Denture Treatment

Although the diagnostic denture technique is used with the demanding denture patient, adjustments following final delivery are minimal. Either the necessary corrections are made before the dentures are completed or the patient's expectations cannot be met and so the dentures are not completed.

If the patient is not satisfied after having said the dentures meet his expectations and

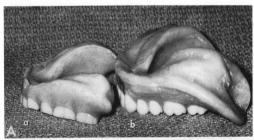
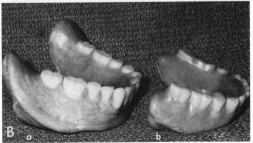

FIGURE 11–103 *A,* The difference in denture form when using the *diagnostic denture technique* as viewed from the tissue surface (a, before; b, after). *B,* The occlusal surface also shows the good coverage achieved using this technique (a, after; b, before).

it was all right to complete them, there are three things to consider. If the problem is related to looseness of the denture, it may be due to a laboratory error (e.g., impression not poured in time, overpolishing). If soreness is the problem, and the functional basing material was comfortable but the hard acrylic resin is not, one should look for occlusal errors, peripheral underextension, or a vertical or centric position that was altered during processing. If a laboratory error has occurred, it can be corrected and the denture reprocessed with acrylic resin. If errors are not found, it might indicate a need for using a laboratory-processed soft liner.* This technique involves placing a new layer of functional basing material† after relieving any undercuts. If the patient is made comfortable by this procedure, a soft liner is indicated, since other errors could not be located. Some indications for a soft liner include thin, nonresilient mucosa, chronic soreness, or extensive undercuts for which surgery may be contraindicated.

When a soft liner is added, the denture is flasked in the normal manner, but a sufficient amount of acrylic resin is removed to allow space for approximately 2 mm of soft liner. This reduction is important, since additional thickness is required for soft liners to provide comfort and allow for some adjustment. The laboratory heat-processed silicone soft liner (Molloplast-b) may be functional for up to several years. The self-cured liner (Mollosil) is softer and may not hold up

*Molloplast-b, Mollosil, Buffalo Dental Manufacturing Co., Brooklyn, N.Y.
†Coe-Comfort, Coe Laboratories, Inc., Chicago, Ill.

as long but can be processed in a shorter time and can be repaired as necessary.

The use of the diagnostic denture technique does not mean that prosthodontic principles such as good impressions, accurate jaw relations, and a correct vertical dimension of occlusion are determined automatically. The dentist must still understand these principles and know what he is looking for, but the patient can help determine the result. Since the ultimate test of dentures is in function, creating the tissue surface of the denture with functional basing is one way of providing the opportunity for such a test. It can make treating the "demanding" patient enjoyable again!

Maxillofacial Prosthetics

Maxillofacial prosthetics involve both intraoral and paraoral (eyes, ears, nose) prostheses for patients with congenital or acquired anomalies. This section covers only a few of the more common intraoral prostheses. This brief overview does not include all the step-by-step procedures. For more detailed information, specific references are listed at the end of the chapter. Even if dentists are not directly involved with maxillofacial prosthetic treatment, they should provide referral and subsequent preventive care as necessary.

Principles of Maxillofacial Prosthetic Therapy

Not only do maxillofacial prosthetic patients require the same thoughtfulness and consideration given to all patients, their greater emotional needs may demand extra consideration. No matter what the anomaly, restoring these patients is both challenging and rewarding. Meeting the expectations of the patient may be difficult or, at times, even impossible. Some patients cannot be rehabilitated to their previous condition or to a condition that others might expect. The limitations of treatment should be made known, not only to the patients themselves but to members of their families. These same limitations should be conveyed to all of those composing the team involved with treatment, including the head and neck surgeon, oral surgeon, radiation therapist, plastic surgeon, orthodontist, speech therapist, nurse, and social worker.

There are many situations that require maxillofacial prosthetics, but the vast majority that the general dentist will be involved with concern cleft palate patients, jaw fracture patients, or cancer patients.

Cleft Lip and Cleft Palate Patients

A cleft may involve the lip, the palate, or both. Usually, during the first 2 to 3 months of life, an initial closure of the cleft lip is performed. This is followed by another surgical procedure at about 12 to 24 months of age to repair the palate. In rare circumstances, the cleft may be inoperable. As the patient grows old enough to begin talking, speech therapy may be indicated. The soft palate must have sufficient length and mobility to contact the posterior and lateral walls of the pharynx and to avoid hypernasality.

As the child becomes older, radiographic evaluation can determine if the soft palate is of sufficient length and if it has adequate mobility to approximate pharyngeal tissues to achieve adequate velopharyngeal closure (Fig. 11–104). If adequate length and mobility are not present, a surgical procedure may be necessary. When feasible, a pharyngeal flap is the method of choice to produce this contact and yet allow air to pass through the nose for breathing (Fig. 11–105). Speech then becomes more intelligible.

It is only in limited situations, such as those in which inadequate velar tissue or excessive scar tissue is evident, that surgery cannot correct the hard or soft tissue defects. For these patients, and some older patients who may not have had the opportunity for treatment as children, an obturator or a speech aid may be the chosen mode of therapy. Obturators should be fabricated

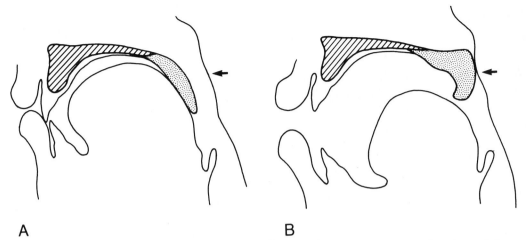

A   B

FIGURE 11–104 *A,* The soft palate of the nonclefted patient at rest. *B,* The soft palate of the nonclefted patient during phonation of the *oooo* sound. (Courtesy Dr. J. Daniel Subtelny, Rochester, N.Y.)

only if, after "team" consultation, it is decided that a prosthesis is the most desirable way to achieve adequate velopharyngeal closure to improve speech and function (Fig. 11–106).

Fracture Patients

Fractures of the maxilla or mandible can occur at any age. Metallic or acrylic resin splints are frequently used to immobilize the fractured segments of the dentulous jaw. When the fractured segments are dislocated, the acrylic resin splint provides a guide to the proper repositioning of the teeth.

Acrylic resin splints are used for the edentulous jaw. When available, an existing denture may be modified to act as a splint (Fig.

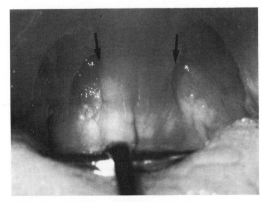

FIGURE 11–105 A pharyngeal flap, which improves phonation (arrows).

11–107). If not, acrylic resin splints, commonly called Gunning splints, are constructed. Splints for both dentulous and edentulous fractured jaws may be in position for 4 to 10 weeks.

Cancer Patients

The number of acquired anomalies, especially as a result of cancer surgery, has been increasing. Approximately one third of all head and neck cancer patients need some type of prosthetic treatment. It is extremely important that the patient be seen by the dentist who is going to provide the prosthetic service *prior* to surgery. Appropriate records must be made before surgical treatment, or the opportunity may be irrevocably lost.

Obtaining diagnostic casts and a centric jaw relation record prior to any surgery is critical. These records allow for a surgical obturator to be fabricated before the surgery is undertaken. It is important to provide some type of obturation, either at the time of surgery (surgical obturator) or at the time of dressing removal, several days after surgery. A long-term obturator may be considered approximately 3 to 9 months following surgery, depending on healing and the prognosis for the patient.

A review of the anatomy of the defect is important (Fig. 11–108). Following the surgical excision of the lesion, the buccal aspect is usually lined with a split-thickness skin

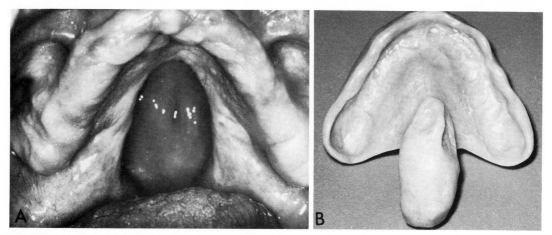

FIGURE 11–106   *A,* An unrepaired cleft palate in an adult patient. *B,* The internal surface of the prosthesis that obturates the defect.

graft. This lining helps to prevent retraction of tissue, inhibits production of granulation tissue, and allows the patient to wear a prosthesis sooner and with more comfort.

No matter which kind of prosthesis is fabricated, the larger the segment of the maxilla that can be retained, especially on the side of the tumor, the better the prognosis. When the incision can be made distal to the cuspid on the side of the tumor rather than down the midline, a real service is performed for the patient, provided that a wide enough excision has been made to remove the tumor completely (Fig. 11–109).

The preservation of any or all teeth on the side opposite the tumor can improve the retention and stability of the prosthesis significantly although a satisfactory prosthesis can be made for the edentulous maxilla. Since

intraoral deficiencies cause speech problems as well as mastication and deglutition difficulties, it must be remembered that the affected patients are frequently depressed following surgery. The sooner a prosthesis is inserted the better.

The lateral border of the tongue and floor of the mouth are two of the most common sites for intraoral cancer. Treatment frequently involves removal of a portion of the mandible. The prognosis is much better when both teeth and mandibular continuity are present. A favorable prognosis decreases

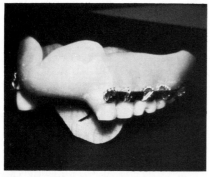

FIGURE 11–107 A complete denture may be used to act as a splint for fractures of the edentulous residual ridges. (Courtesy of Dr. Bejan Iranpour, Rochester, N.Y.)

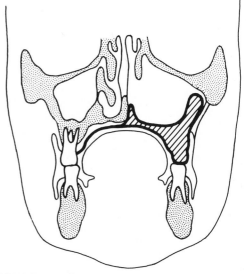

FIGURE 11–108 A diagrammatic cross section of a maxillectomy procedure and of obturation with a prosthesis.

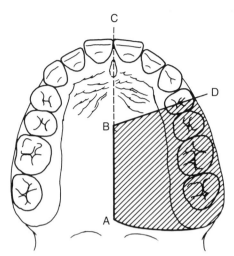

FIGURE 11–109 When tumor location permits, the surgical resection should follow ABD as opposed to ABC. Preservation of even one tooth or of a small segment of the residual ridge located between BCD can increase the stability and the retention of the prosthesis considerably.

somewhat when no teeth remain but the mandible remains continuous. The worst prognosis is made when there is an absence both of teeth and of mandibular continuity. One thing that has improved the prognosis of this last group of patients is the use of a "functional basing" impression technique, which is discussed in the complete denture section. This allows the patient to develop the impression according to his altered physiologic needs. The teeth are not replaced on the posterior aspect of the defect; only a small fingerlike projection is placed to provide additional stability.

Biologic Considerations

Many of the same considerations that apply to other prosthetic patients also apply to the maxillofacial prosthetic patient. However, a frequent complication for many patients who have been treated with radiation for the eradication of cancer is the effect of radiation therapy. Radiation of soft tissue has both immediate and delayed effects. Initially, there is an erythema, then, whitening of the irradiated area intraorally. The epithelium becomes thinner and atrophies, whereas the connective tissue becomes fibrotic and avascular. If some salivary glands are in the path of the irradiation, a diminution of saliva generally occurs along with in-

creased viscosity. Taste may be altered as well. Gradually, over several months, normal color returns to the tissue. The saliva resumes to some extent, depending on the dosage and duration of irradiation and the path of the beam. The more salivary glands involved, the greater the loss of saliva. It is the xerostomic patient who presents a real prosthodontic problem. Taste may take longer to return, and for some patients there may always be a degree of alteration.

The most frequently raised question concerning the irradiated patient is how soon a prosthesis can be placed on irradiated tissue. The concern, of course, is not to induce trauma to irradiated tissue, which might eventually result in osteoradionecrosis. For patients who have worn prostheses prior to irradiation, recent work has shown no greater incidence of osteoradionecrosis with prostheses fabricated 3 to 6 months after treatment than with those delayed for 1 year following surgery. Nonetheless, there may be some patients who should wait a year or longer, particularly for the mandibular prosthesis, when teeth are extracted and radical alveolectomies are performed just prior to radiation treatment.

When possible, the teeth should be in good health *before* irradiation. Hopeless teeth that are severely periodontally involved should be extracted, and other teeth should be restored with temporary or definitive restorations and treated with fluoride before radiation therapy. A fluoridation program before, during, and after the radiation treatment will generally prevent "radiation caries." For all patients, the prosthesis must be carefully constructed and maintained so that there is no undue trauma to the tissue.

Illustrative Techniques
Cleft Lip and Cleft Palate Patients

Prosthetic considerations for these patients involve improvement of speech and restoration of missing teeth and lip support as well as the obturation of any defects.

Speech-Aid Prosthesis. The palatal section of the prosthesis is similar to that of other removable partial dentures except that additional retention is required to support the pharyngeal section. The palatal section is completed first, and once the patient is comfortable with this section, the velar section is attached by welding or using self-curing

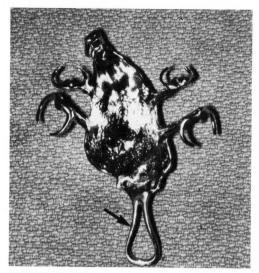

FIGURE 11–110 A speech-aid prosthesis consists of a velar section (arrow) attached to the palatal section of the prosthesis.

resin in order to attach a metal wire for molding the pharyngeal section (Fig. 11–110).

The pharyngeal section of the prosthesis is molded in stages (Fig. 11–111). The posterior wall of the speech bulb is influenced primarily by head posture, speech, and swallowing; the anterior wall is influenced by speech and swallowing; the lateral walls are influenced primarily by head posture and speech. The head posture is incorporated by rotational movements of the head as well as forward, backward, and side-to-side movements. The speech is incorporated by having the patient pronounce the sounds *aaaa, ssss, eeee,* and *oooo*. The *oooo* sound, such as the word "food," is considered to produce maximal soft palate movement.

The patient can then make the *ahhh* sound, which allows direct observation of the soft palate section and obturator to a

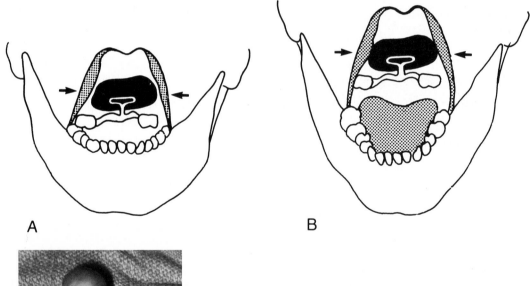

A   B

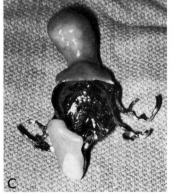

C

FIGURE 11–111 *A* and *B*, The pharyngeal section is molded in the stages explained in the text. It must have enough width to contact the lateral walls of the pharynx in function. (Courtesy of Dr. J. Daniel Subtelny, Rochester, N.Y.) *C*, The completed speech aid is processed in heat-cured acrylic resin.

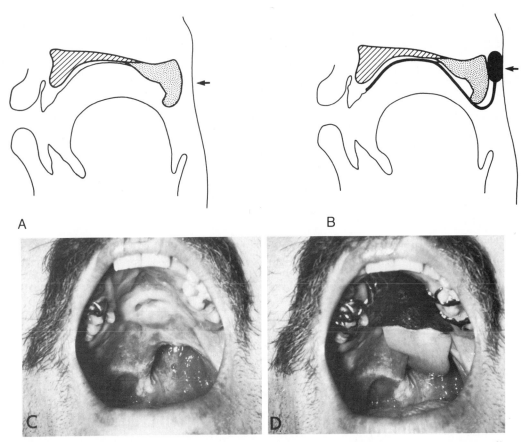

FIGURE 11–112 *A* and *B,* The cleft palate defect without and with the prosthesis, as seen diagrammatically in a lateral view. (Courtesy of Dr. J. Daniel Subtelny, Rochester, N.Y.) *C* and *D,* A patient without and with a speech-aid prosthesis, making the *ahhh* sound to allow direct observation. The velar section can usually be narrower, but additional support was needed with this patient.

limited extent (Fig. 11–112). The velar section of the prosthesis follows the contour of the oral surface of the soft palate at rest. The obturator contacts the posterior wall of the pharynx usually at, or slightly above, the approximate level of the hard palate in the region of maximal pharyngeal muscle activity.

Restoration of Tissue and Obturation of Defects. As the child approaches the preteen years, orthodontic therapy is usually necessary to position the segments of the maxilla properly and to develop proper occlusion. Once the patient enters the retention phase of orthodontics, with teeth in proper alignment, prosthetic rehabilitation is generally needed. Usually some teeth are missing in the region of the cleft. A fixed partial denture is desirable to stabilize the segments following orthodontics. If a large segment of alveolus must be restored, a removable partial denture may be the treatment of choice (Fig. 11–113).

Prior to placement of the fixed partial denture, an alveolar defect may be corrected with a bone graft, eliminating the need for a removable segment on the prosthesis. The abutments may require periodontal surgery in order to lengthen short clinical crowns (Fig. 11–114*B*). Pulpal anatomy should also be evaluated, as it often differs from that of the normal tooth not involved with a cleft palate. Larger defects or bilateral clefts with little or no premaxillary tissue may have to be corrected with a fixed partial denture and a bar bridging the defect with a removable segment that attaches to the bar (Fig. 11–114*C* and *D*).

As a general rule, when the fixed partial denture is indicated, at least two abutments on each side should be included in order to

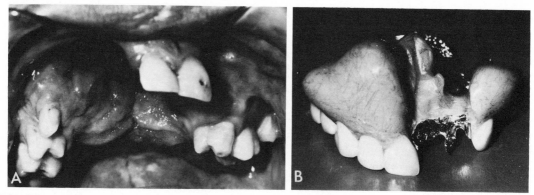

FIGURE 11–113 *A* and *B,* When a large segment of the alveolus is missing, as with this bilateral cleft, the removable partial denture should be used to restore the defect.

provide the necessary stability to each segment. This decision should be based on a thorough examination, including radiographs, to determine the bone support around each of the potential abutments. There may be some situations in which only one abutment is needed on one or both sides of the cleft, although at other times at least three abutments on each side may be necessary. The length of the roots, the size of the cleft, and an esthetic appearance are three other important factors to consider in determining the number of abutments.

Fixed partial dentures are generally not recommended until the patient is 19 or 20 years old. Until this age, following ortho-

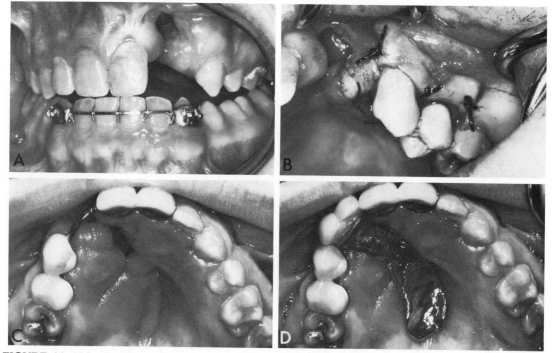

FIGURE 11–114 *A,* Often, the cleft palate patient should have the two segments of the alveolus stabilized with a fixed prosthesis. *B,* If a fixed partial denture is to be used, a gingivectomy may be necessary to provide sufficient length to the clinical crown. *C,* The fixed partial denture, using a bar to allow attachment of a removable segment (mirror view). *D,* The removable segment is in place to obturate a portion of the cleft that could not be corrected surgically (mirror view).

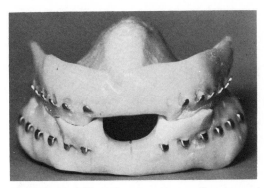

FIGURE 11–115 The Gunning splint is made for the edentulous patient. Metal loops are attached to the acrylic resin to immobilize the fractured segments, and an opening is placed in the anterior for intake of liquids. (Courtesy of Dr. Norman Schaaf, Buffalo, N.Y.)

dontic treatment, the temporary removable prosthesis should be worn day and night to prevent relapse. When teeth are prepared for the fixed partial denture, the two segments must be splinted temporarily at that appointment, again, to prevent any relapse.

Any type of palatal defect that cannot be corrected surgically should have coverage with a palatal prosthesis, no matter what the age of the patient. This not only aids speech but allows for the proper intake of food and liquid.

Fracture Patients

Edentulous Patients. Occasionally the dentist is called upon to make splints to immobilize fractured segments of the mouth. Gunning splints are used to immobilize the segments of edentulous mouths. These splints are generally made of acrylic resin bases and occlusal rims, with the anterior segment from cuspid to cuspid kept open to allow for feeding and breathing while the jaws are immobilized (Fig. 11–115). The surgeon should be consulted in the placement of the loops and holes necessary for immobilization with wires.

Dentulous Patients. Fracture splints for dentulous patients are fabricated somewhat differently. When the fracture is of the mandible, an impression is made of the lower jaw. Sometimes, owing to the limited opening or altered position of the segments, wax trays must be made. The trays should have holes and adhesive* to provide retention for the irreversible hydrocolloid. The resulting stone cast is then cut and reassembled so that the teeth occlude with a cast of the maxilla, made from an impression of that arch. The assembled cast is then sealed together with wax, and a stone base is placed. An acrylic resin splint is constructed by placing

*Hold, William Getz Corp., Chicago, Ill.

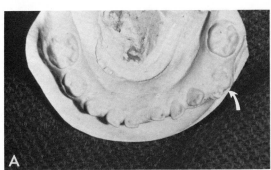

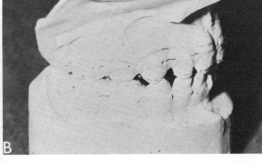

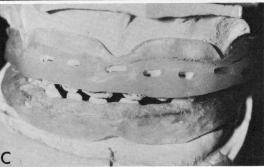

FIGURE 11–116 *A,* An impression and cast is made of the fractured mandible (arrow) of a child. *B,* The cast is sectioned and reassembled to occlude with the opposing arch. *C,* A clear acrylic resin splint is made to immobilize the mandible until the fractured segments have healed. (Courtesy of Dr. Bejan Iranpour, Rochester, N.Y.)

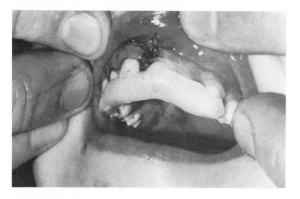

FIGURE 11–117 Another method to provide stabilization of the fractured jaw or repositioning of the jaw is through the use of the interocclusal wafer. (Courtesy of Dr. Bejan Iranpour, Rochester, N.Y.)

wax over the buccal and lingual surfaces of the teeth as well as some of the tissues. The splint is then flasked and packed with clear resin (Fig. 11–116). Fractures of the maxilla are treated in the same manner. The interocclusal wafer is fabricated in a similar manner; it may be used for fractures, implants, and surgical repositioning (Fig. 11–117).

Cancer Patients

The actual prosthetic application for cancer patients is usually related to their need for radiation therapy and surgical treatment.

Radiation Therapy With Prosthetic Aids. Radiation treatment may involve the fabrication of a device called a carrier prosthesis, which can be used to position a known amount and kind of radiation in the same position over several days. In working with the radiation oncologist, the field is delineated, and a wax mold that can be placed intraorally in the same position each time is formed (Fig. 11–118). Once fabricated and

tried-in, the carrier prosthesis is processed in clear acrylic resin (Fig. 11–119). The oncologist has holes placed the exact distance from the tumor, so that a known amount of radiation can be delivered to this location.

The patient must be able to insert and remove the prosthesis so that others are not exposed to the radioactive material unnecessarily. A piece of dental floss may be inserted through the prosthesis for easier removal (Fig. 11–120*B*). The prosthesis may also be used to place or displace the tongue, depending upon whether it should be included in the field of radiation.

There is also a docking prosthesis, which can be used by the radiologist to orient an external radiation beam properly. The docking prosthesis is fabricated out of acrylic resin after it has been oriented in wax initially and placed in the proper position with the help of the radiologist (Fig. 11–121).

Surgical Treatment and Prosthetic Restoration of the Maxilla. Surgical treatment of the maxilla of cancer patients usually in-

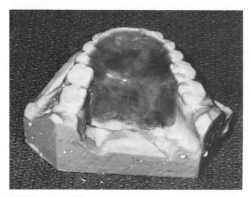

FIGURE 11–118 A radiation carrier prosthesis is made by blocking out undercuts on a cast, duplicating the cast, and waxing up the device.

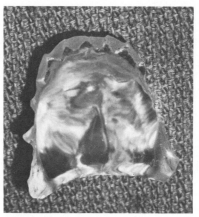

FIGURE 11–119 The carrier, after processing in clear acrylic resin.

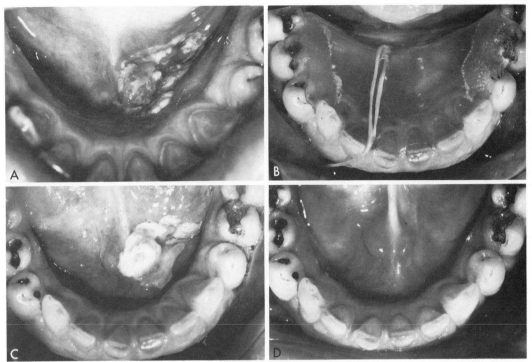

FIGURE 11–120 *A,* A squamous cell carcinoma of the floor of the mouth is seen prior to radiation. *B,* The radiation carrier as it appears intraorally. The dental floss allows the patient to remove the device. *C,* The lesion as it appears 5 days following the radiation treatment. *D,* The lesion is no longer evident 5 weeks after the completion of radiation therapy.

volves some type of obturator (Fig. 11–122). The obturator may be used to close off a small defect of the hard palate, or to replace half the maxilla or even the entire maxilla (Fig. 11–123).

Surgical Obturators. A prosthesis should be fabricated presurgically if adequate time is available. The surgeon can outline the approximate extent of the excision on the diagnostic cast. The surgical prosthesis can

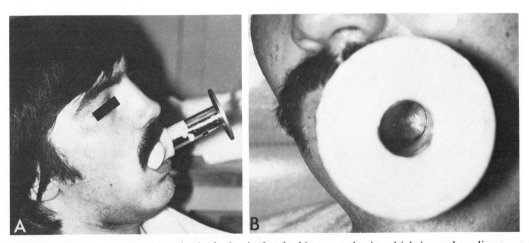

FIGURE 11–121 *A,* Another prosthetic device is the docking prosthesis, which is used to direct external radiation to a specific area intraorally. *B,* The lesion should be visible when looking down the tube. (Courtesy of Dr. Norman Schaaf, Buffalo, N.Y.)

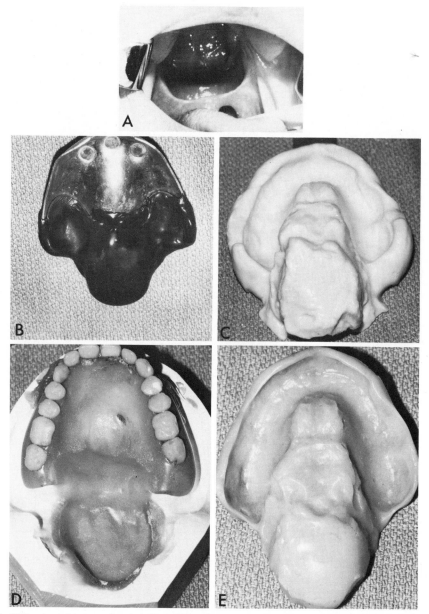

FIGURE 11–122   *A,* A large palatal defect following surgical resection of an adenocystic carcinoma. *B* and *C,* An impression of the area is obtained by modifying a stock tray with compound, and the impression is then made using alginate. *D* and *E,* The interim obturator is made by adding a segment to the existing prosthesis and lining it with a tissue-conditioning material.

then be made by cutting the teeth from the cast in the area of the tumor and replacing only the anterior teeth, if necessary. Wrought wire clasps and self-curing acrylic resin are used so that the prosthesis is ready at the time of surgery (Fig. 11–124). Posterior teeth would only increase trauma to the area of surgery and are not placed on the prosthesis at this time. If time does not allow or

the surgeon prefers not to have the prosthesis inserted at this stage, it can be inserted following dressing removal, generally 7 to 10 days later.

The surgical prosthesis can be modified slightly with a resilient denture liner to provide a better seal of the defect. After a few weeks, the obturator may be built up in height in order to provide additional reten-

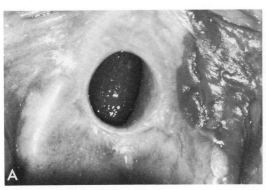 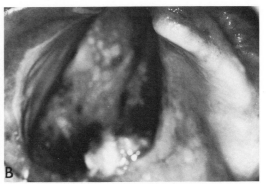

FIGURE 11–123 *A,* A small palatal defect can be obturated with a resilient material in the area of the defect. *B,* Larger defects can be obturated, but retention and stability are somewhat compromised.

tion, improved speech, or better support for the soft tissue. This may be accomplished through the use of resilient lining material if adequate support is available from the obturator; otherwise, modeling compound can be used and then replaced with autopolymerizing acrylic resin (Fig. 11–125).

The patient should be seen within 24 hours after insertion of the prosthesis; further adjustments are made as necessary. The soft liner used for the obturator must be changed periodically so that it does not become too hard or pick up odors from the oral fluids. When healing is complete and the prognosis is favorable, a long-term prosthesis restoring the posterior occlusion can be fabricated.

Definitive or Long-term Obturator. The long-term prosthesis for the partially dentu-

lous patient is fabricated with a cast metal framework, obtaining as much retention and distributing the stress to as many teeth as possible (Fig. 11–126). At times, the tooth immediately adjacent to the defect has minimal bone support and should not be clasped. All retentive features of the periphery of the surgical defect should be used in order to minimize the strain produced by the cantilever effect of such a prosthesis. Scar formation and areas above the skin graft as well as of the anterior and posterior aspects of the surgical margin may provide favorable undercuts, allowing some retentive areas for the prosthesis. All lateral extensions must be compatible with the path of insertion of the cast framework.

The bulb of the prosthesis should be extended superiorly to aid in the resonance of speech but should not be extended so high that the respiratory mucosa is irritated. The

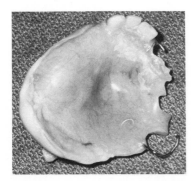

FIGURE 11–124 The anterior teeth that will be removed as a result of the surgery are reduced from the cast and replaced with denture teeth. Wrought wire clasps are used around the most anterior and posterior abutments, and the interim prosthesis is completed with self-curing acrylic resin.

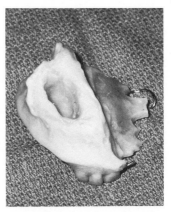

FIGURE 11–125 The interim obturator is built up in layers in the area of the defect, using a functional impression material.

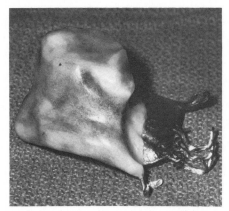

FIGURE 11–126 The definitive obturator is made with a cast chrome-cobalt framework. The bulb portion of the obturator is formed with modeling compound and then refined with a wax at mouth temperature, or other suitable material.

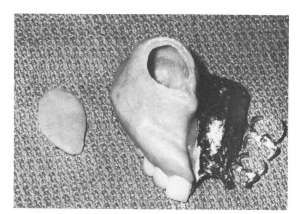

FIGURE 11–127 A hollow-bulb obturator may be used to lighten the weight of the prosthesis. It is then closed by sealing it with a cap.

bulb of the obturator may be hollow and thin-walled in order to decrease its weight. A piece of acrylic resin is then used to close the bulb by sealing the periphery with self-curing resin. (Fig. 11–127). An alternative method is to allow the bulb to be open at the top (Fig. 11–128). It has been shown that this does not adversely affect speech and yet simplifies the fabrication. Obturator contours should allow for easy cleaning and minimize the accumulation of secretions from the nasal cavity.

Although soft liners are used for the bulb of the surgical or treatment prosthesis, heat-cured acrylic resin is generally the material of choice for the definitive prosthesis.

Posterior occlusion should be developed with no lateral interferences, sometimes using nonanatomic teeth to keep lateral stresses to a minimum (Fig. 11–129).

Surgical Treatment and Prosthetic Restoration of the Mandible Once mandibular continuity is lost, such as with the lateral resection, the mandible generally closes with a deviation toward the surgical side (Fig. 11–130A). The use of strong hand pressure on the jaw, for several weeks, may help to provide better alignment (Fig. 11–130B). Pressure should be applied a minimum of four times each day for at least 5 minutes per session. For others, some type of guiding prosthesis may be necessary to retrain the mandible (Fig. 11–130C and D). Some patients require such a prosthesis indefinitely; however, most need it only a short time.

One other factor to consider is that with

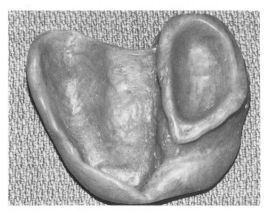

FIGURE 11–128 Another method is to construct an open-bulb obturator.

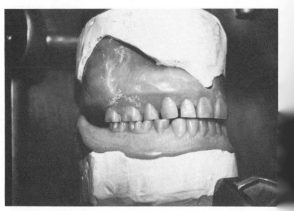

FIGURE 11–129 Nonanatomic teeth are generally used to minimize the forces to the defect.

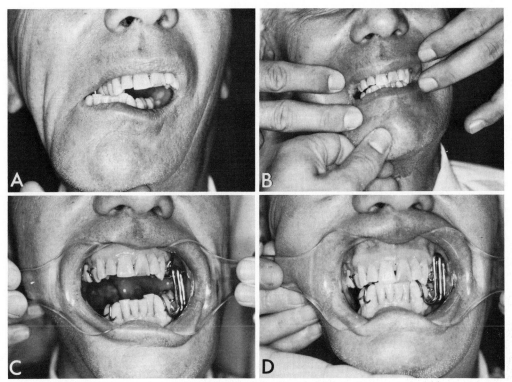

FIGURE 11–130 *A,* When the surgical procedure to the mandible involves a loss of continuity of the arch, the mandible will deviate to the resected side. *B,* Hand pressure may allow the mandible to be retrained to close into occlusion. *C* and *D,* For some, a guide prosthesis may be made of metal with guide bars to help train the mandible to occlude properly, as seen in the open and closed positions. (Courtesy of Dr. Norman Schaaf, Buffalo, N.Y.)

many of these mandibulectomy patients, a portion of the tongue is also removed with the mandible, affecting speech (Fig. 11–131). It has been shown that for those patients whose tongue movement has been restricted and who are unable to contact the palate or maxillary teeth, lowering the palate with an acrylic resin prosthesis can provide a significant speech improvement. The use of speech therapy may also be beneficial for mandibulectomy patients.

Complications in Maxillofacial Prosthetic Treatment

Congenital Anomalies

When using partial or complete overdentures to treat cleft palate patients, frequent recall and re-emphasis of oral hygiene are of paramount importance. The value of a water-free 0.4 per cent SnF_2 gel* must be

stressed for home use and for professional applications.

Another complication for cleft palate patients is the need to make changes in the prosthesis as the patient gets older and growth occurs. Alterations in the removable prosthesis must be made when the patient is developing, and a fixed prosthesis can be fabricated as the late teens or early twenties are reached.

Acquired Anomalies

Cancer patients make up the majority of these patients. One of the most frequent complications is a diminished amount of saliva as a result of irradiation. The potential for dental caries increases greatly as the salivary flow decreases and the oral flora is altered. Water-free 0.4 per cent SnF_2 gel daily as well as regular, periodic professional applications of fluoride must be used to prevent caries, as discussed under complications for overdentures.

*Omnigel, Dunhall Pharmaceuticals, Gravette, Ark.

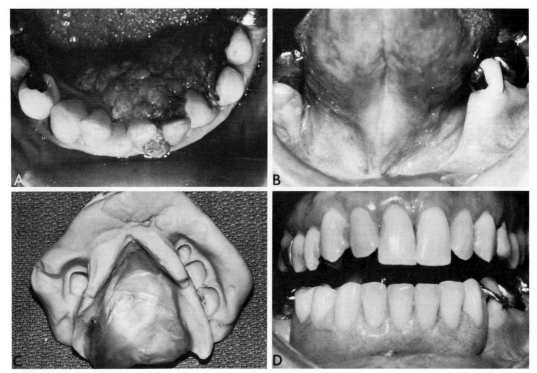

FIGURE 11–131   *A,* A squamous cell carcinoma that has expanded very rapidly (mirror view). *B,* The surgical resection of the carcinoma did not involve a complete loss of continuity of the mandible but did affect tongue mobility. *C,* An impression is made of the defect to construct the metal framework. *D,* Following a functional impression of the surgical area and a try-in, the prosthesis is completed.

The xerostomic patient who needs to wear a removable prosthesis may have soreness and poor retention owing to the dryness of the mouth. A saliva substitute* can be used to alleviate some of the problem. Fortunately, for some of the patients the decrease in saliva is only temporary, and salivary flow will gradually increase depending upon the amount and duration of the irradiation. The prognosis for return of salivary flow can be ascertained best by the radiation oncologist.

Another complication that occurs when using maxillary obturators is the stress placed on the remaining abutment teeth. Because of a cantilever design, greater forces will be placed on abutment teeth. The patient should be advised to modify eating habits by chewing only on the side with the natural teeth or residual ridge support and eating softer foods that require less masticatory force. Although every effort is made to distribute the stresses as uniformly as possible, some

*Orex, King's Dental Specialty Co., Fort Wayne, Ind.

changes may occur, especially if the teeth had reduced periodontal support to begin with. Frequent recall plus refitting or remaking of the prosthesis is needed for these patients.

Osteoradionecrosis is an additional complication. In addition to the obvious component of radiation, some form of trauma is usually present in order for osteoradionecrosis to take place. The prosthesis could produce this undesirable trauma. Therefore, the dentist should know the type, amount, and extent of radiation as well as the amount of denture-bearing surface included in the beam of radiation.

The average dosage for most cancer patients is 5000 to 7000 rads over 6 to 8 weeks. A poor anatomic prognosis in a heavily irradiated region may contraindicate the use of a prosthesis. If the mucosa is inflamed and edematous and the flow of saliva is minimal several months after radiation therapy, it may be best to postpone prosthetic therapy. The time before fabricating a prosthesis following radiation therapy depends on each situation. Some former denture wearers who have had no recent extractions have dentures fabricated 3 months following radiation therapy. During radiation therapy, the existing removable prosthesis should not be worn. Following radiation therapy, the dentures should be evaluated for fit and adjusted accordingly. The occurrence of osteoradionecrosis is much greater in the mandible than the maxilla, so frequently the maxillary prosthesis can be made sooner. This is important in boosting the morale of these patients.

Sound prosthodontic principles should be followed carefully when fabricating a prosthesis for maxillofacial prosthetic patients. However, when making impressions of small defects that might allow particles of material to become lodged, placing a small piece of gauze with Vaseline into the defect can prevent this. A "functional-basing" type of impression can be very useful, since it provides limited pressure on the mucosa, minimizing the chance of osteonecrosis or soft tissue necrosis. A functional method of providing a posterior palatal seal is preferred to altering the master cast. Zinc-oxide impression materials should be avoided because of their potential for tissue irritation.

A possible complication is the chance of recurrence of the primary tumor or of secondary tumor. The importance of frequent recalls cannot be overemphasized. The patient should be seen every 3 to 4 months by the dentist as well as by the physician.

Another potential complication for these patients is the emotional effect that treatment and rehabilitation can have. When the general dentist and others work as a team, the best chances exist to improve the patient's self-image and to enable him to feel confident while working or socializing. When this is accomplished, maxillofacial prosthetics can be one of the most challenging and rewarding areas of prosthodontics.

QUESTIONS

1. A prosthesis should not be worn or fabricated for at least 1 year following radiation therapy for intraoral cancer. True or false?

2. What are the advantages of using the *diagnostic denture technique* for the demanding denture patient?

3. How far should the major connector be from the free gingival margin in the maxilla and the mandible?

4. Why is rigidity such an important component of the removable partial denture?

5. What are the directions of three possible movements of a removable partial denture?

6. How can these movements best be resisted during function by a well-designed removable partial denture?

7. What type of impression material should not be used for the patient who has received intraoral radiation therapy?

8. What types of fluoride should be used and for what time interval in relation to intraoral radiation therapy?

9. How does the fluoride program differ following treatment with an overdenture?

10. What are the advantages and disadvantages of heat-processed record bases?

11. A centric jaw relation record is three-dimensional. How can this be verified and in which dimension might an error be most critical?

12. What is the best height and contour for an overdenture abutment?

13. What are some of the potential complications associated with an overdenture? How can they be prevented?

14. Should only one tooth be saved for an overdenture abutment?

15. What is needed in addition to good clinical technique to treat the prosthodontic patient successfully?

16. The reciprocating, or bracing, arm of a removable partial denture clasp is an important component. Name two ways this can be designed to function properly.

17. What is the best clasp design for a bilateral distal extension removable partial denture?

18. When fabricating a fixed partial denture for a cleft palate patient, how many abutments are usually needed on each side of the cleft?

19. Name some of the conditions in which an overdenture can be used for either congenital or acquired defects.

20. What is the most critical component in the long-term success of any prosthesis involving the natural dentition?

See answers in Appendix.

REFERENCES

General Principles

1. Brewer, A. A.: Prosthodontic research in progress at the school of aerospace medicine. J. Prosthet. Dent., 13:49–69, 1963.
2. Graser, G. N.: Completed bases for removable dentures. J. Prosthet. Dent., 39:232–236, 1978.
3. Roraff, A. R.: Arranging artificial teeth according to anatomic landmarks. J. Prosthet. Dent., 38:120–130, 1977.
4. Shannon, I. L., McCrary, B. R., and Starcke, E. N.: A saliva substitute for use by xerostomic patients undergoing radiotherapy to the head and neck. Oral Surg. 44:656–661, 1977.
5. Swoope, C. C., and Hartsook, E.: Nutrition analysis of prosthodontic patients. J. Prosthet Dent., 38:208–213, 1977.

Removable Partial Dentures

1. Bergman, B., Hugoson, A., and Olsson, C. O.: Caries and periodontal status in patients fitted with removable partial dentures. J. Clin. Periodontol., 4:134–146, 1977.
2. Bertram, U.: A clinical survey of removable partial dentures after ten years usage. J. Dent. Res., 58:151, 1979.
3. Henderson, D., and Steffel, V. L.: McCracken's Removable Partial Prosthodontics, 6th ed. St. Louis, C. V. Mosby Company, 1981.
4. Johnson, D. L., and Stratton, R. J.: Fundamentals of Removable Prosthodontics. Chicago, Quintessence Publishing Company, 1980.
5. King, G. E.: Dual-path design for removable partial dentures. J. Prosthet. Dent. 39:392–395, 1978.
6. Koper, A: An intracoronal semiprecision retainer for removable partial dentures: the Thompson dowel. J. Prosthet. Dent., 30:759–768, 1973.
7. Zarb, G. A., Bergman, B., Clayton, J. A., and MacKay, H. F. (eds.): Prosthodontic Treatment for Partially Edentulous Patients. St. Louis, C. V. Mosby Company, 1978.

Overdentures

1. Brewer, A. A., and Morrow, R. M.: Overdentures, 2nd ed. St. Louis, C. V. Mosby Company, 1980.
2. Crum, R. J., and Rooney, G. E.: Alveolar bone loss in overdentures: a 5-year study. J. Prosthet. Dent., 40:610–613, 1978.
3. Fenton, A. H., and Hahn, N.: Tissue response to overdenture therapy. J. Prosthet. Dent., 40:492–498, 1978.
4. Garver, D. G., and Fenster, R. K.: Vital root retention in humans: a final report. J. Prosthet. Dent., 43:368–373, 1980.
5. Morrow, R. M.: Handbook of Immediate Overdentures. St. Louis, C. V. Mosby Company, 1978.

Complete Dentures

1. Landesman, H. M.: A technique for the delivery of complete dentures. J. Prosthet. Dent., 43:348–351, 1980.
2. Pound, E.: Personalized Denture Procedures. Anaheim, Denar Corporation, 1973.
3. Winkler, S.: Essentials of Complete Denture Prosthodontics. Philadelphia, W. B. Saunders Company, 1979.

Maxillofacial Prosthetics

1. Beumer, J., Curtis, T. A., and Firtell, D. N.: Maxillofacial Rehabilitation. Prosthodontic and Surgical Considerations. St. Louis, C. V. Mosby Company, 1979.
2. Cooper, H. K., Harding, R. L., Krogman, W. M., et al. (eds.): Cleft Palate and Cleft Lip: A Team Approach to Clinical Management and Rehabilitation of the Patient. Philadelphia, W. B. Saunders Company, 1979.
3. Laney, W. R. (ed.): Maxillofacial Prosthetics. Littleton, Mass., PSG Publishing Company, 1979.
4. Rahn, A. O., and Boucher, L. J.: Maxillofacial Prosthetics: Principles and Concepts. Philadelphia, W. B. Saunders Company, 1970.
5. Ramstad, T.: Post-orthodontic retention and post-prosthodontic occlusion in adult complete unilateral and bilateral cleft subjects. Cleft Palate J., 10:34–50, 1973.

DANIEL P. CASULLO

MULTIDISCIPLINARY APPROACH TO THERAPY

It is axiomatic that periodontal health is critical for the long-term preservation of the natural dentition as well as for the success of artificial prostheses. Unfortunately, however, the periodontium is highly susceptible to disease. The integrity of the soft tissues and the attachment apparatus can be compromised by microbial toxins, mechanical irritants, and aberrant occlusal morphology.

Although the production of microbial toxins is most frequently associated with plaque, caries and pulpal disease also generate toxic by-products that can interfere with periodontal health. Mechanical irritants, primarily faulty restorations and malposed teeth, contribute to the initiation and progression of periodontal disease. Aberrations in occlusal morphology associated with extruded, rotated, or poorly inclined teeth can result in the generation of excessive off-axis force, which also contributes to the initiation and progression of periodontal disease.

Because periodontal disease is caused or exacerbated by a multitude of disparate etiologic factors, a *multidisciplinary approach to therapy* is imperative. Restoration of periodontal health often requires more than the conventional periodontal procedures: scaling, root planing, curettage, and surgery. Other treatment modalities must be employed and may be combined or integrated with standard periodontal treatment. The requisite therapy depends on the particular etiology. The following examples are cited to illustrate this concept.

1. Advanced dental caries can lead to severe loss of tooth structure and infringement upon the embrasure space, resulting in soft tissue bunching, enlargement, and edema. Restoration of periodontal health would then require replacement of the destroyed tooth structure in harmony with the periodontal tissues.
2. Extensive dental caries can lead to pulpal disease, which can result in destruction of the attachment apparatus. Restoration of periodontal health would then necessitate root canal therapy.
3. Aberrations in occlusal morphology can lead to interferences and excessive off-axis forces, which can cause destruction of the attachment apparatus. Restoration of periodontal health would therefore require occlusal adjustment, which may involve simple selective grinding or complex tooth movement via adjunctive orthodontic therapy.

Once periodontal health has been reestablished, a more accurate prognosis can be made, and the restorative treatment plan can be finalized. Because of the intimate relationship between the restoration and the periodontium, the restoration can either maintain or jeopardize health. The potential to create an environment conducive to disease is inherent in every restorative procedure: This is one of the ironies of dental treatment.

OBJECTIVES

This chapter considers the restoration and maintenance of periodontal health and demonstrates a number of procedures employed in a multidisciplinary approach to therapy. The following topics have been selected for discussion: (1) the relationship between the

599

periodontium and restorative dentistry, (2) the combination of periodontal surgery with restorative dentistry to regain periodontal health, (3) the principles of strategic extraction for maximal preservation of the attachment apparatus, (4) the implications of the apical migration of marginal tissues (exposing root irregularities and furcations) for restorative dentistry, (5) a consideration of periodontal and pulpal diseases, problems in differential diagnoses, and the effects on tooth viability when communication between the two disease processes occurs, (6) the restoration of the endodontically and periodontally treated tooth, and (7) the combination of adjunctive orthodontic procedures (forced eruption and uprighting inclined molars) with periodontal therapy and restorative dentistry.

The actual biologic and mechanical considerations of most of the procedures, such as periodontics, endodontics, restorative dentistry, and orthodontics, are presented in the various disciplinary chapters. The integration of these dental disciplines and the combination of many procedures that can be applied to general practice are described in this chapter in a multidisciplinary approach to therapy.

RESTORATIVE DENTISTRY AND THE PERIODONTIUM

Restorative dentistry and the periodontium are intimately related. Restorations can re-establish, maintain, or destroy periodontal health. Conversely, periodontal health is necessary for the placement, integrity, and longevity of the restoration. There is an undeniable symbiosis between restorative dentistry and the periodontium.

The gingival sulcus and the interproximal col area (Fig. 12–1) are of particular importance in restorative dentistry. These areas are highly susceptible to inflammatory periodontal disease. Because the sulcus and the col are not keratinized, they have less inherent resistance and greater vulnerability to local irritants.

Although the gingival sulcus and interproximal col are the first areas affected by irritants and are readily visible for an assessment of health, it is the junctional epithelium and connective tissue attachment to the tooth and root that provide the protective

seal against the progression of disease to the underlying attachment apparatus. The restoration of a tooth alters the marginal ridges, crown contours, and interproximal contacts, all of which are intimately related to the vulnerable sulcus, col area, and junctional epithelium. Even the slightest deficiency in the restoration can lead to the accumulation of plaque and debris, initiating an inflammatory response. The inflammatory response is evidenced clinically by sulcular bleeding and ulceration, gingival enlargement, detachment of the junctional epithelium, and the development of pocket depth and radiographically by the dissolution of the crestal lamina dura. These signs are indicative of incipient periodontitis. Extension of this inflammatory process eventually results in advanced periodontitis, with extensive pocket depths, more severe soft tissue destruction, and progressive loss of the attachment apparatus.

Operative Dentistry

In the management of proximal caries, the restoration must not interfere with periodontal health. If inflammation is present, the restoration should contribute to the reversal of the disease process. This means re-establishing marginal integrity, normal interproximal contacts, proper contours, and embrasure space. The re-establishment of correct tooth form facilitates oral hygiene, prevents plaque accumulation and food impaction, and creates a local environment conducive to health.

The restoration should always be as conservative as possible. With minimal decay, an amalgam filling for posterior teeth or a composite resin restoration for anterior teeth is indicated (Fig. 12–2). If partial coverage is required, the amalgam restoration (with a sedative base) should be used provisionally to establish periodontal health. Amalgam is generally the material of choice for temporary restorations. Unlike zinc oxide and eugenol, amalgam does not promote the accumulation of plaque and debris and is stable and reliable throughout any requisite periodontal, endodontic, or orthodontic therapy (Fig. 12–3).

If a supporting cusp has been destroyed, a partial coverage restoration with supragingival margins conserves tooth structure optimally and maintains or enhances periodon-

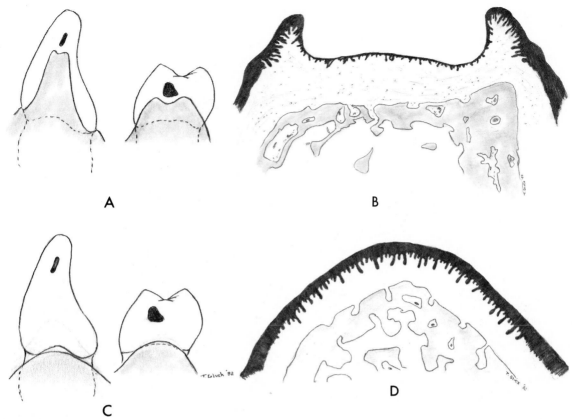

FIGURE 12–1   The Embrasure Space and Interproximal Col. *A,* In a normal, ideal periodontium, the depression of the soft tissue below the contact area (interproximal col area) is created by the buccal and lingual papillae. ***B,*** This diagram represents the histology of the col area. The papillae are covered by keratinized epithelium, and the interproximal col area is covered by a thin, nonkeratinized epithelium. ***C,*** After gingival recession or periodontal therapy, the interproximal col area no longer exists. The soft tissue architecture of the interproximal tissue is rounded or flat. ***D,*** This diagram represents the histology of the interproximal tissue after recession or surgery. It is now keratinized and similar to the external gingival tissues.

tal health without infringement on the soft tissue–crown interface. Concomitant therapy includes (1) isolated scaling and root planing and the re-establishment of proximal crown contour to control inflammation, and (2) isolated selective grinding procedures to eliminate any occlusal interferences that may have resulted from the eruption of the opposing tooth.

Partial coverage restorations are the cast restoration of choice, since the margins are kept coronal to the periodontal tissues. Yet this conservative approach, as the ideal of what is best for the periodontium, can be self-defeating in patients with advanced caries and periodontal disease. The presence of mobile teeth or exposed roots and furcation involvement introduces the need for more extensive treatment procedures using complete rather than partial coverage restorations.

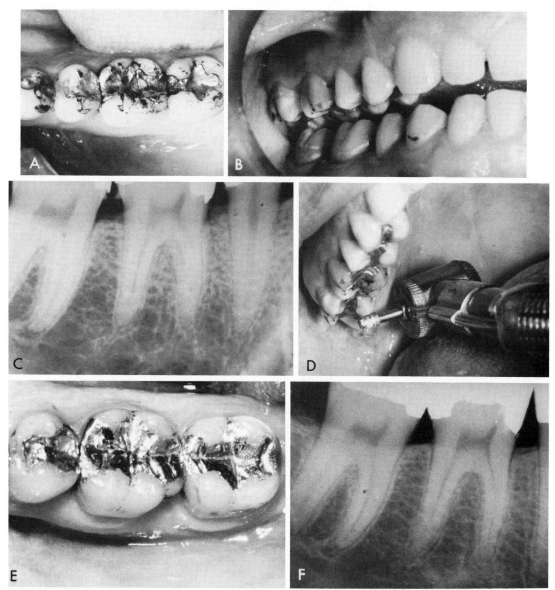

FIGURE 12–2   Combined Operative, Occlusal, and Periodontal Therapy. *A,* This 24-year-old patient's chief complaints were sensitivity to cold and pain on chewing, especially in the mandibular first molar area. The amalgam restorations are cupped out and the first molar MOD restoration is fractured. The soft tissue is edematous and bleeds on probing. *B,* In a left working movement, there are nonworking interferences associated with the maxillary and mandibular first and second molars. *C,* The radiograph shows subgingival calculus, overhanging restorations, and dissolution of the crestal bone. Treatment consists of oral hygiene instruction and scaling and root planing to remove the calculus and reduce the soft tissue inflammation. *D,* Two weeks later, isolated occlusal adjustment was done in conjunction with the placement of new amalgam restorations. The hanging palatal cusp associated with the nonworking interference is adjusted first to remove the interference. *E,* The new amalgam restorations reduce the depth of the central fossae and are occluded with the adjusted maxillary molars. *F,* The 6-month postoperative radiograph shows healing of the marginal bone.

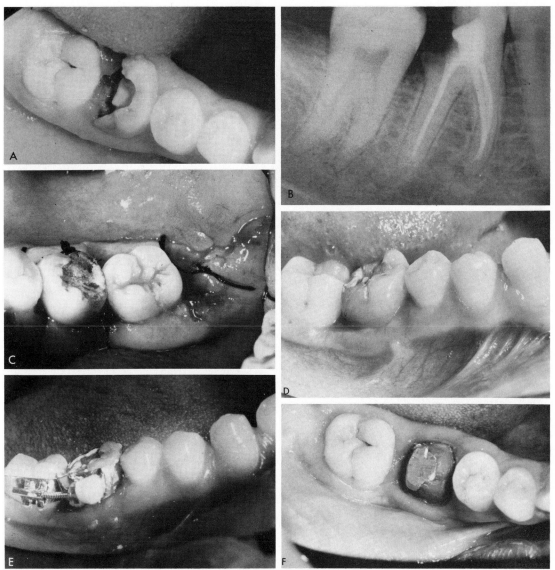

FIGURE 12–3   Combined Restorative, Periodontal, and Adjunctive Orthodontic Therapy. *A,* Severe, long-standing caries has destroyed the entire distal half of this endodontically treated, nonvital mandibular first molar, resulting in mesial drift of the second molar and encroachment on the broken-down tooth and embrasure space. This occlusal view demonstrates the severe soft tissue inflammation, edema, and enlargement caused by food impaction and plaque and calculus accumulation. Note the position of the soft tissue on the crown. *B,* The preoperative radiograph demonstrates the extensive caries relative to the crestal bone, the dissolution of crestal lamina dura, the mesial drift of the second molar, and the healthy periodontium of adjacent teeth. Since the problem is isolated in an otherwise healthy dentition, treatment was instituted to control the soft tissue enlargement and replace lost tooth structure. Tooth movement was then executed to regain an adequate embrasure space and to facilitate placement of a full-crown restoration with adequate crown contours. *C,* Buccal and lingual flaps were raised to gain access to the caries and to reduce the soft tissue enlargement. At this same visit, a temporary amalgam restoration was placed to recreate lost tooth structure that could be maintained during Phase II therapy (adjunctive orthodontics). The soft tissue is sutured in place. *D,* This is a buccal view of soft tissue healing 4 weeks after surgery and operative dentistry. *E,* An open coil-spring is placed to move the second molar distally and open the embrasure space between the first and second molars. *F,* After orthodontic therapy, the tooth is prepared for the provisional full-crown restoration. Note the healing of the sulcular tissue and normal embrasure space.

Illustration continued on following page

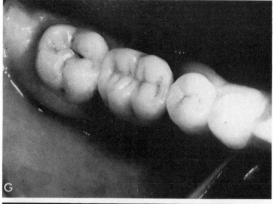

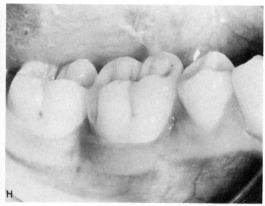

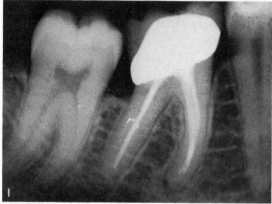

FIGURE 12–3 *Continued* *G,* Occlusal view of the final restoration showing the normal mesiodistal dimension of the first molar. *H,* Buccal view of the final restoration. *I,* This 1-year postoperative radiograph shows the final restoration and healing of the marginal bone.

The full-crown restoration is the most demanding and exacting restoration in restorative dentistry, since it can have the greatest effect on the periodontium. When properly executed, it is an excellent adjunct for achieving and maintaining periodontal health. Because of its importance, the full-crown restoration will be emphasized throughout this chapter.

Provisional Restoration

Long-standing caries can result in the extensive loss of tooth structure and the destruction of the self-protective capacity of the tooth. Loss of normal crown contours associated with advanced caries leads to food impaction and debris and plaque accumulation, resulting in isolated periodontal disease (severe inflammation and gingival enlargement). Similarly, faulty restorations promote the build-up of plaque and debris, insult the vulnerable sulcus and col, and cause an inflammatory response. When placement of a subgingival full-crown restoration is deemed necessary, periodontal health must be restored *first* and tested with a well-fitted provisional restoration (Fig. 12–4).

Although periodontal surgical procedures—soft tissue reduction, osseous reduction, or both—may eventually be required, the *most conservative* method must be employed to control inflammation and to re-evaluate periodontal health. By re-establishing normal crown contours, the provisional restoration promotes the maintenance of periodontal health and the restoration of proper sulcular architecture while protecting the underlying tooth structure and pulp.

The metal band and acrylic provisional restoration is superior to the all-acrylic provisional restoration because the metal band provides optimal strength in the gingival third of the crown for support of the sulcular tissues and provides optimally thin, knifelike margins to prevent food impaction and plaque accumulation. Because the metal band and acrylic provisional restoration creates an environment that is most conducive to health, the soft tissue response is more reliable for predicting the long-term success of the final restoration and for assessing the need for more advanced surgical procedures.

There are other advantages to the metal band provisional restoration: (1) Crown contours can be easily altered, if indicated; (2) it

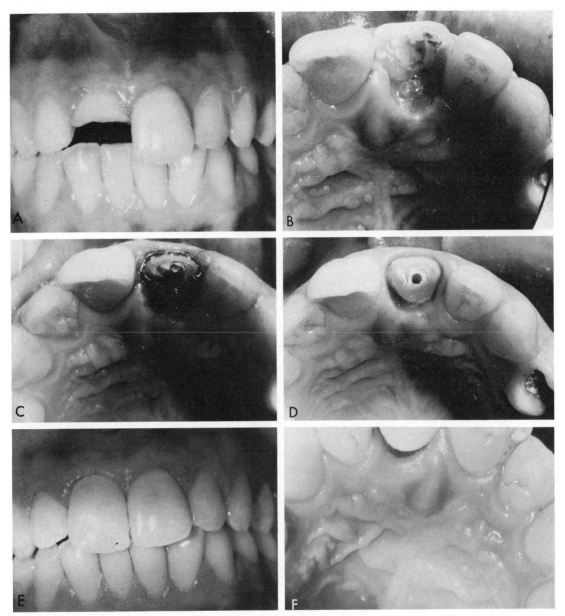

FIGURE 12–4 Combined Restorative and Periodontal Therapy—The Provisional Restoration. A, Fractured right central incisor in a 23-year-old female. The labial view shows a thin, friable soft tissue with its margin at the cementoenamel junction (CEJ). **B,** The fractured tooth structure was sheared off toward the palatal aspect. The question arose as to whether surgery would be necessary to expose sound tooth structure. Note the soft tissue overgrowth. **C,** A gold band and metal post was fitted to the fractured tooth. Since the fracture did not go below the osseous crest, the severe soft tissue response was re-evaluated after fabrication of a gold band and acrylic provisional restoration. **D,** After 8 weeks, the provisional restoration was removed and the soft tissue was evaluated. The sulcular tissue, junctional epithelium, and interproximal tissues returned to a healthy state via the provisional restoration, thus avoiding a surgical procedure. **E,** Labial view of the final restoration. **F,** Palatal view of final restoration.

is easier to repair; (3) it is more stable and durable; and (4) it is easier to fabricate, since once the bands are fitted, a marginal area is established that serves as a guide for devel-

oping and refining crown contours, especially those of the critical gingival third of the tooth. This is of particular importance when establishing healthy sulcular form

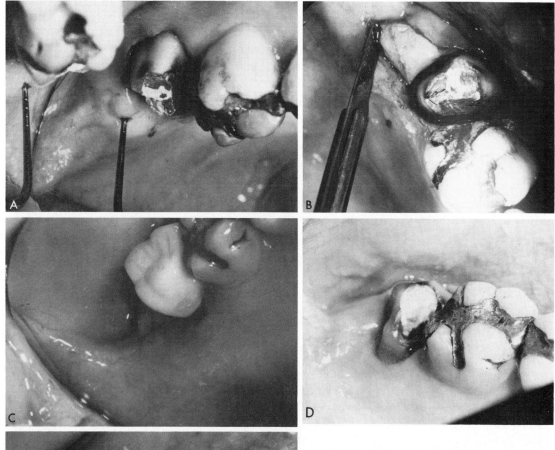

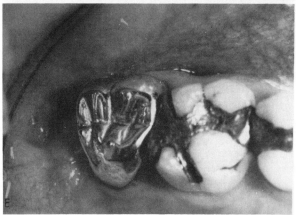

FIGURE 12–5 Concomitant Provisional Fabrication and Soft Tissue Reduction. *A,* The sequence of treatment included preparation of this second molar for a full crown followed by a surgical procedure to eliminate the 10-mm pocket at the distal aspect of the second molar. The periodontal probe is used to determine the soft tissue depth in the tuberosity area. The molar was prepared and the provisional restoration fabricated but not cemented to allow access for the surgical reduction procedure. *B,* The surgical procedure consisted of buccal and lingual inverse beveled incisions, removal of the distal wedge of tissue, and minimal osteoplasty. The tissues were sutured in place to cover all osseous tissue. The provisional restoration was then placed with a minimal wash of cement, making absolutely sure no cement got below the sutured soft tissue. *C,* Two-week postoperative healing. The provisional restoration was tapped off and recemented to ensure an adequate seal and prevent recurrent caries. Six weeks after surgery, the tooth was reprepared and the final impression was taken. The provisional restoration was relined. *D,* Final tooth preparation and soft tissue healing. *E,* Final restoration in place. (In conjunction with Craig Williams, Philadelphia, Pa.)

(depth and width), evaluating the need for further periodontal therapy, and establishing contours for combined procedures (periodontal surgery and provisional restoration fabrication).

After 4 to 6 weeks, the provisional resto-

ration is removed to evaluate the status of the soft tissues. If ulceration and bleeding in the sulcus and col area and gingival enlargement have not been resolved, crown contours and margins of the provisional restoration must be re-examined. The finish line of the full-crown provisional and final restoration should be thin and accurately placed 0.5 mm short of the junctional epithelium. This position is preferred to prevent recurrent caries, alleviate tooth sensitivity, gain retention on broken-down teeth, enhance appearance, and establish optimal soft tissue crown contours as the restoration exits the sulcus.

The crown contours must be evaluated relative to the soft tissue response. The proximal crown contours are generally flat or concave to provide adequate embrasure space for the interdental gingiva and yet must not be too open, which would allow food impaction. The facial and lingual surfaces are generally convex and must be in harmony with the sulcular form. There should be smooth, consistent crown–soft tissue relations as the restoration exits the sulcus.

The contour of the provisional restoration should support the sulcular tissue and should not produce a ledge between the crown and tissue that would increase food and plaque accumulation. The transitional line angle (the area forming the transition between the flat or concave proximal surface and the convex facial or lingual surface) is generally flat or concave.

The ultimate goal of the provisional restoration is to resolve the periodontal prob- lem, yet this is not always possible when dental caries or periodontal disease is extensive. Nonetheless, the provisional restoration will help control the inflammatory disease process and will contribute to the correction of the form and consistency of the soft tissue, so the tissues will be better prepared for surgery.

COMBINED PERIODONTAL AND RESTORATIVE PROCEDURES

Soft Tissue and Osseous Reduction

Soft tissue reduction is indicated in the presence of soft tissue overgrowth and isolated periodontal defects such as the residual pocket depth associated with third molar extraction. Soft tissue reduction via inverse bevel incisions and primary closure is generally the procedure of choice in order to preserve the attached gingiva and control the position of the tissues (Fig. 12–5).

In the process of performing soft tissue reduction, the clinician may discover that an inadequate amount of sound tooth structure remains for the placement of a full-crown restoration: 2 mm for the biologic width (1 mm for connective tissue and 1 mm for junctional epithelium) plus 1 to 2 mm for the crown margin termination, for a total of

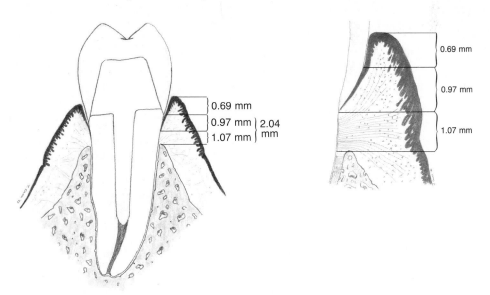

FIGURE 12–6 Diagrammatic Representation of the Biologic Width. The biologic width is the dimension from the crest of aveolar bone to the base of the sulcus (2.04 mm) and includes the connective tissue (1.07 mm) and epithelial (0.97 mm) attachments. (Adapted from Ingber, J. S., Rose, L. F., and Coslet, J. G.: The "biologic width"—A concept in periodontics and restorative dentistry. Alpha Omegan, Vol. 10, No. 3, 1977.)

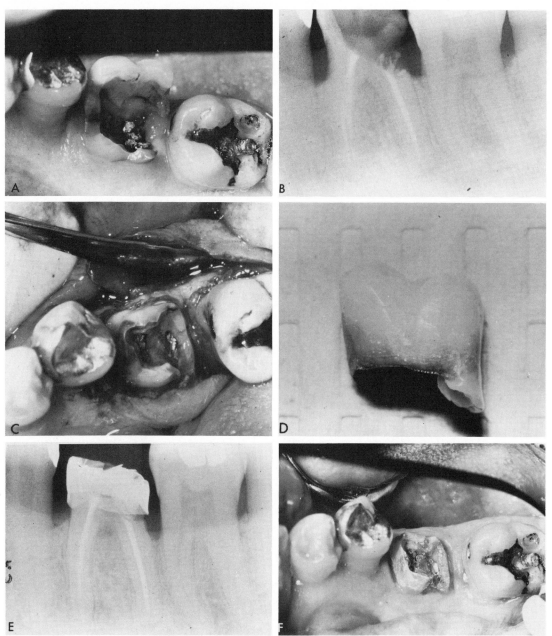

FIGURE 12–7 Concomitant Provisional Fabrication and Osseous Reduction. A, The occlusolingual view of the mandibular first molar shows extensive loss of tooth structure due to dental caries. The caries has left a shell of enamel and root structure. The soft tissue on the distal surface extends into the cavernous opening. **B,** The periapical radiograph shows the caries extending to the osseous crest in the distal surface. There is inadequate tooth structure on which to terminate the margin of a restoration and provide the necessary soft tissue attachment (biologic width). The treatment plan included osseous surgery in conjunction with the fabrication of a provisional restoration, followed by a period of healing, re-evaluation, and final restoration with a post, core, and crown. **C,** The tooth was prepared as well as possible and a metal band and acrylic provisional restoration was fabricated. Osseous surgery was executed at this same visit. Buccal and lingual flaps were raised to gain access to allow reduction of the bone on the distal surface. The tooth structure exposed during the osseous surgery was prepared and covered by relining the metal band and acrylic provisional while the flaps were raised. **D,** The relined provisional restoration.

Illustration continued on opposite page

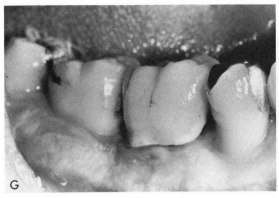
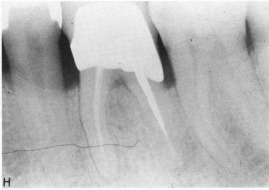

FIGURE 12–7 *Continued E,* This periapical radiograph was taken with the provisional metal band and acrylic crown in place. Note the 3 to 4 mm of exposed tooth structure on the distal surface. *F,* This occlusolingual view shows healing of the interproximal and sulcular tissues 12 weeks after the surgical and restorative therapy. Adequate sound tooth structure is available for the final restoration. *G,* Buccal view of final restoration. *H,* This periapical radiograph of the final restoration in place demonstrates healing of the attachment apparatus, marginal integrity of the restoration, and the individually fitted post in the distal canal.

3 to 4 mm of sound tooth structure (Fig. 12–6). Inadequate tooth structure is frequently found when fractures and caries approach the osseous crest and cannot be detected radiographically.

The surgical procedure provides total access to the visualization of the tooth. Osseous surgery then becomes necessary to gain the requisite 3 to 4 mm of sound tooth structure. The clinician must always be aware of this contingency and be prepared to proceed with osseous surgery. Inadequate reduction or failure to gain adequate tooth structure will cause an infringement on the junctional epithelium and the connective tissue attachment. This will result in a poor soft tissue response and ultimately lead to bone loss and the apical migration of the soft tissue complex.

When osseous reduction is deemed necessary (e.g., when less than 3 to 4 mm of sound tooth structure is above the osseous crest), the consequence of rendering such treatment must be carefully evaluated. The objective of the periodontal surgical procedure is to remove adequate bone from the fractured or decayed tooth in harmony with the attachment apparatus of adjacent teeth (Fig. 12–7). When the problem is localized and isolated to one or two teeth, an inordinate amount of bone removal from adjacent teeth may be necessary to resolve the problem. The surgical procedure can compromise the harmonious soft tissue and osseous form of the quadrant. Forced eruption via adjunctive orthodontic treatment may be more appropriate in such cases (see p. 658).

Concomitant Periodontal Surgery and Placement of the Provisional Restoration

By assessing the extent of pocket formation via probing and by examining the progression of caries relative to the osseous crest via bite-wing radiographs, the clinician can often determine at the outset that surgical procedures will be required regardless of the results of scaling and root planing or provisional restorations. Under such circumstances, execution of surgical procedures and fabrication of the provisional restoration may be done at the same visit. This combined approach affords better access to and control of the operative area, enhancing the clinician's efficiency and easing the dental experience for the patient. In such cases, the provisional restoration must be constructed *first.* It must be accurately formed and well-fitting, with the requisite crown contours and proximal contacts established to enhance healing and to reduce the need for postsurgical relining and correction of the gingival third of the restoration. Since the provisional restoration is completed prior to the surgical procedure, tooth preparation and fabrication of the restoration are not complicated by bleeding and soft tissue flaps. After the provisional restoration has been fabricated, the clinician can reasonably judge whether to execute the surgical procedure at the same sitting. This decision is based on how fatigued and anxious the patient is, on the duration and amount of anesthetic administered, and on time constraints.

Once the provisional restoration has been fabricated, surgery can be postponed with no adverse results. However, the converse is not true. It is important that the teeth be protected optimally following surgery. The accumulation of plaque and debris is a problem in the surgically treated patient. Home care is unavoidably inadequate owing to tissue sensitivity. This creates a local environment that is conducive to the reinitiation of active disease (caries). A deficient provisional restoration increases the potential for the recurrence of disease. An impeccably fabricated provisional restoration must be placed to protect the remaining tooth structure from recurrent caries, to protect the soft tissues from plaque and debris, and to allow reformation of proper sulcular architecture. Therefore, it is imperative that the clinician fabricate a well-fitting, properly contoured provisional restoration before the initiation of surgical procedures.

Mucogingival Surgery

The mucogingival complex comprises (1) the bound-down, keratinized masticatory mucosa or attached gingiva, and (2) the thin, friable, movable alveolar mucosa. In health, the masticatory mucosa adheres tightly to the tooth by means of its junctional epithelium, gingival fiber apparatus, and connective tissue attachment. The nature of this soft tissue crown interface allows for optimal oral hygiene and is essential for the protection of the underlying attachment apparatus.

The integrity of the masticatory mucosa can be compromised by a traumatic insult (e.g., muscle pull, frenum tear, injudicious restorative dentistry, overzealous toothbrushing), or it can be congenitally thin and vulnerable to disease. When this is the case, the entire mucogingival complex is more susceptible to plaque accumulation and its toxic by-products, which can cause inflammation, recession, pocket formation, gingival clefts, fenestrations, dehiscences, bone loss, and crown and root caries.

When the masticatory mucosa has been compromised in some way, the clinician must determine whether an adequate amount of attached gingiva remains or whether surgery is indicated to increase the zone of attached gingiva. In some cases, the decision is straightforward. When the masticatory mucosa is unattached or totally absent and the soft tissue–crown interface has been compromised by recession or inflammation, surgery is required. Determining appropriate treatment in the majority of cases, however, is much more challenging. The judgment is based largely on whether advanced restorative dentistry is planned. This is because restorations involving the subgingival placement of crown margins or requiring concomitant adjunctive orthodontic therapy place greater demands on the natural tissues, especially on the maintenance of the soft tissue–crown interface.

When no restorative therapy is indicated, any questionable or borderline mucogingival problems can be observed for a period of time. Health may be sustained indefinitely; otherwise, surgery can be implemented when the need arises.

When advanced restorative therapy is required, questionable areas of adequate masticatory mucosa must be corrected. The two surgical procedures that can be employed easily in general dentistry are the free gingival graft and the laterally or apically positioned flap. The free gingival graft affords the clinician more latitude, flexibility, and predictability in the decision-making process (Fig. 12–8). This is because the free gingival graft maintains the marginal tissue, and the procedure can be performed at various stages of restorative therapy: (1) at the provisional restoration visit, (2) at the final impression visit, or (3) at the coping or gold try-in visit. (If necessary, the tooth can be reprepared and the impressions retaken.) Moreover, by basing the decision on marginal soft tissue response at different intervals during treatment, unnecessary surgery can be avoided.

The free gingival graft facilitates decision-making because it achieves a predictable result. The clinician can better estimate the new position of the marginal gingiva. Usually, the marginal position is maintained or moves coronally owing to elimination of muscle pull. The free gingival graft, however, does require securing donor tissue, which may be taken from an adjacent eden-

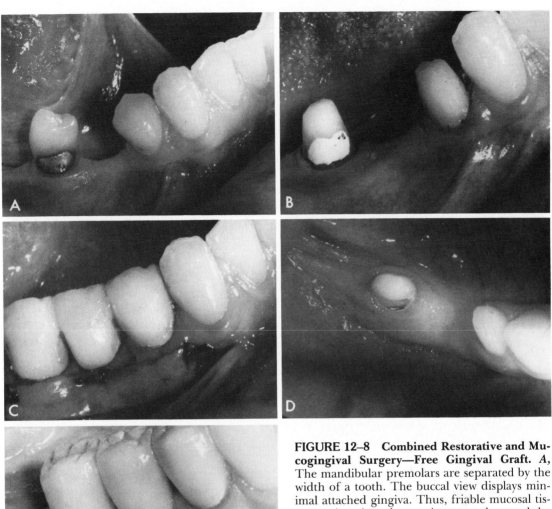

FIGURE 12–8 Combined Restorative and Mucogingival Surgery—Free Gingival Graft. *A,* The mandibular premolars are separated by the width of a tooth. The buccal view displays minimal attached gingiva. Thus, friable mucosal tissue projects into the pontic area and around the second premolars. The treatment plan included a three-unit bridge to replace the missing tooth and a free gingival graft to augment the masticatory mucosa around the abutment teeth and on the edentulous ridge. *B,* The teeth are first prepared for full-crown restorations, and, in this case, the final impressions were taken. *C,* The free gingival graft was taken from the maxillary palatal tissue and sutured in place, followed by cementation of the provisional splint. *D,* The tissues healed uneventfully in 6 weeks, allowing the framework try-in for the final fixed restoration. This occlusal view shows the increased buccolingual dimension of the edentulous ridge. *E,* The final restoration was placed 12 weeks after all the surgical procedures.

tulous ridge or from the hard palate, whichever is more accessible. This procedure is predictable, quick, and easy to perform.

There are distinct advantages to combining restorative and surgical procedures at the same visit. Executing the free gingival graft and fabricating the provisional restoration (or taking the final impressions) at the

same time minimize treatment time, enhance the clinician's efficiency, and minimize traumatic insult to the tissues, thus increasing patient comfort. Combining periodontal and restorative therapy is warranted when all the following conditions have been met: (1) The mucogingival problem is isolated and easy to manage (any periodontal pock-

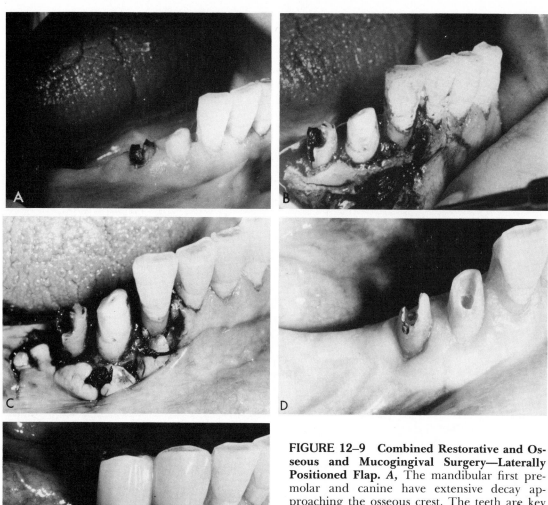

FIGURE 12–9 Combined Restorative and Osseous and Mucogingival Surgery—Laterally Positioned Flap. A, The mandibular first premolar and canine have extensive decay approaching the osseous crest. The teeth are key abutments for a removable partial denture, and, if they can be saved, more extensive restoration will be avoided. **B,** The labial surgical flap reveals a fracture at the distobuccal line angle of the premolar where the pin had been placed. The fracture extended below the osseous crest and required osseous surgery to gain sound tooth structure. **C,** The masticatory mucosa was apically and laterally positioned to protect the labial plate of bone and to maintain the zone of attachment gingiva. **D,** Postoperative healing 3 months after surgery demonstrates adequate tooth structure for the new restoration. **E,** Final restoration in place.

ets, dehiscences, or fenestrations would have been handled separately). (2) All other periodontal therapy to control inflammatory disease has been completed. (3) The junctional epithelium has not been injured or destroyed; as such, the relation of the tooth preparation to the marginal gingiva and the incision for the free gingival graft are totally separated. (4) Adequate time is available to execute therapy effectively.

When severe caries approaches the osseous crest and requires extensive periodontal surgery (a full-thickness flap extending to adjacent teeth and osseous reduction to gain sound tooth structure), the attached masticatory mucosa must be preserved. The apically and laterally positioned flap is an excellent means of preserving and gaining attached gingiva (Fig. 12–9).

Surgical Correction of the Deformed Edentulous Ridge

The configuration of the edentulous ridge is of primary importance in fixed restorative dentistry. The deformed ridge can interfere with the clinician's ability to fabricate and place a restoration that will achieve optimal esthetic appearance, occlusal form and function, and health. An unacceptable appearance of the maxillary anterior region is perhaps the most common problem caused by ridge deformities. It is this area that usually requires surgical correction to meet the esthetic requirements of the patient. Surgical

procedures for the problems to be described must be approached with caution and only after consideration of all other alternatives.

Abnormal ridge dimensions, either inadequate or excessive, often compromise (1) framework design, (2) pontic form, (3) pontic inclination, (4) surface finish, and (5) the pontic ridge interface. These factors, in turn, can cause accumulation of plaque and debris, inflammation, hyperplasia, impeded oral hygiene, ridge resorption, mechanical instability, fractures and flexure of solder joints and cast restorations, and above all, esthetic problems, especially in the maxillary anterior region.

There are two types of ridge deformities that complicate restorative dentistry: the excessively bulky ridge, usually associated with anodontia or early tooth loss before the

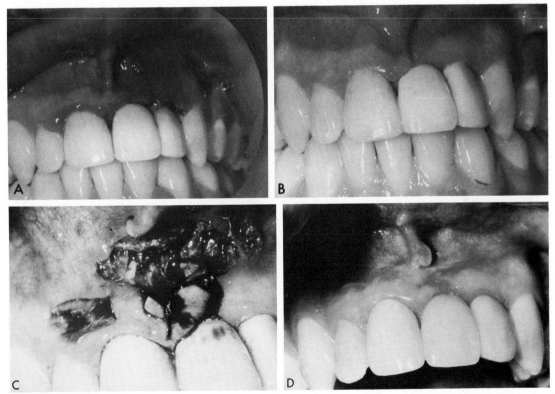

FIGURE 12–10 Management of the Edentulous Ridge—Scaling, Root Planing, and Frenectomy. *A,* The soft tissue around the maxillary three-unit provisional restoration is severely inflamed and edematous. The patient is 22 years old, has poor oral hygiene, poor nutritional habits, and an acute gingival reaction with associated pain and bleeding. ***B,*** After scaling and root planing and oral hygiene reinforcement, the provisional restoration was recontoured. The gingival tissue responded well to therapy. However, the labial frenum is pulling on the marginal tissue and requires a surgical procedure. ***C,*** A frenectomy was performed, and a free gingival graft from the adjacent incisors was placed to eliminate the frenal muscle attachment. ***D,*** Final healing of the soft tissue and the final restoration in place.

eruptive process was completed; and the collapsed ridge, associated with advanced periodontal disease, surgery, pulpal disease, surgical trauma during extraction, traumatic injuries, and trauma caused by ill-fitting removable prostheses. In any case, surgical techniques can restore proper ridge form, so that mechanical problems can be managed. Surgery will allow restoration of proper occlusal form and function, provide an optimal esthetic result, and establish a local environment conducive to health. However, surgical procedures should not be used routinely. Such treatment is warranted only after careful assessment indicates that the desired results cannot be accomplished with more conservative therapy (Fig. 12–10).

The provisional restoration is an integral part of treatment. Its use is essential before, during, and after the surgical phase of therapy. Before surgical procedures are initi-

ated, a provisional prosthesis is fabricated according to the dictates of the deformed ridge. It is placed in the mouth and used as a guide to determine the amount and location of tissue to be excised or added. During the surgery, the provisional restoration is corrected, adapting it to the newly created ridge. If problems persist after surgery, the restoration must be further adjusted (or the soft tissue further reduced or augmented).

The provisional restoration is a valuable adjunct in treatment that involves the extraction of a tooth. Immediate placement of a well-designed provisional splint serves as a guide in the healing and reformation of the tissues, resulting in an optimally shaped concave ridge form, possibly avoiding the need for future corrective surgery.

Technique for Ridge Reduction. When excessive tissue is a problem, surgery is used to reduce the size of the ridge while devel-

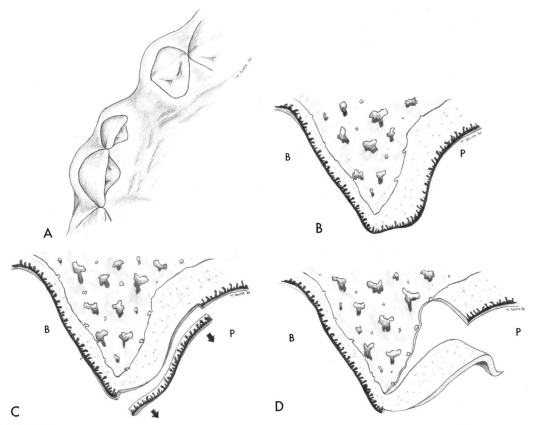

FIGURE 12–11 Diagrammatic Representation of the Connective Tissue Pedicle Graft Procedure (Inward Roll). *A,* Occlusal view of deformed edentulous ridge. *B,* Cross-sectioned view of a deformed edentulous ridge. (Note crestal and labial deformities.) *C,* The surface epithelium of the adjacent palatal tissue is removed first. *D,* The connective tissue pedicle is outlined and dissected from the palate.

Illustration continued on opposite page

oping a concavity to accommodate the ideal convex pontic form. The particular procedure employed depends on whether the deformity is due to an overabundance of soft tissue or bone. This is ascertained by periodontal probing and radiographic analysis of the occlusogingival and buccolingual dimensions of the ridge.

Gingivoplasty or flap procedures may be used for reduction of soft tissue. Surgery must be performed judiciously, leaving between 1.5 and 2 mm of soft tissue to cover the osseous ridge. Combined flap procedures and osseous surgery are used to reduce the bone and to make confluent the hard and soft tissue forms of the ridge and the adjacent teeth.

Technique for Ridge Augmentation. The collapsed ridge may be restored with aug-

mentation procedures. Lost dimension may be regained with (1) the connective tissue pedicle graft (Fig. 12–11), (2) the autogenous connective tissue graft, or (3) the free gingival graft.

The connective tissue pedicle graft is indicated when adequate tissue is available at the maxillary surgical site to achieve the desired increase in the buccolingual and occlusogingival dimensions of the ridge. A de-epithelialized triangular flap is extended from the palate, inverted (rolled) to form a concave configuration, and positioned with a single suture (Fig. 12–12).

The autogenous connective tissue (Fig. 12–13) and the free gingival graft (see p. 189) are indicated when an inadequate amount of tissue is available at the surgical site. The donor tissue used in the autoge-

Text continued on page 621

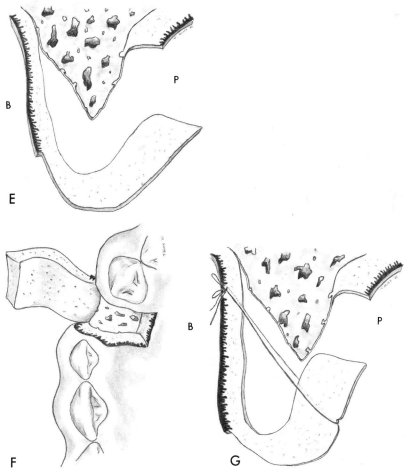

FIGURE 12–11 *Continued E,* The labial pouch is then created by separating the soft tissue from the labial aspect of the edentulous ridge. *F,* Occlusal view of dissected tissue. (Note that the marginal tissue of the adjacent abutment teeth is intact.) *G,* A suture is placed through the labial tissue onto the connective tissue pedicle.

Illustration continued on following page

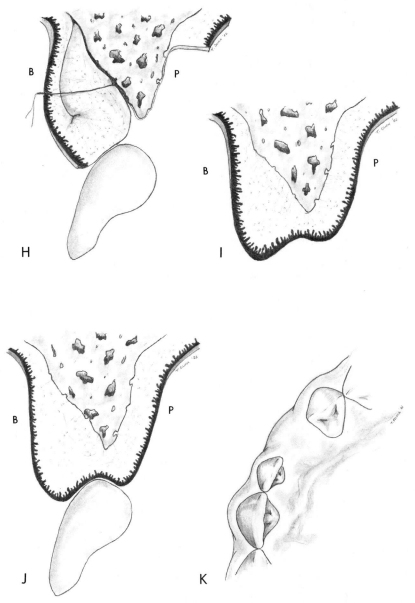

FIGURE 12–11 *Continued H,* The palatal connective tissue is rolled into the labial pouch and positioned with the suture. *I,* The final healing and new dimension of the edentulous ridge. *J,* Ovate pontic form maintains soft tissue form, appearance, and health. *K,* Occlusal view of corrected ridge.

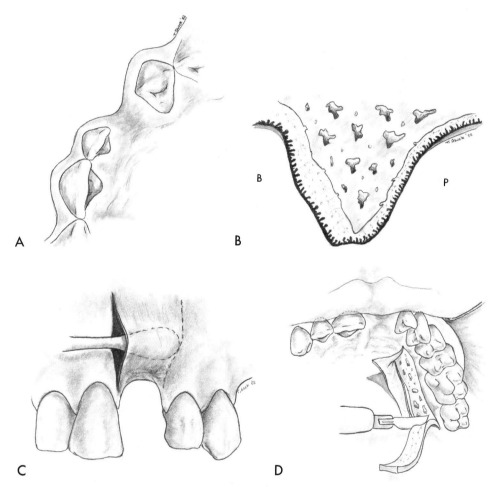

FIGURE 12–12 **Diagrammatic Representation of the Autogenous Connective Tissue Graft Procedure (Pouch).** *A,* Occlusal view of deformed ridge. *B,* Cross-sectional view of a deformed edentulous ridge. (Note inadequate palatal donor tissue). *C,* This labial diagram outlines the pouch created by a vertical incision and dissection of the labial tissue from the ridge. *D,* The donor connective tissue is taken from posterior palatal area. Split-thickness dissection is used to raise the epithelial covering of the palate, the donor connective tissue is removed, and the epithelium is sutured back in place.

Illustration continued on following page

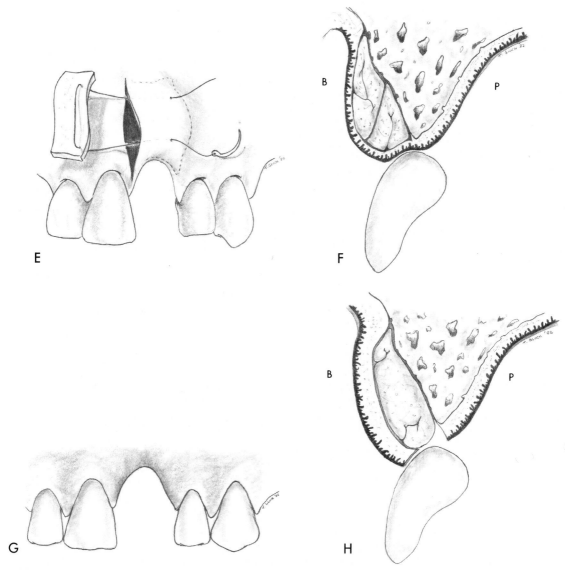

FIGURE 12–12 *Continued E,* A suture is passed from the labial tissue into the free connective tissue. The connective tissue is placed and positioned into the pouch by the suture beneath the epithelium. *F,* This cross-sectional view diagrams the pouch and the connective tissue in place. *G,* Labial view showing deformed ridge with not only inadequate buccolingual dimension but also inadequate apical-occlusal dimension. *H,* This cross-sectioned diagram demonstrates the use of a horizontal incision on the palatal aspect of the edentulous ridge. This allows the tissue to be released, thus accommodating more connective tissue to enhance the ridge augmentation in both a vertical and a horizontal dimension. (Modified from D. Garber, E. Rosenberg, and S. Rosenberg, University of Pennsylvania, Philadelphia, Pa.)

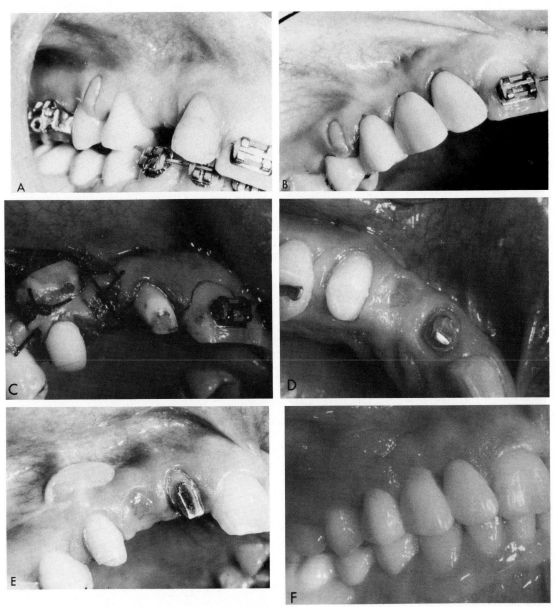

FIGURE 12–13   Management of the Edentulous Ridge—Inward Roll Procedure. A, After tooth movement created space for a canine pontic, the edentulous ridge presented excessive soft tissue in an occlusogingival dimension and inadequate tissue in a buccolingual dimension. The patient's high smile line allowed the deformity to be noticeable. Other isolated gingival problems in the area included muscle attachment over the first premolar and edematous and enlarged interproximal tissues. Note the soft tissue indentation from orthodontic wire over the second bicuspid. The combined procedures planned were tooth preparation of the first premolar and lateral incisor, fabrication of a provisional restoration, correction of the soft tissue problem, and recontouring of the pontic. **B,** The correction of the edentulous ridge required first fabricating the provisional restoration to visualize the extent of the problem and to guide the actual correction. A connective tissue pedicle graft was planned to increase the buccolingual dimension of the collapsed ridge. The surface epithelium, which must be removed from the connective tissue, is to be used as a free gingival graft over the premolar. Open-flap curettage is planned to remove the excessive interproximal tissue. **C,** The connective tissue pedicle graft is sutured in place; the free gingival graft is placed over the premolar and the interdental papilla is also sutured. The pontic of the provisional restoration is adjusted to its ideal form and positioned to help support the newly positioned pedicle graft. **D,** Healing 8 weeks postoperatively. Note the concave ridge form and increased buccolingual dimension. **E,** Buccal view of final healing of all tissue. **F,** Final restoration in place.

619

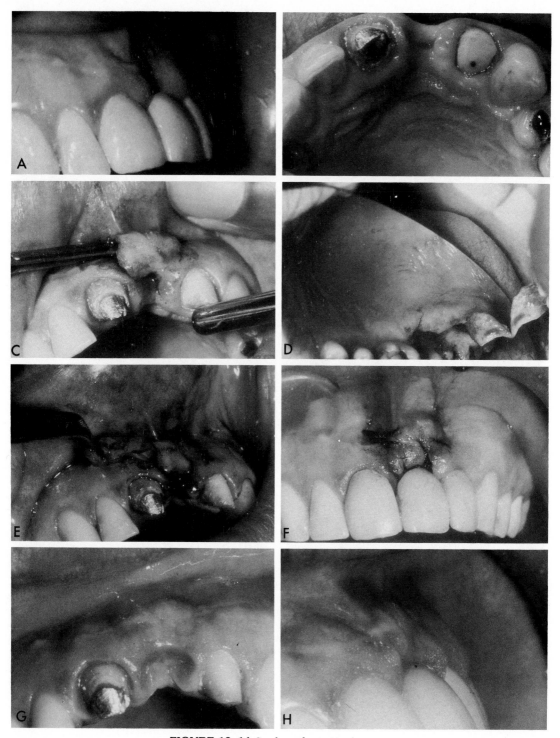

FIGURE 12–14 *See legend on opposite page*

nous connective tissue graft may be taken from the posterior part of the palate. However, if posterior periodontal surgery is required to eliminate pockets, for example, the two surgical procedures should be executed at the same visit. This minimizes the requisite surgery, increases the clinician's efficiency, and minimizes the patient's discomfort. The donor tissue is placed between the periosteum and the flap, or in the pouch, and positioned and stabilized with sutures (Fig. 12–14).

MANAGEMENT OF MULTIROOTED TEETH WITH FURCATION INVOLVEMENTS

The restorative management of multirooted teeth affected by periodontal disease and dental caries can be complex and demanding because of the interdependence of restorative, periodontal, and endodontic therapy. Also, the tenuous environment created by periodontal disease and the concomitant migration of the gingivodental complex contribute to the complexity of successful treatment of furcation problems. The apically positioned periodontium exposes vulnerable areas and surfaces of the teeth that are more susceptible to plaque and calculus accumulation, leading to the acceleration and exacerbation of the disease processes.

Position of the Periodontium

In the restoration of periodontally and endodontically involved teeth, the position of the marginal tissue and the osseous crest relative to the cementoenamel junction is of prime importance. The scars of disease and the requirements of therapy will vary significantly from one position to the next. The extent of apical migration can be described using three anatomic configurations that simplify the explanation of a complex set of circumstances. The marginal tissues may be located at one of three basic positions (Fig. 12–15): Position 1—at the cementoenamel junction; Position 2—1 to 5 mm apical to the cementoenamel junction; and Position 3—more than 5 mm apical to the cementoenamel junction.

At Position 1, the marginal tissues are healthy and properly positioned, the anatomic crown and clinical crown are synonymous, and the sulcular morphology is normal. As the tissues migrate apically to Position 2, however, root surface irregularities, developmental depressions, and cemental surface irregularities become exposed. The sulcus narrows, and the soft tissue thins. When the marginal tissues are more than 5 mm apical to the cementoenamel junction, at Position 3, root surface aberrations become more exaggerated; the furcation, undercuts, and cul-de-sac areas are exposed; the sulcus becomes more narrow; and the tissues are

---

FIGURE 12–14   Management of the Edentulous Ridge—Pouch Procedure. A, This lateral view of the maxillary left central incisor edentulous ridge demonstrates the diminished buccolingual (horizontal) dimension. Note indentation of the labial aspect of the ridge extending into mucobuccal fold. This incisor had extensive endodontic and periodontal involvement, which resulted in loss of the labial plate of bone. The provisional restoration was fabricated at the time of extraction of the central incisor. **B,** This occlusal view shows the decreased buccolingual ridge dimension. The patient had a high smile line, which made the edentulous deformed (collapsed) ridge visible. A procedure was planned to build up the ridge to enhance the esthetic relation of the pontic soft tissue interface. The donor tissue was to consist of connective tissue from the palatal area. **C,** A vertical incision is made to split thickness. Dissection is employed to separate the soft tissue covering the deformed ridge area. A vertical incision is made to create a pouch to receive the connective tissue graft. **D,** The connective tissue graft is taken from the maxillary palatal area. **E,** The donor tissue is being placed into the pouch. **F,** The graft is sutured in place. The provisional restoration is reshaped to ideal pontic form in order to form a template for the edentulous ridge to heal to. **G,** This 3 month postoperative view demonstrates the increase in buccolingual ridge dimension. **H,** One-year postoperatively, the ridge form is maintained. The final restoration is in place. It is extremely important to realize that control of the form and shape of the provisional and final restorations is a key aspect of a successful surgical result.

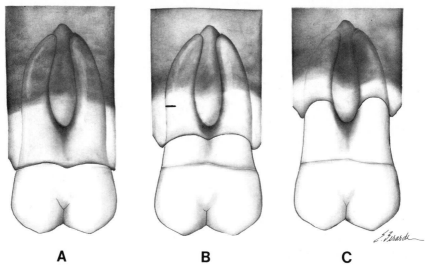

A **B** **C**

FIGURE 12–15 Position of Marginal Tissue to the Cementoenamel Junction. Maxillary first molar describing position of marginal tissue relative to the cementoenamel junction (CEJ). *A,* Position 1. The marginal tissue is at the CEJ and the anatomic and clinical crowns are essentially equal. *B,* Position 2. The marginal tissue is 3 to 5 mm apical to the CEJ. *C,* Position 3. The marginal tissue is more than 5 mm apical to the CEJ. This exposes a major portion of the root surface, and the multirooted teeth furcation areas are accessible. (From Casullo, D.: The integration of endodontics, periodontics, and restorative dentistry in general practice. Part III. Restorative considerations. Compend. Cont. Educ. Gen. Dent., *1* (5):295–316, 1980.

FIGURE 12–16 Tooth and Root Anatomy. For illustrative purposes, the maxillary first molar, mandibular first molar, and maxillary first premolar, the most consistently occurring multi-rooted teeth, will be described herein. Salient anatomic features as they relate to preparation and restoration of these teeth will be highlighted.

Key: PR, Palatal root. MBR, Mesiobuccal root. DBR, Distobuccal root. DR, Distal root. CEJ, Cementoenamel junction. DD, Developmental depression. FR, Furcation. RT, Root trunk. DF, Distal furcation. MF, Mesial furcation. BF, Buccal furcation. D, Distal. B, Buccal.

A, Maxillary Molar. (1) Distal view. Note position of furcation buccopalatally (midway between the buccal and palatal surfaces) and occlusoapically (relative to the mesial and buccal furcation, the distal furcation opening is more apical). (2) Mesial view. Furcation occurs two-thirds the distance between the buccal and palatal surfaces. Note larger buccolingual width of the MBR as compared with the DBR. (3) Buccal view. (4) Cross section through root trunk displaying flat mesial surface and slight buccal concavity of developmental depression. (Note rhomboid shape and wider mesial aspect.) (5) Cross section through furcation. Note root form, position of roots to one another, and trifurcation. Proximal surfaces of the MBR and the DBR are all flat or concave.

B, Maxillary First Premolar. (1) Mesial view. (2) Distal view. Both surfaces display developmental depressions in the root; however, the mesial surface has a DD that extends onto the gingival third of the crown, and the entire DD is more accentuated. The buccal and palatal roots are very similar in form and basically rounded. (3) Cross section through the cementoenamel junction. Note DD on mesial surface only. (4) Cross section through midroot area. Note the more accentuated DD on mesial surface; but a DD is present on the distal surface at this level.

C, Mandibular Molar. (1) Buccal view. Generally the mesial root has a greater curvature and a greater buccolingual width than the distal root. (2) Lingual view. (3) Cross section through the root trunk. Note the concave mesial and rounded distal root surfaces. (4) Cross section through the furcation, displaying the concave nature of the roots within the furcation chamber. This also depicts the entrances to the chamber as narrower than the chamber itself. (From Casullo, D., and Matarazzo, F.: The preparation and restoration of the multi-rooted tooth with furcation involvement. Philadelphia, Cont. Dent. Ed., University of Pa., 1977.)

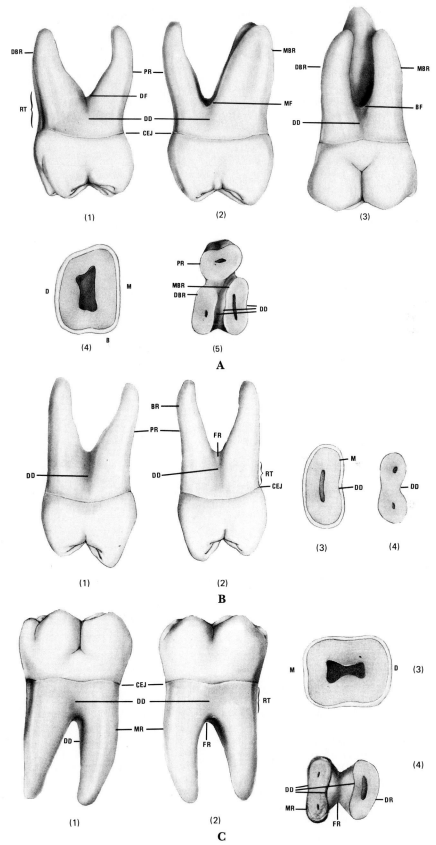

FIGURE 12–16 *See legend on opposite page*

friable. In Position 3, the exposure of the anatomic root, with its irregular surfaces, produces an abrupt and disharmonious architecture conducive to greater plaque retention and possible reinitiation or acceleration of periodontal disease and root caries. If such teeth are further compromised by pulpal disease and root canal therapy, their preparation and restoration become extremely complex and demand an understanding of integrated therapy. Specifically, it is in Positions 2 and 3 that the preparation and restoration of the multirooted tooth and furcation involvement clearly demonstrate the need for a multidisciplinary approach to treatment (Fig. 12–16).

Classification of Furcation Involvements

Furcations are classified according to the extent of bone loss, as evidence by the degree of horizontal penetration (probing) into the chamber (Fig. 12–17): (1) *Class I*—up to 1.5 mm of penetration; (2) *Class II*—more than 1.5 mm of penetration, usually up to 4 or 6 mm; and (3) *Class III*—complete penetration.

Since the range of measurements of horizontal penetration defining a Class II furcation is rather extensive, and thus nonspecific, the more shallow probings will indicate an "incipient" Class II furcation (1.5 to 2.5 mm) or a moderate furcation (2.5 to 4

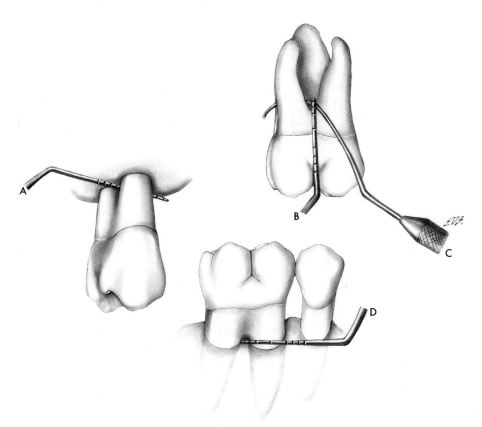

FIGURE 12–17   Three-Dimensional Evaluation of the Furcation Area. *A,* Periodontal probe in place evaluating the depth of the furcation chamber. In this instance, a through-and-through Class III furcation exists. This kind of probing also serves as the basis for classifying furcations periodontally. *B,* Periodontal probe measuring the height of the furcation chamber. It is measured from the roof of the furcation (2.5 mm mark) to the junctional epithelium (not shown). *C,* Nabers probe entering the buccal furcation and exiting the distal furcation. This instrument is specifically designed for exploring the depth of a furcation and in this case depicts a Class III. Because of its shape, it can easily enter mesial or distal furcations with an adjacent tooth present. *D,* Periodontal probe assessing the width of the furcation chamber, which is the distance between the roots. It is an important consideration in developing an optimal interradicular area. (From Casullo, D., and Matarazzo, F.: The preparation and restoration of the multi-rooted tooth with furcation involvement. Cont. Dent. Ed., Vol. 1, No. 1, Philadelphia, University of Pa., 1977.)

mm), and the deeper probings (4 to 6 mm) will indicate a "severe" Class II furcation.

The Class III complete penetration, known as a through-and-through furcation involvement, is assessed clinically by probing and radiographically by its relative radiolucency. Periodontal probing into the furcation is problematic when the furcation is located in a malposed or rotated molar, especially in maxillary teeth. Thus, great care and expertise are needed to obtain an accurate location and assessment.

Another criterion used to help categorize furcations is relative radiopacity. Class I displays a normal degree of radiopacity, Class II may show a diminished degree of radiopacity, and Class III usually manifests a radiolucency.

Evaluation of the Furcation Area

A thorough clinical and radiographic examination of tooth and root anatomy is made, since anatomic form will largely determine the outline of the tooth preparation and the need for tooth sectioning, root removal, and a final restoration. At times, surgical exploratory procedures may be needed to substantiate tentative conclusions, e.g., the extent of periodontal defects, aberrant furcation anatomy, fused roots, fractures, and perforations.

The evaluation begins with the gingival third of the crown and proceeds with all remaining tooth structures encased in the periodontium. The following assessments are made:

1. *Root trunk*—assessment of length and configuration and of the extent of developmental depressions and involutions. (These anatomic factors are assessed clinically and radiographically.) There is a positive correlation between the length of the root trunk, the degree of root divergence, and the spatial dimensions of the furcation chamber. Root divergencies are less severe with a longer root trunk. There is a negative correlation between the length of the trunk and the length of the roots. The longer the root trunk, the farther marginal tissues can migrate apically without exposing the furcation. However, when the furcation is finally exposed in such a tooth, retention of the short roots is questionable and tooth sectioning becomes problematic.

2. *Roots*—evaluation of width (the amount of root structure), location of root depressions and involutions, proximities (relative position of roots of the tooth with those of adjacent teeth), degree of flaring (convergencies and divergencies), and fused roots. These anatomic factors are assessed both clinically and radiographically.

3. *Spatial dimensions of the furcation*—evaluation of the depth, height, and width of the furcation itself. The depth, or horizontal component, of penetration into the furcation chamber provides the basis for the periodontal classification of furcations. The amount of tooth structure exposed coronally (e.g., the roof of the furcation chamber) is an important criterion for the elimination of Class I and Class II (incipient and moderate) furcation involvements by restorative therapy. These spatial dimensions are not the only criteria for assessing one's ability to lessen or eliminate furcation involvements. Height, the vertical component, indicates the degree of bone loss in an apicocoronal direction, applicable primarily to Class II and Class III furcations. Width, or interradicular space, the lateral component, indicates the distance between the roots, which varies according to the particular root configuration. The depth of the furcation chamber is ascertained clinically, whereas the height and width of the chamber, relative to the alveolar bone and adjacent roots, are determined clinically and radiographically.

4. *Location of the furcation*—determination of the location of a furcation by the position of the roots and by the location of its opening. In the maxillary molar teeth, there are three furcation openings: (1) mesial, located two-thirds the distance from the buccal to the palatal surfaces, (2) distal, located midway between the buccal and palatal surfaces, and (3) buccal, located midway between the mesial and distal surfaces. In the mandibular molar teeth, there are two furcation openings: the buccal and the lingual, both located midway between the mesial and distal surfaces. Maxillary furcations, especially mesial and distal, are not readily accessible and therefore complicate tooth preparation and sectioning. Certain cases may require an exploratory flap procedure in order to ascertain the true

relationship between the opening to the furcation and the bone loss around the affected roots.

5. *Gingival architecture*—evaluation of sulcular depth and width, relative thickness of soft tissue, and configuration and location of marginal tissues by clinical examination.

6. *Osseous topography*—assessment of infrabony defects and the position of the osseous crest relative to the roof of the furcation as significant determinants of the adequacy of the embrasure space. Vertical probings must be executed separately for each root to determine the osseous architecture around the individual root.

Goals of Treatment

Treatment of the multirooted tooth with furcation pathology involves a multidisciplined approach. The goals of periodontal therapy are especially relevant, since the practitioner must first improve the periodontal climate before the tooth itself can be prepared and restored. In the management of furcation problems, an initial provisional restoration may be necessary to control the periodontal problem. The goals of treatment are as follows: (1) to restore the mutually protective capacity of the tooth and the periodontium via the establishment of a healthy relationship between the tooth and its gingival and osseous structures; (2) to create a harmonious physiologic occlusion that provides the maximal distribution of occlusal forces; and (3) to maintain health by preventing, eliminating, or minimizing the accumulation of bacterial plaque and debris.

Restoration of Choice

The only restoration that can effectively change the anatomy of an exposed furcation, and thereby alter its influence on health and disease, is the full-crown retainer. This is the restoration of choice based upon its ability: (1) to control, by means of tooth preparation, the entrance of the furcation either by totally eliminating the furcation involvement or by at least minimizing it; (2) to cover the exposed root structure, which is highly susceptible to caries and sensitivity; (3) to establish coronal contours that are conducive to maintenance of gingival health, passively filling and smoothly exiting from the epithelialized gingival sulcus; (4) to modify the occlusal scheme in order to control force direction and dissipation; and (5) to correct deformities in esthetic appearance.

In order to accomplish these treatment goals, the marginal finish line must be placed within the gingival sulcus just short of the junctional epithelium.

Management of Class I and Incipient Class II Furcations

The primary goal of treatment is to eliminate all undercut and cul-de-sac areas that collect plaque and debris. The accomplishment of this goal begins with tooth preparation, which removes the roof of the furcation chamber and establishes a smooth, and continuous surface extending from the base of the furcation to the occlusal aspect of the preparation as well as in a lateral direction (mesiodistally or buccolingually). Because of the minimal amount of tooth structure in this gingival third (e.g., Position 2 or 3), a chamfer or featheredge finish line is used (Figs. 12–18 and 12–19).

Although the gingival architecture is aberrant, the finish line of the tooth preparation that is executed below the soft tissue must follow the configuration of the soft tissues and available tooth structure. The finish line usually rises (coronally) in the furcation area and extends down (apically) on the root surface.

Two common errors associated with the final restoration, overextending and overcontouring, are easily avoided. The crown contour must follow the outline circumscribed by both the marginal tissues and the remaining prepared tooth structure (Fig. 12–20).

Management of Moderate Class II, Severe Class II, and Class III Furcations Without Sectioning

Most moderate and severe Class II furcations can only be minimized, not eliminated, precluding optimal treatment and prognosis. The problems associated with moderate and severe Class II furcation involvements are more exaggerated (Fig. 12–21) than those of Class I because of greater apical migration of the marginal tissues and deeper horizontal probings. Exposure of the furcation chamber, involutions, root conver-

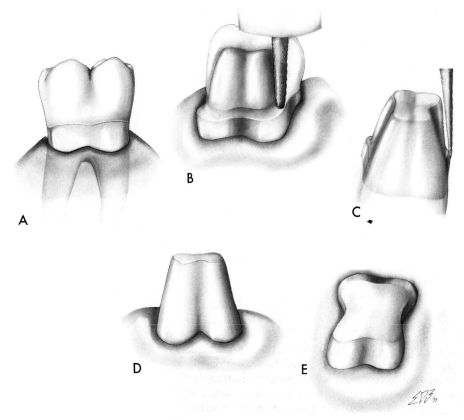

FIGURE 12–18 **Mandibular Molar Preparation. A,** Class I furcation involvement with 2 mm of exposed root surface. **B,** Placement of a shoulder following occlusal reduction. **C,** Removal of the shoulder with a thin tapered diamond stone (210-10P). Note that the point dissects away the shoulder and is within the confines of an area once occupied by tooth structure, thereby minimizing soft tissue laceration. **D,** Buccal view of the final preparation. Note buccal barreling of the furcation to accommodate the interradicular papilla and to eliminate any undercuts in the furcal area. **E,** Occlusal view displaying concave surfaces that mimic the root surface configuration. (From Casullo, D., and Matarazzo, F.: The preparation and restoration of the multi-rooted tooth with furcation involvement. Cont. Dent. Ed., Vol. 1, No. 1, Philadelphia, University of Pa., 1977.)

gencies, root divergencies, aberrant root form, and root surface anomalies are also more severe. More extensive coronal preparation is required to remove tooth structure that impedes access to the furcation area and the roots. Furthermore, the increased exposed spatial dimensions of the furcation chamber (depth, width, and height) make total removal of the chamber roof more unlikely.

The final tooth preparation requires excessive reduction of the coronal aspect of the tooth in order to gain access to the undercut furcation areas and the divergent roots. Upon completion, the finish line established is a featheredge (because of the diminished amount of tooth structure between the outer surface of the root and the root canal) and

terminates at the roof of the chamber and on the lateral root surfaces.

Because of the inconsistent nature of furcation involvement in both Class II and Class III cases, the extent of preparation (barreling) into the furcation to eliminate or to lessen the furcation involvement can be determined only during the actual clinical procedure. Clinical judgment determines the amount of the furcation involvement that can be eliminated relative to the sequelae that may ensue. For example, in barreling deeply into the furcation area, the clinician may decide to stop and accept the remaining furcation involvement or to continue and section the tooth and perform root canal therapy at that time. If the tooth is not sectioned, it usually has a tortuous,

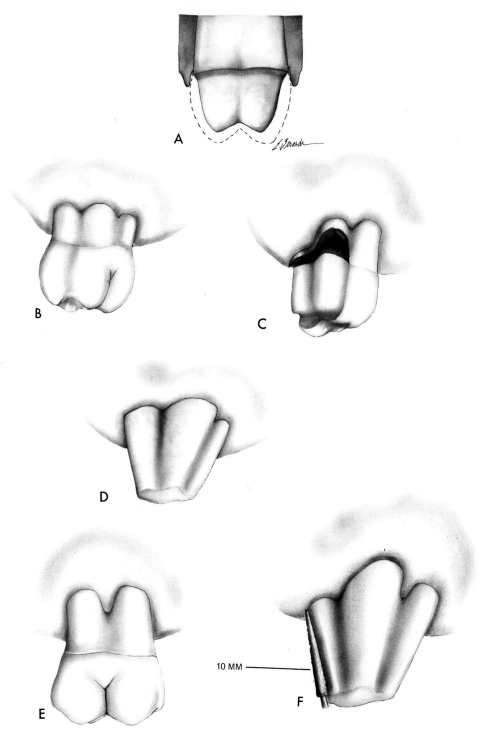

FIGURE 12–19 Tooth Preparation of the Maxillary Molar. *A,* A large chamber or shoulder preparation, which is appropriate for teeth with the marginal tissue at the CEJ (Position 1). ***B,*** Maxillary molar; Class I furcation; soft tissue at Position 2. ***C,*** Placement of a shoulder just above the gingival margin consistently following the gingival outline. ***D,*** Final preparation, after subgingival removal of the shoulder. Note the preparation of the developmental depression. ***E,*** Class II furcation; soft tissue at Position 3. Note increased root and furcation exposure. ***F,*** Final preparation showing an increased concavity into the furcation to remove the furcation roof and eliminate the furcation problem. Note the diamond stone, in place, which is used for subgingival preparation and removal of all coronal tooth structure that may cause undercuts. Also note the smooth, flowing taper (occlusoapically) in the barreled furcation area. (From Casullo, D., and Matarazzo, F.: The preparation and restoration of the multi-rooted tooth with furcation involvement. Cont. Dent. Ed., Vol. 1, No. 1, Philadelphia, University of Pa., 1977.)

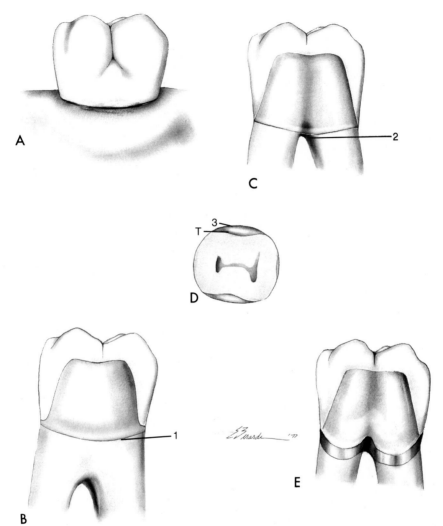

FIGURE 12–20   Restoration of the Mandibular Molar With Class I and Class II Furcations. *A,* Mandibular molar with anatomic crown and clinical crown equal. ***B,*** Restoration relative to the preparation for this tooth. Note preparation with a beveled chamfer finish line. Restoration is uncomplicated and follows the gingival contour, which is a smooth and continuous arc (1). ***C,*** Preparation of the tooth with furcation pathology showing a common mistake of overcontour and overextension of the restoration into the furcation area (2). Laboratory and clinical mistakes can be attributed to following the restorative concepts for the tooth with equal anatomic and clinical crowns. ***D,*** Occlusal view through the trunk of the tooth demonstrating the margin of the restoration (3) extending away from the tooth and trapping the soft tissue (T). ***E,*** Restoration for Class II or Class III unsectioned molar displaying a concavity in the furcation area to allow room for the interradicular tissue. Note the rise and fall of the margin at the furcal area. (From Casullo, D., and Matarazzo, F.: The preparation and restoration of the multirooted tooth with furcation involvement. Cont. Dent. Ed., Vol. 1, No. 1, Philadelphia, University of Pa., 1977.)

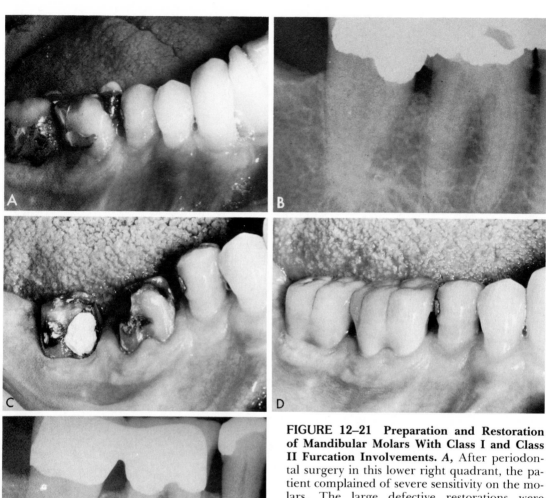

FIGURE 12–21 Preparation and Restoration of Mandibular Molars With Class I and Class II Furcation Involvements. *A,* After periodontal surgery in this lower right quadrant, the patient complained of severe sensitivity on the molars. The large defective restorations were influential in the initial periodontal disease process. The soft tissue and attachment apparatus have been repositioned 3 to 5 mm apical to the CEJ, thus exposing the root trunk of the second molar and the incipient Class II furcation on the first molar. Note the plaque accumulation on these root surfaces. *B,* This radiograph shows intact attachment apparatus, subgingival calculus, and large defective amalgam restorations. The furcation area of the first molar is radiopaque, giving no indication of the incipient Class II involvement. *C,* The teeth were prepared for full-crown restorations in order to recreate normal crown contours, prevent recurrent caries, and manage the sensitivity. Note the flat and concave preparation (barreling) in the furcation area. *D,* The final restorations support the marginal tissue and establish smooth, consistent crown contours as they exit the sulcus. Note the rise and fall of the tissue and the accommodation of the interradicular soft tissue in the furcation area. *E,* Radiograph of the final restorations in place.

long outline form, making final restoration quite complex. The marginal area is extremely undulating and lengthy, and the furcation area must be contoured to house the interradicular soft tissue. When furcation involvement is so extreme as to preclude optimal conventional treatment, tooth sectioning or root removal or both may be indicated.

Management of Furcations by Tooth Sectioning

Unwarranted Use of Tooth Sectioning

Management of the severe Class II or the Class III furcation with sectioning involves a great deal of treatment: endodontic therapy,* tooth sectioning, and root removal in addition to complicated tooth preparation, placement of posts, and fabrication of splinted units with or without telescopes. At times, such extensive treatment is not warranted or possible. This might be true in the following situations: (1) when the requisite treatment is considered excessive relative to the severity of the problems associated with the furcation (in other words, the prognosis for the tooth is good, and further breakdown is judged to be a remote possibility, as in the case of a stable, vital tooth with tight, healthy tissue in the furcation area); (2) when vertical osseous resorption is minimal and the soft tissues are healthy and fill the furcation area, preventing food impaction and plaque accumulation in the furcation area; and (3) when short roots of a multirooted tooth would be unstable when restored or would possibly be extracted during restorative procedures.

In such cases, the clinician is aware of the potential problems of an exposed furcation and makes a decision based on sound clinical judgment. The decision not to section these teeth must be based on evaluating the tissue response to a metal band and acrylic provisional restoration for a period of time. If sectioning is required, it can be executed at the re-evaluation stage of treatment. If it is not required, the furcation is managed with conventional preparation and the tooth is restored with a full crown.

---

*Endodontic treatment is done before tooth sectioning to facilitate both procedures. Gutta percha is the required root-canal filling material.

Contraindications for Tooth Sectioning

Tooth sectioning and root removal procedures may be contraindicated from the outset. This would occur (1) when endodontic therapy is not feasible, (2) when roots are fused or convergencies are extreme, (3) when inadequate tooth structure remains, (4) when the patient is unwilling or uncooperative (poor oral hygiene), and (5) when the patient lacks the requisite finances.

Indications for Tooth Sectioning

The exposure of furcations and root irregularities in the severe Class II and the Class III furcation so compounds the number, type, and extent of problems associated with involved teeth that tooth sectioning and root removal are often the treatment of choice. The combined restorative and endodontic or exodontic techniques with periodontal concepts are directed at enhancing the overall prognosis of a compromised area. The reasons for sectioning a tooth are:

1. *Control of severe caries.* Caries penetrating into the furcation may be controlled by splitting the tooth and treating each segment individually. However, extensive caries on only one root has to be handled by means of the removal of the affected root and the restoration of the remaining root or roots (Fig. 12–22).

2. *Furcation accessibility for self-maintenance.* The tenets of plaque control can be practiced effectively only when the patient has access to all areas of teeth exposed to the oral environment. Severe furcation involvements are unique situations in that although the patient has access to and through the entrance, it is almost impossible to débride the internal walls of the chamber mechanically because of the chamber's anatomic configuration. The result is the creation of a depository for debris and bacterial plaque, which eventually result in further periodontal breakdown or furcation caries. To allow for patient self-management, tooth sectioning is usually the only practical solution (Fig. 12–23).

3. *The benefits of strategic extraction.* Extraction of a portion of a sectioned tooth may be the treatment of choice when the periodontal involvement of an individual root jeopardizes a contiguous tooth or other roots of the same tooth. Expeditious root removal may allow for

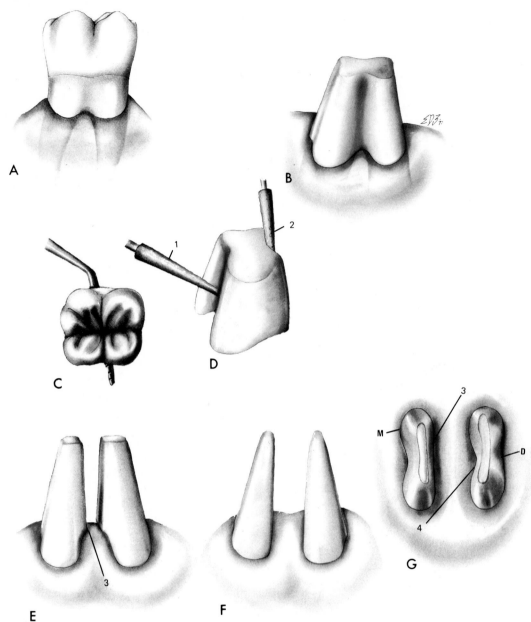

FIGURE 12–22   Hemisection of Lower Molar. *A,* Mandibular molar with Class II furcation. Note greater exposure of the root surface. *B,* Final preparation. *C,* Class III furcation with probe in place. *D,* Thin, pointed diamond stone (1) in place probing furcation entrance to begin sectioning procedure. Once the cut is begun gingivally, the bur is placed upright and moved through the furcation (2). *E,* Completion of the cut through the furcation, which leaves a lip of tooth structure. This represents the remainder of the furcation roof (3). *F,* Buccal view of the final preparation displaying a newly created embrasure, removal of the lip of tooth structure, and the flat proximal surfaces. *G,* Occlusal view of the sectioned mandibular molar displaying a form consistent with the anatomic cross section. The proximal concavity within the furcation should be removed as shown (3) to allow for greater width of the embrasure space mesiodistally and to create an entrance to the chamber as wide as the chamber itself. In certain instances this is not always possible and the entrance may remain narrower (4). (From Casullo, D., and Matarazzo, F.: The preparation and restoration of the multi-rooted tooth with furcation involvement. Cont. Dent. Ed., Vol. 1, No. 1, Philadelphia, University of Pa., 1977.)

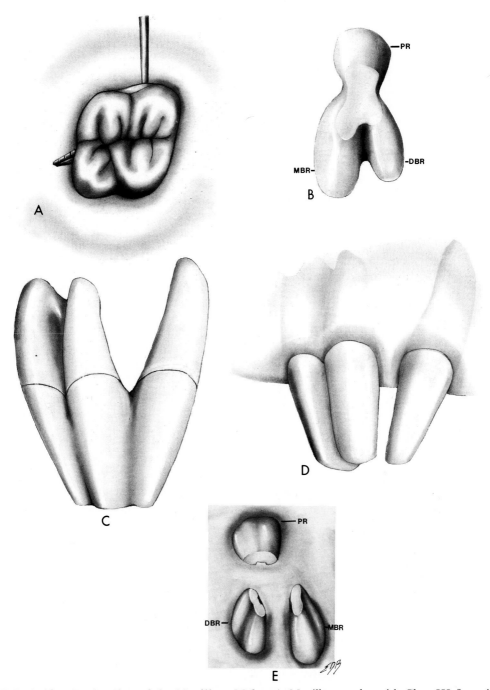

FIGURE 12–23   Hemisection of the Maxillary Molar. *A*, Maxillary molar with Class III furcation. *B*, Preparation of an unsectioned maxillary molar with extensive Class II or Class III furcations. Note the extensive barreling into the furcation and the relative positions of the roots as they relate to the remaining crown structure. *C*, Distal view of the preparation with a feather-edge finish line creating a smooth transition to the root. *D*, Buccal view of the sectioned maxillary molar. *E*, Occlusal view of sectioned maxillary molar.

Key. PR, Palatal root. MBR, Mesiobuccal root. DBR, Distobuccal root. (From Casullo, D., and Matarazzo, F.: The preparation and restoration of the multi-rooted tooth with furcation involvement. Cont. Dent. Ed., Vol. 1, No. 1, Philadelphia, University of Pa., 1977.)

maximal conservation of the interdental bone and obviate the necessity for surgical correction of the periodontal defect. In a high proportion of patients, the surgery required to eliminate an isolated infrabony region may actually result in substantial bone removal from adjacent roots (see Fig. 12–26).

4. *Management of the endodontically compromised situation.* Roots with untreatable canals owing to calcification, broken instruments, or perforations are removed, and the remainder of the tooth is preserved and restored to health.

5. *Control of interdental embrasure.* Tight root proximities are common sequelae of advanced periodontal disease and present a number of obstacles in the restoration and maintenance of the ensuing embrasure. In the case of proximate upper roots (e.g., the distobuccal root of the first molar and the mesiobuccal root of the second molar), removal of one of the roots will usually alleviate the problem, whereas in the lower molar roots, tight root proximities may be treated either by root removal or by root separation with orthodontic therapy in order to widen the interdental or interradicular areas.

Tooth Preparation for Sectioning Roots

The first step in sectioning multirooted teeth is to prepare the tooth as for a full crown. This preparation should precede tooth sectioning in order to arrive at an informed decision that a tooth with a severe Class II or Class III furcation must be sectioned. When sectioning is the original decision, the full-crown preparation is executed to gain access to the furcation, to visualize the root form, and to maintain stability of the roots. The actual tooth sectioning is executed with a thin diamond stone to preserve the remaining root structure and to avoid overcutting the roots. The roots should be completely separated with the diamond stone, not cut halfway and then wedged apart with a surgical elevator. This wedging technique can result in unpredictable separation and root fracture. Following the complete separation of the roots, the interradicular surfaces are prepared to widen the newly created embrasure space (Figs. 12–22 and 12–23).

Restoration of Sectioned Roots

The goal of separating or removing roots is to establish an embrasure space conducive to periodontal health and resistant to dental caries. The clinician is attempting to recreate a discrete entity of the remaining root(s) by transforming the furcational area into an embrasure space that will provide smooth crown contours and adequate room for healthy interdental tissues. The optimal embrasure space must be created by gaining adequate length and width during tooth preparation and restoration. The width of

FIGURE 12–24 Preparation and Restoration of the Mandibular Molar for the Treatment of Dental Caries. *A,* The removal of the crown from this mandibular first molar revealed caries extending to the crestal bone in the furcation area. An exploratory surgical procedure was performed to aid in a decision on treatment of the tooth and its individual roots. It was decided that the roots could be saved with minimal osseous surgery, hemisection of the molar, and restoration of both molars with new full-crown restorations. ***B,*** The left preoperative radiograph demonstrates the extensive dental caries approaching the interradicular osseous crest. The right radiograph was taken during the surgical procedure to evaluate the remaining sound tooth structure after hemisection. The surgical procedure, hemisection, and provisional restoration were completed in one visit. ***C,*** The final healing of the periodontal tissues after surgery and tooth preparation demonstrates soft tissue health and adequate embrasure spaces for the advanced restorative therapy. ***D,*** The final restorations consisted of telescopes with posts and an overcase of porcelain on gold. Telescopes with posts cast as one integral unit were used for maximum retention to replace lost tooth structure and to provide a smooth, even path of insertion of the final restoration. ***E,*** The telescopes in place. Note gingival health. ***F,*** Final porcelain-to-gold restoration. ***G,*** The left radiograph shows the fitting of the post into the roots of the hemisected molar canals. This is a critical and demanding procedure owing to minimal amounts of tooth structure and aberrant root anatomy. The right radiograph shows the final restoration 1 year postoperatively.

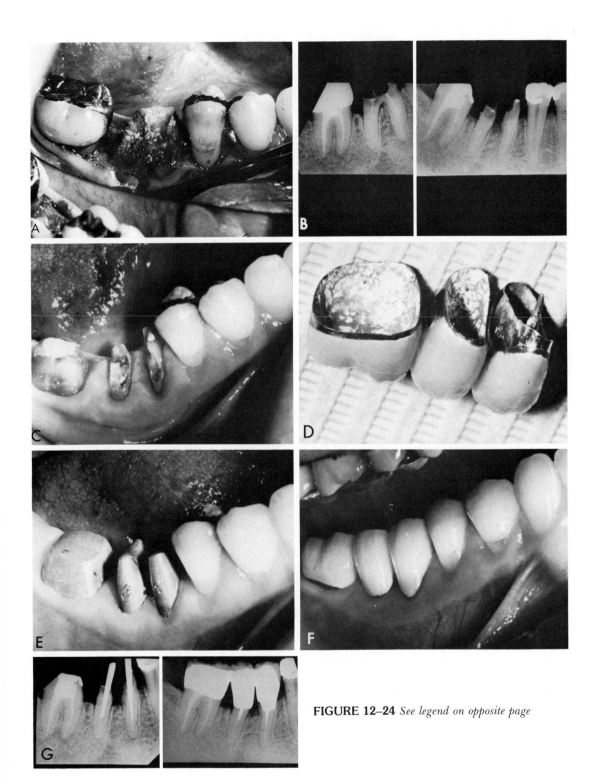

FIGURE 12–24 *See legend on opposite page*

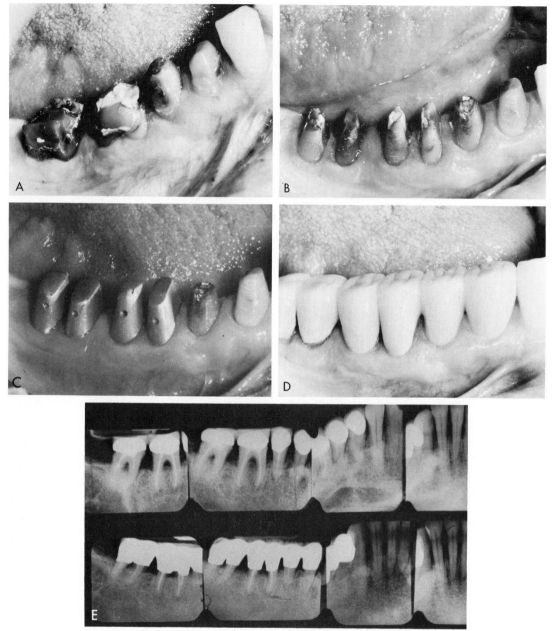

FIGURE 12–25   Preparation and Restoration of the Hemisected Mandibular Molar for the Treatment of Periodontal Disease. *A,* Full-crown restorations were removed from these mandibular posterior teeth. There were through-and-through Class III furcations on both endodontically treated molars. Periodontal and restorative therapy consisted of scaling, root planing, and hemisection of both molars, followed by full-crown restorations. *B,* The final tooth preparations set up a series of premolars with the interradicular space converted to embrasure spaces. *C,* Telescopes were placed on the molar roots to compensate for the irregular and nonparallel root surfaces as well as to protect the root canal–treated roots. Note gingival health. *D,* The final restoration is set up as a series of premolars with embrasure spaces adequate for cleaning but not wide enough to allow lateral food impaction. *E,* The preoperative radiographs (top) show the radiolucent areas associated with Class III furcation involvements. Note the interradicular space of the first molar is wider mesiodistally than that of the second molar. Therefore, the new embrasure space is more accessible in the first molar area. The postoperative radiographs (bottom) show the final restoration of the hemisected molars.

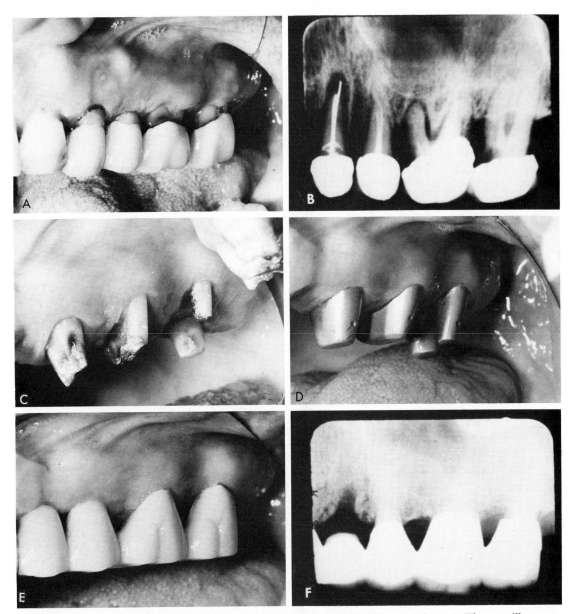

FIGURE 12–26 Preparation and Restoration of Hemisected Maxillary Molars. A, The maxillary posterior quadrant exhibits severe periodontal disease demonstrated by 7- to 10-mm pocket depth, Class III furcation involvements, and secondary occlusal traumatism. **B,** The preoperative radiograph demonstrates failing and inadequate root canal therapy, ill-fitting restorations, advanced periodontal disease, radiolucencies in furcation areas, and extensive root caries. Periodontal therapy consisted of scaling, root planing, home care, open-flap curettage and strategic root removal, and stabilization with a provisional restoration. **C,** The hopelessly diseased mesiobuccal roots of the first and second molars were extracted. The distobuccal and palatal roots of the first molar were left intact, and the palatal and distobuccal roots of the second molar were sectioned. The final tooth preparation of the remaining molar roots and second premolar demonstrates the healed soft tissue, wide embrasure spaces, and root relations. **D,** The final fixed prosthesis included telescopes, which were placed to protect the remaining roots and to provide parallelism. Note gingival health. **E,** The final restoration in place. **F,** The postoperative radiograph demonstrates healing of the attachment apparatus, new embrasure spaces, and relations of remaining roots.

the newly created embrasure is established by adequate proximal tooth preparation and a restoration with flat or concave transitional line angles and proximal surfaces. The length required for an adequate embrasure space can be attained by raising the contact area of the restoration coronally.

The two roots of the mandibular molars are aligned with each other and with other roots and teeth in the quadrant, forming a smooth, continuous arch. The sectioned roots resemble a series of bicuspids and can accommodate a pontic when required.

In the maxilla, there are three roots creating a multitude of alternatives in restoring sectioned or removed roots. The palatal root is not in line with the rest of the teeth in the arch, thus complicating the problem of crown contours and pontic placement. If the palatal root is extracted, the maxillary teeth or roots mimic a lower molar in shape if unsectioned, and if sectioned, behave as two premolars. If the palatal root remains and one of the buccal roots is extracted, pontics are not indicated because of minimal space available and because of the potential for blocking the remaining roots.

Outline of Occlusal Table

All occlusal tables should be designed to direct forces through the long axis of the remaining roots. If the missing root is in direct line mesially and distally with other abutments, then the occlusal table can be maintained consistent and continuous. However, if the palatal root alone remains, it may be advisable to restore the tooth in crossbite and accept the lower buccal cusps out of occlusion. On the other hand, if the palatal root is missing, then the occlusal table should be narrowed and should occlude primarily with the lower buccal cusps (Figs. 12–24 to 12–26).

The multitude of factors and the complex interplay among the various dental disciplines required in the management of multirooted teeth with furcation involvements demonstrates the need for a multidisciplinary approach for successful therapy. The relationship among the various dental disciplines, especially as one can affect the other, must be understood to avoid unwarranted therapy and possible tooth loss. The value of strategic extraction and the complex nature of periodontal and pulpal disease are specific areas that must be understood for successful management of teeth with furcation involvements.

STRATEGIC EXTRACTION

The goal of strategic extraction is maximal preservation of the periodontium (attachment apparatus). Strategic extraction is based on the judgment that the extraction of a root or tooth is indicated for the correction of a localized problem while *enhancing the long-term prognosis* of the entire dentition.

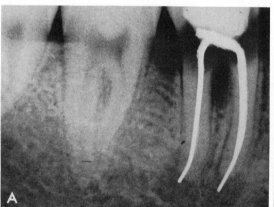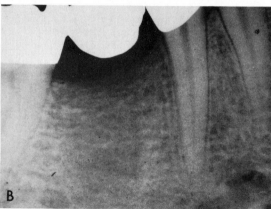

FIGURE 12–27 Strategic Extraction for the Treatment of Dental Caries. *A,* A 20-year-old patient presented with pain and swelling in the mandibular first molar area. Clinically, the internal aspects of the roots were decayed owing to the breakdown and corrosion of the exposed silver points. Surgical procedures were considered too extensive relative to the amount of involvement of adjacent supporting structures. *B,* The tooth was extracted, the bony socket healed, and the supporting bone on the adjacent teeth was preserved. A three-unit bridge was fabricated.

Active disease can result in a severe, isolated defect involving a single tooth. Common examples of such defects are (1) unresolvable infrabony periodontal defects, resulting from periodontal disease or combined pulpal and periodontal disease; (2) severe decay extending below the osseous crest, resulting from long-standing caries (Fig. 12–27); and (3) exposed root proximities and furcations, resulting from periodontal disease. The management of such cases may require treatment that compromises ad-

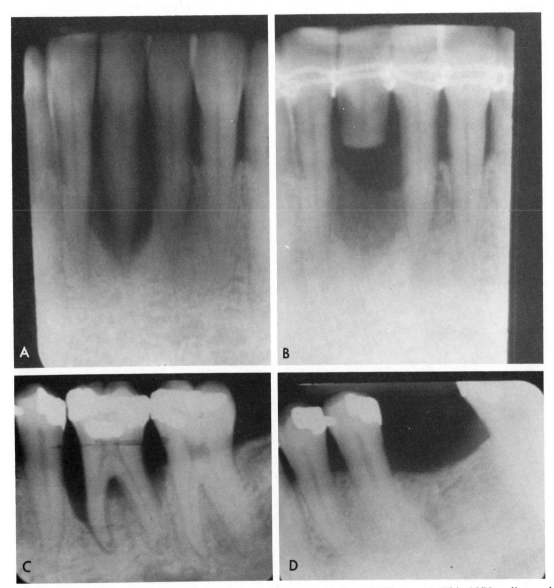

FIGURE 12–28   Strategic Extraction Due to Advanced Periodontal Disease. A, This 1979 radiograph of the left central incisor shows the total loss of attachment apparatus. Clinical periodontal probings confirmed the radiographic picture of bone loss and verified the loss of the labial and lingual plate of bone. **B,** After wire and acrylic ligation of the crown to the adjacent teeth, the root was extracted to allow healing of the attachment apparatus of the adjacent incisors. This 1-year postoperative radiograph shows the healing of the extraction site extending from the adjacent incisors. **C,** This radiograph of the mandibular first molar, obtained from the previous treating dentist, was taken in 1973. **D,** This 1980 radiograph demonstrates the healing and maintenance of the attachment apparatus. The patient is still undergoing Hawley bite plane and periodontal therapy.

Illustration continued on following page

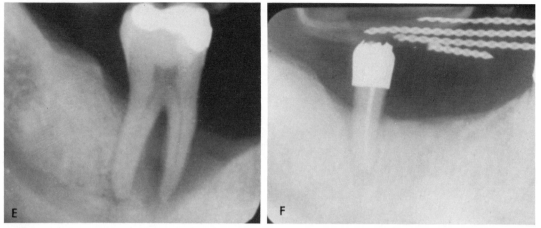

FIGURE 12–28 *Continued* **E,** This radiograph of a lone-standing mandibular second molar demonstrates severe bone loss on all surfaces of the mesial root. The distal root appears to have adequate bone remaining. It was decided to perform endodontics on the distal root, remove the mesial root, and stabilize the distal root with a metal band and acrylic provisional restoration. **F,** This postoperative radiograph was taken 8 months after stabilization in order to re-evaluate the distal root as an abutment for a fixed restoration. Note the healing and favorable prognosis. The final restoration is to be placed.

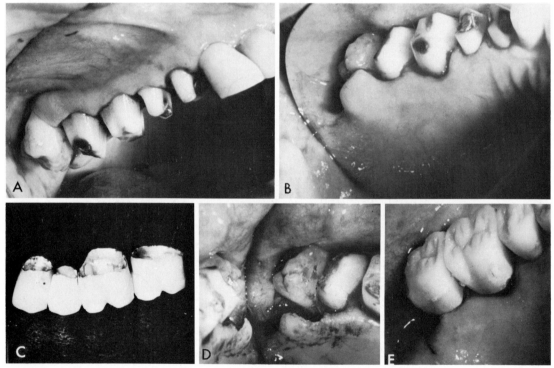

FIGURE 12–29 Strategic Extraction of a Third Molar—Concomitant Restorative and Periodontal Therapy. **A,** The maxillary third molar was retained throughout initial adjunctive orthodontic and periodontal therapy. **B,** The palatal view shows excessive tissue in the tuberosity area that must be reduced to prevent a deep periodontal pocket at the distal aspect of the second molar. **C,** The gold band and acrylic provisional restoration was completed prior to starting the periodontal management of the third molar. **D,** An internal beveled incision was employed to reduce the excessive soft tissue prior to extraction of the third molar. At the time of stabilization with a fixed gold band and acrylic provisional restoration, the third molar was extracted and the soft tissue sutured to cover the tuberosity area. **E,** The provisional restoration was cemented after suturing the soft tissue in place.

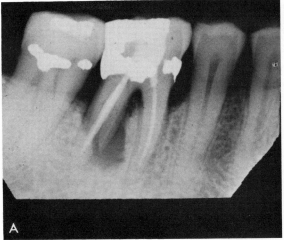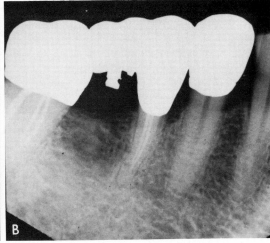

FIGURE 12–30   Strategic Extraction for the Treatment of a Fractured Root. *A,* A long-standing distal root fracture of the mandibular first molar has resulted in isolated and extensive breakdown of the attachment apparatus. The remaining osseous structure is intact and will respond well to therapy. It can be predicted that when the distal root is extracted, the bone will fill in from the osseous crest on the mesial surface of the second molar to the distal aspect of the mesial root of the first molar. *B,* The distal root was extracted and the osseous structure healed as predicted.

jacent structures. Extraction of the involved root (of a multirooted tooth) or of the tooth is a procedure that *predictably* leads to the healing of the pocket and periodontally involved contiguous structures. Therefore, in the long run, strategic extraction may be the more conservative approach to therapy.

To make the appropriate decision, the clinician must first assess the following factors: (1) the extent and severity of the disease process and the defect; (2) the potential of the disease process or the defect or both to destroy adjacent tissues (Fig. 12–28); (3) the extent, complexity, and cost of treatment required to reverse the disease process or correct the defect or both; and (4) the potential of requisite treatment, especially osseous surgery, to create deformities, including exposure of root surfaces and furcations and disruption of occlusal stability and function.

These data must be carefully studied and analyzed in relation to the importance of the involved tooth or root as an individual entity and in relation to the rest of the dentition. This includes a consideration of its esthetic function, its contribution to occlusal stability and function (especially masticatory efficiency), and its role as an abutment at the time of evaluation or in the future; the amount of attachment apparatus that can predictably be regenerated after extraction and healing; and the conservative nature of

the surgical procedure, which does not compromise contiguous structures.

Strategic extraction is the treatment of choice when the clinician can determine that the surgical removal of a root or tooth will improve the long-term, overall prognosis of the entire dentition. Strategic extraction is also indicated for hopeless teeth, that is, teeth that present with defects that no form of therapy can ameliorate. This usually means teeth or roots with root canals destroyed by vertical fractures, perforations, or extensive root resorption (internal or external) (Figs. 12–29 and 12–30).

PULPAL AND PERIODONTAL DISEASE: DIFFERENTIAL DIAGNOSIS AND TREATMENT

Thus far, this chapter has focused on the interrelationship between restorative dentistry and the periodontium, specifically the gingival tissues and the marginal crest of bone. The focus of the following section is the attachment apparatus, with special emphasis on the differential diagnosis between periodontal and pulpal disease and on the destruction of the attachment apparatus wrought by communicating periodontal and pulpal disease.

First, one must address the question of differential diagnosis. Primary periodontal disease can cause secondary pulpal involvement. Conversely, primary pulpal disease can cause secondary periodontal involvement. Signs of the secondary disease process can easily be mistaken for signs of the primary disease process. Consequently, the differential diagnosis of periodontal and pulpal disease is often problematic.

An accurate diagnosis of disease is critical for determining the proper treatment and sequence of therapy. When a diagnosis is premature or incorrect, unnecessary treatment might be rendered, and failure to execute the requisite treatment will result in the perpetuation and possible exacerbation of the primary disease process and deformity. However, with the systematic collection and interpretation of appropriate clinical and radiographic data, the diagnostic process is greatly facilitated. Communicating periodontal and pulpal disease can involve a single tooth. Initially, the diseases may be discrete entities, but owing to the progressive nature of both disease processes, communication eventually occurs. This communication increases the virulence and destructive potential of both diseases, resulting in the acceleration of the breakdown of the attachment apparatus and in extreme bone loss. However, the situation is not hopeless, and such teeth need not be condemned to extraction. The reversal of the disease processes, reformation of normal anatomy, and restoration of the teeth are possible. The key to the successful management of such cases is establishing an accurate diagnosis, since the diagnosis dictates the requisite treatment and proper sequence of therapy.

Classification of Disease

Periodontal disease and pulpal disease (as primary and secondary disease processes) have been divided into five classes:

Class I, Division I: Pulpal involvement (transient hyperemia, pulpitis, and partial necrosis).

Class I, Division II: Pulpal disease (total necrosis).

Class II: Pulpal disease with secondary periodontal involvement (total necrosis with isolated destruction of the attachment apparatus).

Class III: Periodontal disease (periodontitis).

Class IV: Periodontal disease with secondary pulpal involvement (periodontitis or occlusal traumatism *or both* with transient hyperemia or pulpitis).

Class V: Communicating pulpal and periodontal disease (total necrosis with periodontitis or occlusal traumatism or both).

Table 12–1 outlines the significant signs and symptoms associated with each class along with the treatment procedures usually indicated to resolve each problem. As such, the table is a valuable tool for differential diagnosis and treatment planning.

Pulpal disease is caused by an interference with cellular metabolism or with vascular supply. This can result from extensive caries, excessive occlusal forces, traumatic injury, or exposure of the dental tubules.

Class I, Division I

With a Class I, Division I pulpal involvement (hyperemia or pulpitis), the tooth exhibits sensitivity to cold and responds erratically to the electric pulp test. Radiographically, no periapical radiolucency is apparent, although there may be evidence of a widened periodontal ligament space and loss of definition and continuity of the lamina dura around the root, which are signs of occlusal traumatism.

Because the results of the pulp test are erratic and therefore unreliable and because the tooth responds to cold, the clinician must proceed cautiously with treatment, making the assumption that the condition is, in fact, reversible. This means using the most conservative and reversible approach to therapy to manage any recognizable local etiological factors. Restorative treatment may be instituted to eliminate occlusal interferences. (Interferences can occur when the tooth is extruded as a result of inflammation of the periapical tissues secondary to the pulpal involvement.)

The status of the tooth is monitored after treatment. An irreversible pulpitis or necrosis can occur at any time during or after therapy. The confined and limited pulpal tissue cannot tolerate constant traumatic or inflammatory insult; thus the disease process cannot always be arrested and necrosis avoided. If signs and symptoms persist, endodontics may be required.

TABLE 12–1.   Classification of primary and secondary periodontal and pulpal disease according to signs and symptoms and standard treatment

Class	Division	Disease Entity and Definition	Tooth Vitality	Hot	Cold	Sensitivity Percussion	Pain	Pockets	Radiographs	Calculus	Standard Treatment
I	I	Pulpal involvement or disease (transient hyperemia, pulpitis, or partial necrosis)	Response to pulp test is erratic	No	Yes	Yes	Erratic (can be severe)	None	No periapical radiolucency	No	Restorative dentistry and/or selective grinding; possible endodontics
I	II	Pulpal disease (total necrosis)	Nonvital	Yes	No	Yes	Erratic (can be severe)	None	Isolated, lateral, or periapical radiolucency	No	Endodontics only
II	II	Pulpal disease with secondary periodontal involvement (total necrosis with isolated destruction of the attachment apparatus)	Nonvital	Yes	No	Yes	Erratic (can be severe)	Sinus track, fistula, or blowout (extensive)	Isolated, lateral, or periapical radiolucency from apex to sulcus	No (possible minimal deposits)	Endodontics only; possible minimal periodontics
III		Periodontitis	Vital	No	Yes	No	No	Moderate	Moderate bone loss from crest down	Yes	Periodontics only
IV		Periodontal disease with secondary pulpal involvement (periodontitis and/or occlusal traumatism with transient hyperemia or pulpitis)	Vital (but response to pulp test may be erratic)	No	Yes	Yes	No (except during an acute exacerbation)	Extensive	Extensive bone loss from crest down, approaching or beyond the apex with or without signs or generalized occlusal traumatism	Yes	Periodontics only; possible selective grinding and/or endodontics
V		Communicating pulpal and periodontal diseases (total necrosis with periodontitis and/or occlusal traumatism)	Nonvital	Erratic	No	Yes	Erratic (can be severe)	Extreme	Extreme and diffuse bone loss	Yes	Endodontics, periodontics, and occlusal therapy (stabilization via selective grinding and/or restorative dentistry)

Class I, Division II

Depending on the severity, duration, and frequency of the particular etiology, hyperemia or pulpitis can lead to pulpal necrosis, classified as Class I, Division II pulpal disease. The Class I, Division II is differentiated from the Class I, Division I when the tooth tests nonvital, shows no response to cold, and displays a radiolucency that may be isolated or diffuse, lateral or periapical. The radiolucency is confined by bone in the attachment apparatus, emanating from the apex and extending coronally along the root, sometimes into the furcation area of a multirooted tooth. Treatment is straightforward, involving routine root canal therapy.

Class II

When pulpitis or pulpal necrosis is left unattended, suppurative and toxic materials build up and create pressure on the surrounding tissues. This results in the passage of these materials through the periapical foramen, the accessory canals if present, and the dentinal tubules into the attachment apparatus, by which they escape to the oral cavity via the path of least resistance in the alveolar bone or periodontal ligament, causing destruction of the attachment apparatus. This condition is classified as Class II pulpal disease with secondary periodontal involvement.

Destruction of the bone is evidenced clinically by periodontal probing, suppuration, and swelling. Radiographically, injury to the attachment apparatus is manifested by a periapical radiolucency that is isolated to the involved tooth and diffuse in nature. The depth and width of probings, the extent of suppuration, the degree of radiographic diffusion, and the configuration of the radiolucency vary. There are three basic periodontal defects: (1) fistula pointing into the mucobuccal fold, (2) sinus track, and (3) "blowout."

Fistula Pointing into the Mucobuccal Fold. The most common Class II defect is a fistula pointing into the mucobuccal fold. Swelling is evident in this area or on the lingual or palatal aspect of the tooth. The radiolucency emanates from the apex and extends coronally along the root, but generally not beyond its midpoint. Since the marginal bone and sulcus are completely intact, there are no significant periodontal pockets; therefore, differential diagnosis is not difficult. The problem is endodontic in nature, so routine root canal therapy alone is indicated.

Sinus Track. Destruction of the attachment apparatus can create an isolated, narrow sinus track that extends from the apex to the sulcular area. Probing reveals an intact sulcus that ends abruptly and leads into the sinus track, which can extend to the

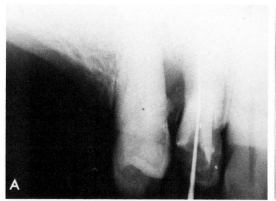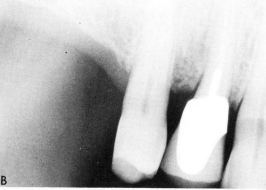

FIGURE 12–31 Class II Pulpal Disease With Secondary Periodontal Involvement. *A,* This radiograph of the maxillary first premolar demonstrates a severe periodontal defect on the distal surface. The pocket probed 10 mm on the direct distal surface, the tooth tested nonvital, and the remaining dentition was periodontally intact. Treatment was approached cautiously to see if the periodontal defect was of pulpal origin (Class II pulpal disease with secondary periodontal involvement). ***B,*** The postoperative radiograph demonstrates complete healing following endodontic and minimal periodontal therapy (closed scaling and root planing). Complete periodontal healing occurred in 12 weeks. (In conjunction with Gerald Weger, Philadelphia, Pa.)

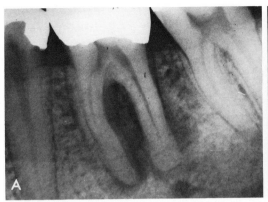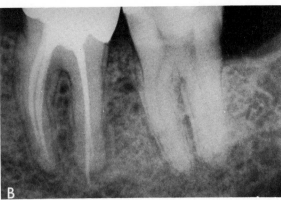

FIGURE 12–32 *A,* The bone loss about the lower molar extends from the apex of the tooth to the furcation area. Clinically, there was swelling in the mucobuccal fold, acute suppuration, and extensive periodontal probing into the furcation area. The lesion, therefore, appeared to be a periodontal problem (Class III), but the large restoration, the isolated nature of the defect, and the nonvital status of the tooth led to a diagnosis of pulpal disease with secondary periodontal involvement (Class II). *B,* Only endodontic therapy was performed. One year later, the tissues have healed completely, and the periodontal ligament space and lamina dura are well defined. (Endodontic therapy by Dr. Irwin Freedman, Haddonfield, N.J.)

apex of the root. Periodontal probing usually reveals the defect to be 1 to 2 mm in width. Depending on the width of the track and its position relative to the roots, the periapical radiograph may show destruction of the attachment apparatus along the lateral aspect of the root.

Root canal therapy, along with scaling and root planing to eliminate plaque and calculus deposits, is instituted as soon as possible. Generally, this type of lesion closes and heals quite dramatically in 1 to 2 weeks. If resolution of the problem fails to occur, as evidenced by continued suppuration and bleeding, open-flap curettage may be indicated to remove calculus that may have extended into the defect.

Blowout. Pulpal disease has the potential to destroy a considerable amount of the attachment apparatus, including the cortical plate of bone, resulting in a "blowout." Periodontal probing indicates a rather wide osseous crater and detachment of the junctional epithelium and connective tissue. The radiographs confirm the clinical findings. Because this condition is usually acute, suppuration is extensive.

Conservative treatment and a well-organized sequence of therapy are crucial in the management of blowouts. Routine root canal therapy in conjunction with scaling and root planing to remove calculus and plaque should promote maximal healing, obviating the need for periodontal surgery (Figs. 12–31 and 12–32).

Because bone loss is considerable, the healing period usually extends 3 to 6 months, during which time any soft tissue inflammation must be controlled. If periodontal disease persists, as evidenced by pocket depths, suppuration, and bleeding, surgery may be required. Premature surgery can destroy tissue that might otherwise have the capacity for regeneration.

Class III

The primary etiology of Class III periodontitis is microbial toxins. The progression of disease depends on the dynamic interplay of all local etiologic factors and the resistance of the individual patient. Inflammation results in bone loss on the periosteal side of the alveolus and in the interdental crest of the alveolus.

The destruction of the attachment apparatus is manifested radiographically by a radiolucency that emanates from the marginal crest and extends apically along the root. The clinical signs of Class III periodontitis include extensive pockets, minimal mobility, plaque and calculus deposits, gingival recession, and soft tissue inflammation and edema. Treatment involves appropriate periodontal therapy according to the severity of the disease.

Class II pulpal disease with secondary periodontal involvement (sinus track and blowout) can be mistaken for Class III periodontitis. This is especially true when the periodontitis involves a developmental anomaly of the attachment apparatus, such as a cervical enamel projection, a palatogingival groove, or an enamel pearl, which creates an environment conducive to the initiation and progression of periodontal disease. When periodontal disease is associated with these anomalies, the defect is isolated and circumscribed, thus mimicking a fistula, sinus track, or blowout secondary to pulpal disease.

In order to differentiate between Class II pulpal disease and Class III periodontitis, it must be recognized that the configuration of the infrabony defect is different. In Class II pulpal disease, the defect is wider at the apex; in Class III periodontitis, it is wider at the crest. Another factor in distinguishing between Class II pulpal disease and Class III periodontitis, is tooth vitality. In Class II pulpal disease, the tooth tests nonvital, whereas in Class III periodontitis, the tooth tests vital.

The treatment of routine, generalized Class III periodontitis is standard, comprising scaling and root planing. However, when the periodontitis is limited to a single tooth associated with a developmental anomaly, treatment becomes more complex. First, it is imperative to make the correct diagnosis, recognizing that the defect is periodontal and *not pulpal*. This point cannot be overemphasized. The basic problem is of periodontal origin; thus, root canal therapy is contraindicated.

Management of a deformity associated with a cervical enamel projection, a palatogingival groove, or an enamel pearl involves periodontal therapy only. The anomaly is removed by odontoplasty, whereas plaque, calculus, suppuration, and inflammation are controlled with definitive scaling and root planing. The prognosis is contigent on the location, configuration, and dimensions of the anatomic deformity and on the relative depth of its extension into the attachment apparatus. If the defect is severe and long-standing, the pulp may eventually become necrotic, and root canal therapy is then required. However, it must be recognized that the endodontic treatment rendered will not resolve the periodontal defect.

Class IV

Periodontal disease can cause inflammation of the pulp—hyperemia, or pulpitis, a condition classified as a Class IV periodontal disease with secondary pulpal involvement. The periodontal disease is defined as periodontitis or occlusal traumatism or a combination of the two disease processes. The periodontitis, however, is more advanced than in the Class III situation, manifested clinically by extreme mobility, by more extensive pocket probings, and by tenacious calculus adhering to root surfaces.

When the radiographic signs associated with occlusal traumatism with secondary pulpal involvement (widened periodontal ligament space, loss of continuity of the lamina dura, and root and osseous resorption) are manifested at the apex of the root, Class IV periodontal disease can be confused with Class I, Division II pulpal disease or with Class II pulpal disease. But teeth with pulpal disease test nonvital, frequently have large restorations, and manifest isolated radiographic signs of occlusal traumatism (Fig. 12–33).

The suppuration, pocket probings, and bone loss characteristic of Class II pulpal disease with secondary periodontal involvement, Class III advanced periodontitis, and Class IV periodontitis with secondary pulpal involvement can complicate diagnosis. Differential diagnosis, however, need not be problematic. Unlike Class IV periodontitis with secondary pulpal involvement, Class II pulpal disease with secondary periodontal involvement involves a nonvital tooth in an environment in which signs of generalized periodontitis are absent. Class IV periodontal disease with secondary pulpal involvement must also be distinguished from Class III periodontitis. With a Class IV disease process, the tooth exhibits sensitivity to percussion as a result of pulpal inflammation and radiographically manifests bone loss approaching the apex.

With Class IV disease, the most conservative treatment is employed, aimed at the elimination of local etiological factors. This includes scaling and root planing and occlusal adjustment (selective grinding, Hawley bite plane therapy, nightguard therapy, or stabilization), when indicated. Frequent evaluations during and after a healing period of 3 to 6 months are required to monitor the status of the pulp. Constant traumatic or inflammatory insult can so compromise the pulp that necrosis will result, necessitating root canal therapy. This complication can develop at any point during or after treatment.

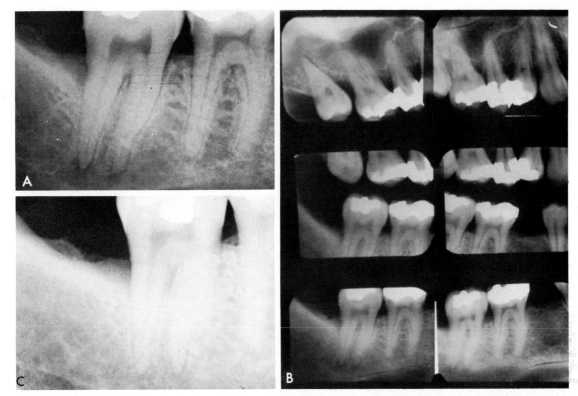

FIGURE 12–33   Class IV Periodontal Disease With Secondary Pulpal Involvement. *A,* This periapical radiograph of a mandibular second molar shows radiolucencies on both roots, calculus near the cementoenamel junction, and an hourglass configuration of the periodontal ligament on the mesial root. The clinical symptoms were sensitivity to cold and percussion. The tooth tested vital. *B,* Full-mouth radiographs were taken, because it was important to survey the entire dentition and to identify all etiologic factors in establishing a correct diagnosis. The films show severe occlusal trauma associated with the maxillary third molar and a periapical radiolucency on the mandibular second molar. Because the radiographic picture of pulpal necrosis can be similar to that of occlusal trauma, further diagnostic tests were conducted. The mandibular molar tested vital and was not sensitive to heat. In addition, these two terminal teeth were involved in a protrusive and nonworking interference. The diagnosis was periodontitis with severe occlusal traumatism (Class IV). The treatment consisted of scaling and root planing, occlusal adjustment, and Hawley bite plane therapy. *C,* This single periapical radiograph shows a close-up view of the healing of the periapical radiolucencies associated with occlusal traumatism (24 months postoperatively).

Class V

When concomitant pulpal disease and periodontal disease (periodontitis with occlusal traumatism) are severe and of long duration, they may communicate, producing an accelerated disease process with extensive destruction of the attachment apparatus. The resultant deformity is known as an "endo-perio" lesion (see Fig. 12–37). This lesion is evidenced radiographically by a single, extremely diffuse defect, showing generalized bone loss from the marginal crest extending apically and from the apex extending coronally. Clinically, periodontal probings are extreme, approaching or moving beyond the apex of the root, and mobility is severe.

Because progression of the disease process is so advanced, the prognosis is questionable. The clinician must determine whether an attempt should be made to salvage the involved tooth. This decision is based on patient desires and on the strategic importance of the tooth.

Root canal therapy is initiated first. Then, periodontal therapy (scaling, root planing, and curettage) and occlusal therapy (selective grinding and stabilization via temporary splinting in conjunction with a Hawley bite plane) are instituted. Stabilization is important to support questionable, periodontally weak teeth and to manage extreme mobility.

The healing period ranges from 2 to 6 months. Frequent evaluations are made to determine whether favorable osseous changes have occurred, whether mobility has decreased, whether soft tissue inflammation has been controlled, and whether undetected complications, such as root fractures, have become evident. Each root of molar teeth is assessed individually.

If a periodontal defect associated with a single root of a multirooted tooth has not healed, tooth sectioning and root removal may be indicated. Strategic extraction, which promotes the maximum regeneration of the osseous tissue by socket healing, may be the treatment of choice. Root removal is also appropriate because a periodontally and endodontically involved root has the potential to jeopardize the viability of contiguous roots in the same tooth or in adjacent teeth. Routine periodontal therapy (scaling and

root planing) is usually precluded by inaccessibility and in any case would not be likely to resolve the problem. Osseous surgery often results in a substantial amount of bone removal from adjacent roots and thus constitutes excessive treatment for an isolated defect. Root removal eliminates the deformity while retaining an optimal amount of osseous structure.

Anatomic Considerations
Structures Relevant in Differential Diagnosis

The cervical enamel projection, palatogingival groove, and enamel pearl are all developmental anomalies of the teeth that can contribute to the initiation and progression of periodontal disease. They are of importance in the differential diagnosis between the periodontal defects resulting from pure Class III periodontitis or Class IV periodontal disease with secondary pulpal involvement, and those resulting from pulpal

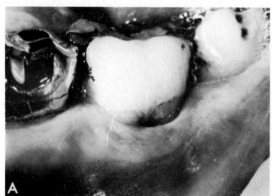

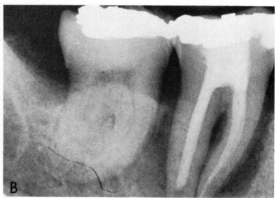

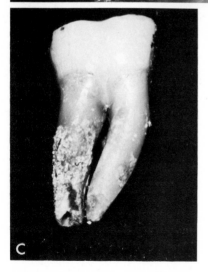

FIGURE 12–34   Cervical Enamel Projection. A, A 54-year-old patient presented with a history of recurrent abscesses associated with the mandibular second molar. Periodontal probing in the furcation area revealed a cervical enamel projection associated with 10-mm pocket depths, heavy subgingival plaque, and calculus. **B,** Endodontics had been completed on this tooth 4 years previously. The radiograph revealed a severe periodontal lesion, poor root canal therapy, and osseous and root resorption. The tooth was extracted. **C,** The extracted tooth demonstrates the cervical enamel projection extending from the CEJ to the furcation area, extensive calculus accumulation, and root resorption at the apex. (Courtesy of Dr. Murray Rabinowitz, Seattle, Wash.)

disease causing secondary periodontal involvement (Class II).

A cervical enamel projection is an enamel structure that extends apically into the furcation area of multirooted teeth. It usually occurs on mandibular molars and creates a nidus for plaque and calculus, increasing the likelihood of the initiation of periodontal disease. Moreover, because the cervical enamel projection is covered by junctional epithelium instead of connective tissue fibers, the periodontium is less resistant to microbial toxins (Fig. 12–34).

A palatogingival groove is an invagination of the root, usually found in maxillary incisors, especially lateral incisors. It originates

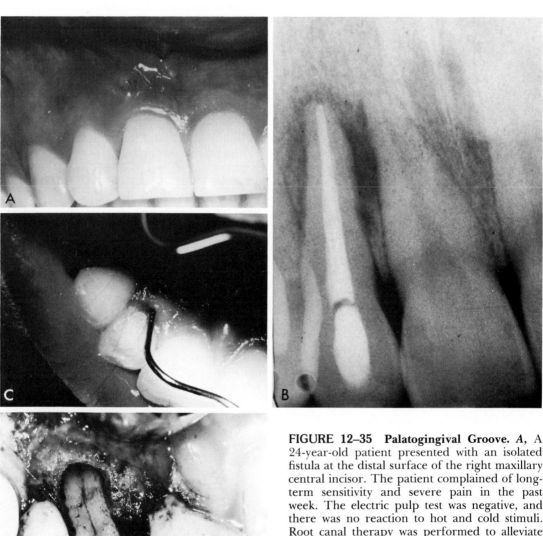

FIGURE 12–35 **Palatogingival Groove.** *A,* A 24-year-old patient presented with an isolated fistula at the distal surface of the right maxillary central incisor. The patient complained of long-term sensitivity and severe pain in the past week. The electric pulp test was negative, and there was no reaction to hot and cold stimuli. Root canal therapy was performed to alleviate the patient's symptoms. *B,* The single periapical radiograph shows a radiolucency extending along the mesial lateral surface of the lateral incisor. *C,* Periodontal probing revealed a severe 10-mm defect on the palatal aspect of the lateral incisor as well as a palatogingival groove. *D,* A surgical exploratory procedure was executed to visualize the extent of the groove. It extended the length of the root. An attempt was made to reshape the root surface. The fistulous tract persisted for a long period of time after these procedures. Therefore, the tooth was scheduled for strategic extraction followed by fabrication of a provisional restoration. (Courtesy of Drs. Willis Cardot and Richard Kaufman, Philadelphia, Pa.)

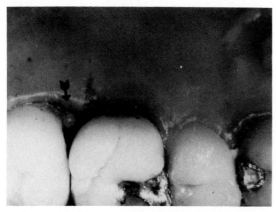

FIGURE 12–36 Enamel Pearl. Enamel pearl at the mesial aspect of CEJ (arrow) of the second molar is associated with isolated periodontal disease. Treatment consists of odontoplasty to remove the enamel pearl and conventional periodontal therapy.

in the cingulum area and extends apically, sometimes along the entire length of the root. The palatogingival groove compromises the integrity of the junctional epithelium and especially the connective tissue attachment to the root surface. This results in increased plaque and calculus accumulation and increased susceptibility to periodontal disease (Fig. 12–35).

An enamel pearl is an enamel structure usually located on the lateral root surface below the cementoenamel junction. This aberrant topography provides a site for plaque and calculus to collect, making the development of periodontal disease more likely (Fig. 12–36).

Structures Relevant in the Healing Capabilities of Tissues

The vascular supply to the pulp and periodontium has a major impact on the healing capabilities of these tissues. The pulp derives its vascular supply primarily from a limited number of capillaries, whereas the vascular supply of the periodontium comes from a broad network of anastomosing vessels that communicate with major vessels throughout the alveolar bone. The blood vessels of the periodontium are larger and more numerous than those entering the pulp. Because of its extensive vascular supply, the periodontium can survive disease better and respond more readily to treatment than can the dental pulp.

In general, when pulpal disease affects the periodontium, the secondary periodontal problem is reversible, whereas when periodontitis and occlusal traumatism affect the pulp, the secondary pulpal problem is usually irreversible. However, the likelihood for resolution of a secondary disease process is naturally dependent on the severity and duration of the primary disease process and its effect on the specific tissues.

Structures Relevant in the Communication of Disease

The periapical foramen, dentinal tubules, and accessory canals all are passages or openings that connect the dental pulp and periodontium. Capillaries arising in the alveolus in the apical area of the tooth travel from the periodontal ligament, through the periapical foramen, where they enter the pulp. When the vascular supply to the pulp is destroyed, owing to a pulpitis or necrosis, the patent foramen becomes a portal for toxic elements to pass to the attachment apparatus.

When periodontal disease or therapy results in the apical repositioning of the periodontium, the exposure of root surfaces, and the loss of cementum, dentinal tubules become exposed, and contact is established with the external environment. Plaque, saliva, and microbial toxins can now be transported to the pulp. This often elicits a pulpal response and tooth sensitivity. (Dentinal tubules rarely, if ever, communicate disease from the pulp to the periodontium.)

Accessory canals are developmental anomalies located along the root surface and in furcation areas. They arise during root formation, when blood vessels traverse the epithelial root sheath and enter the papilla. Absence of accessory canals is not unusual, as growth of the epithelial diaphragm can obliterate the vessels. Accessory canals are patent pathways with the capacity to communicate disease from the pulp to the periodontium or to communicate disease from the periodontium to the pulp.

RESTORATION OF THE ENDODONTICALLY TREATED TOOTH

In the restoration of the endodontically treated tooth, the goal of treatment is to re-establish lost tooth structure and the self-protective capacity of the tooth in an effort to prevent fracture and the recurrence of disease. The restoration should be accomplished with the most logical, simple, and predictable treatment procedures, keeping in mind that overinstrumentation can result in unwarranted tooth loss. There are a myriad of restorative options available: amalgam, cast partial coverage restorations, full crowns, telescopes, posts, posts and cores, tooth-lengthening procedures, and adjunctive orthodontics. Unfortunately, the mechanical factors of retention have been overemphasized and are frequently considered the first priority in the restoration of the endodontically treated tooth. This is especially true of posts and cores, in which numerical guidelines of length and prefabricated shapes have been established as the main criteria for their use.

Restorative treatment of the endodontically treated tooth must be based on sound clinical judgment and on assessment of all biologic, mechanical, and functional requirements of the individual tooth and the entire dentition as well as on the financial resources of the patient.

Considerations for Restorative Treatment

To select the most appropriate treatment, the clinician must recognize, understand, and interrelate anatomic factors, occlusal considerations, the extent and type of destruction wrought by disease, and patient resources. Anatomic factors include (1) the amount, shape, and width of remaining tooth structure; (2) the relationship of the periodontal gingival and osseous structure to the cementoenamel junction; (3) the exposure of roots, furcations, convolutions, and developmental depressions; (4) the size and configurations of roots (curvatures); and (5) the presence of accessory canals, cervical enamel projections, and palatogingival grooves.

Occlusal considerations include (1) the anterior tooth position and the role of the anterior teeth in supporting all protrusive and lateral-protrusive tooth-contacting movements and disarticulation of posterior teeth; (2) the posterior tooth position and the role of the posterior teeth in supporting the occlusal vertical dimension and being free of interference in all protrusive and lateral-

protrusive movements; (3) the presence of parafunctional forces; (4) the presence of interferences; and (5) the design and role of the final restoration in the dental arches.

The extent and type of destruction wrought by disease include (1) dental caries, periodontal disease, and pulpal disease that have been eliminated and their effect on the remaining tooth structure; (2) the injured and weakened periodontium and tooth structure that remains; (3) an evaluation of the healed disease process; and (4) an overall evaluation of the resistance of the patient to disease and of the future prognosis of the restoration.

It must be clearly understood that numerous factors influence the mechanical (restorative) phase of therapy. There are no absolute rules. Each tooth must be considered on its own and with the conditions present in the individual patient's dentition in mind. The restoration of the endodontically treated tooth will be discussed in view of the materials available and the factors that influence their use.

Operative Dentistry: Amalgam and Composite Resin

Routine operative dentistry may be employed on an endodontically treated tooth that is basically intact if dental caries has not destroyed marginal ridges or extensive amounts of tooth structure and if periodontal disease has not compromised the attachment apparatus, increasing the likelihood of fracture. The intact anterior tooth with a lingual access cavity usually requires placement of a prefabricated or cast post followed by a composite resin. A post is usually placed because during protrusive and lateral-protrusive tooth contacting movements, the anterior teeth receive horizontal, off-axis forces. The support gained from the post serves to protect the tooth from root fracture.

When an endodontically treated posterior tooth is structurally intact (only occlusal access has been made, with no unsupported tooth structure) and the occlusal scheme is favorable, with no off-axis forces associated with protrusive and lateral-protrusive tooth contacting movements, routine operative dentistry with an amalgam restoration may be the only treatment required.

Cast Partial Coverage Restorations

An onlay or three-quarter crown is usually the minimal restoration of choice for the endodontically treated posterior tooth that has been structurally compromised. There must be sufficient remaining tooth structure to satisfy the internal and external retentive needs of this restoration. The cast restoration enhances the resistance of the tooth to fracture, since it covers and protects all cusps, especially centric supporting cusps (palatal of the upper and buccal of the lower). The onlay maintains maximal tooth structure and preserves periodontal health via use of supragingival margins. When the tooth is essentially intact and the external tooth preparation is minimal, placement of a post could be executed easily if the occlusal forces and position in the dental arch require it.

If posterior teeth such as the maxillary first and second premolars help support lateral-protrusive movements (group function), thus receiving off-axis forces, the onlay must be designed with an adequate thickness of metal to protect the tooth from fracture and the restoration from flexure. Placement of a post is also indicated in this situation.

At times, partial coverage restorations are not the treatment of choice. The full-crown restoration is the preferred treatment when the patient is highly susceptible to caries or when the self-protective capacity of the soft tissue–crown interface has been lost because of root and furcation exposure or when excessive tooth structure has been lost. Additionally, if the attachment apparatus has been compromised extensively and if the teeth are mobile, splinting with full crowns may be required. Finally, cast gold, partial coverage restorations are not indicated on lower posterior teeth if the patient's appearance is a major consideration.

Full-Crown Restoration: Preparation, Post Consideration, and Final Restoration

A full-crown restoration is indicated when a minimal amount of tooth structure remains or when the alveolar bone and gingiva have migrated apically as a result of periodontal disease and treatment, and the self-protective capacity of the tooth–soft tissue interface has been lost. Repositioning of the marginal tissue exposes tortuous root morphology, complicating tooth and root preparation.

It is the external surface of the root, not only the clinical crown, that must be prepared for the restoration. The external surface of the root is exposed and is no longer protected by encasement in bone. Yet, preparation for a post involves the internal root surface. Although crown preparation is done on the external surface and post preparation is internal, both procedures involve the same structure, the root, and the limited dimensions and irregular form and shape of the roots complicate both operations. What appears to be an abundance of root structure actually represents dead space, the chamber of the root canal and furcation, obstructed from view by external root surfaces.

The amount and configuration of remaining tooth structure determine the extent and complexity of tooth preparation for the full-crown restoration. When the marginal tissues are repositioned apically, exposure of tooth and root surfaces does two things: (1) It functionally increases the length of the tooth and amount of tooth structure to be prepared, and (2) it confronts the clinician with a highly irregular, undulating, and unpredictable surface. Tooth preparation becomes more time-consuming and complex and requires sound clinical judgment. The finish line on the root should take the form of a chamfer or featheredge in order to preserve the maximal amount of remaining tooth structure.

This full-crown restoration is the most demanding and difficult to execute. Not only must it replace the excessive amounts of lost or prepared tooth structure, it must also reestablish crown contours that are conducive to optimal periodontal health and occlusal function.

Post and Cores

Perhaps the most critical aspect of restoring the root canal–treated tooth is whether or not to use a post and core. Often a post and core is absolutely essential to restore a tooth and allow it to function in its normal capacity. Yet, overzealous instrumentation and unwarranted use of the post and core can lead to total destruction of the tooth. The clinical decision to place a post and core requires the careful assessment of all anatomic, occlusal, and mechanical factors of the individual tooth and restoration.

Anatomic considerations for a post and core begin with the clinical assessment of the position of the marginal tissue and osseous crest. When the clinical crown and anatomic crown are equal, the periodontium is intact and the roots are encased in bone. External tooth preparation involves the anatomic crown and internal root preparation involves the anatomic root. At Position 1 (Fig. 12–15), a post would terminate in the middle one third of the root, which has the greatest bulk of root structure. All restorative procedures are straightforward and simple in this case.

When the marginal tissues have migrated apically (Position 2 or 3), disharmonious root architecture becomes exposed and more extensive loss of external tooth structure occurs, resulting in a more delicate and difficult situation. The internal and external root forms and shapes become more aberrant and unpredictable as loss of supporting structure increases. The clinician is faced with minimal root structure, extensive undercuts, depressions, and nonparallel roots. As the need for retention via post and cores increases, the risk of perforation and root fracture becomes greater.

Occlusal stability and function on an individual tooth or a complex restoration must be distributed evenly in all functional and parafunctional tooth-contacting movements. A post and core or splinted units are not substitutes for optimal occlusal relationships. In fixed prostheses, especially in cross-arch stabilization, terminal abutments must be protected from contralateral occlusal forces in functional and parafunctional movements.

When the attachment apparatus reforms and heals after extensive, long-standing pulpal and periodontal disease (Class II and Class V), the tissues (tooth and periodontal) are usually structurally weak and susceptible to disease. Placement of a post and core involves an additional risk. The instrumentation required to clean out the canal can result in the dislodgement of the apical or lateral seal. This loss of seal establishes communication with the external environment (oral cavity) and may induce the recurrence of a disease process, especially if accessory canals are present. Additionally, the already thin root structures may be weakened and eroded by the toxic products of disease. This structural damage could lead easily to fracture or root perforation.

Communicating pulpal and periodontal disease (Class V) (Fig. 12–37) is a good example of a disease process that has an enormous destructive potential, that involves a prodigious amount of therapy for healing and resolution, and that can break down at any time. The risk of disturbing this healed, quiescent environment with internal tooth preparation must be weighed in relation to the retentive and supportive needs of the restoration. Many times the clinician may have no choice but to be assertive in fulfilling these mechanical requirements in face of all the risk and possible damage that can occur with the use of a post and core.

Post and Core Fabrication

The post and core is a mechanical device that comes in many shapes, forms, and combinations of materials. The post helps prevent root fracture by internally reinforcing the tooth and root. It also provides for retention of the core, which replaces lost tooth structure, blocks out undercuts, and provides the body and parallel walls for the internal and external retention of the restoration.

Cast metal and wrought gold wire, in conjunction with a cast core, are the most reliable and durable materials available for post and core fabrication. Unstable materials, such as resin and amalgam, in conjunction with posts are inadequate in these tenuous situations.

The configuration of the post may be predetermined, or it may be determined by the individual requirements of the particular root anatomy. Use of predetermined posts may involve a prefabricated metal post, intended to be used with or without a core, or a post made from a plastic pattern and then cast with a core. In this case, the shape of the post dictates the shape of the canal. Most canals are irregular in shape, whereas prefabricated posts are uniform. Instruments and posts should not be forced into the canals, nor should canals be overinstrumented to provide for insertion of a post that represents the manufacturer's ideal but does not conform to the anatomic shape of the root canal. This increases the chance of tooth fracture and root perforation, especially when roots are narrow, root curvature is extreme, walls are thin or fragile, and access is difficult. Posterior teeth with aberrant root anatomy and minimal root structure should be approached with caution. Rarely should they be prepared to receive a prefabricated, preformed post.

Nevertheless, use of prefabricated, preformed posts can be routine in the restoration of maxillary anterior teeth. In the protrusive and lateral-protrusive movements associated with anterior tooth guidance, the maxillary anterior teeth are subjected to horizontal force application by the mandibular teeth. Since the maxillary anterior teeth have straight canals and an abundance of tooth structure, they can accommodate the manufacturer's predetermined post shape and size more readily, and the incidence of perforation is rare. But of even greater significance is that the root anatomy of maxillary anterior teeth can easily accommodate the placement of posts of maximal width and length, so the desired protection from occlusal forces and root fractures is optimal.

The individually shaped post or post and core may be made from a Duralay pattern

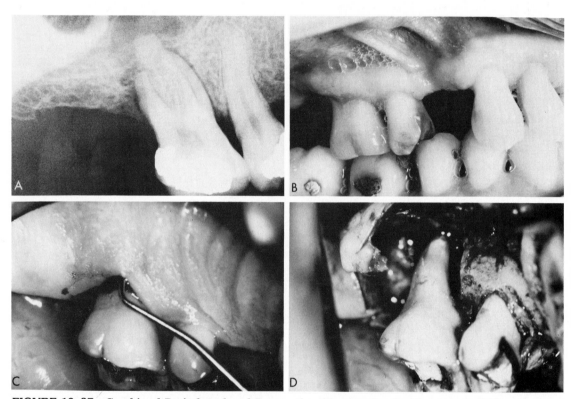

FIGURE 12–37   Combined Periodontal and Restorative Therapy for the Treatment of Class V Communicating Pulpal and Periodontal Disease. *A,* This radiograph of a maxillary terminal molar exhibits a widened periodontal ligament space, extended periapical radiolucencies, and severe bone loss. The patient presented with severe pain, swelling, and suppuration. Clinically, extensive subgingival and supragingival calculus, deep periodontal pockets, and a severe mobility (depressible tooth) were present. The tooth tested nonvital. The diagnosis was Class V, combined pulpal-periodontal disease with severe occlusal traumatism. The resultant prognosis was questionable. ***B,*** Clinically, only two posterior teeth support the vertical dimension of occlusion on the right side. It is extremely important to retain the involved maxillary terminal molar so that arch integrity can be restored and a fixed restoration can be placed. Each root of this tooth must be evaluated separately to arrive at the appropriate treatment decision. ***C,*** A periodontal probe is in place on the palatal root. It extends 10 mm, and both the mesial and the distal furcations have Class III involvements; the buccal furcation is not involved. The prognosis for the palatal root is hopeless, but the two buccal roots, especially the mesiobuccal root, have a favorable prognosis. The treatment will consist of scaling and root planing, stabilization with a bite plane, endodontics, palatal root removal, and a provisional splint, followed by re-evaluation after a 6-month healing period and final periodontal and restorative therapy. ***D,*** A palatal flap discloses the extensive destruction of the palatal plate of bone and a severe osseous crater in the furcation area. The bone on the palatal aspect of the buccal root is found to be intact on probing.

Illustration continued on opposite page

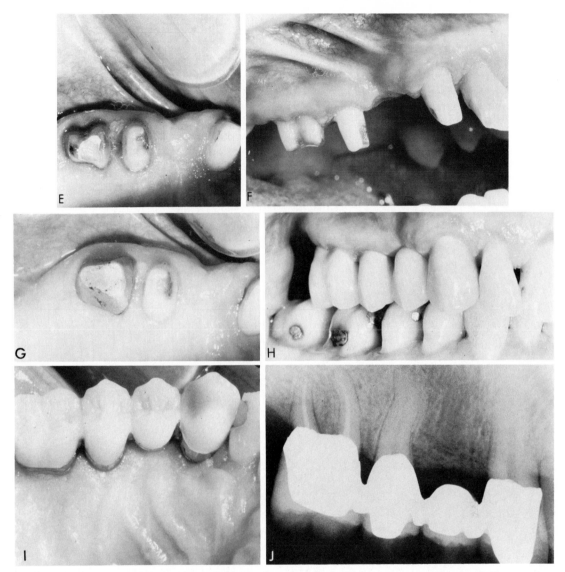

FIGURE 12–37 *Continued E,* After all planned periodontal therapy was completed, all disease processes reversed, and the mouth restored to health, the teeth were reprepared for the final restoration. The maxillary molar consisted of the two buccal roots; the outline form of the preparation mimics that of a lower molar. Note the flat mesial surface and barreling into the palatal and buccal furcation areas as well as the healing of the palatal tissue. *F,* The buccal view of the final preparation demonstrates the mesial inclination of the premolar and canine relative to the first molar. This results in a different path of insertion for the planned porcelain-to-gold restoration. *G,* This occlusal view of the molar reveals a telescope in place to protect the endodontically treated roots from fracture and to provide a smooth path of insertion for the final restoration. *H,* The final prosthesis is in place, maintaining arch integrity and helping to support the vertical dimension of occlusion. *I,* The final restoration is seen from the palatal aspect. *J,* The supporting bone has healed and the disease processes have been reversed. Because the pulp, periodontium, and occlusion are all intimately related via the attachment apparatus, radiographic signs of healing are important to consider when establishing a prognosis and evaluating the success of therapy. (Periodontic therapy by Dr. Albert Konikoff, Norfolk, Va.)

and then cast, or it may be an individually shaped wrought gold wire that is cast with a core. The form of the post is dictated by the form of the canals and the degree of reten-

tion required. Because of conformity in anatomic shape and size, insertion of the post should not present difficulties and should require only a minimal amount of preparation and instrumentation. Consequently, the individually shaped post is a relatively safe and conservative procedure, as the post is fabricated to fit the canal.

The individually shaped wrought gold wire is an excellent material for post fabrication. The wrought gold wire is specifically shaped to fit the individual canal and, once fitted, is never changed, thus avoiding the problem of dimensional stability seen with cast posts. The individually shaped gold wire is indicated for teeth with aberrant and poor root form, internal root undercuts, a minimal amount of root or tooth structure or both, or sectioned roots (Figs. 12–6 and 12–24).

Root Canal Preparation for a Post and Core

The preparation of the internal aspect of the roots for a post and core is routine and simple when the marginal tissue and osseous crest are at Positions 1 and 2. As the tissue is displaced apically (Position 3) and the external tooth preparation and the internal root preparation are on the same walls, extreme caution must be employed. Not only is the root structure minimal, but the aberrant root curvatures are involved in the preparation (Fig. 12–38).

The canal should be prepared first by removal of gutta percha with heated hand in-

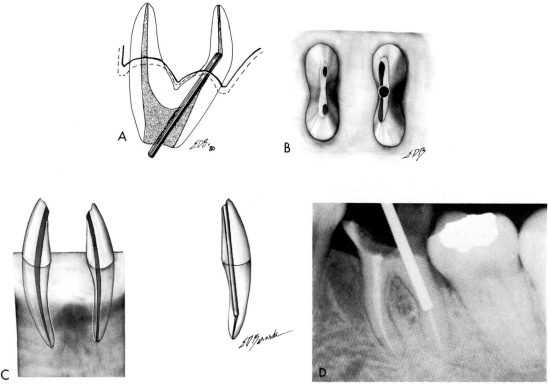

FIGURE 12–38 Molar Root Preparation and Post Fabrication. Post preparation and restoration of posterior teeth should be approached cautiously owing to unpredictable root anatomy. *A,* A narrow post is placed in a palatal root with accentuated curvature and form. The curvature on the buccal aspect and the thinness of the palatal aspect of this palatal root must be allowed for. *B,* Occlusal view of cross section of mesial and distal roots of a mandibular molar. The distal root is commonly used for post preparation and restoration. The middle of this root has a post placed in it. This is the area of the severest developmental depression. *C,* Buccal view of sectioned roots of a mandibular molar. The straight post in the curved distal root is shown. Note post proximity to the mesial external surface of the distal root. The developmental depression and root curvature are common anatomic forms for mandibular molar roots, and must be approached cautiously in post preparation. *D,* A radiograph of overpreparation of a distal root of a mandibular molar. The post approaches the external mesial root surface aspect at the middle one third of the root. (From Casullo, D.: The integration of endodontics, periodontics and restorative dentistry in general practice. Part III. Restorative considerations. Compend. Cont. Educ. Gen. Dent., *1* (5):295–316, 1980.)

struments and then by minimal preparation with Peeso reamers, Gates-Gliddon burs, or both. These instruments follow the path of least resistance and minimize the risk of perforation. The length and width of the post should be determined by the anatomy of the roots, the retention required, and lateral stability, rather than by a preconceived idea of shape and form or by a universal ratio. Instruments should not be forced into the canal. If the clinician has problems with instrumentation of a canal, he should discontinue the preparation and allow the anatomy of the canal to dictate the form and length of the post restoration (see Additional Aids for Retention).

It can happen, though, that the clinician is confronted with a "Hobson's choice"; the retentive needs demand placement of a post and core, but the anatomy precludes the extension of the post deep enough into the canal to gain the requisite retention. In such cases, use of the telescopic restoration cast in conjunction with the individually shaped post, a chamfer or featheredge finish line and parallel walls may successfully manage the problem.

Telescopic Restoration

The telescopic restoration builds up lost tooth or root structure, provides full circumferential external support and protection for the remaining tooth structure, provides external retention and smooth contours for the overcasting, protects against crown or root fractures, and can correct parallelism problems. The telescope may be used in conjunction with a cast post for optimal retention and for protection against root fractures. The telescope with or without a post is ideally suited for management and protection of sectioned roots, which have an absolute minimal amount of remaining tooth structure and are generally not parallel to each other or to other teeth (Fig. 12–39).

The telescope is an excellent mechanism for protecting endodontically treated teeth that have had advanced periodontal disease, pulpal disease, or both (Classes II, IV, and V) and do not require a post for retention and protection from fracture. When the osseous structure and marginal tissue are at Position 2 or 3, it may be impossible to place a post to extend adequately below the osseous crest for support and prevention of root fracture. If a post were so placed, it

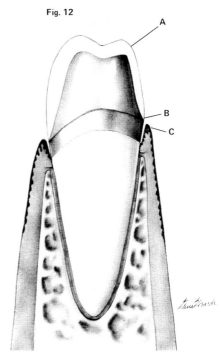

Fig. 12

FIGURE 12–39 Telescopic Restoration. Three important aspects of the telescope must be considered. **A,** Coronal aspect. The walls of the telescope must be machined to be as parallel as possible to each other and to the other abutments. Clinically, the coronal portion should end at the gingival margin to prevent placement of two gold margins subgingivally, while providing maximum length for retention. An objective in the porcelain-to-gold restorations is that, coronally, the telescope should approach the same height of the other abutments to provide an even thickness of material in the porcelain-to-gold overcast. **B,** Finish line. A chamfer or feather edge finish line should be placed to accept the overcast. It should be supragingival unless esthetics is a consideration. **C,** Gingival collar. The portion beneath the overcast finish line that extends subgingivally must be compatible with the sulcular tissue. (From Casullo, D.: The integration of endodontics, periodontics and restorative dentistry in General Practice. Part III. Restorative considerations. Compend. Cont. Educ. Gen. Dent., 1 (5):295–316, 1980.)

would enter the apical one third of the root, which is highly vulnerable to fracture or perforation because of its anatomic limitations and aberrations.

Additional Aids for Retention

Although the placement of auxiliary pins, screw posts, and excessively long or wide posts has the potential to enhance retention of a restoration, the use of such devices must be approached with caution. The risk of perforation or fracture relative to the expected increase in retention usually militates against their use. There is, however, another way to increase retention: to increase the length of the tooth via periodontal surgery or placement of a chamfer or featheredge finish line as close to the junctional epithelium as possible. The repositioning of the periodontium with osseous surgery to gain sound tooth structure increases the length of the clinical crown, thus increasing the retention of a restoration. When the remaining tooth structure is inadequate for a restoration and inadequate for retention, it is imperative that the tissues be repositioned surgically to gain crown length so that the restoration can be terminated on sound tooth structure.

Use of a chamfer or featheredge finish line placed as close as possible to the functional epithelium (ideally 0.5 mm) provides for maximal length and for maximal parallelism of the external walls, thus enhancing retention of the restoration. These two procedures are safe, predictable, and effective for increasing retention of a restoration.

While restorative therapy may be involved at the beginning and at the end of endodontic and periodontal therapy, its proper execution is necessary for the establishment and maintenance of health in the involved tissues. This requires a thorough understanding of pulpal and periodontal disease, dental and periodontal morphology, and the interrelationship between the dental disciplines required to accomplish the goals of treatment. The final restoration of the destroyed tooth structure is a difficult task that must be approached cautiously, yet be adequately done to overcome the severe deformity created by the advanced disease processes.

COMBINED ADJUNCTIVE ORTHODONTIC, PERIODONTAL, AND RESTORATIVE THERAPY

Adjunctive orthodontics for the adult patient is a therapeutic modality aimed toward the establishment of health or the elimination of the patient's complaints that are associated with malposed teeth (See Chapter 7, Orthodontics in General Practice). Based on the definition of a physiologic occlusion pre-

sented in Chapter 8, malposed teeth and malocclusions per se are not pathologic. As such, adjunctive orthodontic therapy is not executed to achieve the ideal occlusion. Yet, when disease is associated with a malposed tooth or malocclusion contributes to disease, orthodontic therapy is executed to set up a healthy, functional, therapeutic occlusion.

Malocclusions that contribute to the perpetuation of active disease or compromise the esthetic needs of the patient requiring full-banded orthodontic therapy should be managed by the orthodontic specialist. Although the actual mechanics of tooth movement are executed by the orthodontist, the general practitioner must (1) ensure that soft tissue inflammation and occlusal forces are controlled prior to and during orthodontic treatment, and (2) ensure that the final tooth position is adequate for requisite restorative and occlusal therapy.

In general practice, adjunctive orthodontic therapy is indicated for the management of a localized problem in the adult dentition. Tooth movement procedures are instituted in conjunction with periodontal and occlusal therapy usually combined with restorative dentistry (temporary or permanent stabilization) to maintain the corrected tooth position and set up a stable therapeutic occlusion.

Indications for Adjunctive Orthodontic Therapy

Adjunctive orthodontic therapy in adults is warranted for various reasons and is usually viewed from a combined periodontal, occlusal, and restorative perspective. Anterior spacing is a common esthetic concern of the adult patient and must be approached with caution. Periodontal problems that can be managed by adjunctive orthodontic therapy include (1) osseous and gingival defects, and (2) open and collapsed contacts associated with dental caries and food impaction. Occlusal problems include (1) malposed teeth with poor mesiodistal and buccolingual landmark relations that receive off-axis occlusal forces (Fig. 12–40), (2) aberrant planes of occlusion, (3) an exaggerated curve of Spee associated with occlusal traumatism, and (4) malocclusions that are influential in the etiology of periodontal and occlusal disease (such as Class II, Division I malocclusion). Restorative problems include (1) nonparallel abutment teeth, (2) inadequate embrasure

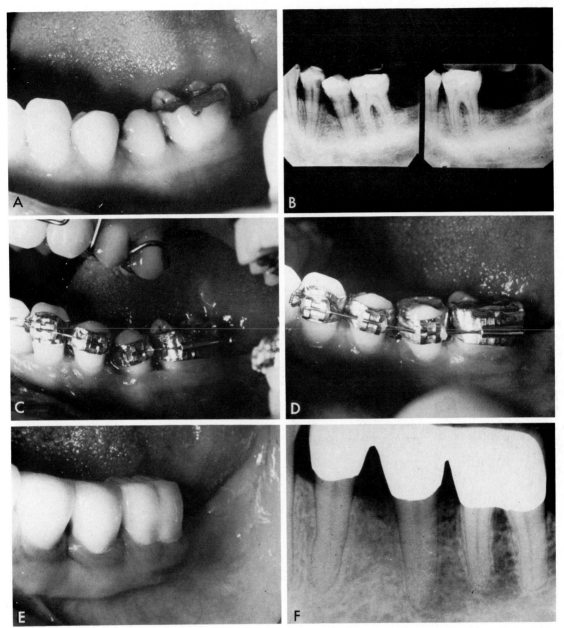

FIGURE 12–40   Combined Molar Uprighting and Forced Eruption for the Treatment of Periodontal Disease. *A,* This 42-year-old female presented with a chief complaint of severe pain in the lower right quadrant, inability to chew, and general discomfort with her bite. The teeth in this quadrant have drifted mesially owing to uneven marginal ridges and poor contact relations. ***B,*** The preoperative radiographs substantiate clinical probings of a Class II molar furcation involvement and infrabone defects around the second bicuspid. Deep caries is present on the distal surface of the first premolar, associated with the mesial migration of the teeth. Treatment included scaling, root planing, caries control and adjunctive orthodontics followed by provisional restoration, periodontal reevaluation for surgery, and final restorative therapy. ***C,*** Bands have been placed as well as a Hawley bite plane to execute the adjunctive orthodontics. The goal of adjunctive orthodontics is to level the osseous crest by leveling and aligning the teeth. A combination of forced eruption and uprighting is required to facilitate periodontal and restorative therapy. ***D,*** Leveling and aligning the teeth in this posterior quadrant took 5 months. The teeth were stabilized for 4 months and re-evaluated for further periodontal therapy. ***E,*** The final restoration was completed after placement of a free gingival graft. ***F,*** Final radiograph 2 years postoperatively showing healing in the attachment apparatus and crestal bone. No osseous surgery was required.

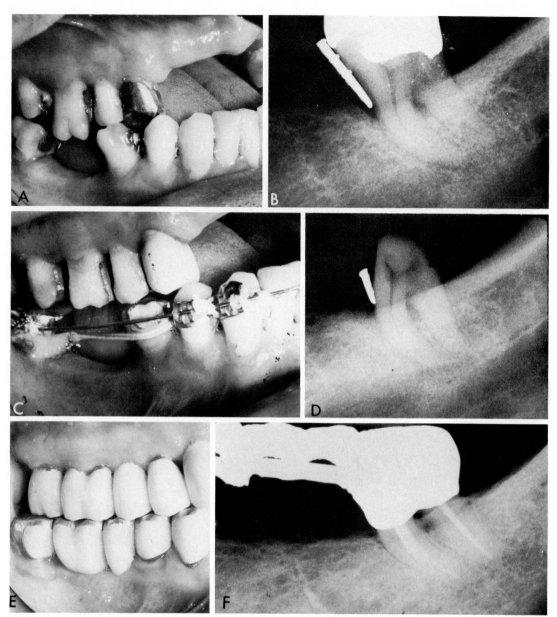

FIGURE 12–41 Uprighting the Mesially Inclined Second Molar. *A,* The mesially inclined mandibular second molar creates a protrusive and lateral-protrusive interference. It is very mobile, has a Class II furcation involvement, and has a 7-mm pocket depth on its mesial aspect. Note the crossbite relation, the extruded maxillary molar, and the poor occlusal relations in the arch. *B,* The preoperative radiograph shows a 3-mm infrabony defect on the mesial surface and a radiolucency in the furcation area. Treatment consisted of scaling, root planing, caries control, Hawley bite plane, occlusal adjustment, uprighting of the molar, and stabilization with a fixed splint. *C,* Mandibular appliance in place to upright the second molar. The goal of adjunctive orthodontics is to lessen the mesial defect on the second molar, to redirect forces along the long axis of the tooth, to eliminate all interferences, and to facilitate fixed restorative dentistry. *D,* After uprighting, the molar was stabilized with a provisional restoration for 3 months. The reevaluation radiograph shows healing of the mesial defect. *E,* The final restoration in place. *F,* This 3-year postoperative radiograph shows the final restoration and maintenance of periodontal health in the attachment apparatus.

Illustration continued on opposite page

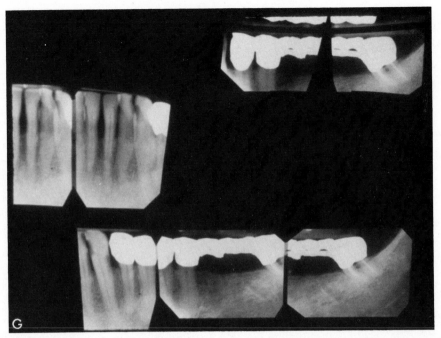

FIGURE 12–41 *Continued G,* Ten-year postoperative radiographs demonstrate maintenance of periodontal health in the attachment apparatus. The Class II furcation was present from the very beginning of treatment and has changed minimally, if at all.

or pontic space, and (3) severely decayed or fractured teeth.

Two very common adjunctive orthodontic procedures (requiring periodontal, occlusal, and restorative therapy) that can and should be executed by the general practitioner are (1) the uprighting of a mesially inclined molar, and (2) the forced eruption of a severely decayed, fractured, or periodontally involved tooth.

Uprighting the Mesially Inclined Molar

In general practice, it is the periodontally involved malposed posterior tooth, most commonly the mesially inclined mandibular second molar with a mesial osseous defect, that requires orthodontic uprighting (Fig. 12–41). The mesially inclined molar and distally inclined premolars usually are associated with incorrect (buccolingual or mesiodistal) landmark relations, open contacts, extruded opposing teeth, uneven marginal ridges, and a deformed plane of occlusion, curve of Spee, and transverse curve. Loss of arch continuity along with disruption of arch rhythmicity leads to interferences and the possible initiation or exacerbation of parafunctional habits. Both generate exces-

sive, off-axis occlusal forces. In addition, the aberrant occlusal morphology interferes with access for proper oral hygiene, resulting in plaque accumulation, calculus formation, and food impaction. This retention of debris and accompanying destructive occlusal force application can induce and accelerate periodontal disease, occlusal traumatism, caries, and pulpal involvement.

Uprighting the molar and repositioning the premolar will re-establish proper landmark relations and occlusal function, thus creating improved conditions for sustained health. Moreover, changing the local gingival and osseous topography can improve or eliminate soft tissue and osseous defects associated with the malposed tooth.

The presence of a malposed tooth also causes problems with parallelism. When abutment teeth are not parallel, a number of complications for restorations arise: (1) establishing an adequate path of insertion for the prosthesis, (2) placing an esthetically contoured pontic or retainer, (3) establishing an appropriate embrasure space, and (4) gaining sufficient access for tooth preparation.

If parallelism of abutments (Fig. 12–42) is not established by orthodontically repositioning the tooth, the following problems

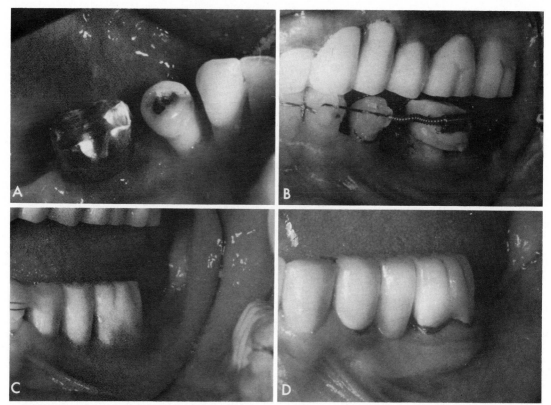

FIGURE 12–42   Adjunctive Orthodontics for the Treatment of Periodontal Disease and To Facilitate Restorative Dentistry. *A,* This occlusolingual view shows the mesial migration of a mandibular first molar and distal drift of the first premolar as a result of a loss of arch integrity, advanced periodontal disease, and occlusal traumatism. Adjunctive orthodontics was planned to alleviate periodontal defects, to provide adequate mesiodistal dimension for a pontic, to redirect forces along the long axis of the abutment teeth, and to facilitate parallelism for a fixed partial denture. ***B,*** The buccal view shows the open coil-spring in place to move the premolar mesially and the molar distally. Adjunctive orthodontics followed scaling and root planing and insertion of a Hawley bite plane. Other planned treatment included stabilization with a provisional restoration, periodontal re-evaluation, surgical therapy, and final restorative treatment. ***C,*** The provisional restoration stabilizes the repositioned teeth and re-establishes optimal occlusal relations. The inadequate masticatory mucosa in the areas of the first molar and edentulous ridge required the placement of a free gingival graft. ***D,*** The final restoration is placed after all disease is eliminated and health is established in all areas. Note the healing of the mucogingival complex.

may result: (1) pulpal exposure during tooth preparation, (2) poor tooth preparation and ill-fitting restoration, (3) impingement on the soft tissues and poor contour, (4) incomplete seating of the restoration, (5) poor oral hygiene, and (6) failure of the restoration with subsequent tooth loss.

A primary factor that must be considered before adjunctive orthodontic therapy is instituted is the patient's commitment to final stabilization, which usually means a fixed prosthesis. A-splints may be acceptable when arch continuity is intact and when any additional requisite occlusal adjustments can be managed by selective grinding. Otherwise, the fixed restoration is the treatment of choice. It is durable and long-lasting, re-establishes arch rhythmicity, stabilizes occlusal relations, redirects forces vertically, supports the occlusal vertical dimension optimally (functionally effective occlusal tables), and restores teeth with minimal tooth structure (resulting from disease or the constant leveling required during tooth movement to prevent interferences). Moreover, adequate interarch and intra-arch space must be available. These clinical assessments require a thorough occlusal examination and a careful evaluation of study casts mounted on an articulator.

Concomitant Periodontal Therapy

The forces induced during tooth movement procedures are functionally equivalent to those associated with parafunction and interferences. Consequently, adjunctive orthodontic therapy can lead to iatrogenic bone loss if inflammation is not controlled throughout treatment. Thus, before orthodontic treatment is initiated, efforts must be made to control any inflammatory process, even if it requires open-flap curettage to gain access to furcations, deep defects, or roots covered with tenacious calculus. Thereafter, frequent monitoring and scaling and root planing are indicated. When a severe osseous defect is cleaned out prior to orthodontic banding, scaling and root planing must be done throughout active tooth movement. Instrumentation must not proceed beyond the junctional epithelium to avoid infringing on the tissues of the infrabony structures, which would have an adverse effect on their healing potential. Injury caused by overinstrumentation could compromise regenerative capabilities of the tissues. Oral hygiene must be exemplary.

Concomitant Occlusal Therapy: Hawley Bite Plane and Selective Grinding

It is imperative that all excessive, off-axis occlusal forces be eliminated during tooth movement procedures to protect tissues already receiving a traumatic insult as a result of orthodontic therapy. The Hawley bite plane disarticulates the posterior teeth, and it effectively eliminates interferences and controls forces generated during parafunctional activity. The bite plane is useful for two other reasons: It facilitates tooth movement by allowing free, unimpeded movement, and it facilitates the establishment of the retruded contact position along the terminal hinge axis by providing for rest of the muscles of mastication.

Concomitant Selective Grinding

As the malposed tooth is uprighted, it can become an interference. Consequently, the crown must be leveled continually by selective grinding. Constant removal of tooth structure can result in the loss of orientation of the axial inclination of the crown. To regain orientation, the positions of the abutment teeth, as identified radiographically, are used as guides.

Provisional Restoration

Upon completion of adjunctive orthodontic treatment (usually in 2 to 6 months), placement of a metal band and acrylic provisional restoration is indicated for temporary stabilization, protection, and optimal tissue healing. Tooth preparation for the provisional restoration is done conservatively, establishing the finish line at, or just below, the marginal tissues. (The teeth will subsequently be reprepared and the finish line repositioned for the final restoration.) This cautious approach is necessary to avoid insulting the tissues, which are in the tenuous process of maturing. Overpreparation into the healing attachment apparatus could result in irreparable damage and loss of osseous tissue. Final maturity is usually achieved about 3 months after stabilization.

Re-evaluation of Therapy

The final evaluation (clinical and radiographic) of tooth position must consider all the periodontal, mechanical, and occlusal problems associated with malposed teeth. Periodontally, the soft tissue should be level, free of food impaction, and accessible for oral hygiene care. The infrabony osseous defect should have been ameliorated or eliminated. Mechanically, the teeth should have adequate embrasure or pontic space and parallelism for a fixed restoration. Occlusally, the teeth should have correct buccolingual landmarks, correct axial inclination for optimal force distribution along their long axes, and a consistent plane of occlusion and curve of Spee.

The orthodontic correction of a malposed molar and any tooth malpositioned in the quadrant generally requires the placement of a fixed prosthesis. The final occlusal correction of buccolingual landmarks, the curve of Spee, and plane of occlusion often cannot be totally or adequately corrected without the fixed prosthesis. Interarch tooth relations (extruded molars) must be corrected by selective grinding, a cast restoration, or both. The entire therapeutic correction must

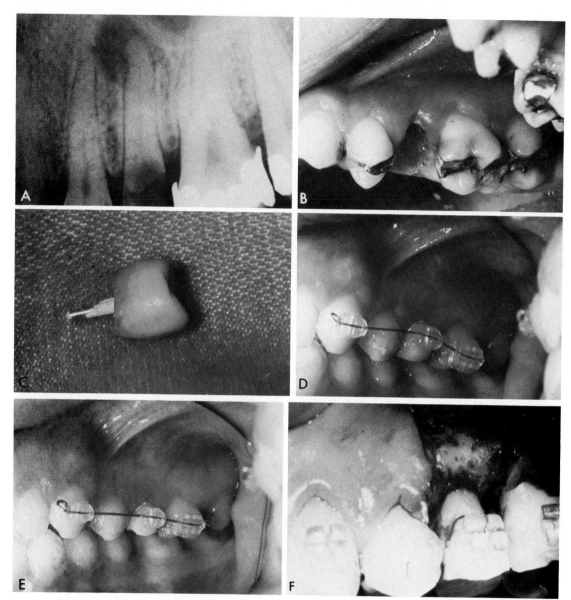

FIGURE 12–43 Forced Eruption for the Treatment of Extensive Caries. *A,* The preoperative radiograph shows the maxillary second premolar decayed to and below the osseous crest as well as a large periapical radiolucency. The patient would like to save this tooth and is willing to go through the complex therapy required. Osseous surgery would require extensive reduction of supporting bone from adjacent teeth and is not a reasonable alternative. ***B,*** Clinically, the crown is completely destroyed by caries, the soft tissue is inflamed, and there is no sound tooth structure coronal to the osseous crest. Treatment required to save this severely decayed tooth included endodontics, fabrication of a provisional restoration with a post, adjunctive orthodontics, isolated periodontal surgery, and final restorative therapy. ***C,*** After endodontics was completed, a gold band and acrylic provisional restoration with a post was fabricated. ***D,*** The provisional restoration was cemented in place, and orthodontic brackets were placed on the tooth to erupt the bicuspid a required 4 to 5 mm. ***E,*** Eight weeks after initial tooth movement, the tooth is extruded adequately and the periodontium has accompanied the tooth. Note the leveling of the brackets. ***F,*** Isolated periodontal surgery was executed to reposition the periodontium of this one tooth at a level in harmony with the quadrant and to gain the required tooth structure for a final restoration.

Illustration continued on opposite page

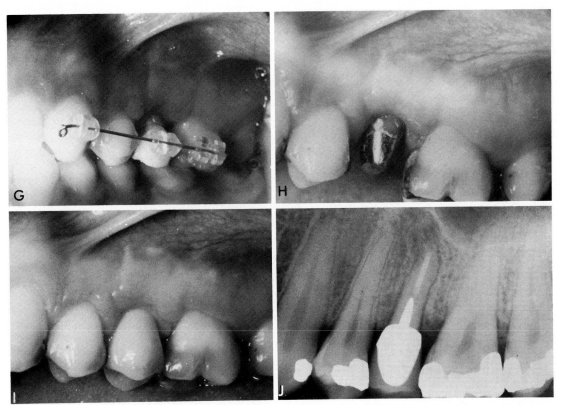

FIGURE 12–43 *Continued* **G,** A passive arch wire is in place to stabilize the tooth during and after surgery. Note new position of marginal tissue 1 week after surgery. **H,** This buccal view shows the healing of the periodontal tissues in harmony with the adjacent teeth. A post and core has been fabricated. **I,** Final restoration in place. **J,** The 1-year postoperative radiograph shows the healing of the periapical lesion with the final restoration in place.

be evaluated and achieved with the provisional restoration. If any further periodontal, mechanical, or occlusal correction is required, it must be executed prior to placement of the final restoration.

If osseous surgery is required for any remaining defects, it should be executed after a period of stabilization (4 to 6 months) in order to allow maximal healing of the attachment apparatus. If mucogingival correction such as a free gingival graft is required, it can be executed 6 weeks after stabilization.

Forced Eruption

When osseous surgery is required to eliminate an isolated periodontal infrabony defect and to gain adequate sound tooth structure for the placement of a restoration on teeth associated with extensive caries, severe fractures, or root canal perforations, orthodontic forced eruption may be employed (Fig. 12–43). During forced eruption, the tooth, *along with* its attachment apparatus, is moved in an occlusal direction. Extruding the tooth and its periodontal structures often obviates the necessity of involving the osseous structures and furcation areas of adjacent teeth during the surgical procedure, thus protecting furcation areas and their adjacent attachment apparatus.

In the case of an isolated infrabony defect (Fig. 12–41), the osseous structure associated with the defect levels out, and the adjacent bone creates an angular defect on that same tooth. Periodontal surgery usually includes leveling of the created angular crest and any remaining infrabony defect and soft tissue deformities.

When forced eruption is executed to facilitate the removal of bone to get below caries or a fracture, the tooth is extruded to gain the required 4 mm of sound tooth structure. When the bone is intact and the decay or fracture is at the osseous crest, the tooth must be extruded at least 4 mm, creating an isolated soft tissue and osseous defect. Periodontal surgery can then be executed on that one tooth, avoiding osseous reduction on adjacent teeth.

The decision to use this adjunctive orthodontic procedure must take into account the subsequent therapy required, which can be quite extensive, complex, and costly. Teeth that must be treated with forced eruption to treat caries or a fracture also require endodontic therapy and a metal band and acrylic provisional restoration with a post for retention. After the tooth has been erupted, the osseous surgery is done, the provisional restoration is relined, or a new band is placed. Following complete healing, the final post and core and full-crown restoration are fabricated.

When the objective is to eliminate a periodontal defect, usually only orthodontic therapy and osseous surgery are required. At times, however, a full-crown restoration, or splinting, is necessary. This is the case when excessive selective grinding is required to allow the eruption and when splinting is required because of a compromised attachment apparatus. Many factors are involved in determining whether such therapy is justified. The most important, perhaps, are the commitment, attitude, and financial resources of the patient and the strategic importance of the tooth as a possible future abutment and in maintaining arch rhythmicity and continuity. Strategic extraction should be considered.

Esthetic Problems

The complaints of adult patients concerning esthetic appearance usually involve anterior tooth problems that cannot be resolved with simple adjunctive orthodontic therapy. Advanced restorative dentistry or full orthodontic correction (usually by a specialist) or both are often required. This is the case when the esthetic deformity is a result of severe, long-standing disease, for example, flaring of the maxillary anterior teeth due to posterior bite collapse or severe tongue thrust. In the case of posterior bite collapse, the anterior spacing cannot be resolved until the posterior occlusion is reestablished to support the occlusal vertical dimension. This is also the case when dissatisfaction with appearance involves a developmental problem, for example, a severe malocclusion or an inter- or intra-arch dental-skeletal disparity.

The general practitioner should attempt to manage *isolated* esthetic deformities only and should manage them only when the requisite orthodontic treatment is not excessive in relation to the extent of the deformity and only when prevention of posttreatment relapse can be reasonably assured. Examples of esthetic problems that might fulfill these criteria are rotations and diastemas not associated with posterior bite collapse. The complexity, limitations, and possible relapse of esthetic corrections must be explained to the adult patient.

All adjunctive orthodontic procedures require strict attention to basic principles ranging from the mechanics of tooth movement to control of periodontal inflammation and occlusal traumatism and the final stabilization and restoration. Failure to apply the basic principles outlined can lead to disastrous and frustrating results. If the patient is not monitored throughout active tooth movement, severe and irreversible periodontal damage can occur.

ETCHED CAST METAL RESIN-BONDED RESTORATIONS

The periodontal, orthodontic, and occlusal stabilization of teeth with and without a mechanical replacement for missing teeth has long been an area of concern among dental specialists and generalists. For example, an important therapeutic modality for patients with advanced periodontal disease and secondary occlusal trauma is the establishment of arch integrity by means of fixed stabilization. Even in a healthy periodontium, early or isolated tooth loss will require a system of stabilization to facilitate the health of the mouth and the long-term maintenance of proper occlusion. Likewise, in orthodontic situations involving the adult patient, fixed stabilization is often necessary to maintain final tooth position and to establish correct occlusal relations. In these and in related situations, the dental profession has sought an uncomplicated, noninvasive, reversible, yet inexpensive mechanism to stabilize loose teeth (Fig. 12–44), replace missing teeth (Fig. 12–45), retain orthodontically positioned teeth (Fig. 12–46), and ameliorate excessive occlusal forces (Fig. 12–47). With new developments in microfilled composite resins and etching of nonprecious metals, an innovative, conservative, and du-

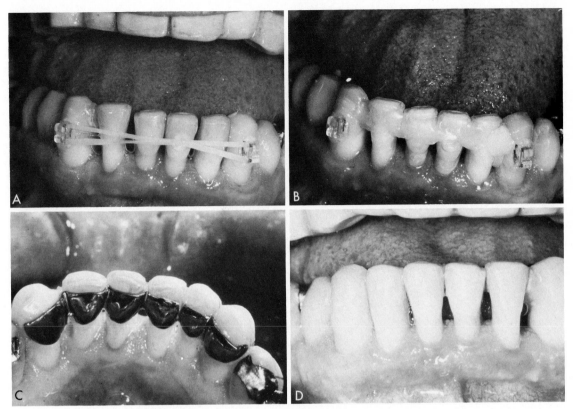

FIGURE 12–44   Lower Anterior Ligation. *A,* The labial view of the flared lower incisors shows an elastic band extending from canine to canine. *B,* Once the teeth were together, they were stabilized on the labial aspect with light-cured composite resin. The brackets were removed from the canines; then a rubber base impression was taken to fabricate a canine-to-canine etched cast metal resin-bonded retainer. *C,* The lingual view shows the retainer in place after 12 months. The supragingival margins, and the open embrasures of the well-adapted restoration allow easy maintenance and home care. *D,* The labial view one month postoperatively shows maintenance of the tooth position and periodontal health. (In conjunction with J. G. Coslet, and D. W. Cohen, Philadelphia, Pa.)

rable adjunct for therapy has evolved. The cast metal resin-bonded restoration is a thin, rigid casting that is contoured, highly polished, and attached to the etched enamel surface of teeth by means of a microfilled composite resin.

Advantages

The conservation of tooth structure and the reversible nature of the acid-etched metal resin-bonded retainer are its most impressive advantages. Since there is no need for excessive tooth preparation into dentin, a simple and maintainable restoration can result. To the patient, this means fewer and less tedious clinical procedures with minimal expense. To the practitioner, the retention of supragingival margins, the lack of dentin

or pulpal involvement, and the maintenance of enamel means that (1) a greater amount of natural tooth structure remains, (2), gingival irritation is significantly lessened, (3) the need for anesthesia is reduced, and (4) the medically, physically, or financially compromised patient can be treated. Thus, because of improvements in composite resins and metal alloys and in the practice of etching alloy and enamel surfaces, a thin, rigid, retentive, and durable restoration results.

Contraindications

Short or worn anatomic crowns and teeth with exposed root surface requiring contour in the gingival third make patients unsuitable candidates for the acid-etching resin-bonded technique, because inadequate en-

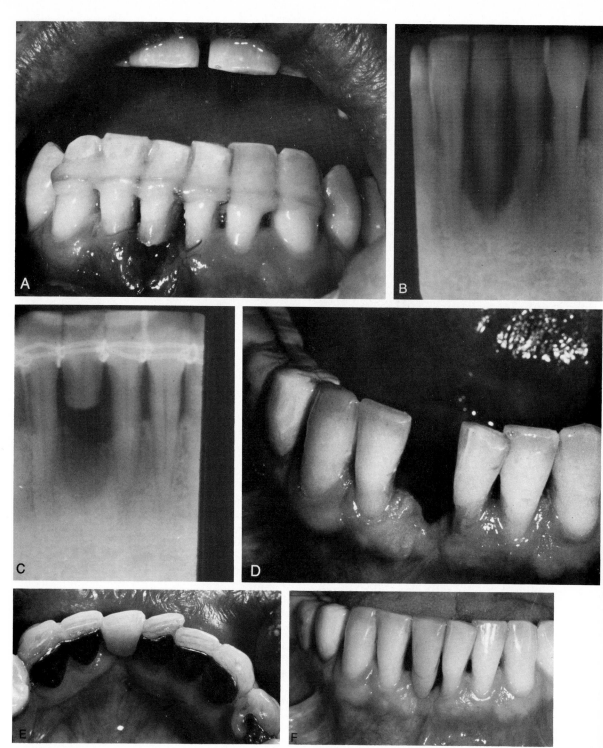

FIGURE 12–45 Lower Anterior Tooth Replacement, and Stabilization. *A,* The mandibular anterior teeth were ligated with extracoronal wire and acrylic. The root of the lower left central incisor was then extracted. ***B,*** The preoperative radiograph shows the isolated severe periodontal defect jeopardizing the adjacent teeth. ***C,*** The postoperative radiograph demonstrates healing of the attachment apparatus. ***D,*** The extracoronal wire and acrylic ligation are removed after 16 months to allow the impressions for the etched cast metal resin-bonded retainer to be taken. The teeth must be religated between visits. ***E,*** The lingual view shows the final restoration in place. ***F,*** The labial view shows the esthetic result, maintenance of soft tissue health and open embrasures and the retention of tooth positions.

668

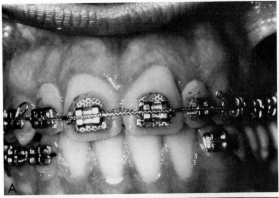

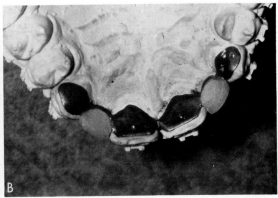

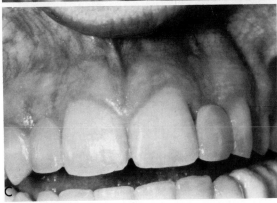

FIGURE 12–46 Maxillary Upper Anterior Orthodontic Stabilization. *A,* The labial view shows the final tooth position of the central incisors. The lateral incisors are congenitally missing. Denture teeth have been placed on the arch wire as an interim measure. *B,* The working cast is fabricated and the etched cast metal resin-bonded retainer is fabricated. The restoration will maintain the orthodontic correction and replace the congenitally missing lateral incisors. *C,* The labial view of the final restoration in place. (In conjunction with R. L. Vanarsdall, Philadelphia, Pa.)

amel surface does not allow enough area for proper bonding and the restoration does not correct poor crown contours. Therefore, mottled enamel, very large restorations, or amelogenesis imperfecta will negate the use of resin-bonded retainers. Food impaction and stagnation can be a problem overcome only by scrupulous home care, so considerable judgment should be exercised in choosing a proper candidate for this procedure.

Although the restoration can correct isolated occlusal problems such as excessive occlusal forces associated with protrusive and lateral-protrusive interferences, its use is contraindicated in situations involving poor occlusal relations of teeth. Contraindications for the use of an acid etched metal resin-bonded retainer also include situations involving poor occlusal relation, such as posterior bite collapse, deep overbite, long edentulous spans, and of course, circumstances of excessive occlusal force. Excessive force generated to the restoration or the abutment teeth will cause displacement or fracture of the framework or the abutment teeth. The practitioner must be able to anticipate whether the application of extra material (on the lingual aspect of the maxillary anterior teeth, for example) will cause insurmountable problems or will serve to correct an occlusal defect.

Occlusal Considerations

The acid etched resin-bonded retainer can be used to correct inadequate anterior guidance and to relieve or eliminate excessive posterior tooth contacts associated with protrusive or lateral-protrusive movement by the build-up of the lingual surfaces of the canines. Posterior retainers can be used to shallow out the central fossa, allowing the opposing cusp to be shortened and thus eliminating unwanted posterior tooth interferences or contacts. The bonded retainer should be analyzed regularly to prevent the development of poor tooth contact and deleterious occlusal force should be adjusted if necessary.

Stability and favorable occlusal relations of teeth make success of the acid-etched metal resin-bonded restoration more predictable. Excessively mobile teeth or teeth that have been orthodontically positioned present a greater degree of difficulty because of the temporary stabilization required between

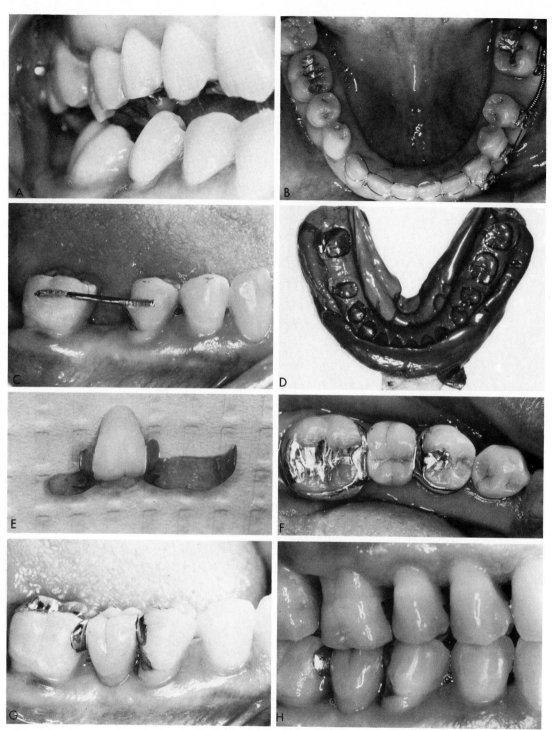

FIGURE 12–47   Mandibular Posterior Restoration. *A,* This right buccal view shows an aberrant plane of occlusion associated with a missing mandibular molar. *B,* The mesially inclined mandibular right molar was uprighted. *C,* Immediate stabilization was achieved with heavy wire and composite resin. *D,* The final impression was taken with rubber base. *E,* The final restoration, with extensive lingual extensions, occlusal rest, and buccal extensions. *F,* The occlusal view of the final restoration in place shows the occlusal rest, and the extension of the lingual and buccal arms. *G,* The buccal view of the mandibular restoration. *H,* The buccal view of the occlusal relations of the teeth. The aberrant plane of occlusion has been corrected as have been all occlusal interferences. (Courtesy of Dr. Ed Katz, University of Pennsylvania.)

670

visits. The interim stabilization must be rigid yet must avoid the surfaces involved in the restoration. Since the materials used are combinations of acrylic and metal in thin proportions, the interim stabilization has a tendency to break, causing relapse of orthodontically moved teeth or further movement of mobile teeth. In such situations, the metal framework may no longer fit and will require remaking.

Mechanical Design

The design of both anterior and posterior restorations are dictated by four factors: (1) enamel surface available, (2) esthetic considerations, (3) position of the gingival tissue, and (4) occlusal relations of the teeth. The general guidelines as applied to each individual patient are based on the presence of enough enamel to retain the restoration, the probability of a satisfactory esthetic result, optimal gingival and periodontal health, and occlusal contacts of teeth in the maximum intercuspal position and in protrusive and lateral-protrusive movements.

Design of the Anterior Restoration. Once the fundamental requirements for the restoration are observed clinically, the sequence of designing an acid-etched metal resin-bonded restoration begins with a study cast mounted on an articulator. On maxillary restorations, incisal clearance and anterior guidance must be sufficient to provide room for the cast retainer. The lingual aspect of the involved tooth structure must provide a smooth and precise path of insertion for the restoration. When required, lingual dimples should be placed on the lingual aspect of the anterior teeth incisal to the cingulum. These dimples and the interproximal surfaces provide a definite and absolute seat for the restoration on the abutment teeth.

The interproximal surfaces of the restoration should extend as far as possible between the teeth to achieve a "gripping" of the tooth. The interproximal extension is dictated by adequate embrasure space for oral hygiene and esthetic result. The tooth surface adjacent to an edentulous span should be prepared with a guide plane to be covered by metal to enhance enamel surface area and the positive path of insertion. Esthetic considerations will determine the extent of this guide plane.

The height of contour of the cingulum is the ideal position to terminate the gingival finish line. The incisal finish line is determined by the occlusion and the incisal translucency of the teeth. The thinner the incisal edges, the greater the chance of the framework creating a gray or even black appearance of the teeth.

Design of the Posterior Restoration. The framework design of the etched cast metal resin-bonded restoration for posterior teeth demands less esthetically but more functionally. It can be designed to correct nonworking and protrusive interferences by shallowing out central fossa, thus allowing occlusal adjustment of the centric supporting cusp (buccal cusps of the mandibular and palatal cusps of the maxillary teeth). Aberrations in arch rythmicity and form can be corrected with combined occlusal adjustment by selective grinding, adjunctive orthodontic therapy, and placement of the etched cast metal resin-bonded retainer.

The posterior restoration should be kept above the gingival wherever possible, include an occlusal rest on each tooth adjacent to an edentulous space, and have both a lingual and a buccal extension beyond the transitional line angle. Guide planes should be prepared on the proximal surfaces to enhance the path of insertion and to allow a smooth flow of the restoration from the buccal to the lingual aspect.

This curvilinear design should be at least 180 degrees and should allow for an occlusal apical path of insertion. If necessary, minimal preparation of the buccal and lingual heights of contour permits a consistent path of insertion and allows the creation of a knifelike finish line in the gingival extension of the restoration. Teeth with a short clinical crown may require new gingival contours or subgingival margins or may preclude the use of the restoration altogether.

Clinical Procedures

The final impression for the retainer is taken with an irreversible elastic impression material such as rubber base or hydrocolloid. The working model is then poured in a high temperature investment material. The outline of the framework should be simple and may be drawn directly on the working model. The design goals of the anterior framework are (1) to cover as much enamel surface as possible, (2) to extend metal interproximally as much as possible, (3) to avoid the gingival one third of the tooth, and (4) to include any necessary mechanical rests into the enamel. Anterior teeth with thin incisal edges require a framework design ending at least 1 mm apical to the incisal edge in order to prevent an unpleasant gray color.

Laboratory Procedures

Inlay wax is used directly on the refractory model. No separating medium is employed, and the wax is kept as thin as possible (0.35 mm to 0.55 mm). The model with the wax-up is cut down to the smallest size possible. The wax-up and the refractory model are invested, the wax is burned out, and the nonprecious metal is cast into the investment. Following these steps, the metal framework is then broken out and cleaned, and procelain is applied. After a try-in to verify fit, color, contour, and occlusion, the restoration is returned to the laboratory, where the portion of the framework that contacts enamel is etched with 10 percent sulfuric acid. The restoration is then cleansed and kept isolated from contact with contaminants.

Insertion

The procedure for inserting an acid-etched cast restoration is outlined by Livaditis (1980); however, a short summary is provided here.

1. Abutment teeth should be isolated.
2. A mechanical prophylaxis of the enamel surfaces using either a rubber cup or a bristle brush is performed to remove microbial contaminants and the pellicle layer. Care must be used not to traumatize the gingiva and cause bleeding.
3. The dried and isolated teeth are etched with a 37 to 50 percent solution of phosphoric acid, which is gently swabbed over the prepared surface. Vigorous rubbing with the solution with serve only to break or disrupt the enamel rods and to weaken the final retention. Etching time is 1 to 1.5 minutes, and the individual teeth are washed in water for 10 to 45 seconds. If the tooth surface does not appear chalky white following acid application, or if contamination with saliva or blood occurs, then the tooth must be retreated.
4. The etched surface of the metal must not be contaminated by touching it with the fingers.

5. Unfilled resin is applied to both the etched surface of the cast restoration and the prepared enamel surface. The unfilled resin enters the microscopically roughened surfaces more effectively than the larger particles of the filled resin material. Following placement of the sealant, equal parts of the filled resin are mixed and applied liberally over the retentive areas of the casting, and the restoration is firmly set in place.
6. Excess resin material is removed with an explorer and a scaler during the setting of the microfilled resin.
7. The occlusion and final seating of the restoration are checked.
8. All margins are finished and polished.

Conclusion

The etched cast metal resin-bonded retainer (restoration) is one of the most recent and innovative developments in restorative dentistry. The new and unique combination of materials (microfilled resin and nonprecious metal) provides the profession with a versatile, rigid, and conservative mechanism for tooth replacement and stabilization while allowing for the conservation of natural tooth structure and the preservation of healthy tissues. The restoration provides a useful adjunct in treating complex cases that involve the integration of multiple treatment modalities. The conservative nature of this restoration, however, requires strict attention to detail. The profession should proceed with cautious optimism, looking forward to newer and better materials as it tests the application of the etched metal resin-bonded retainer in restorative therapy.

SUMMARY

The multidisciplinary approach to dental therapy described in this chapter presents periodontics as the common denominator. In treating dental caries or other dental diseases or in evaluating the complaints of a patient with a healthy periodontium, the clinician must execute all therapy with utmost respect for the presence of periodontal health.

Throughout this chapter, individual and combined periodontal, restorative, endodontic, orthodontic, and oral surgical considerations and procedures have been presented to demonstrate a multidisciplinary approach to therapy. The combined periodontal, restorative, endodontic, orthodontic, and oral surgical (strategic extraction) procedures are directed toward the elimination or control of active disease and the correction of deformities created by active disease or are influential in other treatment modalities.

These procedures, which integrate the various dental disciplines, can be done by the general practitioner alone or in conjunction with the specialist. The treatment of choice and its sequence are at the discretion of the individual practitioner. Yet successful resolution of clinical problems requires an astute understanding of diagnosis, treatment planning, and the symbiotic relationship between restored dentition, periodontium, dental pulp, and occlusion. The time sequence, logistic combinations, and integration of the various procedures are critical in effecting a final evaluation of dental health. The multidisciplinary approach and the procedures discussed in the chapter should, it is to be hoped, provide a more effective and efficient method of practicing for the clinician as well as a basis for expansion and innovation of other combinations of procedures.

QUESTIONS

1. The gingival sulcus and col area are fully keratinized. True or false?

2. The finish line for the full-crown restoration is placed just short of the junctional epithelium to
    a. gain retention on broken-down teeth
    b. establish optimal crown contours
    c. prevent recurrent caries
    d. all of the above

3. The biologic width is approximately 2 mm in length and consists of
    a. osseous structure
    b. gingival connective tissue
    c. junctional epithelium (epithelial attachment)
    d. none of the above

4. The partial-coverage restoration is the restoration of choice to
    a. treat and control advanced periodontal disease and occlusal trauma
    b. treat rampant caries
    c. treat broken-down teeth or isolated caries involving a supporting cusp
    d. all of the above

5. The optimal provisional full-crown restoration should
    a. be a prefabricated stainless-steel crown
    b. provide a template for the final restoration and establish periodontal health and therapeutic occlusal relations
    c. be fabricated with supragingival margins
    d. be all of the above

6. The provisional restoration is an important adjunct in periodontal therapy. It can be used
    a. to determine if periodontal health can be achieved without surgery when badly broken-down teeth or carious lesions are a cause of periodontal disease
    b. to re-establish soft tissue health in cases of poor contours and food impaction
    c. to set up an environment more amenable to periodontal surgical procedures and soft tissue control
    d. all of the above

7. When dental caries extends close to or below the osseous crest, a periodontal surgical procedure is required to
    a. provide approximately 1 mm of tooth structure for the connective tissue attachment

b. provide 1 mm of tooth structure for the epithelial attachment (junctional epithelium)

c. provide 1 to 2 mm of tooth structure to end a restoration

d. provide all of the above, including approximately 4 mm of tooth structure

8. Bound-down masticatory mucosa (attached gingiva) is an important protective barrier for the underlying attachment apparatus.

a. It should always be 2 mm wide.

b. It should always come up to the cementoenamel junction of the tooth.

c. It should always be executed when full-crown restorations are done.

d. It should always be evaluated in light of many variables.

9. The free gingival graft is an excellent procedure for gaining bound-down masticatory mucosa (attached gingiva) because

a. it can maintain or ameliorate the position of the marginal gingiva when subgingival restorations are employed

b. it is very predictable

c. it is easy to perform

d. all of the above

10. The management of edentulous ridges by periodontal surgical procedures

a. is an important part of treatment planning and must be approached judiciously

b. can be executed very simply in any part of the mouth

c. should be employed in all compromised edentulous ridges

d. all of the above

11. The restoration of choice in treatment of multirooted teeth with furcation involvement is

a. the three-quarter crown

b. the amalgam restoration

c. the full crown

d. none of the above

12. All mandibular molars with Class II furcation involvements that require full-crown restorations should be sectioned. True or false?

13. The principle of strategic extraction is

a. the extraction of teeth because of inadequate finances

b. the extraction of all teeth with furcation involvements

c. the extraction of teeth in order to maximize and preserve the periodontal tissues (attachment apparatus)

d. the extraction of all third molars

14. Pulpal and periodontal disease are separate and distant and do not affect common tissues. True or false?

15. The palatogingival groove is an anatomic anomaly found

a. on most teeth

b. on maxillary incisors

c. on mandibular incisors

d. on mandibular molars

16. Class II communicating pulpal and periodontal disease is characterized by

a. necrotic (nonvital) pulp

b. extensive pocket depth

c. extreme mobility patterns

d. all of the above

17. Restorative dentistry of teeth ravaged by advanced pulpal and periodontal disease must include

a. posts and cores

b. amalgam and auxiliary pins

c. advanced periodontal surgery

d. sound clinical judgment and an assessment of the extent of disease

18. When the mesially inclined molar is uprighted, the treatment includes
    a. periodontal management
    b. occlusal adjustment
    c. planned stabilization
    d. all of the above

19. The method of choice for stabilizing the uprighted molar is usually determined after tooth movement. True or false?

20. The basis for the multidisciplinary approach to therapy as described in this chapter is
    a. restorative dentistry
    b. orthodontics
    c. periodontics
    d. endodontics

21. The greatest advantage of the acid-etched resin-bonded retainer is
    a. the ease of fabrication
    b. the conservation of tooth structure
    c. the inexpensive cost
    d. all of the above

22. The acid-etched resin-bonded retainer should not be included in the occlusal relations of teeth. True or false?

23. Orthodontically positioned teeth and loose teeth can be stabilized with the acid-etched resin-bonded retainer. True or false?

24. Minimal tooth (enamel) preparation may be required to provide a positive and precise insertion of the acid-etched cast metal resin-bonded retainer. True or false?

25. Inadequate or weakened enamel surface is a consideration for not employing the acid-etched resin-bonded retainer. True or false?

See answers in Appendix.

SUGGESTED READINGS

Endodontic, Periodontic, and Restorative Dentistry

1. Album, M. M., and Loyd, R. W.: Technique for restoring endodontically treated anterior teeth with precision posts and porcelain-bonded-to-gold crowns. J. Am. Dent. Assoc., *93*:591, 1976.
2. Amsterdam, M.: Discussion: Periodontics-endodontics. Trans. Int. Conf. Endod., *5*:12, 1973.
3. Amsterdam, M.: Periodontal prosthesis. Twenty-five years in retrospect. Alpha Omegan, *67*(3):8, 1974.
4. Baraban, D. J.: The restoration of pulpless teeth. Dent. Clin. North Am., 1967, p. 633.
5. Bender, I. B., and Seltzer, S.: The effect of periodontal disease on the pulp. Oral Surg., *33*:458, 1972.
6. Bergenholtz, G., and Lindhe, J.: Effect of soluble plaque factors on inflammatory reactions in the dental pulp. Scand. J. Dent. Res., *83*:153, 1975.
7. Blair, H. A.: Relationships between endodontics and periodontics. J. Periodontol., *43*:209, 1972.
8. Casullo, D.: The integration of endodontics, periodontics and restorative dentistry in general practice. Part I. Diagnosis. Compend. Contin. Ed. Gen. Dent., *1*(2):137, 1980.
9. Casullo, D.: The integration of endodontics, periodontics and restorative dentistry in general practice. Part II. Sequence of therapy. Compend. Contin. Ed. Gen. Dent., *1*(4):268, 1980.
10. Casullo, D.: The integration of endodontics, periodontics and restorative dentistry in general prac-

tice. Part III. Restorative considerations. Compend. Contin. Ed. Gen. Dent., *1*(5):295, 1980.
11. Chacker, F.: The endodontic-periodontic continuum. Dent. Clin. North Am., *18*:393, 1974.
12. Colman, H. L.: Restoration of endodontically treated teeth. Dent. Clin. North Am., *23*:647, 1979.
13. Endo, J.: The use of the telescopic crown. NACDLJ, April, 1970.
14. Frank, A. L.: Protective coronal coverage of the pulpless tooth. J. Am. Dent. Assoc., *59*:895, 1959.
15. Goldman, H. M., and Cohen, D. W.: The infrabony pocket: Classification and treatment. J. Periodontol., *29*:272, 1958.
16. Gregory, W. B., et al.: Periodontal disease, bacteria, and pulpal histopathology. Oral Surg., *37*:257, 1974.
17. Harrington, G. W.: The perio-endo question—differential diagnosis. Dent. Clin. North Am., *23*:673, 1979.
18. Hiatt, W. H.: Periodontal pocket elimination by combined endodontic-periodontic therapy. J. Periodontol., *1*:152, 1963.
19. Hiatt, W. H.: Pulpal periodontal disease. J. Periodontol., *48*(9):598, 1977.
20. Johnson, J. K., Schwartz, N. L., and Blackwell, R. T.: Evaluation and restoration of endodontically treated posterior teeth. J. Am. Dent. Assoc., *93*:597, 1976.
21. Mazur, B., and Massler, M.: Influence of periodontal disease on the dental pulp. Oral Surg., *17*:592, 1964.
22. Oliet, S., and Pollack, S.: Classification and treat-

ment of endo-perio involved teeth. Bull. Phila. Cty. Dent. Soc., *34*:12, 1968.

23. Prichard, J.: Regeneration of bone following periodontal therapy. Oral Surg., *10*:247, 1957.
24. Prichard, J.: The infrabony technique as a predictable procedure. J. Periodontol., *28*:202, 1957.
25. Prichard, J., and Feder, M.: A modern adaptation of the telescopic principle in periodontal prosthesis. J. Periodontol, *33*:360, 1962.
26. Rosen, H.: Operative procedures on mutilated endodontically treated teeth. J. Prosthet. Dent., *11*:973, 1961.
27. Rubach, W. C., and Mitchell, D. F.: Pulp reactions in periodontal disease. IADR, *41*:39, 1963.
28. Shillingburg, H. T., Fisher, D. W., and Dewhirst, R. B.: Restoration of endodontically treated posterior teeth. J. Prosthet. Dent., *24*:401, 1970.
29. Simon, J. H., Glick, D. H., and Frank, A. L.: The relationship of endodontic-periodontic lesions. J. Periodontol, *43*:202, 1972.
30. Stahl, S. S.: The influence of pulpal necrosis on gingival reattachment potential. J. Periodontol., *34*:371, 1963.
31. Stahl, S. S.: Pathogenesis of inflammatory lesions in pulp and periodontal tissues. J. Periodontol., *4*:190, 1966.
32. Stallard, R. E.: Periodontic-endodontic relationships. Oral Surg., *34*:314, 1972.
33. Turner, P. S.: Periodontic-endodontic lesions and their management. J. Can. Dent. Assoc., *42*(10):506, 1976.

Adjunctive Orthodontics, Periodontics, and Restorative Dentistry

1. Ackerman, J. L., and Profitt, W. R.: The characteristics of malocclusion: A modern approach to classification and diagnosis. Am. J. Orthod., *56*:433, 1969.
2. Berlinger, A.: Ligatures, Splints, Bite Planes and Pyramids. Philadelphia, J. B. Lippincott Co., 1964.
3. Bernstein, M.: Orthodontics in periodontal and prosthetics therapy. J. Periodontol., *40*:577, 1969.
4. Bien, S. M.: Orthodontic procedures in the treatment of periodontal disease. Int. Dent. J., *3*:78, 1952.
5. Brown, I. S.: Effect of orthodontic therapy on periodontal defects. J. Periodontol., *44*:742, 1973.
6. Goldstein, M. C.: Orthodontics in crown and bridge and periodontal therapy. Dent. Clin. North Am., 1964, p. 449.
7. Goldstein, M. C.: Adult orthodontics and the general practitioner. J. Can. Dent. Assoc., *24*:26, 1958.
8. Hirshfeld, J.: The individual missing tooth: A factor in dental and periodontal disease. J. Am. Dent. Assoc., *24*:67, 1937.
9. Ingber, J. S.: Forced eruption: II. A method of treating non-restorable teeth—periodontal and restorative considerations. J. Periodontol., *47*:203, 1976.
10. Ingber, J. S.: Forced eruption: I. A method of treating isolated one and two wall infrabony osseous defects—Rationale and case report. J. Periodontol. *45*:199, 1974.
11. Marks, M. H.: Tooth movement in periodontal therapy. *In* H. Goldman and D. W. Cohen (eds.): Periodontal Therapy, 6th ed. St. Louis, The C. V. Mosby Co., 1980, Chapter 21, pp. 564–627.
12. Marks, M. H., and Corn, H.: Adult tooth movement: Alteration of the occlusal vertical dimension preparatory to tooth movement. Alpha Omegan, *10*:54, 1977.
13. Marks, M. H., and Corn, H.: The integration of adult tooth movement into a comprehensive periodontal treatment program. *In* H. L. Ward (ed.): A Periodontal Point of View. Springfield, Ill., Charles C Thomas, Publisher, 1973, Chapter 5, pp. 75–96.
14. Marks, M. H., and Corn, H.: The role of tooth movement in periodontal therapy. Dent. Clin. North Am., *13*:229, 1969.
15. Reitan, K.: Clinical and histologic observations on tooth movement during and after orthodontic treatment. Am. J. Orthod., *53*:721, 1967.
16. Vanarsdall, R. L.: Uprighting the inclined mandibular molar in preparation for restorative treatment. Contin. Dent. Ed., Univ. of Pa., Vol. 1, No. 2, 1977.

Periodontal and Restorative Therapy

1. Abrams, L.: Augmentation of the deformed residual edentulous ridge for fixed prosthesis. Compend. Contin. Educ. Gen. Dent., *1*(3):205, 1980.
2. Amsterdam, M., and Fox, L.: Provisional splinting, principles and techniques. Dent. Clin. North Am., 1959, p. 73.
3. Braden, B. E.: Deep distal pockets adjacent to terminal teeth. Dent. Clin. North Am., *13*:161, 1969.
4. Corn, H.: Mucogingival surgery and associated problems. In H. M. Goldman, and D. W. Cohen (eds.): Periodontal Therapy, 4th ed. St. Louis, The C. V. Mosby Co., 1968.
5. Corn, H.: Edentulous area pedicle grafts in mucogingival surgery. Periodontics, *2*:229, 1964.
6. Coslet, J. G., Vanarsdall, R. L., and Weisgold, A.: Diagnosis and classification of delayed passive eruption of the dentogingival junction in the adult. Alpha Omegan, Scientific Issue, 10:24, 1977.
7. Eissman, H. J., Radke, R. A., and Noble, W. H.: Physiological design criteria for fixed dental restorations. Dent. Clin. North Am., *15*:3, 1971.
8. Garber, D., and Rosenberg, E.: The edentulous ridge in fixed prosthodontics. Compend. Cont. Ed. Gen. Dent., *2*(4):212, 1981.
9. Garguilo, A. W., Wentz, F. M., and Orban, B.: Dimensions of the dentogingival junction in humans. J. Periodontol., *32*:261, 1961.
10. Ingber, J. S., Rose, L. F., and Coslet, J. G.: "The biologic width"—A concept in periodontics and restorative dentistry. Alpha Omegan, Scientific Issue, 10:62, 1977.
11. Kraus, B., Jordan, R., and Abrams, L.: Dental Anatomy and Occlusion. A Study of the Masticatory System. Baltimore, Williams & Wilkins Co., 1969.
12. Langer, B., and Calagna, L.: The subepithelial connective tissue graft. J. Prosthet. Dent., *44*:363, 1980.
13. Loe, H., and Ainamo, J.: Anatomical characteristics of gingivae—A clinical and microscopic study of free and attached gingivae. J. Periodontol., *37*:5, 1966.
14. Ochsenbein, C., and Ross, S. E.: A re-evaluation of osseous surgery. Dent. Clin. North Am., *13*:87, 1969.

15. Phillips, R., and Castaldi, C.: Proximal contour of Class II amalgam restorations made with various matrix band techniques. J. Am. Dent. Assoc., *53*:391, 1956.
16. Prichard, J., and Feder, M.: A modern adaptation of the telescopic principle in periodontal prostheses. J. Periodontol., *33*:360, 1962.
17. Richey, B., and Orban, B.: The crest of the interdental alveolar septa. J. Periodontol., *24*(2):75, 1953.
18. Robinson, R. E.: The distal wedge operation. Periodontics, *4*:256, 1966.
19. Rosenberg, E., Garber, D., and Evian, C.: Tooth lengthening procedures. Compend. Cont. Ed. Gen. Dent., *1*(3):61, 1980.
20. Stein, R. S.: Pontic-residual ridge relationships: A research report. J. Prosthet. Dent., *16*:283, 1966.
21. Weisgold, A.: Contours of the full crown restoration. Alpha Omegan, *70*(3):77, 1977.
22. Weisgold, A., and Feder, M.: Tooth preparation in fixed prosthesis. Part I. Compend. Cont. Ed. Gen. Dent., *1*(6):375, 1980.

The Management of the Multirooted Tooth With Furcation Involvement

1. Abrams, L., and Trachtenberg, D.: Hemisection—technique and restoration. Dent. Clin. North Am., *18*(2):415, 1974.
2. Amsterdam, M., and Rossman, S. R.: Technique of hemisection of multirooted teeth. Alpha Omegan, *53*:4, 1960.
3. Casullo, D., and Matarazzo, F.: The preparation and restoration of the multirooted tooth with furcation involvement. Cont. Dent. Ed., Univ. of Pa., Vol. 1, No. 1, 1977.

The Etched Cast Metal Resin-Bonded Restoration

1. Amsterdam, M.: Periodontal Prosthesis—Twenty-five years in retrospect. Alpha Omegan, *67*:8, 1974.
2. Bounocore, M. G.: A simple method of increasing the adhesions of acrylic filling materials to enamel surfaces. J. Dent. Res., *34*:849, 1955.
3. Howe, D. F., and Dencchy, G. E.: Anterior fixed partial dentures utilizing the acid-etch technique and a cast metal framework. J. Prosthet. Dent. *37*:28, 1977.
4. Livaditis, G. J.: Cast metal resin-bonded retainers for posterior teeth. J. Am. Dent. Assoc., *101*:926, 1980.
5. Livaditis, G. J.: Resin-bonded cast restorations: clinical study. Int. J. Periodont. Rest..Dent., *4*:71, 1981.
6. McCaughlin, G.: Composite bonding of etched metal anterior splints: Compend. Cont. Dent. Ed., University of Pennsylvania, *2*:279–283, 1981.
7. Rochette, A. L.: Attachment of a splint to enamel of lower anterior teeth. J. Prosthet. Dent., *33*:418, 1973.
8. Thompson, V. P., Del Castillo, E., and Livaditis, G. J.: Resin bond to electrolytically etched non-precious alloys for resin-bonded prosthesis. J. Dent. Res., *60*(Special Issue A):377, 1981.
9. Wood, M.: Etched casting resin-bonded retainers: An improved technique for periodontal splinting. Int. J. Periodont. Rest. Dent., *4*:9, 1982.

APPENDIX

Answers

Chapter 1.   The Prevention of Dental Caries

1. The reversal of a carious lesion occurs when the surface of a tooth that is diagnosed as carious at one appointment is found to be sound, or noncarious, at a later appointment. It is now felt that initial lesions, which are undergoing demineralization but have not yet cavitated, may, under the proper conditions, revert to a clinically sound state. Such lesions would be considered to have remineralized.

2. The principal area of demineralization of the "white spot," or early carious lesion, occurs beneath, rather than at, the enamel surface. Thus, it is possible to diagnose lesions at this early stage and attempt to arrest or remineralize them before they cavitate.

3. In the presence of fluoride ions, remineralization is accelerated. Additionally, fluoride is deposited in the demineralized tissue as remineralization occurs. Thus, remineralized enamel, which contains more fluoride than adjacent sound enamel, can actually be more chemically resistant to acid attack.

4. Fluoride protects both pit and fissure (occlusal) surfaces and smooth surfaces against caries. However, it appears to be least protective for occlusal surfaces. Sealants are specifically designed to prevent pit and fissure caries, especially of the occlusal surfaces. If an occlusal sealant is intact, the surface will not decay.

5. The base of most sealant systems is the reaction product of bisphenol A and glycidyl methacrylate. Through common usage, this material is called by the acronym BIS-GMA. It is also the base formulation in most currently marketed anterior restorative composite materials. Differences between commercial sealants include:
    a. The method of polymerization
    b. Whether they are unfilled or contain filler particles
    c. Whether they are clear, tinted, or opaque

6. Sealants may be used on *sound* occlusal surfaces after considering such factors as the caries status of the proximal surfaces, the occlusal morphology, tooth age, general caries activity in the patient's mouth, and whether the patient is using other caries-preventive methods. Sealants should not be used on *carious* occlusal surfaces. Generally, sealants should be used on *questionable* occlusal surfaces provided the proximal surfaces of the teeth being treated are sound.

7. The steps in sealant application are:
    a. Select tooth to be sealed
    b. Provide prophylaxis of occlusal surfaces with a slurry of flour of pumice
    c. Rinse
    d. Isolate and air dry occlusal surface
    e. Acid etch for 60 seconds with phosphoric acid
    f. Rinse and thoroughly dry

679

g. Apply sealant (This step will vary depending on whether an auto-polymerizing or ultraviolet light polymerizing sealant is used.)

h. Check the hardened sealant visually and with an explorer

It is critical that the tooth be dry and saliva-free immediately before the sealant is applied. Saliva should not be allowed to touch the tooth surface once the tooth has been acid etched. Water or saliva can contaminate the etched tooth surface and result in a poor bond between the sealant and tooth. The sealant will be poorly retained and will fail.

8. The three compounds available for topical fluoride treatments in the United States are:

a. Sodium fluoride (NaF)

b. Stannous fluoride (SnF_2)

c. Acidulated phosphate fluoride (APF)—an acidifed buffered sodium fluoride

APF is popular because (1) its taste can be masked with flavoring agents so that it is acceptable to most patients, (2) it possesses a long shelf life, (3) it is available in gels for use in a convenient gel-tray application, and (4) it does not cause gingival reactions or stain the teeth.

9. The steps in topical fluoride application using a gel-tray procedure are:

a. Provide prophylaxis of all tooth surfaces with a fluoride-containing prophylaxis paste

b. Floss the proximal surfaces of the teeth with unwaxed dental floss

c. Prepare disposable trays to fit the patient's maxillary and mandibular teeth

d. Place gel in the trays and apply to the air-dried maxillary and mandibular teeth for 4 minutes. Use saliva ejector

e. Instruct patient not to eat or drink for 30 minutes

For patients in fluoride-deficient communities, professional topical fluoride applications should be performed twice a year. If caries activity is especially high, treatments may be performed more frequently.

10. Caries inhibition by professionally administered topical fluoride treatments to children residing in fluoride-defi-

cient areas is generally accepted to be between 30 and 40 per cent. Evidence is lacking that this treatment significantly reduces caries in groups of children who are already receiving the benefits of community water fluoridation. However, individual patients who demonstrate a high caries activity, despite a history of communal water fluoridation, should receive topic fluoride treatments.

11. The sequence for applying occlusal sealants and topical fluoride at the same visit is:

a. Provide prophylaxis of all tooth surfaces with a slurry of flour of pumice

b. Apply sealants following usual procedure

c. Apply topical fluoride

If the topical fluoride is applied between the etching and sealant application steps, the fluoride-enamel reaction products may adversely affect bonding. The sealant will be poorly retained and will fail.

12. *Nutrition* is the process by which food is ingested and assimilated by the body in order to promote the growth and repair of tissues. *Diet* is what a person eats or drinks. A person's diet may have a local effect on the erupted teeth and is the more important determinant of caries causation.

13. The four factors of the diet that determine cariogenicity follow:

a. Type of carbohydrate. Sucrose, or common table sugar, which is a disaccharide composed of glucose and fructose, is considered to be the most cariogenic sugar in the human diet.

b. Form of carbohydate. A sticky form of sugar requires a prolonged oral clearance time and is considered to be very cariogenic.

c. Frequency of carbohydrate ingestion. Frequent snacking of carbohydrate foods is believed to be associated with high caries attack rates in individuals.

d. Amount of carbohydrate. A "threshold level" of sugar in the diet may be necessary to produce caries. Rampant caries may be associated with a saturation level of dietary sugar.

TABLE 1–12 Daily Dietary Fluoride Supplement Schedule

Fluoride in Water (ppm)	Age		
	Birth to 24 Mos.	*25 to 36 Mos.*	*37 Mos. to 13 Yrs.*
Less than 0.3	0.25 mg F	0.50 mg F	1.00 mg F
0.3 to 0.7	0.0 mg F	0.25 mg F	0.50 mg F
Greater than 0.7	0.0 mg F	0.0 mg F	0.0 mg F

Note: A 2.2 mg NaF tablet provides 1.0 mg F.
Modified from Ripa, L. W.: The role of the pediatrician in dental caries detection and prevention. Pediatrics, *54*:176–182, 1974.

14. For patients with a high caries incidence, especially those with rampant caries, special dietary counseling is necessary. For most other patients, a single session explaining the pertinent food-caries relationships should suffice.

15. Dentifrices accepted by the American Dental Association and their active ingredients are:
    a. Aim (sodium monofluorophosphate)
    b. Aquafresh (sodium monofluorophosphate)
    c. Colgate with MFP Fluoride (sodium monofluorophosphate)
    d. Crest (sodium fluoride)
    e. Macleans' Fluoride (sodium monofluorophosphate)

16. The three methods of fluoride self-application are:
    a. Toothbrushing (*without* a dentifrice)
    b. Mouthrinsing
    c. Using custom mouthtrays
    The method most often used in a school-based program and most convenient for home use is fluoride mouthrinsing. The highest caries reductions have been obtained with the daily use of self-applied gel trays over a long period of time. In a fluoride-deficient community, use of fluoride gel trays during two school years resulted in caries reductions of 64 to 67 per cent.

17. Self-applied fluoride methods are indicated for caries-active patients and those with special caries problems, such as nursing bottle caries, rampant caries, and root caries. Self-applied fluorides are also indicated for individuals who are going into a potentially more caries-susceptible status. This includes patients undergoing orthodontic therapy, when the teeth are difficult to clean, and patients with xerostomia. Self-application brushing methods are recommended for a preschool child, mouthrinsing for a child of school age, and mouthtrays for adolescents and adults.

18. A fluoride rinse is swished and expectorated. An oral fluoride rinse supplement may be swished and swallowed. On teaspoonful (5 ml) of an oral rinse supplement having a concentration of 0.044 per cent NaF will provide 1 mg of fluoride when swallowed.

19. The daily dietary fluoride supplement schedule is as shown in Table 1–12 repeated above.

20. Dietary fluoride supplements should be started at birth, since all of the primary teeth and some of the permanent teeth (first molars) are forming. Fluoride supplements should be continued until all permanent teeth (exclusive of third molars) have erupted. In most patients, this will be until 13 years of age. There is little evidence that prenatal fluoride supplements are beneficial, and it is not recommended that they be prescribed during pregnancy.

Chapter 2. Pedodontics in General Practice

1. The "tell, show, and do" technique is a method whereby procedures are introduced to the child in a manner that gains the child's acceptance. In words appropriate for the child's age, the child is told what is to be done and is shown briefly how the procedure is to be performed, followed immediately by performance of the procedure.

2. In the hand over mouth exercise, the dentist places his or her hand firmly over the child's mouth to muffle noise

but does not obstruct the airway by covering the nose.

3. The very young child can be managed with oral administration of chloral hydrate alone or together with promethazine. The older child may be managed with hydroxyzine, diazepam, or a combination of meperidine and promethazine. Drug dosages are somewhat arbitrary and are usually based on body weight. Approximate dosages are as follows:

> Chloral hydrate—25 mg/lb
> Hydroxyzine—0.5 mg/lb
> Diazepam—0.15 mg/lb
> Promethazine—0.5 mg/lb
> Meperidine—1.0 mg/lb

4. Only essential radiographs should be taken. When contacts between posterior teeth are open and there is no clinical abnormality, no radiographs are necessary. If the contacts between posterior teeth are closed, then bite-wing radiographs are indicated. Other appropriate radiographs should be taken if an abnormality is suspected.

5. A 3-year-old child should be taught the scrub technique of toothbrushing. However, children of that age lack the manual dexterity to properly clean the teeth and parents should assist with toothbrushing each night following the child's attempt to do so.

6. The inferior alveolar block injection is used to anesthetize mandibular permanent molars, and infiltration techniques are used for maxillary molars.

7. A modified technique is used to lessen any pain associated with the palatal injection. Following maxillary infiltration buccal to the tooth, a few drops of solution are injected in the interdental papilla from the buccal to the palatal aspect, followed by injection of the palatal tissues, which have become anesthetized.

8. For efficient practice, a minimal number of teeth should be isolated. When a Class I restoration is being placed, single tooth isolation is sufficient. When a Class II restoration is performed, the teeth on either side of the restoration are isolated, and where possible, the clamp is placed on the tooth distal to the tooth receiving the restoration.

9. The contact area determines the exten-sion of the proximal box, buccolingually and gingivally. The buccal, lingual, and gingival walls are extended so that the tip of an explorer can just reach all margins. Pulpal extension should be just past the dentinoenamel junction (1 to 1½ mm from the tooth surface).

10. Circumferential reduction should be performed on the proximal surfaces; however, little if any preparation should be performed on the buccal or lingual surfaces. The cervical bulge should be maintained to provide retention for the crown.

11. The enamel at the fracture edge is beveled slightly with a suitable bur, in order to remove loose enamel rods and provide a better edge for the restoration.

12. Indirect pulp treatment is indicated for those lesions that radiographically approximate the pulp with a possibility of exposure if all caries is removed.

13. The presence of a parulis usually indicates necrosis of the pulp, and, consequently, either a pulpectomy or an extraction should be performed.

14. The formocresol pulpotomy procedure is indicated in a tooth with vital pulp in the pulp canals. Furcation involvement usually indicates necrosis of the pulp, and, consequently, the formocresol pulpotomy procedure is not indicated, but the tooth should be treated with a complete pulpectomy or extraction.

15. Apexification is performed whenever immature permanent teeth with incompletely formed apices become nonvital. The canal is instrumented 1 mm short of the apex and a mixture of calcium hydroxide is placed. Following closure of the apex, the canal is instrumented and sealed with gutta percha in the usual manner.

16. Anterior teeth are pushed apically and then slightly rotated mesially and distally. Molar teeth are pushed apically and then bucally and lingually.

17. Frequently, the pulps of injured teeth are in "a state of shock" and give false-negative responses to vitality tests. Endodontic treatment should not be performed unless other signs or symptoms of disease are present.

18. Generally, intruded teeth should be allowed to re-erupt. A primary tooth se-

verely intruded so as to impinge on the developing permanent tooth should be extracted.

19. A splint is easily constructed by bonding a slightly curved .030 stainless-steel wire with the acid-teeth technique to the mobile tooth and to abutment teeth.

Composite material is placed on top of the wire bonding it to the tooth surfaces.

20. The yellow color in the crown usually indicates that reparative dentin has filled the pulp chamber. Vitality is frequently maintained and no treatment is necessary, unless the pulp becomes nonvital.

Chapter 3.   Oral Medicine in General Practice

1. False.
2. False.
3. 140/90.
4. Management of stress.
5. Congestive heart failure. Pulmonary edema.
6. Postural hypotension—sudden drop in blood pressure when moving quickly from a supine to an erect position. Orthopnea—difficulty in breathing when supine.
7. Tranquilizers in treating hypertension.
8. True.
9. Six months.
10. Three minutes.
11. False.
12. Control of blood glucose levels.
13. True.
14. Too much.
15. Prevention of cross infection.
16. False.
17. False.
18. Hypertension, diabetes, heart disease.
19. Hypertension, diabetes, myocardial infarction.
20. False.

Chapter 4.   Diagnosis and Treatment Planning in General Practice

1. b, e
2. a, b, c, d, e
3. a, b, c, e
4. a, c
5. a, b, c
6. c
7. a
8. a, b, c, d, e
9. b, c, d
10. a, b, c, d, e
11. c
12. b
13. a, b
14. a
15. a
16. c
17. a, b, c, d
18. c, d
19. b, c
20. a, b, d, e
21. a, b, c
22. a, b, c, d
23. c, d, e
24. a, b, c, d, e

Chapter 5.   Periodontics

1. c
2. a
3. d
4. d
5. d
6. b
7. d
8. d
9. c
10. a
11. c
12. b
13. d
14. d
15. a
16. c
17. c
18. c
19. c
20. d

Chapter 6. Endodontics in General Practice

1. There is no correlation between clinical symptoms and the state of the pulp.
2. Incomplete fracture.
3. Maxillary sinusitis.
4. The maxillary first premolar has two roots. The pulp of one root is vital and hyperreactive. The pulp of the second root is necrotic, and an apical periodontitis has developed.
5. Root canal infection.
6. It is impossible to radiographically distinguish between the two. A definite diagnosis can be made only under microscopy.
7. To promote healing of pulpal inflammation and to prevent external irritants from reaching the pulp.
8. By application of a cavity varnish prior to the insertion of the amalgam restoration.
9. Eighty to 90 per cent.
10. The exposed pulp must be free of inflammation, calcium hydroxide must be used as capping material, and the pulp must be sealed off from the oral environment, bacteria-tight, during the repair phase.
11. Thirty to 40 per cent.
12. Experimental as well as long-term follow-up studies have shown that this is optimal treatment.
13. You ignore the misadventure and obturate the root canal at the optimal level, 1 to 2 mm coronal to the radiographic apex.
14. It is an apical plug made of dentin chips from the root canal walls that serves as a biologically well-tolerated interface between obturating material and pulpal and periapical tissues.
15. As a result of the normal instrumentation procedures, dentin chips will often obturate the pulpal ends of lateral and accessory canals.
16. A vital pulp is not infected, and there are no biologic reasons why the root canal should not be obturated immediately after pulpectomy and canal instrumentation.
17. There are several reasons, but the most important is to obtain a bacteria-free root canal before obturation.
18. A traditional root canal medicament is used because of its antimicrobial effect. Calcium hydroxide has an antimicrobial effect but in addition has beneficial effects on periapical repair (anti-inflammatory effect, induction of hard tissue formation, and so on).
19. The apical part (1 to 5 mm) of the root canal is given a circular shape with known diameter by means of rotating instruments. A gutta-percha point with the same diameter as the instrument used last will then fit in this part of the canal like a cork in a bottle and with a cement will give a bacteria-tight apical seal. Farther coronally, where the canal is not standardized, additional gutta-percha points are used to seal the canal at all levels.
20. Inadequate seal of the root canal.

Chapter 7. Orthodontics in General Practice

1. Two different groups of patients requiring orthodontic treatment fit particularly well into general practice. The first are adults who need tooth movement to facilitate and perhaps make possible other dental treatment, as, for instance, in conjunction with fixed prosthodontics or periodontal care. Producing ideal occlusion through major orthodontic tooth movement is not the treatment objective for many such adult patients.

   The second major group who are potential candidates for orthodontic treatment within the framework of general practice are children with fixed-dentition space problems. A conscientious general practitioner can provide an important service by working with the children in his practice who have less severe problems that are amenable to relatively simple treatment procedures.
2. About 15 per cent of all children could receive a satisfactory occlusal result from preventive and interceptive treatment alone. Since this is the type of treatment that can be reasonably provided in general practice, it appears that approximately one child patient in

six in the typical general practice might be a candidate for some mixed-dentition orthodontic treatment.

3. There is relatively more mandibular than maxillary growth at the time of the adolescent growth spurt. Since the great majority of skeletal jaw discrepancies are Class II, the fact that the mandible tends to grow later than the maxilla can be very helpful.

4. It is now apparent that the soft tissue development lags behind the growth of the face. In the postadolescent period there is a noticeable amount of nose growth, especially in males. There are also hard and soft tissue changes at the chin, again predominantly in males. The vertical growth of the lips also lags behind the vertical growth of the face but is ultimately of a greater magnitude than the vertical skeletal development. This results in an increased incidence of competent lips in the postadolescent age group. The thickness of the lips also decreases in the postadolescent period and is more noticeable in females than males.

5. Patients who have maxillary retrusion and Class III skeletal relationships are hard to evaluate by this technique. This is probably due to the lack of attention to the maxillary skeletal position. Patients with long lower face height are also difficult to evaluate. It would probably be wise to request an orthodontic consultation for those patients with vertical discrepancies in order to accurately evaluate the underlying skeletal relationships.

6. Several assumptions made by the dentist completing a space analysis must be recognized as such. One assumption is that all permanent teeth are forming and that the unerupted teeth have a size correlating with the erupted incisors. Another assumption is that prediction tables will apply to the patient under examination. Differences in ethnic backgrounds make application of these prediction tables very risky. The size of the dental arches measured on the casts is considered to be stable and unchanging. This means that the dentist should assume that all growth in the mandible will occur away from the alveolar ridge and that the incisors are in a fixed position.

7. If incisors are highly protrusive, it may be desirable to retract them to a less protrusive position. This will mean arranging them along the perimeter of a smaller arc and thus will decrease the amount of available space, thereby increasing the crowding.

8. Eruption of the permanent tooth usually takes place when its root is approximately one-half to two-thirds completed. To predict when the permanent successor will erupt after a primary tooth has been lost prematurely, two factors may be used as a guide: the degree of completion of the root of the permanent successor (as above) and the amount of alveolar bone overlying the permanent successor. Early removal of a primary tooth will accelerate the eruption of the permanent successor (1) if the permanent tooth is within 12 months of normal eruption, as determined by its degree of root formation, or (2) if periapical infection or other causes have resulted in the destruction of much of the alveolar bone overlying the permanent tooth. The general rule is that loss of an overlying primary tooth 6 to 12 months early will accelerate the eruption of the permanent tooth. If, however, a primary tooth is lost prematurely at a time when its permanent successor is not well formed and is nowhere near alveolar emergence, the eruption of the permanent successor may be delayed rather than accelerated.

9. The two major variables that determine the response to orthodontic force are the duration of the force and its magnitude. Duration is controlled by the wearing time of a removable appliance or by the amount of time a spring is active. Light force applied continuously is quite effective in producing tooth movement, because the periodontal membrane is constantly kept in a state leading to the production of bony changes. With this type of force, tooth movement continues without frequent appliance adjustments.

10. Anchorage may be defined as the resistance areas (teeth or other structures) against which a relative force will be placed as teeth are moved. Retention is the ability to keep an appliance firmly in place in the mouth when the active

compounds are engaged to move the desired teeth.

11. The longer a primary tooth has been missing, the greater the incidence and amount of space closure. Closure is more rapid during the first 6 months following tooth loss in either arch and occurs more rapidly in the maxillary arch than in the mandibular arch. Posterior space closure has been noted before and after eruption of first permanent molars. Although space closure is multidirectional, it occurs predominantly from the posterior in the maxillary arch and predominantly from the anterior in the mandibular arch.

12. If no orthodontic treatment is available, and if the space discrepancy is greater than 10 mm, there will probably be a net benefit to the patient from serial extraction procedures alone.

13. Disking or selective removal of primary incisors, canines, and molars will help reduce faciolingual irregularity if space is available. On the other hand, rotational changes are not as successfully resolved by selective removal of primary teeth.

14. When only the dental structures are at fault, the constriction may be unilateral or bilateral. Dental crossbites usually involve teeth with axial inclinations that are not consistent with the rest of the dentition. Crossbites in the primary and mixed dentitions are best treated when they are discovered. There are several reliable appliances to correct posterior dental crossbites: the W-arch, the quad helix, or cross elastics. By contrast, a posterior skeletal crossbite should be approached by opening the maxillary midpalatal suture. Expansion of the maxilla by opening the midpalatal suture has routinely been referred to as rapid maxillary expansion or more grapically as "palate splitting." The technique calls for fitting a jack-screw appliance firmly to the teeth, separating the two halves of the maxilla at the rate of 0.5 to 1.0 mm per day, and then holding the expansion for 8 to 12 weeks while the open suture fills in with new bone.

15. If a child has good vertical skeletal jaw relationships, an anterior open bite is quite likely to close spontaneously. If there is a vertical growth problem, the open bite may persist. It is true that the longer an anterior open bite persists, the more difficult it is to correct and the more likely that there is a significant skeletal component. The anterior open bites that have a good chance for spontaneous correction or correction with simple treatment usually resolve by 10 years of age. It is probably good judgment to refer open bite patients older than 10 years of age to an orthodontist, since a difficult problem of malocclusion probably exists in these patients.

16. For a maxillary excess, headgear therapy to restrain the maxilla is indicated. A functional appliance is probably more suitable to facilitate growth for severe mandibular deficiencies.

17. The difference is that growth is no longer available, so that changes in both the horizontal and the vertical dimensions must be made within the existing skeletal configuration.

18. The canine and premolars in the quadrant in which the uprighting is to be done are banded and stabilized with a relatively stiff passive wire, ligated to brackets on these teeth. A segment of rectangular wire is then formed into an uprighting spring so the coil is compressed when the anterior arm of the spring is engaged. Finally, a coil spring is compressed between the molar tooth and the premolar adjacent to it to complete the uprighting.

19. When neither the orthodontist nor the surgeon can treat a problem alone. Severe open bites, mandibular deficiency, crossbite, and maxillary protrusion are commonly treated by orthognathic surgery.

20. The two types of complications encountered most often in orthodontic treatment are problems of increased susceptibility to other types of dental disease because of the orthodontic treatment and problems due to orthodontic tooth movement itself. Of the two, problems relating to caries and gingival inflammation occurring during orthodontic treatment are much more common.

Chapter 8. Occlusion in General Practice

1.	b	11.	d
2.	c	12.	c
3.	False	13.	b
4.	d	14.	b
5.	b	15.	d
6.	False	16.	b
7.	False	17.	a
8.	c	18.	a
9.	d	19.	False
10.	c	20.	d

Chapter 9. Restorative Dentistry in General Practice

1. A complete diagnostic work-up for a complex restorative dentistry patient includes the following: a full-mouth panoramic x-ray, full-mouth periapical x-rays, bite-wing x-rays, mounted diagnostic casts, periodontal charting, charting of existing restorations, examination of temporomandibular joints, vitalometer tests, and examination of the soft tissue lesions.

2. Pin and amalgam build-ups should be used before final tooth preparation in any build-up situation in which high caries probability is observed. Amalgam restorations offer more cariostatic activity than do composite restorations.

3. Pin and composite build-ups should be used before final tooth preparation whenever high caries susceptibility is not suspected and addition of a small amount of parallel preparation structure is required.

4. Bases other than simple CaOH preparations are not necessary under amalgam or composite cores. Approximately 0.5 mm of low calcium–release CaOH paste is recommended on deep areas under amalgam or composite cores.

5. Occlusal equilibration is indicated before all complex restorative dentistry therapy to allow the development of an occlusal scheme that does not have interferences and that will have the optimal possibility for prolonged health.

6. Intracoronal restorations should be included in complex restorative dentistry if teeth are not destroyed to the degree that more comprehensive restorations are necessary.

7. Fear may be lessened in patients requiring extensive therapy by proper education before therapy, use of sedatives before treatment, hypnosis, a positive attitude toward treatment outcome, and confident reinforcement about the desirability of the treatment.

8. Margins for crown preparations should be placed supragingivally, unless one or more of the following conditions demand subgingival margins: esthetic considerations, short clinical crown length, caries, old restorations, dentin sensitivity, and physiologic or psychologic inhibition of proper oral hygiene.

9. Water spray should be used during gross cutting procedures in restorative dentistry. Dry cutting may be accomplished on small final procedures.

10. Stainless-steel posts and amalgam build-ups have been shown to be adequate in strength and can be compared favorably with cast post-and-core restorations.

11. Onlay restorations offer the following advantages over full crowns: less gingival irritation, the same esthetic appearance as the original teeth, and less extensive tooth structure removal.

12. Porcelain-fused-to-metal crowns require removal of tooth structure on the facial surfaces to allow for adequate porcelain thickness and an optimal esthetic result.

13. Rehabilitation of the dentition on one side of the mouth at a time (1) allows the patient to chew on the opposite side during treatment, (2) allows maintenance of the original vertical dimension of occlusion, (3) allows the anatomy and function of the rehabilitated

side to be adjusted and formed to the best possible relationship, and (4) allows accomplishment of a rehabilitation in a manner that is financially affordable to many people.

14. Rehabilitation of the dentition on one side of the mouth at a time does not allow changing of the vertical dimension of occlusion, and it usually requires more appointments than does treating all of the teeth at one time.

15. Rehabilitation of one quadrant at one time does not offer an optimal situation for contouring occlusal surfaces and occlusion.

16. Rehabilitation of all the posterior dentition at one time (1) requires the patient to be in temporary restorations for a significant period of time, (2) may not allow optimal recording of the original vertical dimension of occlusion, and (3) often introduces many variables that can cause significant occlusal disharmony and necessitate remaking of the crowns.

17. Rehabilitation of all the posterior dentition at one time allows optimal redevelopment of an occlusal scheme at any vertical dimension of occlusion, and it also offers an optimal opportunity for ensuring an esthetic result.

18. The following steps are required for rehabilitation of one side of the mouth at one time:
   a. Radiographic survey
   b. Fabrication and mounting of diagnostic casts
   c. Diagnosis and occlusal analysis
   d. Treatment planning
   e. Initial adjustment of gross occlusal interferences
   f. Preliminary rebuilding of dental structures with amalgam or composite cores
   g. Occlusal correction
   h. Preparation of teeth for extra-

coronal restorations (preferably one quadrant or one side of the mouth at a time)
   i. Fabrication of working casts from full-arch impressions
   j. Interocclusal records and mounting of casts in a semiadjustable articulator (Whip-Mix or other)
   k. Trimming and waxing of dies
   l. Try-in of castings for checking of proximal contacts, color, occlusion, contour, and margins.
   m. Remounting and adjusting of occlusion if necessary
   n. Cementation
   o. Repetition of procedures for the alternate side of the mouth

19. The following steps are required for rehabilitation of all the posterior teeth at one time:
   a–g. Same as a–g, Answer No. 18
   h. Preparation of teeth for extracoronal restorations (by quadrants or more)
   i. Temporary restorations made
   j. Full-arch working casts mounted in a fully adjustable or a semiadjustable articulator
   k. Fabrication of castings from full-mouth occlusion concept
   l. Try-in restorations for checking of proximal contacts, color, occlusion, contour, and margins.
   m. Fabrication of remount casts with acrylic matrix
   n. Occlusal correction of castings on remount casts in the articulator
   o. Cementation of finished restorations

20. A typical ideal treatment plan should first involve diagnostic activities with periodontics and preliminary restorative dentistry at the same time, endodontics if required, final fixed prosthodontics and restorative dentistry, and removable prosthodontics as required.

Chapter 10.   Oral Surgery in General Practice

1. Drape the unit table with a sterile towel that is large enough to extend over the edges of the table. This facilitates moving the table without touching unprotected surfaces of the table. Cover the light handle with a sterile towel or aluminum foil. Wipe the arms of the chair and all adjustment levers or buttons with 70 per cent isopropyl alcohol. Autoclave other equipment and supplies or use prepackaged sterile disposable materials. (For further details, see the

section, Preparation for Oral Surgery: Preparations of Office Equipment).

2. The panoramic radiograph is a screening tool. It distorts some structures, only one plane is "in focus," and some superimposition of images of contralateral structures exists. This results in the distortion of root shapes and lengths as well as some extreme variations in radiolucency and radiopacity.

3. The advantages of intravenous sedation over oral sedation are as follows:
   a. Doubt about how much drug reaches the circulating blood is eliminated.
   b. A small portion may be administered as a test dose. If a reaction occurs, administration can be stopped with only a small amount of drug having been given, and an IV pathway is present should other medication be required to counter the reaction to the tested drug.
   c. The patient does not come to the office groggy or possibly unaffected by the oral medication.
   d. The patient receives only sufficient drug to achieve the desired level of sedation.
   e. The desired level of sedation is achieved rapidly.

4. The dose of epinephrine for managing an anaphylactic reaction or a cardiovascular collapse is 0.3 to 0.5 mg administered intravenously or intramuscularly (0.3 to 0.5 ml of 1:1000 solution).

5. To manage the patient giving a history of allergic reaction to local anesthesia:
   a. Obtain a description of the event from the patient.
   b. Call the person who administered the anesthetic for his description and interpretation of the event.
   c. If the patient knows the exact drug used, select an anesthetic from a different chemical grouping.
   d. Be prepared to treat an anaphylactic reaction even if you suspect the described event was not a true allergic response and you elect to proceed with administration of the same or another class of local anesthetic.
   e. If you cannot satisfy yourself regarding the patient's allergic status, refer him to an allergist. Do not attempt skin tests in your office.

6. The risks associated with the administration of antibiotics include the possible development of: allergic reaction, resistant strains of organisms, moniliasis, enterocolitis, pneumonia, deafness, stained teeth, superinfections, agranulocytosis.

   Different antibiotics have different risks, and careful thought must be given to the selection of the appropriate drug and what the risks are in relation to the severity of the infection or the possibility of systemic reaction.

7. Factors of importance in flap reflection include
   a. Appropriate design to assure a good blood supply to the flap.
   b. Design of the flap so that the line of closure will be supported by bone if the surgery will leave a defect with unsupported mucosa.
   c. Adequate size to minimize stretching of the flap and tearing of tissue.
   d. Clean, sharp cuts perpendicular to the surface.
   e. Careful dissection along a surgical plane, such as subperiosteally or along fascial planes.
   f. Extreme gentleness in retraction.

8. Early removal of third molars is a service to patients because with removal, periodontal problems and caries associated with food impaction accompanying eruption of the teeth are avoided. Early removal is less traumatic, the patients tolerate the surgery and recovery periods better, and complicating systemic problems should removal of such teeth be required 20 to 30 years later are avoided.

9. In surgery for removal of third molars, one must keep in mind the location of the lingual nerve and the inferior alveolar canal and the thinness of the bone between the apices of impacted teeth and the floor of the mouth.

10. Multiple biopsy specimens from the same lesion are placed in separate specimen bottles containing 10 per cent neutral formalin or other fixative recommended by the pathologist. Each is identified by a special number or letter that corresponds to a number or letter

indicating locations on a diagram of the lesion. Description of the characteristics of each location biopsied or of unusual features encountered during surgery should accompany each specimen. The "map" of the lesion, indicating biopsy sites, should also be recorded in the patient's record.

11. Three essentials in emergency care of patients with fractured jaws are (1) an adequate airway, (2) control of bleeding, and (3) the comfort of the patient.

12. To reduce a fibrous tuberosity, an elliptical incision is made along the alveolar crest, extending distally from the second molar region to the mucogingival junction. The two incisions forming the elipse converge at the alveolar crest. The wedge of fibrous tissue is removed, and the surface mucosa is undermined with incisions extending from the anterior pole to the posterior pole of the elipse. The incisions are carried to bone on both the palatal and buccal sides. The wedges of fibrous tissue are then elevated from the bone and removed. The thinned mucosal flaps are pressed to the ridge, and if they overlap, the tissue is trimmed so that the mucosa can be sutured and closely adapted to the alveolar crest. (Drawings are shown in Figures 10–23 and 10–24).

13. The technique that uses the transposition of mucosal and periosteal flaps to deepen the mandibular vestibule has the following advantages: (1) It can be done as an office procedure; (2) it does not require grafts. (3) Splints are not necessary.

14. The lingual gingival crevice or alveolar crest incisions are used in reflecting mandibular lingual flaps. This is because incisions made through the mandibular lingual mucosa are difficult to suture. In addition, such incisions heal slowly and are unusually uncomfortable. The thinness of the mucosa also contributes to dehiscence and exposure of bone.

15. Prior to definitive surgery on bony lytic lesions, aspiration should be carried out to determine the contents of the lesion. If frank, bright blood is easily aspirated, one should suspect a vascular lesion, which might produce uncontrollable bleeding that could be fatal.

16. Differentiation of cellulitis and an abscess is not always easy because of the similarity of signs and symptoms. Cellulitis generally produces diffuse swelling that is very firm. An abscess, because of necrosis and the pocketing of pus, feels fluctuant when palpated. The fluctuance may not be a prominent feature, and frequently careful palpation is required to locate a point of fluctuance that will also be a point of greater tenderness.

17. The patient described is in good health and does not have a very elevated temperature. In view of the circumstances described, the tooth could be extracted immediately using local anesthesia. If the patient is quite apprehensive, IV sedation may also be used and has an added advantage in that the intravenous fluid may alleviate the dehydration associated with avoiding food and fluids because of pain. Dehydration is frequently accompanied by an elevated temperature. Tooth removal provides drainage for pus via the tooth socket. If one has detected fluctuance in the buccal vestibule and it is not relieved by the extraction, an incision should be made in the vestibule, penetrating to bone, and a drain should be placed and sutured to the tissue margin.

Antibiotics are not necessary for the patient described in the question. The patient should receive a prescription for an analgesic compound containing 30 mg of codeine. (The history does not describe any allergies or sensitivities to these drugs.) The patient should be contacted in 12 hours or seen early the next day to ascertain that symptoms have abated and swelling is relieved. If the condition has not improved, the patient should receive additional evaluation and be started on an antibiotic such as penicillin V, 500 mg every 4 hours. The drain, if placed, is generally removed in 2 days.

18. The dressing in a "dry socket" does the following: (1) It serves as a carrier and a reservoir for medication. Eugenol is a standard agent in most dressings; it is mildly antiseptic and anesthetic. (2) It helps occlude the space to prevent accumulation of debris. (3) It acts as a "drain."

19. When evaluating the potential for

transplanting an unerupted third molar to a first molar location, one must determine (1) that one half to two thirds of the roots is developed, (2) that the mesiodistal measurement is not greater than the space that will be available after the first molar is removed, and (3) that the removal of the first molar and of the third molar will not result in bone loss that will put the second molar in jeopardy, and (4) that the third molar will not be damaged in the procedure.

20. The symptoms of pain and malaise and the signs of fever and swelling, induration, redness, lymphadenopathy, and fluctuance are similar in both children and adults. Children respond differently to infection as follows: They are very labile in their physiologic response to infection, so they make dramatic changes from health to sickness and the reverse. Dramatic change in body temperature is an example.

In children, the larger marrow spaces and the presence of developing teeth facilitate the spread of infection in bone. The size of the face and jaws permits spontaneous drainage of abscesses buccally into the buccal space and occasionally onto the face, because the root apices are above (in the maxilla) or below (in the mandible) the insertion of the buccinator muscle.

Chapter 11. Prosthodontics in General Practice

1. False. There are some circumstances, such as for patients who have previously worn a prosthesis before irradiation, in which a prosthesis may be worn 3 to 6 months following the completion of radiation therapy. This is particularly true for the maxillary prosthesis (which is supported by tissue with a good blood supply) and can be psychologically important to the patient because of improved appearance.
2. The advantages of the diagnostic denture technique include the following:
   a. The dentist does not have to say the new dentures will be better than the ones the patient is presently using. The patient will be the one to decide *before* the new dentures are completed.
   b. Necessary adjustments and changes may be made before the dentures are completed.
   c. If the patient's expectations cannot be met, either the dentist or the patient may decide to discontinue treatment.
3. The superior edge of the lingual bar should be kept a minimum of 3 mm away from the free gingival margin for the mandible. The palatal major connector usually can be a minimum of 6 mm from the free gingival margin.
4. A rigid major connector allows forces to be distributed throughout the arch when the patient closes on the distal extension base or swallows. This avoids undue stress being concentrated in any one area.
5. The distal extension removable partial denture may move around vertical, horizontal, and perpendicular axes.
6. Vertical forces toward the mucosa can best be resisted using an altered cast impression technique and good basal seat extensions. Vertical forces away from the mucosa are counteracted by indirect rests.

A rigid major connector is very important in resisting horizontal forces, such as those that occur during swallowing.

The third movement, around the perpendicular axis, can occur when mastication occurs on only one side. Movement can be minimized by chewing bilaterally, which also provides a bilaterally balanced occlusion.
7. Zinc-oxide impression materials should be avoided because of their potential for tissue irritation following radiation therapy.
8. Following intraoral radiation therapy, a water-free 0.4 per cent SnF_2 gel should be used nightly. The gel can be carried directly to the tooth surfaces with a toothbrush, swished for 10 seconds, and held for 1 minute before expectorating. No further rinsing is done.
9. A water-free 0.4 per cent SnF_2 gel can be applied to the indentations of a wet overdenture usually in the morning, following cleansing of the dentures.

Professional applications should be given on a 6-month basis, using APF (acidulated phosphate-fluoride) (0.31 per cent F, pH 4.0) followed by 0.4 per cent SnF_2 solution.* Two 1-minute rinses with APF should be followed by two 1-minute rinses with SnF_2.

10. Advantages of completed bases are as follows:

    a. They allow for an evaluation of the fit of the final denture before making a centric jaw relation record.

    b. A more accurate maxillomandibular relation can be made, since the bases are stable and retentive.

    c. The greatest deformation in the acrylic resin is released before making the centric jaw registration, not after.

    d. During the try-in appointment, both dentist and patient are more comfortable because the completed bases are more retentive.

    e. The need to remount at the delivery appointment can be eliminated, since the artificial stone is removed from the denture after the second processing, *before* the occlusion is adjusted on the articulator.

    Disadvantages of the completed bases involve a slight increase in time and cost initially, but this can be made up at insertion, when the need to remount the dentures can be eliminated if verification of the jaw relation is accomplished using heat-processed bases.

11. An accurate method to verify centric jaw relation is through the use of three sets of metal points, called Centric Check Points,† that allow an error to be seen in either the horizontal plane (anteroposteriorly or mediolaterally) or in the vertical plane. An error in the vertical plane is probably most critical, since the teeth would not contact on both sides simultaneously.

12. At this time, no one contour has proven to be better than another. A rounded, or dome, shape allows for more natural placement of the artificial tooth and a greater bulk of acrylic resin in the region of the abutment. This will help to minimize the fracture of the overden-

ture in the region. The height of the overdenture abutment depends upon the mobility and periodontal support of the tooth. A firm tooth with fair to good periodontal support may be kept 2 to 3 mm above the gingiva, whereas a tooth with more mobility and minimal periodontal support should be reduced to, or only slightly above, the level of the gingiva.

13. Complications related to the use of overdentures can involve dental caries, periodontal disease, fracture of the overdenture, and tooth wear. Periodontal disease can best be prevented by making sure that the patient is capable of and motivated to provide good plaque control. Regular recalls are a must.

    Dental caries can best be prevented through the use of fluoride. A water-free 0.4 per cent SnF_2 gel* applied into the indentations of the wet overdenture once a day is beneficial as a decay-preventive measure.

    Professional applications of fluoride should be given on a 6-month basis, using APF (0.31 per cent F, pH 4.0) followed by 0.4 per cent SnF_2 solution.* Two 1-minute rinses with APF should be followed by two 1-minute rinses with SnF_2.

    Fracture of the overdenture can be minimized by reducing the abutments adequately, so they have no sharp edges. Use of a high-strength acrylic resin† (Lucitone 199) can also help to prevent fractures. A third method is to incorporate a metal substructure into the overdenture to reinforce thin sections and reduce wear in susceptible areas.

    Wear of the overdenture abutment has also been noted as a potential complication. Daily topical application of fluoride can harden the tooth surface. A second method is to use a coping fabricated in a non-precious alloy.

14. Although it is better to have teeth for overdenture abutments on both sides of the arch, even one tooth can be helpful to the patient.

15. Getting to know the patient is an espe-

---

*Dunhall Pharmaceuticals, Inc., Gravette, Ark.
†Teledyne Hanau, Buffalo, N.Y.

---

*Dunhall Pharmaceuticals, Inc., Gravette, Ark.
†L. D. Caulk Co., Milford, Del.

cially important consideration in prosthodontics. Differentiating between the "accepting" patient and the "demanding" patient can allow the method of treatment to be altered accordingly. Extreme care and thoughtfulness with the difficult prosthodontic patient may mean the difference between success or failure.

16. Having the reciprocating arm at the same level as the retentive arm is a critical component in the design of a removable partial denture. This may be accomplished by recontouring the tooth or by providing a vertical or horizontal clasp reciprocating surface. A wide, horizontal reciprocating arm could function properly without having to cross the free gingival margin or necessitate recontouring the lingual undercut of an abutment tooth.

17. To date, no one particular clasp has been found to be superior to all other clasps when used with the bilateral distal extension removable partial denture. The relationship of the clasp to the gingiva, the amount of undercut it is placed into, and the proper functioning of the reciprocating arm may be more important. The other "critical components" mentioned in the chapter

also play a significant role in the long-term prognosis of the prosthesis.

18. As a general rule, when the fixed partial denture is indicated for the cleft palate patient, at least two abutments on each side of the cleft should be included. This will provide the necessary stability to each segment. The final decision should be based upon a thorough examination, including radiographs, to determine the bone support around each of the potential abutments.

19. Overdentures can be used for such congenital defects as cleft palate, oligodontia, microdontia, amelogenesis imperfecta, cleidocranial dysostosis, and prognathic mandible. Acquired defects resulting from trauma, erosion, and abrasion may also be considered for treatment with overdentures.

20. One of the most critical components in the long-term success of any prosthesis involving the natural dentition is oral hygiene. Even the best prosthesis can fail if a high plaque index is present, and a poorly designed prosthesis will fail even sooner. The periodontium should be brought to the optimum level of health and then maintained through daily oral hygiene and regular recall appointments.

Chapter 12.   Multidisciplinary Approach to Therapy

1.	False		14.	False
2.	d		15.	b
3.	b, c		16.	d
4.	c		17.	c
5.	b		18.	d
6.	d		19.	False
7.	d		20.	c
8.	d		21.	b
9.	d		22.	False
10.	a		23.	True
11.	c		24.	True
12.	False		25.	True
13.	c			

INDEX

Note: Page numbers in italics refer to illustrations; page numbers followed by t refer to tables